# Kidney Transplantation

AF393646

Andrzej Baranski

# Kidney Transplantation

## Step-by-Step Surgical Techniques

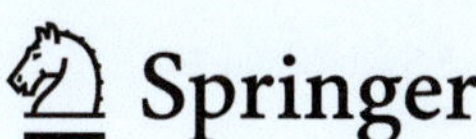 Springer

Andrzej Baranski
Abdominal Organ Transplant Centre,
Department of Surgery
Leiden University Medical Center
Leiden, The Netherlands

ISBN 978-3-030-75888-2        ISBN 978-3-030-75886-8    (eBook)
https://doi.org/10.1007/978-3-030-75886-8

© The Editor(s) (if applicable) and The Author(s), under exclusive license to Springer Nature Switzerland AG 2023
This work is subject to copyright. All rights are solely and exclusively licensed by the Publisher, whether the whole or part of the material is concerned, specifically the rights of translation, reprinting, reuse of illustrations, recitation, broadcasting, reproduction on microfilms or in any other physical way, and transmission or information storage and retrieval, electronic adaptation, computer software, or by similar or dissimilar methodology now known or hereafter developed.
The use of general descriptive names, registered names, trademarks, service marks, etc. in this publication does not imply, even in the absence of a specific statement, that such names are exempt from the relevant protective laws and regulations and therefore free for general use.
The publisher, the authors, and the editors are safe to assume that the advice and information in this book are believed to be true and accurate at the date of publication. Neither the publisher nor the authors or the editors give a warranty, expressed or implied, with respect to the material contained herein or for any errors or omissions that may have been made. The publisher remains neutral with regard to jurisdictional claims in published maps and institutional affiliations.

This Springer imprint is published by the registered company Springer Nature Switzerland AG
The registered company address is: Gewerbestrasse 11, 6330 Cham, Switzerland

*This book is dedicated to my wife Ewa Anna Baranski-Szczepanowska and my daughter Julia Monika Baranska, who are my dearest and the most important and special persons in my life.*

# Foreword to the Polish Edition by Professor Przemysław Pisarski

More than 60 years have passed since the first successful kidney transplant. In the history of the world, we have experienced flights into space, the fall of communism, the birth of the Internet and an explosion in the progress of medicine. One of its fields is transplantology, the branch of medicine that studies the issues in organ transplantation. The roots of organ transplantation date back to the third century after Christ and its patrons—Cosmas and Damian. Over the past few decades, it has undergone very significant changes. They concern not only the surgical side, but also the whole of its multidisciplinary character. The multilayered nature of transplantology has generated advances in immunology, anesthesiology, surgery, infectious diseases, and internal medicine: Andrzej Baranski's book is very welcome and I predict that it will enjoy great popularity. This book consists of eight very carefully prepared chapters. The first is about the anatomy and physiology of the urinary system. Further on, there is talk about surgical techniques and—as the author himself emphasizes—"non-laparoscopic technique of kidney retrieval for kidney transplantation from living donors". History shows that the ability to open donation is also important to know how to react early and to move from laparoscopic to open donation without exposing the donor to unnecessary risks. Chapter 3, which is quite extensive, I call "jewelry". The author emphasizes the importance of the transport and preparation of the kidney before transplantation (divided into right and left kidney preparation). In the same chapter the author describes possible anatomical abnormalities which the surgeon might face during kidney preparing (benching) and transplantation with the technical errors that are not so rarely encountered. Chapter 4 consistently presents not only surgical access during the first and subsequent transplants, but also kidney transplants with anatomical anomalies. The book is crowned by the author's priceless experience in the treatment of surgical complications after kidney transplantation. Renal failure of the organ and irreversible return to dialysis mean retreat from immunosuppression and the necessity of kidney removal (graftectomy). The guidelines for selecting a recipient for transplantation closes a perfect whole.

In conclusion, I would like to congratulate the PZWL and Springer publishing houses on its decision to issue this publication and thank you for the honor of writing a preface to it.

Prof. Dr. Med. Przemysław Pisarski<br>
Department of Organ Transplantation<br>
Center for Surgery<br>
University of Freiburg<br>
Freiburg, Germany

# Preface

I started kidney transplantation in the 1980s in Poland at the Medical University in Warsaw. I then continued my training in abdominal organ procurement and transplantation at the Catholic University of Leuven—University Hospital Saint-Luc in Brussels, Belgium and at the Leiden University Medical Center in Leiden, the Netherlands. During more than 30 years of my work as a transplant surgeon, I have visited various world transplant centers in Great Britain, France, Hungary, the USA, Saudi Arabia, South Korea, China and Japan. During my travels to foreign centers, I have been systematically acquainted with various surgical techniques regarding kidney, pancreas and liver procurement, benching and transplantation. My experience gained during everyday practice and my visits to other centers as well as everyday conversations with residents and colleagues allowed me to develop my own surgical thoughts on these transplantation techniques.

At the Transplant Centers of Leiden University Medical Center, we transplant an average of 130–160 kidneys from deceased and living donors every year. Our department is one of the oldest transplant centers and has been implementing programs for retrieving and transplanting kidneys from living donors since 1966. The number of kidney donations and transplantations that we have carried out from living donors has been increasing steadily and for over the last ten years had remained stable at 75–85 transplants per year. At Leiden, in addition to kidney, pancreas and liver transplantation, pancreatic islet isolation and transplantation are also performed.

This book is devoted solely to the topic of kidney transplantation and is probably one of the few publications in the world presenting step by step with explanation the various kidney procurement, preparation (benching) and transplantation surgical techniques.

I have devoted a lot of space to detailed descriptions of surgical techniques and difficult cases, as well as descriptions of developing decision-making plans. I present rich illustrative material including many photos taken during surgery and drawings which facilitate understanding of the subjects which allows for faster mastering of the relevant surgical techniques.

I realize that some surgical techniques are very difficult to understand especially for a young surgeon. All the comprehensive cases which I present were performed by me and/or my colleagues. The surgical treatment plans and decision-making emerged out of many difficult multidisciplinary discussions.

The first version of this book was written by me in Polish for a Polish editor PZWL and published in 2017. In Poland this book enjoyed and still enjoys great success among transplant surgeons. Photos from this book which I have shown at many conventions and workshops all over the world have aroused great interest among the young surgical transplant generation with requests to publish the book in English.

In this very personal book, I have attempted to pass on all my surgical achievements after 30 years of work. In short, I tried to create a book that I hope will serve a generation of surgeons to improve their skills in kidney retrieval, preparation and transplantation. This book is devoted also to these young, talented and ambitious transplant surgeons to whom I would like to convey the following message: that only through hard and systematic work supported by a continuous process of skills improvement will you be able to rise to the greatest heights of surgery which will enable you to perform organ procurement and transplantation in human beings.

Leiden, The Netherlands
May 2022

Andrzej Baranski

# Acknowledgments

I would like to thank my surgical colleagues at the Transplant Center—Department of Surgery at the University Medical Center in Leiden, the Netherlands for helping with decision-making, operating plans, assistance in operations and for all actions and changes which were taken to enable our "Small Transplant Ward" to function better.

People who I especially thank are:

Dr. A. M. F. Schaapherder—transplant surgeon, (Sandro)
Dr. J. Dubbeld—transplant surgeon, (Jeroen)
Dr. A. E. Braat—transplant surgeon, (Dries)
Dr. Hwai-Ding Lam—transplant surgeon, (David)
Dr. V. A. L. Huurman—transplant surgeon, (Volkert)
Dr. W. N. Nijboer—transplant surgeon, (Mijntje)
Dr. D. K. de Vries—transplant surgeon, (Dorottya)
Mrs. A. Haasnoot—physician assistant, (Ada)
Mrs. R. F. J. Muiselaar—physician assistant, (Robin)
Prof. Dr. I. P. J. Alwayn—transplant surgeon, Head of Department (Ian)

With this book, I would also like to thank all the anesthetists, scrub and circulating nurses and also the transplant coordinators for their extraordinary help, understanding and for the wonderful moments which we have spent together in and outside the operating room.

All the drawings in this book were made by my daughter, Julia Monika Baranska, and my wife Ewa Anna Baranski-Szczepanowska to whom I would like to express my sincere thanks for their help and support in writing this book.

# Contents

# Chapter 1
# Basic Anatomy of the Kidney, Ureters and the Urinary Bladder, and Their Functions

## 1.1 Kidney Anatomy

The kidney is a pair of bean-shaped organs situated in the retroperitoneal space on the left and right side of the vertebral column in the upper abdomen. In a human body kidneys are surrounded by adipose tissue. The amount of body fat surrounding each kidney depends on the age and body weight of the person. The right kidney is situated slightly lower than the left kidney. The cause of the lower position of the right kidney is the liver, which with its mass pushes the right kidney downwards and thus does not allow it to move towards the right dome of the diaphragm. The kidneys lie at the height of the last two thoracic vertebrae and the first three lumbar vertebrae. The right kidney is located from the twelfth thoracic vertebra to the third lumbar vertebra (Th12-L3). The left kidney lies slightly higher, from the eleventh thoracic to the second lumbar vertebra (Th11-L2). The difference in the level of the position of both kidneys is about 1.5–3.0 cm. Each kidney, but only on its anterior surface, is covered with the peritoneum, to which the different abdominal organs adhere [1–10].

The following organs adhere to the anterior surface of the right kidney (Fig. 1.1):

- right suprarenal gland area;
- liver–hepatic area (segment VI);
- duodenum area (descending part);
- small intestine jejunum loops;
- hepatic flexure of the colon.

The following organs adhere to the anterior surface of the left kidney (Fig. 1.2):

- area of left suprarenal gland;
- stomach area;
- splenic area;
- pancreas area (pancreas body/tail);

© The Author(s), under exclusive license to Springer Nature Switzerland AG 2023
A. Baranski, *Kidney Transplantation*,
https://doi.org/10.1007/978-3-030-75886-8_1

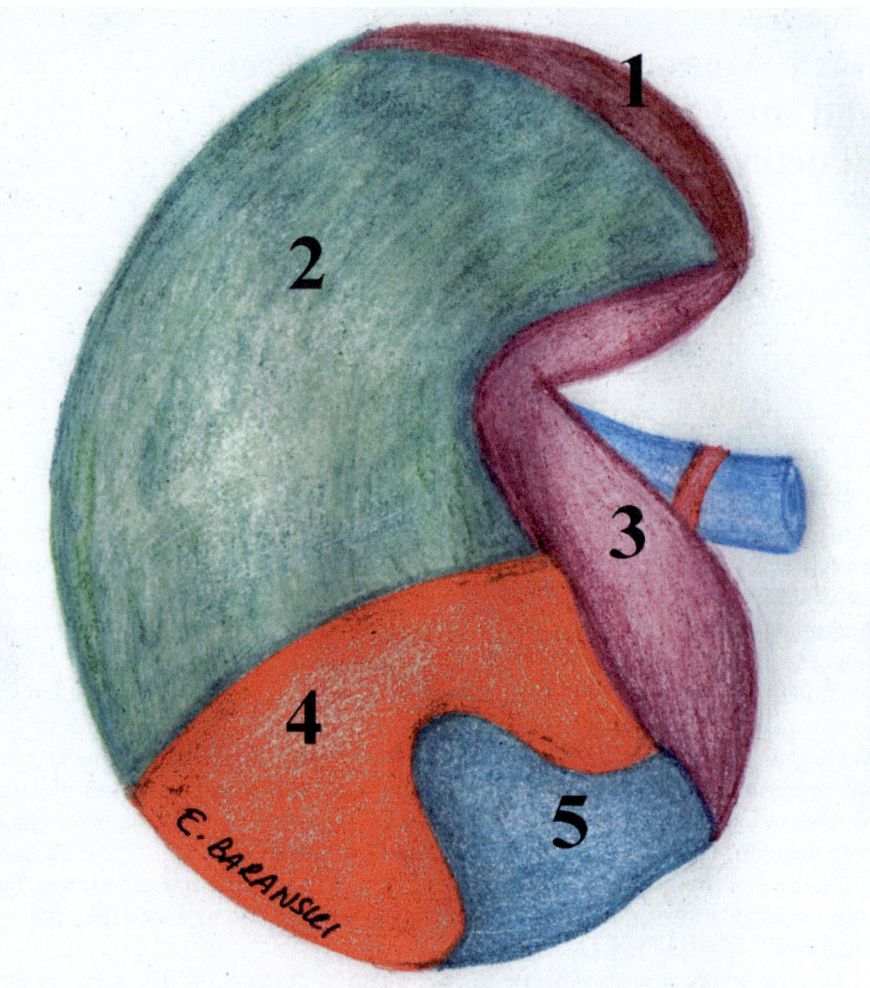

**Fig. 1.1** The adjacent areas of organs to the front surface of the right kidney. 1—Suprarenal gland, 2—Hepatic area (segment VI), 3—Duodenal area (second descending part), 4—Hepatic flexure of the colon, 5—Jejunum loops of small intestine

- splenic flexure of the colon area;
- loops of the small intestine (jejunal area).

The posterior surfaces of both kidneys are adjacent to the diaphragm, quadratus lumborum muscle, major lumbar muscle, transverse abdominal muscle (right kidney) and the beginning of the aponeurosis of the transverse abdominal muscle (lateral side of left kidney) (Fig. 1.3). The average mass of a single kidney is 120–200 g. The kidney of an adult man weighs about 150 g and that of an adult female about 135 g. The longitudinal dimension of the kidney is between 8 and 12 cm, the

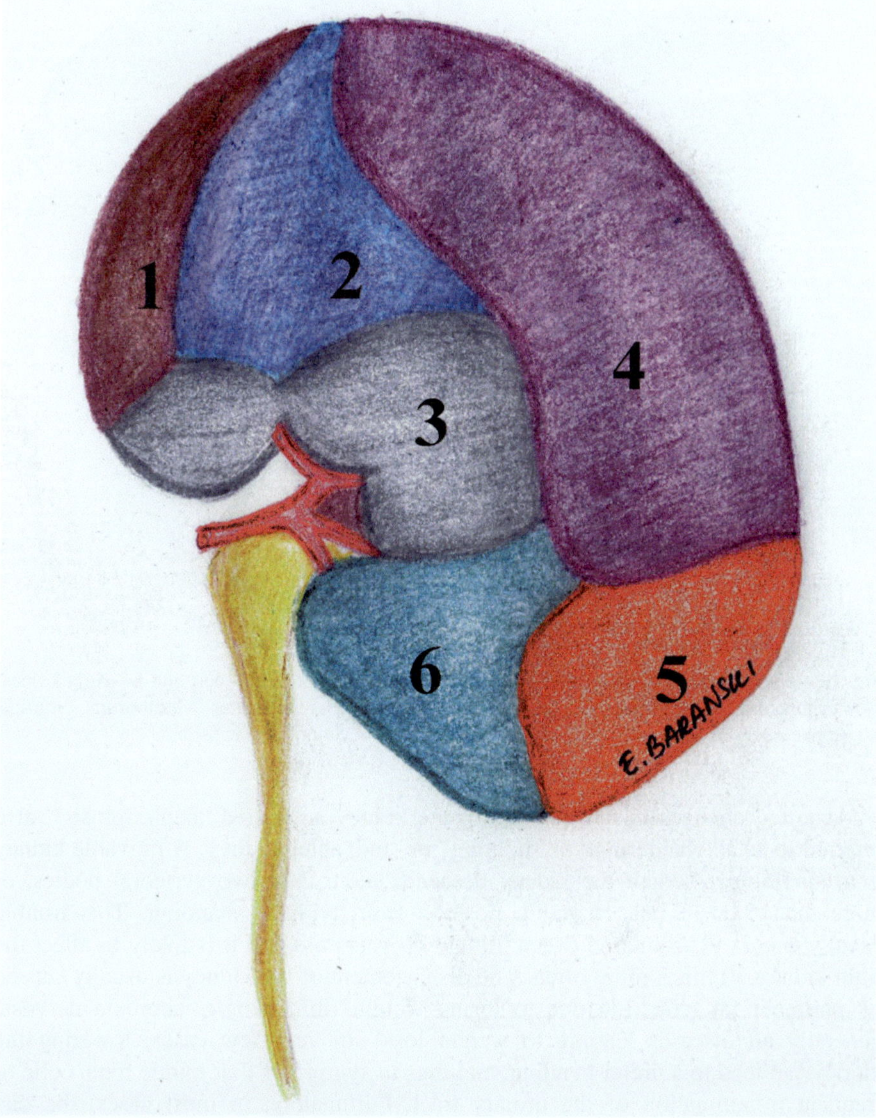



**Fig. 1.2** The adjacent areas of organs to the front surface of the left kidney. 1—Suprarenal gland left, 2—Stomach area, 3—Pancreatic area (body/tail), 4—Splenic area, 5—Splenic flexure of the colon, 6—Jejunum loops of the small intestine

transverse dimension between 5 and 6 cm, and the thickness is between 3 and 4 cm. The left kidney may be slightly longer than the right kidney while the right kidney may be more round due to radiological diagnosis—such as computed tomography and magnetic resonance imaging which give the impression that the right kidney is smaller, but more bellied, compared to the left kidney [10, 11].

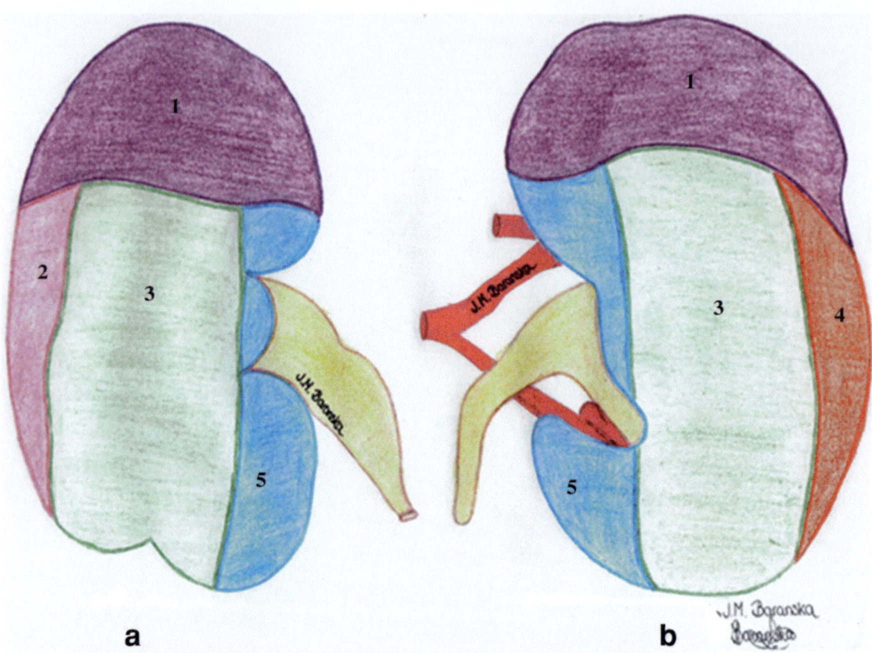

**Fig. 1.3** The adjacent areas of organs to the posterior surface of the **a**—left and **b**—right kidney: 1—Diaphragm, 2—Transverse abdominal muscle, 3—Quadratus lumborum muscle, 4—Aponeurosis of the transverse abdominal muscle, 5—Major lumbar psoas

Acquired changes in the position of the kidney are called "nephroptosis", also referred to as a "wandering" or "floating" or "movable" kidney. A movable kidney is a condition in which the kidney descends more than two vertebral bodies, or more than 5 cm, when changing position from lying to standing. This trouble usually occurs in women between 20 and 40 years old and it is likely to affect the right kidney 30 times more often. The displacement of the kidney is usually caused by perirenal fat reduction due to losing weight (thin people, anorexia nervosa, generally all diseases leading to weight loss). In very few cases, lowering the kidney can lead to a ureter bending, and thus to symptoms that mimic renal colic or frequent inflammation of the urinary tract. Fortunately, in most cases, the displacement of the kidneys or one kidney downward does not cause any discomfort or disease and is usually diagnosed accidentally during radiological examinations. The wandering, movable or floating kidney in most people functions properly, which means that it does not cause any ailments. Generally speaking, the nephroptosis of the kidney is not a contraindication to its possible retrieval and transplantation from living and/or deceased donors [1–4].

## 1.2   The Most Common Congenital Anomalies of the Kidney and Urinary Tract

### *1.2.1   Anomalies of the Collecting System*

The duplex collecting system or duplication of the renal collecting system is recognized in approximately 1:4000 pregnancies and is more frequent in females
(Fig. 1.4a). It disproportionately affects the left kidney and is bilateral in 15–20% of
cases. Complete duplication or double/duplicated ureters have two separate pelvicalyceal systems and two ureters that enter the bladder at different points.
Duplication of the renal collecting system is the most common congenital anomaly
of the urinary tract. A complete or incomplete duplication of the pelvicalyceal
system and ureter has different clinical manifestations depending on the height of
fusion [3, 11–13].

An incomplete duplication has two collecting systems that merge between the
ureteropelvic junction and the urinary bladder, resulting in a single ostium in the
bladder (Fig. 1.4b). This definition includes the following anomalies. A bifid and
single ureter. A bifid ureter means that the affected kidney has two separate
pelvicalyceal systems and two ureters that join together into one ureter before
emptying into the urinary bladder (Y-shaped ureter) (Fig. 1.4c) and [11–14].

An ectopic ureter (see Fig. 1.4d) is a ureter that does not connect properly to the
bladder and drains somewhere outside of it. In boys the ectopic ureter usually drains
into the urethra close to the prostate and in girls into the reproductive organs or
urethra (Fig. 1.4d) [13–15].

In the rare case of inverted Y-ureteral duplication, two ureters fuse before
entering the kidney (Fig. 1.4e).

A ureterocele is an abnormal dilation of the terminal portion of the ureter, which
bulges into the urinary bladder or extends to the bladder neck and the urethra; it
often appears balloon-shaped on cystoscopy or ultrasound examination of the urinary bladder. It is simply a swelling limited to the end of the ureter as it enters into
the bladder. The swollen area prevents urine from moving freely into the bladder.
The urine collects in the ureter and stretches its walls so that it expands like a water
balloon. A ureterocele can also cause urine to flow backward from the bladder to
the kidney, which is called vesicoyreteral reflux (VUR) [12, 15].

Using kidneys with anomalies of the collecting system for transplantation is
sometimes a highly demanding surgical procedure, but in high volume kidney
transplant centers and with a good kidney with anomalies of the collecting system it
should not be a contraindication for living and deceased donation [11–18].

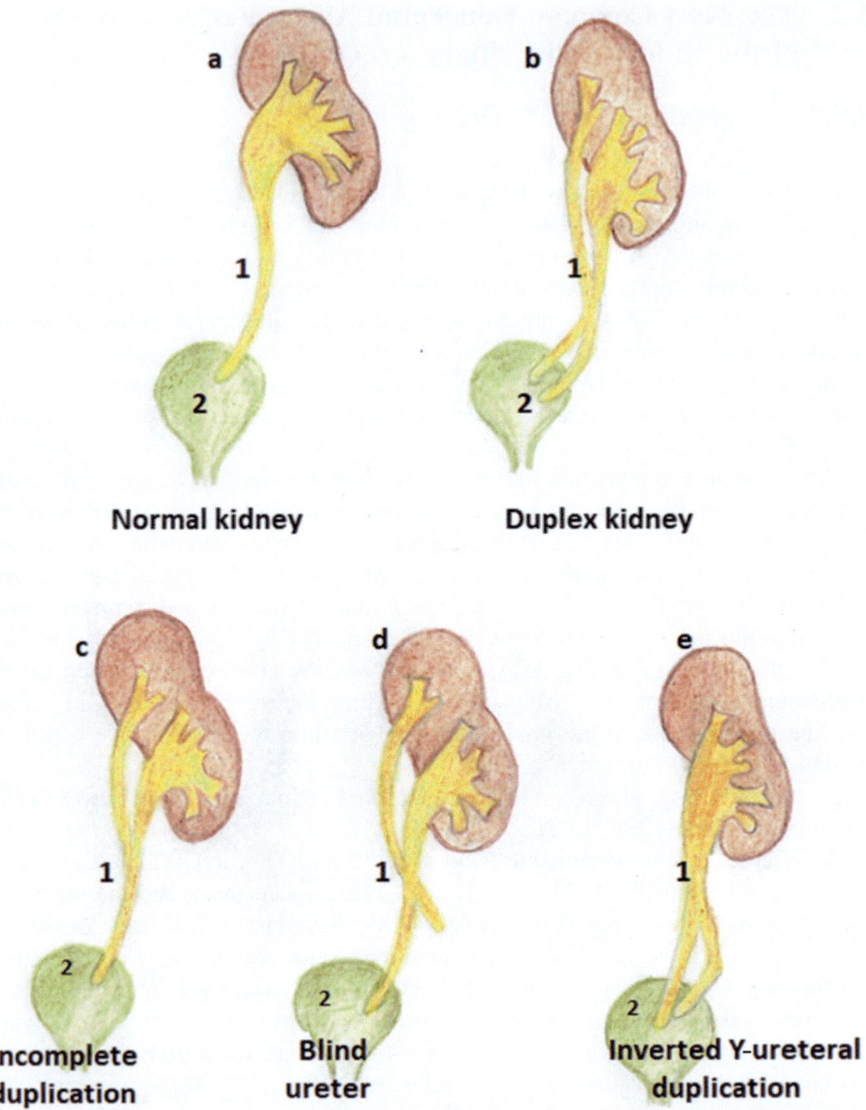


**Fig. 1.4** Classification of duplex kidney anatomy. Compared with a normal kidney (**a**), complete duplication produces a duplex kidney with two poles that drain into two ureters (**b**). Incomplete duplication leads to a Y-shaped ureter (**c**). Blind ureters do not drain into the bladder (**d**). In the rare case of inverted Y-ureteral duplication, two ureters fuse before entering the kidney (**e**), 1— Ureter(s), 2—Urinary bladder (drawing by E. A. Baranski based on [17] https://doi.org/10.12688/f1000research.19826.1)

## 1.2.2   *Malformation of the Renal Parenchyma*

Renal dysgenesis is a broad term which can include any form of underdevelopment of the kidneys [5, 12, 13, 15].

A. Renal agenesis is a medical condition in which one (unilateral) or both (bilateral) fetal kidneys fail to develop. It is a genetic disorder characterized by a failure of the kidney(s) to develop in a fetus. The absence of the kidney(s) and the ureter(s) occurs more often in men than in women. The kidney and the ureter do not develop because of the complete lack of stimulating signals for the differentiation of embryological structures that cause the kidney to grow.
B. Renal hypoplasia (RH) is an abnormality that a person is born with in which one or both of the kidneys are smaller than normal (hypoplastic) but with normal structure. Disease severity depends on whether RH is unilateral or bilateral and on the degree of reduction in the number of nephrons.
C. Renal dysplasia (RD) is an abnormal development of the kidney that results in a nonfunctional kidney. RD is a form of renal malformation in which the kidney (s) are present but their development is abnormal and incomplete. RD can be unilateral or bilateral, segmental and/or variable. Renal parenchyma consists of disorganized nephrons, a reduced number of nephrons and abnormal cells. Unilateral RD is usually asymptomatic. Bilateral RD leads to early renal insufficiency. Examples are polycystic kidney disease, multi-cystic dysplastic kidneys, obstructive cystic dysplasia and medullary sponge kidney.
D. Renal aplasia or agenesis of the kidney is an anatomical anomaly where one of the kidneys together with the ureter is completely absent [11–18].

## 1.2.3   *Congenital Solitary Kidney*

The definition of a "congenital solitary kidney" is that of a person was born with one or two kidneys, but only one of which is functioning in the body. The absence or severe anomalies of the contralateral kidney are caused by an abnormal development due to—for example—renal aplasia, severe RD or RH. A congenital solitary kidney is often asymptomatic and diagnosed during prenatal ultrasound screening. A congenital solitary kidney is usually hypertrophic to compensate for the contralateral kidney and can be responsible for a higher incidence or risk of vesicoureteral reflux, hypertension, renal insufficiency and progression to end-stage renal disease [11–18].

### *1.2.4   Anomalies of Kidney Migration*

The horseshoe kidney is also known as a "ren arcuatus" in Latin, or as a renal fusion or super kidney. The horseshoe kidney is the most common type of fusion anomaly, initially described during autopsies by da Carpi performed in 1522: they are characterized by abnormalities in position, rotation and vascular supply. A horseshoe kidney occurs in about 1 in 500 children during fetal development as the kidneys move into their normal position. Horseshoe kidneys are identified as having functioning renal masses present on both sides of the vertebral column, fused together with ureters that remain uncrossed from the renal hilum to the urinary bladder. The isthmus connecting the two renal masses may be positioned in the midline or laterally, resulting in an asymmetric horseshoe kidney. In more than 90% of cases, fusion occurs at the lower poles (Fig. 1.5), although fusion may occur at the upper pole in a minority of cases. The horseshoe kidney in contrast to

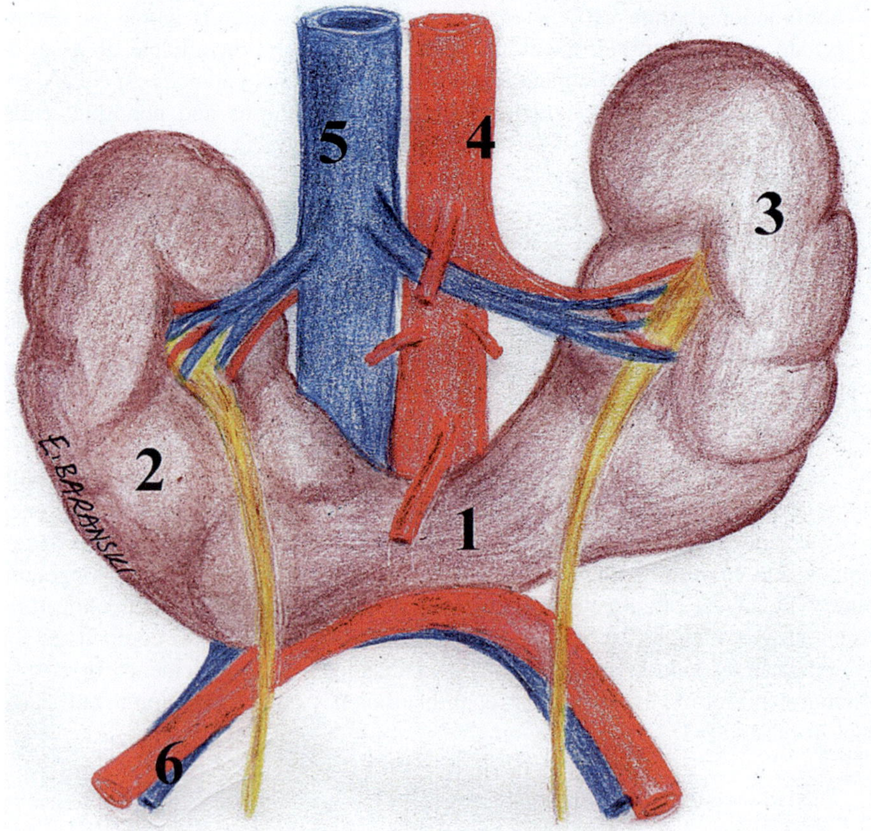

**Fig. 1.5**  Horseshoe kidney. 1—Isthmus connection of two to one renal mass of the lower poles of the kidneys, 2—Right side of the horseshoe kidney ("right kidney"), 3—Left side of the horseshoe kidney ("left kidney"), 4—Abdominal aorta, 5—Inferior vena cava, 6—Right iliac vessels. In about 30% of cases there are constrictions or complete obstruction of pelvic-ureteral connections and also in about 30% of cases horseshoe kidneys are supplied with single arteries

the normal kidney is usually positioned lower. In 30% of the cases, the lower poles of the kidneys are supplied by single renal arteries, in other cases, the vascularization of the horseshoe kidney is very complex and the arterial blood supply consists of a network of small renal arteries deriving from the abdominal aorta, common iliac arteries, the inferior mesenteric artery or the median sacral artery. In about 30% of cases of the horseshoe kidney, there are disorders of the outflow of urine due to the narrowing or closure of the renal pelvis–ureter connections, well known as a ureteropelvic junction. When it comes to using the horseshoe kidney for transplantation, it is generally believed that as soon as the anatomical structure of the kidney allows, it can be donated, procured and transplanted. So far, few descriptions have appeared, because only about 40 cases of successful horseshoe kidney transplantations have been done throughout the world. In most cases, the kidney was taken in its entirety and during preparation for the transplant, it was usually separated into two kidneys, cutting the tissues at the site of the growth of its lower poles and thus obtaining two kidneys for transplantation [1–4, 19–28].

If the anatomy of the kidney does not allow it to be divided and the venous and arterial blood supply is not complicated—for example due to the common renal pelvis system—the kidney is transplanted in its entirety. In the literature only a few cases of successful transplantation of the horseshoe kidney have been described worldwide. In this book, I will not accurately describe the procedures for the retrieval and preparation of the horseshoe kidney for transplantation for several reasons. The first reason is that my personal experience with such a kidney is small as it is only based on one procedure. The second reason is that I believe that the horseshoe kidney is always a big challenge for the surgeon and besides that a high risk for the recipient. If we decide to transplant such a kidney it is necessary to bear in mind, first of all, the safety and benefit of the recipient of this kidney. I would like to warn young surgical adepts not to think that the procurement, benching and transplantation of the horseshoe kidney is a simple operation. If you decide to perform such an operation ask a very experienced surgeon from one of the high volume centers to help and/or guide you or send this kidney to them [19–28].

Renal dystopia or renal ectopia is the displacement of the kidney within the retroperitoneum and crossed dystopia is when both kidneys are located on the same side of the vertebral column [1–4, 29, 30]. The ectopic kidney is also called a 'pancake kidney' and is more common on the left side. Several alternative forms are described, such as a sigmoid-shaped kidney mass with the pelvis of the cranial kidney passing medially while that of the caudal kidney emerges laterally, or makes an L-shape with the caudal kidney lying horizontally or lastly as a renal lump. Nephrolithiasis and hydronephrosis due to pelviureteric junction obstruction are more common in the crossed ectopic kidney [14] and may influence any decision to separate the two kidneys. Developmental vertebral and sacral anomalies are commonly associated with crossed ectopic kidneys.

Retrieval: The lower part may have an arterial supply from the ipsilateral or contralateral common iliac artery [5, 30].

Malrotation is abnormal renal rotation, in particular toward anomalous orientation of the renal hilum. It may occur unilaterally or bilaterally. It is almost always an asymptomatic incidental finding [1–4].


### *1.2.5   Kidney Function*

The four mechanisms which are used in every kidney and which lead to the conversion of blood into urine are filtration, reabsorption, secretion and excretion. The nephron is a structural and functional unit which consists of three parts: a renal corpuscle, renal tubules connecting tubules and a collecting duct system. Each nephron connects to a collecting duct. The collecting ducts are shared by nephrons and for this reason are not taken into consideration as part of a single nephron [1–4, 6].

The renal corpuscle is located in the renal cortex and composed of two structures: the glomerulus and the Bowman's capsule. A renal corpuscle is also known as a Malpighian corpuscle, named after Marcello Malpighi (1628–1694), an Italian physician and biologist from the University of Padua [3, 4].

The renal tubule portion of a nephron is a long, convoluted structure that emerges from the glomerulus. It can be divided into three parts based on function. The first part is called the proximal convoluted tubule (PCT), due to its proximity to the glomerulus. The second part is called the loop of Henle, or the nephritic loop, because it forms a loop with descending and ascending limbs and goes through the renal medulla. The third part of the renal tubule is called the distal convoluted tubule (DCT); this part is also restricted to the renal cortex (Fig. 1.6).

The connecting tubule is the last part of the nephron and connects with and empties its filtrate into collecting ducts that line the medullary pyramids.

The collecting duct system of the kidney consists of a series of tubules and ducts that physically connect nephrons to a minor calyx or directly to the renal pelvis. The collecting ducts accommodate contents from multiple nephrons, fusing together as they enter the papillae of the renal medulla. Urine leaves the medullary collecting ducts through the renal papillae, emptying into the renal calyces, the renal pelvis and finally into the bladder via the ureter(s). A properly functioning human kidney is composed of 1–1.5 million nephrons; 20–25% good functioning and undamaged nephrons are needed by a person to survive without dialysis [1–6].

The basic functions of the kidney are [1, 2, 4]:

A. Secretory: in principle the removal from the blood substances harmful to our health, such as creatinine and urea, uric acid, toxins and drugs, as well as substances taken by the body in excess.

B. Regulatory: which consists in maintaining the balance of the body by affecting the volume and composition of body fluids and osmotic pressure, as well as regulating the acid–base balance by concentrating urine and regenerating the carbonate buffer.

C. Reabsorption: of substances necessary for the body, such as glucose, amino acids, organic acids, phosphates.

D. Hormonal: when the kidneys secrete renin acts on angiotensinogen, which is made in the liver and converts it to angiotensin I. Angiotensin converting enzyme (ACE) converts angiotensin I to angiotensin II. Angiotensin II raises blood pressure by constricting blood vessels. It also triggers the release of the mineralocorticoid aldosterone from the adrenal cortex, which in turn stimulates the renal tubules to reabsorb more sodium. Angiotensin II also triggers the release of anti-diuretic hormone (ADH) from the hypothalamus, leading to water retention in the kidneys.

E. Production within the kidney under the influence of a parathyroid hormone active form of vitamin D—1.25-hydroxycholecalciferol—and within the native substance of certain forms of prostaglandin and kallikrein. Prostaglandins together and the kallikrein-kinin system constitute a major vasodepressor system.

F. Maintaining the water–electrolyte balance by controlling secretion into the urine and the reabsorption of electrolytes. These are the following electrolytes. Sodium (Na+), important for the proper functioning of muscles (99% of ions are absorbed by the kidneys back into the body). Potassium (K+), important for muscle function, neurons and blood volume regulation (absorbed back at 60–80%). Chlorine (Cl−), regulates the pH of the blood, "watches" over the proper conduction of nerve impulses in neurons and muscle cells, and absorbed by the kidneys at 90%. Calcium (Ca+), in the human body calcium is one of the most important electrolytes, which occurs in striated and cardiac muscle. Calcium reabsorption helps Parathyroid Hormone (PTH) through its effects on bone, kidney and intestine. Calcium is absorbed at 90%, magnesium (Mg+) is absorbed by the kidney at almost 100%. Magnesium is necessary for the proper synthesis of about 300 enzymes that interact with phosphate compounds such as ATP, ADP, DNA and RNA (Fig. 1.6) [3, 5, 6].

At the level of the kidney, there are several hormones that are not produced in the kidneys but which help to control their function:

G. Antidiuretic hormone (ADH) (vasopressin), produced by hypothalamus cells, responsible for the resorption of water from the urine, which causes its high density.

H. Angiotensin II, a hormone produced in the liver, responsible in the kidney for the absorption of sodium and chlorine.

I. Aldosterone, produced by the adrenal cortex, responsible at the level of the kidney for the absorption of sodium and chlorine and the excretion of potassium.

J. ANP—atrial natriuretic peptide—is produced by the walls of the atrium of the heart under the influence of high concentrations of sodium ions, a large amount of extracellular fluid or a large amount of blood; it inhibits the resorption of

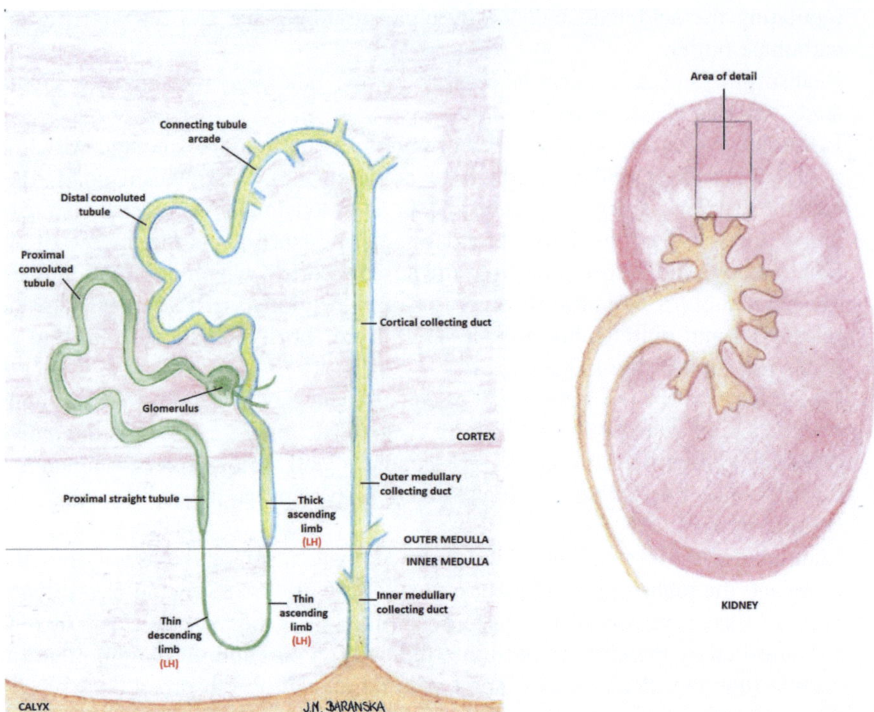


**Fig. 1.6** Microscopic anatomy of the kidney. Anatomy of nephron. LH—loop of Henle. Reabsorption in the nephron: Proximal Convoluted Tubule: amino acids—100%, glucose—100%, water—70%, sodium—70%, potassium—70%, calcium—70%, phosphate—70%, urea—50%, magnesium 30%. Proximal Straight Tubule: phosphate—15%. Thick Ascending Limb: magnesium —60%, sodium—25%, calcium 25%, potassium—20%, Distal convoluted tubule: calcium—8%, sodium—5%, magnesium—5%, water and urea—unstable, Collecting duct (cortical, medullary, inner): sodium 3%, water and urea unstable. Calyx and urinary bladder: phosphate- 15%, magnesium —5%, potassium—1–100% (variable), calcium—1%, sodium—1%, water and urea unstable

sodium and water ions, mainly in the kidney tubules, and leads to their increased urinary excretion, causes an acceleration of urine production, inhibits the renin–angiotensin–aldosterone (RAA) system by stimulating prostaglandin synthesis and reducing ADH release.

Summary: the seven functions of the kidneys:
A—controlling ACID–base balance.
W—controlling WATER balance.
E—maintaining ELECTROLYTE balance.
T—removing TOXINS and waste products from the body.
B—controlling BLOOD PRESSURE.
E—producing the hormone ERYTHROPOIETIN.
D—activating vitamin D [1–6].

## 1.3   Blood Flow Through the Kidney—Glomerular Filtration [1–6]

In this section, I would like to recall some of the most important information on glomerular flow rate (GFR) that the surgeon should bear in mind. GFR is the value of filtration that is now the basis for determining kidney function in terms of their suitability for procurement and transplantation. The blood supply to the kidneys is very rich and the blood flow is relatively large. Every minute 0.8–1.2 L of blood passes through them, that is 20% of the blood pumped through the heart, although the kidneys alone represent no more than 0.1–0.5% of the weight of an adult human [4–6]. Approximately 10% of the volume of blood flowing through the kidneys is filtered through the renal glomeruli, which means that the GFR is correctly about 80–120 ml/min. This is a very important indicator of normal kidney function or the degree of their failure, damage or disability. During the day, about 150 L of glomerular filtrate is formed, which undergoes major changes in the renal tubules, and about 1.5 L of urine (1% of glomerular filtrate).

The amount of glomerular filtration can be approximately estimated from the serum creatinine concentration using appropriate formulae.

The simplest of them has the form:

$$\text{GFR (ml/min)} = 100/\text{serum creatinine (mg/dl)}$$

One of the most commonly used patterns by doctors is the Cockcroft and Gault equation:

$$\text{GFR (ml/min)} = (140 - \text{age [years]}) \times \text{body weight [kg]}/72 \\ \times \text{serum creatinine (mg/dl)}$$

For a woman, the result obtained should be multiplied by 0.85.

Regarding kidney dysfunction, it is worth recalling the classification of the five stages of chronic kidney disease (CKD), where at each stage a glomerular filtration rate is determined.

- stage 1—normal or high GFR (GFR > 90 ml/min)
- stage 2—early CKD (GFR = 60–89 ml/min)
- stage 3—moderate CKD (GFR = 30–59 ml/min)
- stage 4—severe CKD (GFR = 15–29 ml/min)
- stage 5—end stage CKD (GFR < 15 ml/min).

The end stage of renal disease occurs in the fifth stage of CKD with a GFR index of 15 ml/min or lower. In this case, dialysis or kidney transplantation is necessary to keep the patient alive [1–6].

We are all aware that in every country in the world there is an increase in the number of people waiting for a kidney transplant. The waiting list are everywhere growing and mortality is increasing accordingly In recent years, the criteria for acceptance of kidneys for transplantation have been changed. The influence of the donor risk factors as a body mass index, donor age, active smoking, arterial hypertension glomerular flirtation rate (GFR) of 80 ml/min are not absolute contraindication for kidney donation. In 1999, Eurotransplant established the European Senior Transplant Program matching donors and recipients over 60 years of age. To help many older dialysis patients above 60 years of age with persistent kidney failure, different types of "old for old" programs have been developed worldwide. Kidneys from donors over 60 years of age with a good function—this means a good GFR—are therefore transplanted as a single organ to recipients of the same age group. Kidneys from older donors with low glomerular filtration do not enable the recipient to become independent of dialysis when one of the kidneys of these donors is transplanted. For old kidney recipients with kidney insufficiency the only way to become independent of dialysis is by the transplantation of two kidneys which results in an increasing number of well-functioning and filtering nephrons. The kidneys come in most cases from donors with a GFR of less than 80 ml/min, with advanced atherosclerotic lesions at the level of glomerular arteries and often with concomitant other diseases, such as diabetes and hypertension [1–6].

## 1.4   Renal Arteries

The renal arteries arise on both sides of the abdominal aorta. The right renal artery courses inferiorly and passes posteriorly to the inferior vena cava (IVC) and the right renal vein to reach the renal hilum. The left renal artery is much shorter and arises slightly more superiorly to the right main renal artery. The left renal artery courses more horizontally, posterior to the left renal vein, to enter the renal hilum. In most cases renal arteries arise from the abdominal aorta inferior to the orifice of the superior mesenteric artery (SMA). Sometimes the renal arteries arise from the abdominal aorta at the level of or above the SMA. The renal artery on one or both sides may arise from the bifurcation of the aorta or from the common and internal iliac arteries, the inferior mesenteric artery (IMA), middle sacral artery or a common intercostal-renal trunk. The right artery may cross in front of instead of behind the IVC. The right and left renal arteries were reported to be at the same level in about 30% of cases, while the right was higher in 47% and the left was higher in about 23% of cases. A single renal artery on one side and multiple (two, three or four) renal arteries on the other is not unusual. There were no reported sex (gender) or race related differences. The average length of the renal artery, counting from the aorta to its branching, is 25–26 mm; in some cases, every renal artery can be divided into numerous branches as soon as it leaves the aorta [29–43]. The average length of the right renal artery ranges from 0.5 to 8.0 cm (it is longer than the left renal artery). The external diameter of the renal artery is 6–8 mm and the internal diameter, depending on the method of measurement, ranges from $5.04 \pm 0.74$ mm during ultrasound to $5.68 \pm 1.19$ mm during classical arteriography. The right renal artery usually moves away from the aorta more in front and slightly lower than the left. The left renal artery runs backwards from the pancreas body and splenic vein, is crossed by the IMA and in most cases is positioned just below and behind the upper pole of the renal vein. Each single renal artery gives off the following branches: a superior one called the inferior adrenal artery to the suprarenal gland, an inferior branch called the ureteral branch to the renal pelvis, and the upper ureter and the renal capsular artery. The ureteral branch is divided into the inferior and superior branch. The inferior branch supplies the upper ureter above the ureteropelvic junction with the testicular or ovarian artery, and the upper one supplies the anterior surface of the renal pelvis. It should be noted that in front of renal hilum, the branches of the main renal artery arise less than 1.5–2.0 cm from the abdominal aorta of the patients who are being evaluated as possible donors, because these early branches may make it impossible to perform not only a kidney donation, but also an arterial anastomosis during the kidney transplantation. Considering the division pattern, a common variant is when the main renal artery divides before it reaches the renal hilum. This condition is named the extra-hilar branching. Normally, early branching of the renal artery should take place within 1.5 cm of the renal ostium of the abdominal aorta. It is essential to identify any pre-hilar branching that occurs within 2 cm of the exit of the renal artery from the abdominal aorta, since most surgeons require at least a 2 cm length of renal artery before hilar branching to guarantee satisfactory control and anastomosis. According to [30] early branching of the left renal arteries (<2 cm from the aorta) is present in 21% of cases whereas early branching of the right renal arteries is present in 15% of individuals [29, 30]. Each renal artery, which reaches the renal hilum, divides into an anterior and posterior branch and these branches divide into segmental arteries which supply the five renal vascular segments of the kidney, such as the apical (superior), anterior superior, anterior inferior (middle), caudal and posterior. The apical and anterior segments form the majority of the anterior surface of the kidney, the posterior segment forms most of the posterior surface of the kidney, and the apical and inferior vascular segments form the anterior and posterior segments of the kidney (Fig. 1.7). Considering the division pattern, a common variant is when the main renal artery divides before it reaches the renal hilum [29, 30]. When there are two or more arteries with a separate origin, the vessel with the greatest diameter is considered as the main renal artery and the rest are branded as accessory or aberrant (supernumerary). Additional arteries can, in turn, be divided into two categories according to how they attain the kidney: hilar (entering at the hilum (accessory)) and polar (reaching at the pole (aberrant)). Renal arteries are, as a rule, the single vessels protruding on the right and left side of the abdominal aorta. The presence of a single renal artery on the right and left side of the abdominal aorta is found in about 70% of the human population, the remaining 30% has more than one renal artery. According to [38] when there were many accessory renal arteries, the

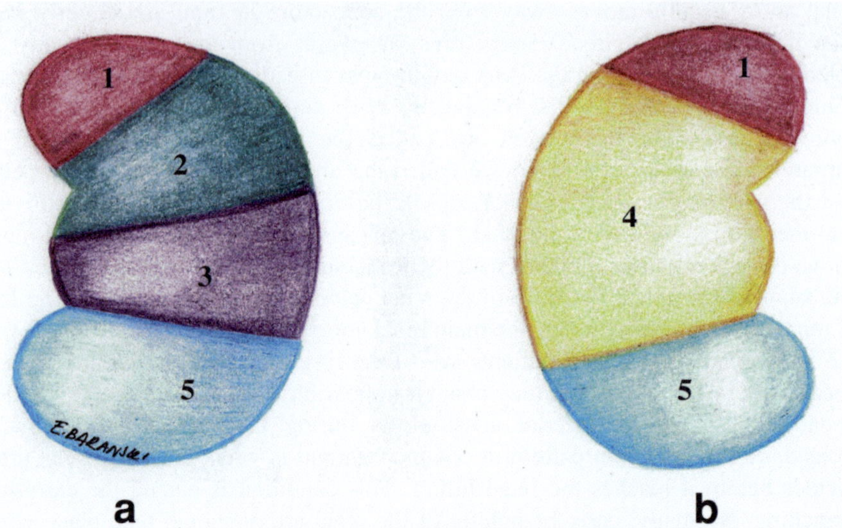


**Fig. 1.7** Left kidney. **a**—Anterior surface of the left kidney. **b**—Posterior surface of the left kidney. The kidney is divided into five vascular segments: 1—Apical (20%), 2—Superior (33%), 3—Middle (40%), 4—Posterior (13%) and 5—Inferior (47%). The superior and middle segments make up the majority of the anterior surface of the kidney, the posterior segments make up the majority of the posterior surface of the kidney and the apical and inferior segments make up the anterior and posterior surfaces

superior accessory renal artery is a separate segment artery and the inferior accessory artery is a separate lower segmental artery. About 10% of the population has multiple renal arteries that enter the kidney through its hilum (accessory) and about 20% enter the kidney parenchyma by passing its hilum (aberrant). Additional renal arteries occur unilaterally three times more often than on both sides. The renal and accessory renal arteries may branch off from the abdominal aorta, as well as from the common, external and internal iliac arteries, the lower mesenteric artery and the medial sacral artery. Both the right main renal artery and the accessory renal artery can run in front of the anterior surface of the IVC (Fig. 1.8). Classically, the renal arteries to the right kidney run behind the IVC, adjacent to its posterior wall. Accessory renal arteries reaching the kidney outside its hilum usually depart from the aorta or the main trunk of the renal artery. Accessory renal arteries are more common on the left side of the abdominal aorta than on the right. Arterial vessels supplying the kidneys show a high anatomical variability in their course, which is found in almost 40% of the human population. A single renal artery to each kidney is present in about 70% of individuals [2]. The division of the main renal artery at

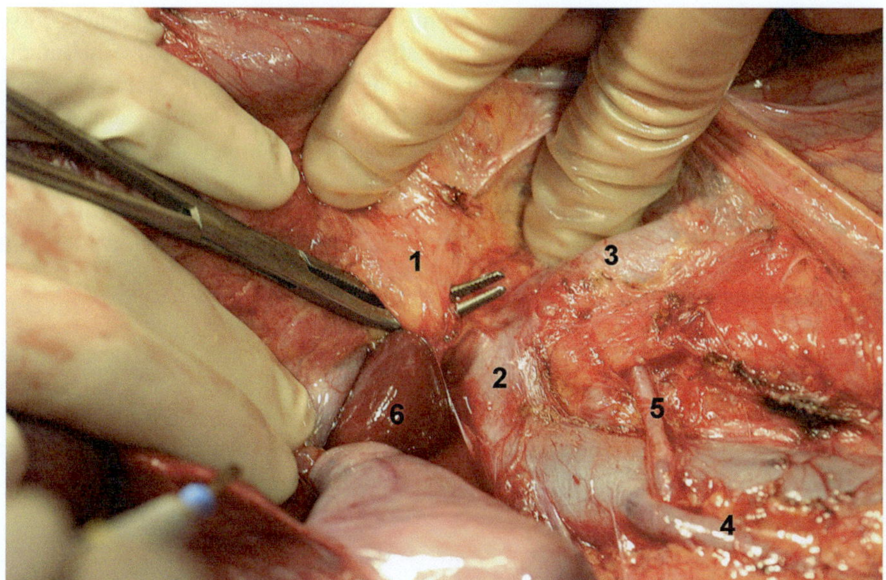

**Fig. 1.8** Classically, the renal arteries run behind the posterior wall of the IVC. Both the right main renal artery and the right additional renal artery may run on the anterior surface of the IVC. 1—Plexus celiacus, 2—IVC, 3—Left renal vein with normal course, 4—Right gonadal vein, 5—Abnormal course of the renal artery on the anterior surface of the IVC under gonadal vein, 6—Caudate lobe of the liver

the level of the kidney hilum occurs in almost 60% of people. In about 15% of the human population, the renal artery after departing from the aorta divides in the initial or middle part of the main renal artery. Various arteries can move away from the renal arteries, for example: the upper diaphragm, additional hepatic, central and lower adrenal, nuclear or ovarian, as well as arteries leaving the pancreas, colon and lumbar arteries. Sometimes an accessory renal artery is responsible for the arterial supply of the upper pole of the kidney which departs from the diaphragm artery [29–43].

Renal arteries abound with arteries and anatomical anomalies. As for the number of arteries, there is a high variability, as the kidneys can be supplied by one, two, three or even more arteries, while accessory renal arteries can move away from different arteries throughout the abdomen. Multiple arteries may coexist with other uretero-vascular variations such as double or multiple renal veins on the same side, or on the opposite side, double or multiple ureters on the same side or on the opposite side, or persistence of the fetal renal lobulation on the adult kidney [29].

The number of renal arteries and their unusual and sometimes unexpected course should stimulate the surgeon to continuously improve his knowledge about the human anatomy and alertness when retrieving the kidneys for transplantation deriving from living, donation after circulatory death or brain death donors. Especially the living donor kidney requires a very thorough screening before donation—regarding not only their function but also their vessels—if we want to transplant them without complications. About 20% of the cardiac output to supply kidneys, which represents less than 100th of the total body weight, flows through the renal arteries to both kidneys [3, 5, 28–39].

**Warning!**
The number, size and location of the renal arteries and veins, advanced arteriosclerosis or other pathologies of the renal vascular wall may be a contraindication to kidney donation and transplantation.

Remember that if the renal vascularization if very abnormal and complicated, it can become a contraindication for kidney donation and transplantation.

## 1.5   Renal Veins and IVC Abnormalities

### 1.5.1   Renal Veins

The renal veins are blood vessels that return blood to the heart from the kidney. Each kidney is drained by its own renal vein(s) (the right and left renal vein). Each renal vein drains into a vena cava inferior (VCI), which carries blood directly to the heart. The right renal vein is 2–4 cm long, the left 4–11 cm. The left renal vein crosses the abdominal aorta, usually on its front wall, just 1.0–1.5 cm below the beginning of the SMA. In most cases, the left renal vein runs horizontally and passes into the IVC slightly higher than the right renal vein. The VCI is found in most cases to the right side of the abdominal aorta; the left renal vein is longer than the right. Depending on sex, the following veins join to the left renal vein: testicular, ovarian, inferior diaphragm vein which drains blood into the left adrenal vein, and in 65.2% of the population the lumbar vein. When the left renal vein has a normal course and passes into the IVC, it runs along the anterior wall of the abdominal aorta (Fig. 1.8, 3–Left renal vein with normal course), the ovarian or testicular vein and adrenal vein always pass into it in 100% and the renal-lumbar vein in 65.2% of cases. A right double renal vein or duplication of the right renal vein occurs in 29% of the population (Figs. 1.9 and 1.10); three right renal veins (Fig. 1.11) are rare and occur in about approximately 9.7% of the population. Venous branches on the right side very rarely enter into the right renal vein, the ovarian or testicular vein enter into the right renal vein in only 3.22% of cases. The kidneys' purified blood flows through the renal veins in the direction of the inferior vena, in order to then be transported to the right atrium of the heart [2, 3, 30, 39–52].

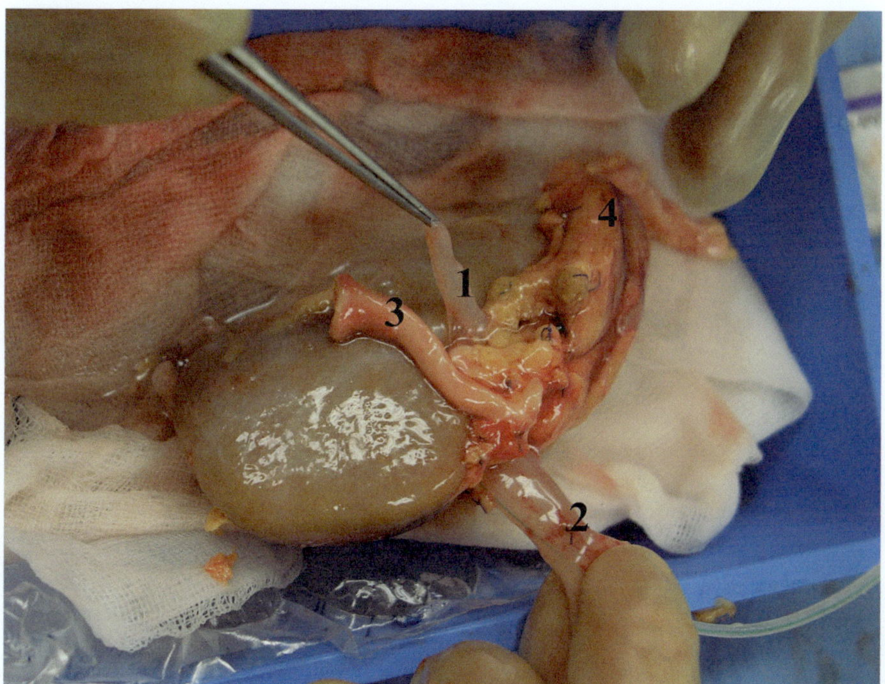

**Fig. 1.9** Double right renal vein—occurs in 29% of the population. 1 and 2—Renal veins, 3—Right renal artery, 4—Ureter

On the left side, the left renal vein which runs behind the abdominal aorta is called a retro-aortic. A retro-aortic left renal vein is located between the aorta and the lumbar vertebrae and drains blood in most of the cases into the IVC or left common iliac vein. The presence of this variant should be suspected when the left renal vein is not found at its physiological location, that is between the posterior wall of the superior mesenteric artery and the anterior wall of the aorta (Fig. 1.12a —2, b—Type I A). The left renal vein with a retro-aortic course occurs with a frequency reported of 0.5 to 3.6%. According to the place of its drainage into the IVC, we can distinguish four types of retro-aortic left renal veins: I—it passes beyond the aorta and flows into the lower main vein at the same height as the normal renal vein (orthotopic position), II—it has a retro-aortic course and escapes into the IVC at the level of L4–L5, III—before exiting the kidney it is distributed and runs both at the back and front of the abdominal aorta, IV—it enters into the common left iliac vein. There are three different anomalies where the left renal vein passes behind the aorta [53–56].

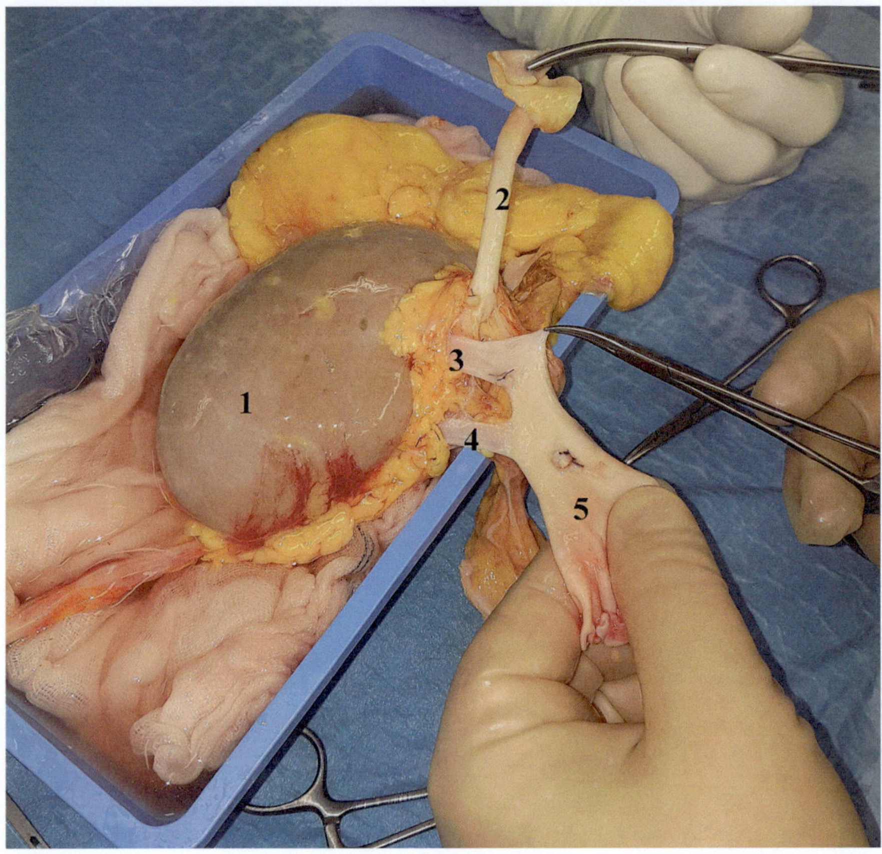

**Fig. 1.10** Right double renal vein—occurs in 29% of the population. 1—Right kidney, 2—Right renal artery, 3 and 4—Two renal veins from the right kidney, 5—Inferior vena cava

The retro-aortic left renal vein passes behind the aorta but is otherwise at the same level as an anterior placed vein would be expected, as mentioned above (Fig. 1.12a—2, b—A).

The oblique retro-aortic left renal vein passes obliquely behind the aorta to enter the IVC on the left side above the confluence of the common iliac veins (Fig. 1.12B) [29].

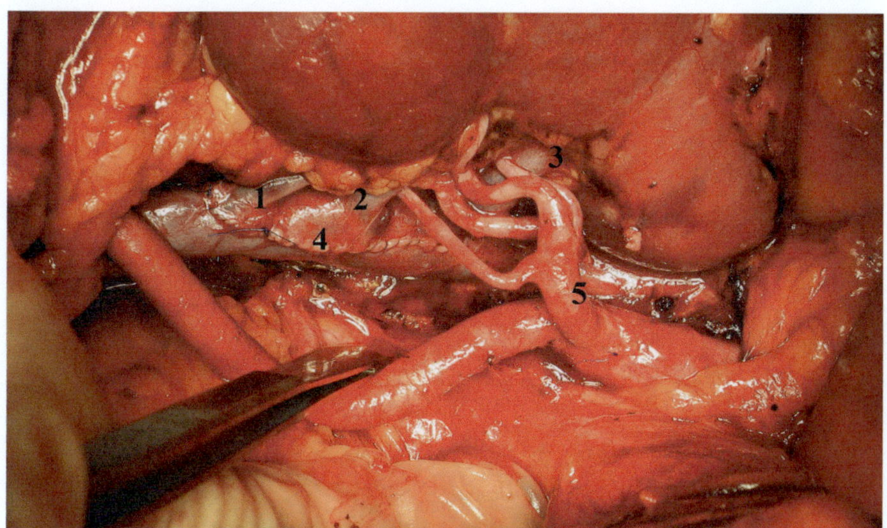

**Fig. 1.11** The three renal veins are very rare in about 9.7% of the population. Transplanted right kidney with three veins on a patch from the IVC. 1, 2 and 3—Three veins to the right kidney, 4—IVC patch, 5—The main trunk of the right renal artery

Regarding the circum-aortic left renal vein (Fig. 1.12, bottom drawing C), the most common abnormality is the presence of an additional tributary, which originates from the main left renal vein at the left lateral edge of the aorta and passes obliquely to the IVC; the two renal veins, thus, encircle the aorta. Based on my experience, there is often a lower pole artery to the right kidney passing in front of the cava associated with this anomaly [29]. The most common urological symptom of retro-aortic left renal vein is hematuria. The major etiology of urological symptoms is compression of the left renal vein between the abdominal aorta and vertebrae: the so-called posterior nutcracker syndrome [29].

Bergman et al. [33, 34] in their articles on renal vascular anatomy, based on the study of human corpses, concluded that the renal veins have less variation in their number and places of departure than renal arteries. Renal veins are usually single vessels, but may divide into several vessels at the exit of the kidney. The renal veins show less variation than the renal arteries and the right renal vein may be double or multiple, even though the left renal vein is usually single [30, 33, 34, 39–52].

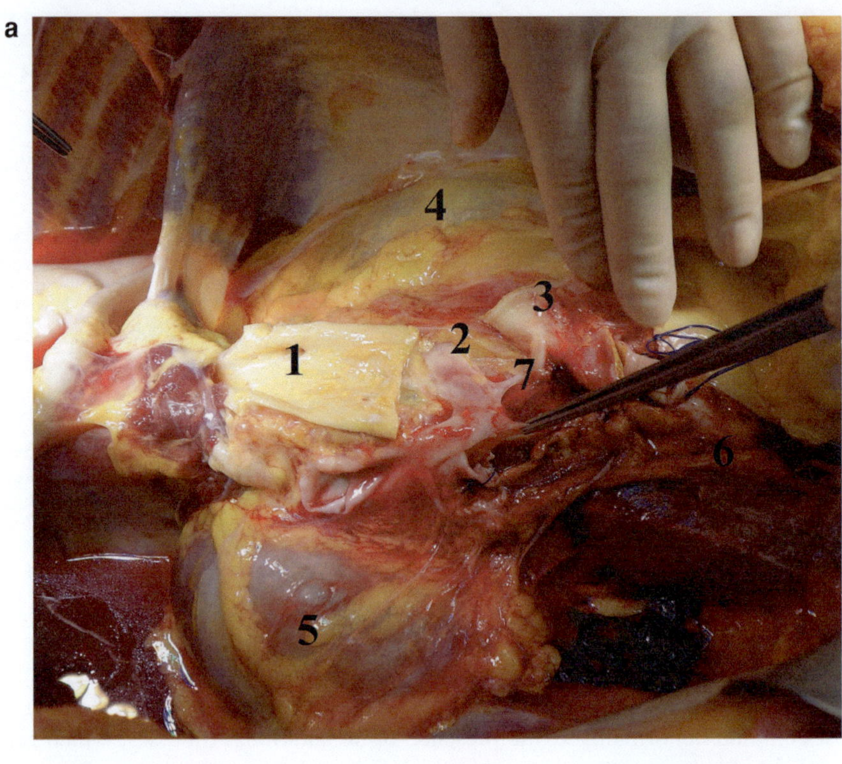

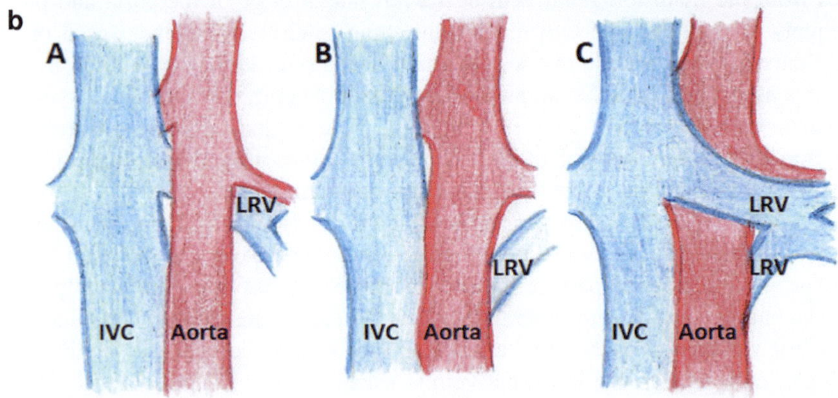



**Fig. 1.12** (**a**) **Top picture:** Retro-aortic course of the left renal vein, 1—Open anterior wall of the abdominal aorta—visible opening of the left renal artery, 2—Left renal vein with preaortic course, 3—Cut posterior wall of the aorta to expose the aortic course of the left renal vein, 4—Left kidney, 5—Right kidney, 6—Right kidney's ureter, 7—One of the very thin branches reaching the left renal vein. (**b**) **Bottom drawing:** Left renal vein anomalies: A—retro-aortic (Type I), B—oblique retro-aortic (Type II), and C—circum-aortic (Type III) (drawing by E. A. Baranski based on [56] https://doi.org/10.1111/ajt.13310)

### *1.5.2  The Most Common Anomalies of IVC*

(a) The absence (agenesis) of the inferior vena cava—a rare anomaly. However, lower extremity tropic ulcer with or without prior deep vein thrombosis (DVT) seems to be a consistent finding in later stages of this condition.

(b) Duplication of IVC occurs as a result of persistence of both supracardinal veins forming duplicated infrarenal IVC. The right and left IVC is observed in a prevalence of 0.2–3.0% of the population—in this case the left IVC usually enters into the left renal vein, which crosses anteriorly to the aorta in the normal fashion to join the right IVC. The IVC may lie on the left side, crossing to the right at the level of the left renal vein. Alternatively, the main IVC may lie in the normal position, but there is a left-sided IVC, often much smaller, which persists, draining the left iliac veins to the left renal vein. Less commonly, a double IVC exists, but with both lying to the right, or partly behind, the aorta [58, 59]. The presence of these IVC anomalies should not affect retrieval or implantation, but knowledge of them will aid recognition (Fig. 1.12 bottom drawing B and C). A left-sided IVC is a rare anatomical variation that has significant surgical implications. Preoperative identification with imaging modalities is critical in preventing unexpected surgical complications.

(c) Left-sided location of the IVC is observed in about 0.4–0.5% of the population. The typical endpoint of a left-sided IVC is at the level of the left renal vein, where it crosses anteriorly to the aorta to form a normal right-sided (Fig. 1.13 top picture—4, 5, 6, bottom drawing—A and B) IVC. A left-sided IVC is a rare anatomical variation that has significant surgical implications. Preoperative identification with imaging modalities is critical in preventing unexpected surgical complications.

Anatomical anomalies occur in the complex process of embryogenesis, which takes place in between the sixth and tenth weeks of gestation. In the embryogenesis of the IVC, three pairs of venous systems are involved: the posterior, subcardinal and supracardinal veins. The subcardinal veins form a part of the IVC, renal veins and gonadal veins The supracardinal veins form part of the IVC, the intercostal veins, hemiazygos vein and azygos vein. Most of the anomalies of the IVC are asymptomatic. However, cases of venous thrombosis and pulmonary embolism due to IVC anomaly have been reported in the literature. Variations of the IVC and thus the unusual location of the renal veins can sometimes make it difficult to procure kidneys from living and/or deceased donors, as well as the decision to transplant them. Preoperative identification with imaging modalities is critical in preventing unexpected surgical complications [59, 60].

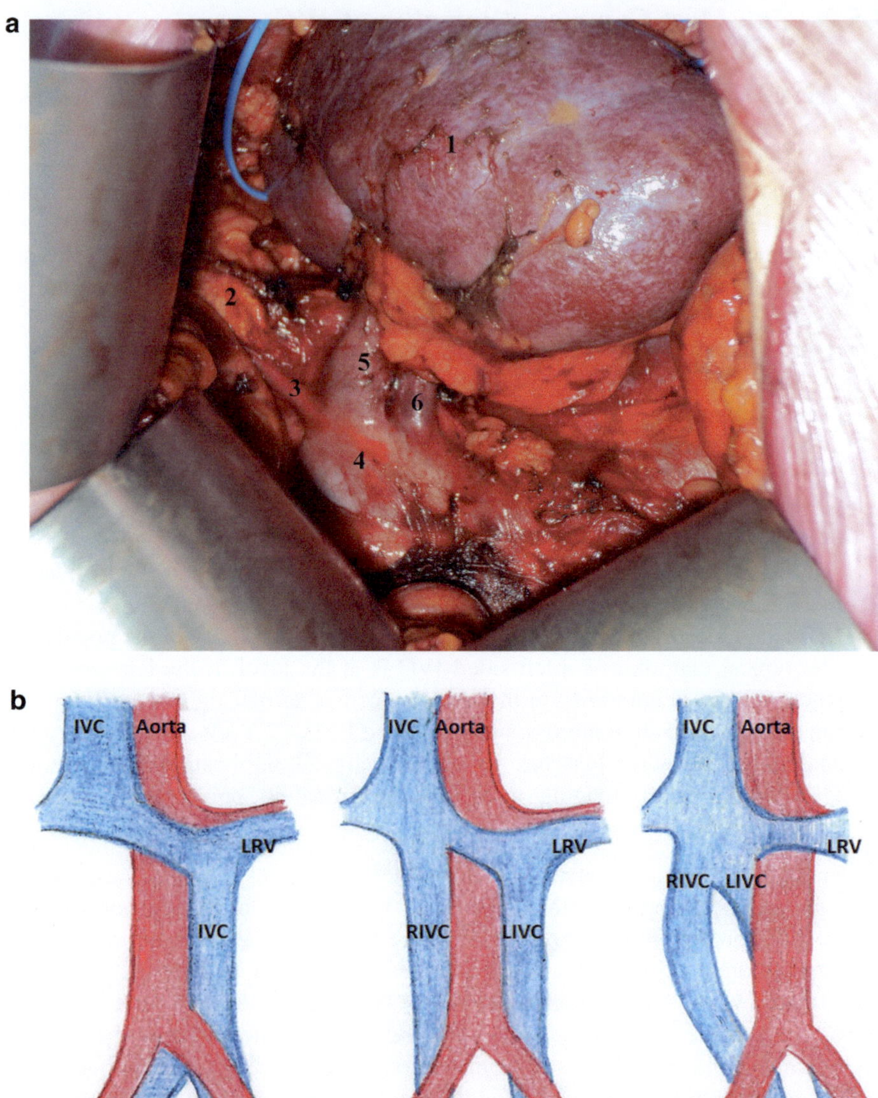


**Fig. 1.13** (**a**) **Top picture:** Left-sided location of the IVC. Picture taken during left kidney donation from a living donor. This anomaly is very rare and applies to about 0.5% of the human population. 1—Left kidney, 2—Left adrenal gland, 3—Adrenal vein, 4—IVC, 5 and 6—Two left renal veins. (**b**) **Bottom drawing:** Anomalies of the IVC: A—Left sided, B—Duplicated and present on the right and left side of abdominal aorta, C—Duplicated branches on the right side— right side double IVC (drawing by E. A. Baranski based on [56] https://doi.org/10.1111/ajt.13310)

### *1.5.3  Renal Lymphatic Vessels*

We begin with three plexuses, around the renal tubules, under the renal capsule and in the perirenal fat. Collecting vessels from the intrarenal plexus form four or five trunks which follow the renal vein to the end in the lateral aortic nodes. The perirenal plexus drains directly into the same nodes [2, 3]. Renal lymphatic vessels of the right kidney drain into lymph nodes located between the IVC and aorta lateral paracaval nodes and anterior and posterior IVC lymph nodes. They also drain towards the diaphragm and downward to the common iliac lymph nodes. The lymphatics of the left kidney drain into the lateral paraaortic lymph nodes. They also drain upward towards the diaphragm and downward to the lymph nodes associated with the IMA [2, 3].

## 1.6  Ureter—Anatomy, Structure, Function and Vascularization

Ureters arise as a continuation of the renal pelvis and terminate in the pelvic cavity. The ureter is thin, its diameter is about 3–4 mm and is about 26–30 cm long. It is mostly located on both sides of the vertebral column and it connects the kidneys to the urinary bladder. The muscular layers of the ureters contract and cause consequently peristaltic waves which are responsible for moving the urine from the kidney into the urinary bladder. The ureters begin at the ureteropelvic junction (UPJ), which lies posteriorly to the renal vein and the artery in the hilum. Afterwards they travel extraperitoneally on the posterior side of the abdominal cavity and terminate in the urinary bladder mouths, which are part of the bladder triangle [2–6, 9, 10]. The blood supply to the ureter is segmental (Fig. 1.14). The upper ureters closest to the kidneys receive blood directly from the renal arteries. The middle part is supplied by the common iliac arteries, branches from the abdominal aorta and the gonadal arteries. The most distal part of the ureter receives blood from branches of the internal iliac artery. The ureter process over the common iliac arteries, showing the anatomical landmark of the bifurcation of the common iliac vessels into internal and external. The arterial supply will course along the ureter longitudinally creating a plexus of anastomosing vessels. This is of clinical significance because it allows safe mobilization of the ureter during surgery when proper exposure from surrounding structures is crucial [2–5, 9, 10].

The venous and lymphatic drainage of the ureter mirrors that of the arterial supply. The lymphatic drainage is to the internal, external and common iliac nodes. The lymphatic drainage of the left ureter is primarily to the left para-aortic lymph nodes while the drainage of the right ureter primarily drains to the right pericaval and inter-aortocaval lymph nodes.

There are three specific areas of narrowing along the ureter. The first is the UPJ. This is the area where the renal pelvis becomes narrower into the proximal

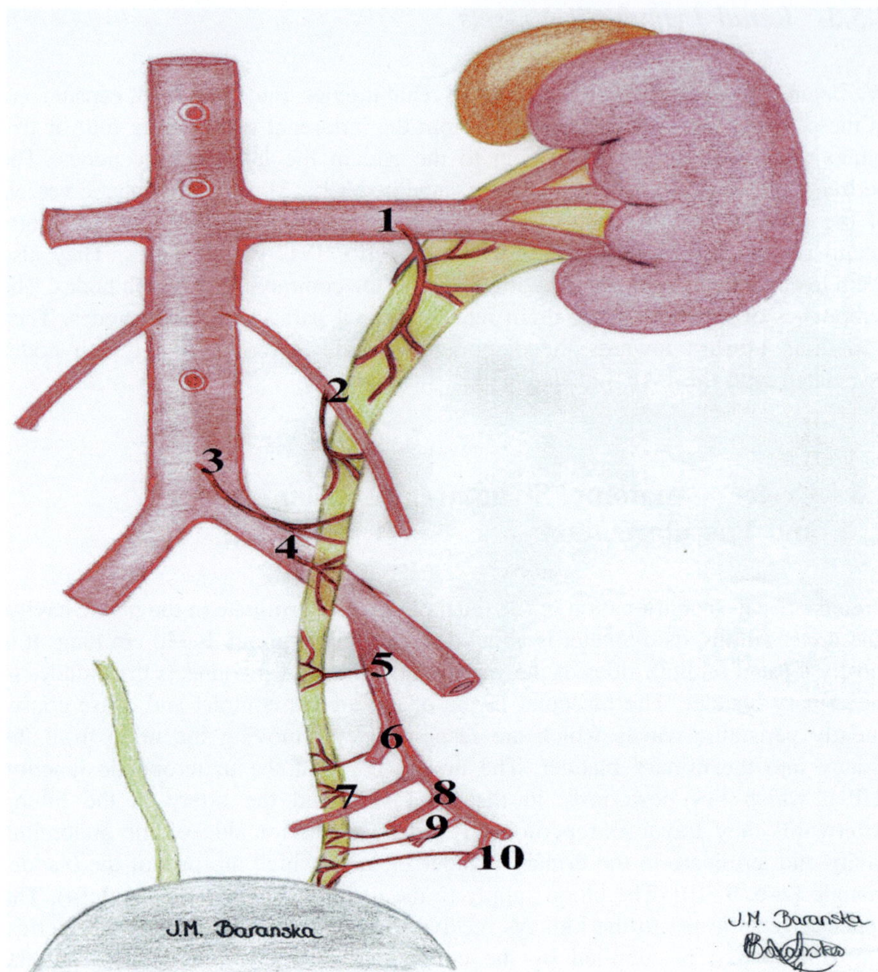

Fig. 1.14  Blood supply of ureter. 1—Renal artery, 2—Gonadal artery, 3—Abdominal Aorta, 4—Common iliac artery, 5—Internal iliac artery, 6—Superior vesical artery, 7—Uterine artery in female, 8—Middle rectal artery in male, 9—Vaginal artery in female, 10—Inferior vesical artery

ureter. The second region of narrowing occurs where the ureter crosses the iliac vessels (pelvic brim). The narrowing is due to the extrinsic compression of the iliac vessels on the ureter and the angle of the ureter as it enters the pelvis. The ureterovesical junction at the intravesical course (0.5–1.0 cm) with diameter 3–4 mm or UVJ is the third site of ureteral narrowing. A retrospective study of 94 patients presenting to the emergency department for colic found that 60.6% of stones were located at the UVJ [3, 5].

Always check the kidneys for stones before (via an echo), during the kidney procurement and inspection.

The ureters have specific anatomic relationships depending upon the side of the body. The right ureter lies in close relationship to the ascending colon, cecum and appendix. The left ureter is close to the descending and sigmoid colon.

The nomenclature of the ureter is based on its anatomic relationship to surrounding structures. The abdominal ureter is the segment of the ureter that extends from the renal pelvis to the iliac vessels. The pelvic ureter extends from the iliac vessels to the bladder. There is an alternative method of ureteral nomenclature: upper, middle and lower segments. The upper ureter extends from the renal pelvis to the upper border of the sacrum. The middle ureter continues from the upper to lower borders of the sacrum. The distal ureter continues from the lower border of the sacrum to the bladder.

In the middle region, at the level of the fourth lumbar vertebra (L4), the ureters cross the gonadal vessels—testicular in men, ovarian in women. The most common causes of ureteral injury are iatrogenic. The overall incidence of iatrogenic ureteral injury varies between 0.5 and 10%. The most common type of procedure responsible for iatrogenic injury to the ureter is a hysterectomy.

For a double ureter—the incidence found on autopsy is 0.3–2.5% [61]. The presence of this condition, if unknown preoperatively, can greatly compromise the outcome of conduit surgery. Careful examination of preoperative imaging studies is essential for the recognition and management of the duplicated ureter.

Pacemaker cells that initiate renal pelvic and ureteric peristalsis are situated in calyces. These allow coordinated peristalsis of the ureter about six times per minute. Ureteral peristalsis also persists after transplantation or denervation, the spontaneous activity also occurs in the ureteral segments isolated in vitro. Normal antegrade peristalsis also continues after cutting a piece of the ureter and turning it in the intersecting direction, i.e. peristaltis of the ureter always takes place from the renal pelvis to the end of the ureter. These findings lead to the conclusion that ureteral peristalsis is not dependent on innervation [2–4].

## 1.7  Urinary Bladder—Position, Anatomy, Function and Arterial Blood Supply

### 1.7.1  The Position of the Bladder

The bladder is located in the smaller pelvis, retroperitoneally, posterior to the symphysis pubis. In men it lies between the symphysis and rectum, and in women between the symphysis and vagina [2–5, 9, 10, 61].

### 1.7.2   Anatomy

The anatomical structure of the bladder includes: the apex (apex vesicae), the body (corpus vesicae) and the bottom (fundus vesicae). The top of the bladder faces up and forward and the bottom faces back and down. From the inside, the bladder wall is made up of the mucosa, submucosa, three-layer muscle and connective tissue adventitia. From the top the bladder is covered with the parietal peritoneum. The first inner layer, the mucosa, is folded with the exception of the area known as the "trigone of the bladder", which does not have a submucosa [2–6].

### 1.7.3   Function

When empty, the bladder is about the size and shape of a pear but the shape and size of the bladder depends on the degree of its filling. Urine is made in the kidneys and travels down through two tubes called ureters to the urinary bladder. The bladder stores urine, allowing urination to be infrequent and controlled. The bladder is lined by layers of muscle tissue that stretch to hold urine. The normal capacity of the bladder is 400–600 ml. During urination, the bladder muscles squeeze, by two sphincters and the valves open to allow urine to flow out. Urine exits the bladder into the urethra, which carries urine out of the body. Because it passes through the penis, the urethra is longer in men (20 cm) than in women (3.5 cm). A central nervous system response is usually triggered when the volume reaches 400 ml and is perceived as the sensation of bladder fullness and the need to void [2, 3, 8].

With an empty bladder, its wall may be up to 1.5 cm thick, while when the bladder is full, the wall thickness is reduced to 0.3–0.4 cm. When the bladder contains a small amount of urine, the epithelial cells overlap due to their mobility, which allows the bladder wall and mucosa to be significantly stretched while filling, preventing it from being damaged. The walls of the bladder stretch a lot and in pathological conditions such as an enlarged prostate or obstruction of the urethra, the bladder can hold up to 2–3 L of urine. The empty bladder is completely hidden in the lesser pelvis behind the symphysis pubis, in front of the uterus in women and in front of the rectum in men. When the bladder is empty, its walls are sunken and the distance and thereby the space between them is significantly reduced. As urine collects, the bladder walls diverge and stretch and the most stretchy front part rises to form a bulge. The bladder then takes a spherical or, more precisely, oval shape, extending beyond the higher edge of the symphysis and touching the anterior abdominal wall. The inside surface of the bladder that can be examined by cystoscopy is yellow and pink; with an empty bladder it is very crosswise folded, while with a full bladder it is completely smooth. There are three openings at the bottom of the bladder: one in front—the inner opening of the urethra, and two in the back (left and right)—urethral openings. The muscle layers of the bladder are very well developed and form the detrusor muscle whose contractions are essential for effective urination. Around the inner opening of the urethra is the bladder sphincter muscle, which relaxes during the act of urinating, allowing urine to flow from the bladder into the urethra (this muscle is voluntarily controlled). The outer layer of the bladder is the connective tissue that covers the bladder in areas devoid of the parietal peritoneum. The peritoneum is adjacent to the upper and posterior surfaces of the bladder and the outer membrane is absent there [2, 3, 5, 9].

Arterial vascularization of the urinary bladder comes from the following arteries: internal vaginal in women, superior vesicular in men. In fact, the urinary bladder is vascularized by the superior bladder arteries (which depart from the umbilical arteries, which in turn depart from the internal iliac arteries) and the inferior bladder arteries, which depart directly from the internal iliac arteries. The arterial blood supply of the urinary bladder consists mainly of the superior and inferior vesical arteries which directly or indirectly arise from the internal iliac artery. The veins drain into the internal iliac vein. The lymphatic vessels carry the lymph to the various iliac nodes [2–6].

## 1.8   Conclusion

Perfect command of the basic knowledge of the anatomy and physiology of the human urinary system is a good start to develop your interest in the procurement and transplantation of human kidneys.

## References


1. Harrison's Principles of Internal Medicine Twelfth Edition, Part Eight, Disorders of the Kidney and Urinary Tract, Sections 220–234, vol. 2, International Edition, McGraw-Hill, 1991. p. 1131–212.
2. Gray's Anatomy, The Anatomical Basis of Clinical Practice, Thirty Ninth Edition, Editor in Chief Susan Standring, Section 7, Chapter 91 Kidney, Chapter 92 Ureter, Chapter 93, Pages Bladder Elsevier, Churchill, Livingstone; 2005.
3. Skandalakis JE. Scandalakis's surgical anatomy. The embryologic and anatomic basis of modern surgery. Chapter 23 Kidneys and Ureters 1291–1344, Chapter 24–Urinary Bladder 1345–1377, Volume 2, Paschalidis Medical Publication Ltd., 2004.
4. Lote CJ. Principles of renal physiology, 5th ed. Springer;2012. p. 21.
5. Cheuck L, Hoening DM, Ghiraldi EM. Kidney anatomy. Medscape Reference. Oct. 04, 2013. https://emedicine.medscape.com/article/1948775-overview.
6. Dimke H, Hoenderop JG, Bindels RJ. Hereditary tubular transport disorders: implications for renal handling of Ca2+ and Mg2+. Clin Sci. 2009;118(1):1–18.
7. Coffin A, Boulay-Coletta I, Sebbag-Sfez D, Zins M. Radioanatomy of the retroperitoneal space. Diagn Interv Imaging. 2015;96(2):171–86.
8. Tirkes T, Sandrasegaran K, Patel AA, Hollar MA, Tejada JG, Tann M, Akisik FM, Lappas JC. Peritoneal and retroperitoneal anatomy and its relevance for cross-sectional imaging. Radiographics. 2012;32(2):437–51.

9. Megha R, Wehrle CJ, Kashyap S, Leslie SW. StatPearls [Internet]. StatPearls Publishing; Treasure Island (FL): Sep 27, 2020. Anatomy, Abdomen and Pelvis, Adrenal Glands (Suprarenal Glands).
10. Soriano RM, Penfold D, Leslie SW. Anatomy, abdomen and pelvis, kidneys. StatPearls. Treasure Island (FL): StatPearls Publishing; 2020.
11. Toka HR, Toka O, Hariri A, Nguyen HT. Congenital anomalies of kidney and urinary trac. Semin Nephrol. 2010;30(4):374–86.
12. Maria M. Rodriguez; congenital anomalies of the kidney and the urinary tract (CAKUT). Fetal Pediatr Pathol. 2014;33(5–6):293–320.
13. Rosenblum ND, Mattoo TK, Baskin LS, Kim MS. Overview of congenital anomalies of the kidney and urinary tract (CAKUT). In: Post TW, editor. UpToDate. Waltham, MA: UpToDate. https://www.uptodate.com/contents/overview-of-congenital-anomalies-of-the-kidney-and-urinary-tract-cakut. Last updated: August 29, 2016.
14. Shaikh N, Hoberman A. Urinary tract infections in infants older than one month and young children: acute management, imaging, and prognosis. In: Post TW, editor. UpToDate. Waltham, MA: UpToDate. https://www.uptodate.com/contents/urinary-tract-infections-in-infants-older-than-one-month-and-young-children-acute-management-imaging-and-prognosis. Last updated: March 27, 2018.
15. Ishiwa S, Sato M, Morisada N, Nishi K, Kanamori T, Okutsu M, Ogura M, Sako M, Kosuga M, Kamei K, Ito S, Nozu K, Iijima K, Ishikura K. Association between the clinical presentation of congenital anomalies of the kidney and urinary tract (CAKUT) and gene mutations: an analysis of 66 patients at a single institution. Pediatr Nephrol. 2019;34(8): 1457–64.
16. Addison OL. Congenital abnormalities of the urinary tract. Postgrad Med J. 1935;380–9.
17. Kozlov VM, Schedl A. Duplex kidney formation: developmental mechanisms and genetic predisposition [version 1; peer review: 2 approved], F1000 Research 2020, 9 (F1000 Faculty Rev):2 Last updated: 06 Jan 2020.
18. Neild GH. Primary renal disease in young adults with renal failure. Nephrol Dial Transplant. 2010;25:1025–32.
19. Natsis K, Piagkou M, Skotsimara A, Protogerou V, Tsitouridis I, Skandalakis P. Horseshoe kidney: a review of anatomy and pathology. Surg Radiol Anat. 2014;36(6):517–26.
20. Cook WA, Stephens FD. Fused kidneys: morphologic study and theory of embryogenesis. Birth Defects Orig Artic Ser. 1977;13(5):327–40.
21. Glodny B, Petersen J, Hofmann KJ, Schenk C, Herwig R, Trieb T, Koppelstaetter C, Steingruber I, Rehder P. Kidney fusion anomalies revisited: clinical and radiological analysis of 209 cases of crossed fused ectopia and horseshoe kidney. BJU Int. 2009;103(2):224–35.
22. Kirkpatrick JJ, Leslie SW. Horseshoe kidney. [Updated 2020 Aug 12]. In: StatPearls [Internet]. Treasure Island (FL): StatPearls Publishing; 2020. https://www.ncbi.nlm.nih.gov/books/NBK431105/
23. Stroosma OB, Scheltinga MR, Stubenitsky BM, Kootstra G. Horseshoe kidney transplantation: an overview. Clin Transplant. 2000;14(6):515–9.
24. David RS. Horseshoe kidney: a report of one family. Br Med J. 1974;4(5944):571–2.
25. Glenn JF. Analysis of 51 patients with horseshoe kidney. N Engl J Med. 1959;01(261):684–7.
26. Boatman DL, Kölln CP, Flocks RH. Congenital anomalies associated with horseshoe kidney. J Urol. 1972;107(2):205–7.
27. Lallas CD, Pak RW, Pagnani C, Hubosky SG, Yanke BV, Keeley FX, Bagley DH. The minimally invasive management of ureteropelvic junction obstruction in horseshoe kidneys. World J Urol. 2011;29(1):91–5.
28. Foster JT, Morrissey PE. Segmental renal ischemia following transplantation of horseshoe kidney as separate allografts. Case Rep Transplant. 2013;1–3.
29. Watson CJE, Harper SJF. Anatomical variation and its management in transplantation. Am J Transplant. 2015;15:1459–71.
30. Raman SS, Pojchamarnwiputh S, Muangsomboon K, Schulam PG, Gritsch HA, Lu DS. Surgically relevant normal and variant renal parenchymal and vascular anatomy in

preoperative 16-MDCT evaluation of potential laparoscopic renal donors. AJR Am J Roentgenol. 2007;188(1):105–14.

31. Shimada K, Ohashi I, Sakai Y, et al. An unusual renal vascular anomaly: common origin of arteries to the lower poles demonstrated by a computed tomography angiography using 16-slice multidetector computed tomography. Acta Radiol. 2006;47(3):332–4.

32. Asala SA, Asumbuko-Kahamba NM, Bidmos MA. An unusual origin of supernumerary renal arteries: case report. East Afr Med J. 2001;78(2):686–7.

33. Bergman RA, Thompson SA, Afifi AK, Saadeh FA. Compendium of human anatomic variation: catalog, atlas and world literature. Baltimore: Urban & Schwarzenberg; 1988.

34. Bergman RA, Cassell MD, Sahinoglu K, Heidger PM Jr. Human doubled renal and testicular arteries. Ann Anat. 1992;174(4):313–5.

35. Topaz O, Topaz A, Polkampally PR, et al. Origin of a common trunk for the inferior phrenic arteries from the right renal artery: a new anatomic vascular variant with clinical implications. Cardiovasc Revasc Med. 2010;11(1):57–62.

36. Benedetti E, Troppmann C, Gillingham K, et al. Short-and long-term outcomes of kidney transplants with multiple renal arteries. Ann Surg. 1995;221(4):406–14.

37. Sykes D. The arterial supply of the human kidney with special reference to accessory renal arteries. Br J Surg. 1963;50(222):368–74.

38. Mir NS, Ul Hassan A, Rangrez R, Sajad Hami S, Sabia, Tabish SA, Masarat IM, Rasool Z. Bilateral duplication of renal vessels: anatomical, medical and surgical perspective. Int J Health Sci. 2008;2(2) (Jumad'a Thani 1429H).

39. Bakheit MA, Motabagani MA. Anomalies of the renal, phrenic, suprarenal arteries. Saudi Med J. 2004;25(3):376–8.

40. Loukas M, Aparicio S, Beck A, et al. Rare case of right accessory renal artery originating as a common trunk with the inferior mesenteric artery: a case report. Clin Anat. 2005;18(7):530–5.

41. Baptista-Silva JCC, Verissimo MC, Castro MJ, et al. Anatomical study of the renal veins observed during 342 living-donor nephrectomies. Sao Paulo Med J. 1997;115:1456–9.

42. Santangelo M, Spinosa G, Grassia S, et al. In situ elongation patch in right kidney transplantation. Transplant Proc. 2008;40(6):1871–2.

43. Santiago-Delpin EA, Gonzalez Z. Successful renal vein reconstruction with a polyte-trafluoroethylene vascular graft in kidney transplantation. Am J Surg. 1985;149:310–1.

44. Sarin PK, Dhanda R, Siwach V, et al. Bridging of renal arteries: a simple technique for the management of double arteries in living donor renal allograft transplantation. Transplant Proc. 2003;35(1):35–6.

45. Satyapal KS. The renal veins: a review. Eur J Anat. 2003;1:43–52.

46. Rajan KS, Tripta S, Gupta R. Retro-aortic left renal vein with left suprarenal vein draining into inferior vena cava. IJAV. 2010;3:134–7.

47. Karaman B, Koplay M, Qzturk E. et al. Retroaortic left renal vein: multidetector computed tomography angiography findings and its clinical importance. Acta Radiol. 2007;48.

48. Arslan H, Etlik O, Cevlan K, et al. Incidence of retro-aortic left renal vein and its relationship with varicocele. Eur Radiol. 2005;15:1717–20.

49. Nam JK, Park SW, Lee SD, et al. The clinical significance of a retro-aortic left renal vein. Korean J Urol. 2010;51:276–80.

50. Hsieh L, Tiao W-M, Chou Y-H, Tiu C-M. Retroaortic left renal vein: three case reports. J Med Ultrasound. 2012;20(2):115–8.

51. Senecail B, Bobeuf J, Forlodou P, Nonent M. Two rare anomalies of the left renal vein. Surg Radiol Anat. 2003;25:465–7.

52. Surucu HS, Erbil KM, Tastan C, Yener N. Anomalous veins of the retroperitoneum: clinical considerations. Surg Radiol Anat. 2001;23:443–5.

53. Satyapal KS, Kalideen JM, Haffejee AA, et al. Left renal vein variations. Surg Radiol Anat. 1999;21:77–81.

54. Cocheteux B, Mounier-Vehier C, Gaxotte V, et al. Rare variations in renal anatomy and blood supply: CT appearances and embryologic background. A pictorial essay. Eur Radiol. 2001;11:779–86.

55. Hsieh CL, Tiao WM, Chou YH, Tiu CM. Retroaortic left renal vein: three case reports. J Ultrasound Med. 2012;20:115–8.
56. Andrade FM, Rocha RP, Pereira HM, et al. A rare variation of the retro-aortic left renal vein with anastomotic a fluent from inferior mesenteric vein. Int J Morphol. 2005;23:5–8.
57. Watson CJE, Harper SJF. Am J Transplant 2015;15(6):1459–71. https://doi.org/10.1111/ajt. 13310
58. Babu CS, Lalwani R, Kumar I. Right double inferior vena cava (IVC) with preaortic iliac confluence: case report and review of literature. J Clin Diagn Res. 2014;8(2):130–2.
59. Sahin H, Pekcevik Y, Aslaner R. Double Inferior vena cava (IVC) with intrahepatic interruption hemiazygos vein, continuation and intrahepatic venues: shunt: a rare variant of IVC anomalies. Vasc Endovasc Surg. 2017;51(1):38–42.
60. Ghandour A, Karuppasamy K, Rajiah P. Congenital anomalies of the superior vena cava: embryological correlation, imaging perspectives, and clinical relevance. Can Assoc Radiolol J. 2017;68(4):456–62.
61. Tublin M, Nelson JB, Borhani AA, Furlan A, Heller MT, Squires J. Ureteropelvic duplications. In: Imaging in urology. Elsevier; 2018. p. 82–3.

# Chapter 2
# Non-Laparoscopic Kidney Procurement Techniques from Living and Deceased Donors

## 2.1  Introduction

In the Transplant Centre in Leiden, the Netherlands where I work, patients who want to donate a kidney to their loved ones can choose from two surgical methods of kidney donation: the mini-incision Non-Muscle-Splitting Mini Open Donor Nephrectomy (MINI) surgical technique during which the skin incision is made along the lateral side of the abdominal rectus muscle starting about 2–3 cm below the costal arch for about 10 cm (extraperitoneal approach) or a laparoscopic donor nephrectomy (LDN) in which kidney procurement in our clinic is performing according to international standards through an intraperitoneal approach [1]. In a polyclinic which is specially designed for this purpose, each donor, recipient and their families who have successfully passed the screening have a discussion with the transplant surgeon and nephrologist. However, in this discussion the surgeon and nephrologist carefully explain each surgical technique's advantages and disadvantages; the final choice is left to the kidney donor. From my experience, I can say that most patients immediately choose—after a short surgical explanation—one of these two surgical methods of donation, though there are also patients who want to think a little bit longer about the methods and discuss it at home with their family and/or the recipient. For the living kidney donors who need a period of time for consideration, we advise them to inform the hospital about their decision no later than two weeks before the surgery. In case of questions concerning the surgical procedure they can make another appointment with a transplant coordinator or surgeon in the form of a telephone consultation or a direct polyclinic visit to have a "face to face" conversation with a surgeon. In this chapter I will not describe the surgical techniques of laparoscopic kidney procurement from a living donor, because I have no experience in this subject, but I will describe the open method. At the Leiden University Medical Center we performed more than 400 kidney donations to the great satisfaction of the donors and recipients. Our centre has been using

© The Author(s), under exclusive license to Springer Nature Switzerland AG 2023

A. Baranski, *Kidney Transplantation*,
https://doi.org/10.1007/978-3-030-75886-8_2

MINI (Mini Incision Non-Muscle-Splitting Mini Open Donor Nephrectomy) as a surgical technique since 1997. The MINI technique is unique due its non-muscle splitting, retroperitoneal approach through the anterior abdominal wall. For more than a decade, this technique has been used in parallel to full LDN in our center. I would now like to quote very briefly (at the time of writing, not yet published) the results of the study carried out by doctor L. J. M. Habets under the supervision of Dr. V. A. L. Huurman from our department, in which they compare MINI and LDN surgical techniques performed over a period of nine years. The aim of this study was to assess the results and safety of the MINI technique for donors when compared to the current gold standard of LDN in short-term ($< 30$ day) complications, as graded by the Clavien–Dindo Classification. All living kidney donors at the Leiden University Medical Center (LUMC) between 2011 and 2019 were analyzed (642 donors: 287 MINI and 355 LDN). Earlier open nephrectomy procedures were excluded to minimize time-related effects. In a multiple regression analysis, MINI was not associated with higher Clavien–Dindo classification complications or prolonged hospital stays. The MINI technique was associated with more blood loss ($275 \pm 382$ ml vs LDN $136 \pm 201$ ml, $p \leq 0.001$) but also with shorter operating times ($175 \pm 40$ min vs LDN $187 \pm 41$ min, $p \leq 0.001$) and shorter warm ischemic times ($100 \pm 56$ s vs. LDN $296 \pm 117$ s, $p \leq 0.001$). One-year post-operative kidney function (eGFR) was not significantly different between MINI and LDN donors ($57.1$ vs. $56.6$ ml/min/$1.73$ m$^2$, $p = 0.648$) [1, 51]. However, I try to be objective and neutral in my judgments, I am not an advocate for the laparoscopy method. Although this method has dominated almost the "whole market" of kidney donation from living donors worldwide, it has not only advantages—as it sometimes seems—but also (unfortunately) many disadvantages. In 1997, when we started the living kidney donation and transplant program at LUMC, it had already been in existence in Leiden for a very long time. The first kidney donation and transplantation from a living donor in the Netherlands was performed in Leiden in 1966. The only problem was that donation was still carried out using anterolateral oblique or posterior lumbotomy incision, which did not encourage potential donors. If you want to describe the whole situation in a few words, you could say that the kidney was donated to someone who was very important to the donor and who was not frightened by not only the quite high risk of major surgery, but also the scarring following the kidney removal. When the family transplant program was born in the 1960s, the need for such transplants was lower and the waiting time for a cadaver kidney transplant was much shorter. The living donation and transplant operations were therefore performed irregularly and society was at that time—generally speaking—very cautious about the living kidney donation. In the 1990s the number of dialyzed patients increased sharply and thus the number of patients awaiting transplantation increased. Unfortunately the number of deceased donors did not increase, which contributed to the fact that the demand for kidney transplantation increased significantly. The waiting time for a kidney transplant increased for this reason to more than five years for unimmunized patients and for highly immunized patients it became almost unpredictable. The mortality rate of those on the waiting list for transplantation began to increase dramatically. The only logical move for the Dutch Transplant Society together with the Dutch Transplant Foundation and the Dutch Government was to start a strong campaign for family donation among patients and in the media. After about three to four months of a very intense campaign, people slowy began to contact hospitals with questions and to ask about the conditions which they must fulfill in order to donate their kidney to their loved ones. At that time we—as transplant surgeons— were looking for the best surgical methods for the donation, so that we would no longer have to scare off any donor with huge incisions and a long hospital stay.

In the 1990s, three surgical techniques were popular for removing kidneys from living donors: The minimally invasive method, in which a kidney is removed through a small incision; the laparoscopic method; and the traditional large incision through the back (dorsal lumbotomy). Laparoscopic donor kidney nephrectomy was becoming increasingly popular, but the number of complications and other inconveniences associated with this method at the time meant that we eventually decided to start a programme using a specially developed small incision mini invasive surgical technique (MINI) with extra-peritoneal access. Finally, we decided in our center to choose the open retroperitoneal, minimally invasive surgical technique (MINI) as our standard for living kidney donation. Six months after incorporating this method, we were assured of good results and the safety of the donor and the recipient on the operating table. When we used the professional abdominal retractor from the LUMC Medical Devices Department with specially modified blades, the method seemed not very complicated, easy to learn, though challenging because of the small incision. However, it provides the possibility of donation with more than one renal vessel. The MINI-method which we have chosen was and is in my personal opinion a fast method which is not only well tolerated by the donor, but also safe for him or her. We have to remember that living related kidney donation and transplantation consists of two operations with two aims. There is the so-called donor wish to survive and the recipient wish to obtain the best kidney that will start working immediately in order to avoid further dialysis. To speak briefly, the kidney donor and recipient have to be satisfied after the operation. After 20 years of experience in donation and transplanting kidneys from living donors, I will try to create a definition of a successful or even ideal vision of a living related kidney transplant program. Usually after a living related kidney transplant neither the donor, the recipient, nor their families ask about the method of surgery, the size of the incision or how long the surgery took. In most cases (99%), the donors are very pleased that they survived the operation. They ask about the quality of the donated kidney and the kidney recipient, whether the kidney has been transplanted with success and whether it has taken up its function (urine secretion and blood filtration) and whether everything went as expected. The recipient is interested in whether the donor survived or had complications, about new kidney function and how soon he or she will be able to go home. As I have already mentioned, we took the first kidney out using this method in April 1997.

For more than ten years we have been offering potential kidney donors two surgical techniques—i.e. the laparoscopic technique and the open kidney technique —and have been presenting them with the pros and cons in a neutral and fair way. From one to ten years ago, many people chose the retroperitoneal access. But nowadays, after my careful observations for the last 20 years, I am not really able to tell if there any significant differences—in terms of the length of stay in the hospital, the length of convalescence, the amount of pain medications used and so on—in the groups of patients who were operated via one or the other technique. However, if we look at the "financial picture" there is one big difference: the price of the procedure. This is incomparably higher if the kidney is taken from a living donor by the laparoscopic method and it is even more expensive when removed by a robot. The other differences are related to the duration of the operation which is much shorter in the case of the method of open kidney donation with many vessels, and the time of the first warm ischemia (the time from the closing of the renal artery to the beginning of the kidney rinsing) which is much shorter in the case of the open method (60–150 s vs. 240–400 s) [1, 51]. Conversations with potential kidney donors provided me with a lot to think about how medical companies shape the market. Various popular scientific journals, articles, interviews, films and on social media convince the population and thus also current and past donors to choose extremely expensive surgery. It is understood that young people (especially young women) choose the laparoscopic method for cosmetic reasons because of the small scar due to a cut of a few centimeters though it can be hidden behind underwear. However, I would like to quote an article written by my colleagues from Rotterdam in this regard. From May 2001 to September 2004 data on all living kidney donations and transplantations were collected. Fifty-one donors underwent mini-incision, muscle-splitting open donor nephrectomy (MIDN) and 49 donors underwent laparoscopic donor nephrectomy (LDN). The median incision length in MIDN was 10.5 cm. In two patients LDN was converted to open. MIDN resulted in significantly shorter warm ischemia and operation time (2.5 vs. 6.5 min and 157 vs. 240 min respectively). During MIDN, donors had more blood loss (200 vs. 120 ml, P = 0.02). Disposables used for MIDN were cheaper (328 vs. 1784 euros). In the LDN group four (8%) major intra-operative and two (4%) major postoperative complications occurred versus no major complications in the MIDN group. Morphine requirement, pain and nausea perception and time to dietary intake did not significantly differ between the groups. Following MIDN, donors were discharged later (four vs. three days, P = 0.02). Transplantation of kidneys pro-cured by either approach led to a similar decline in serum creatinine throughout the first year. One-year graft survival was 100% following MIDN and 86% following LDN (P = 0.005) [29].

In this chapter I would like to share with readers my knowledge about the surgical techniques that I performed and checked myself, and which I and my team of surgeons invented and modified. This method is probably a compilation of older, previously existing surgical techniques, but which have been significantly modified by our team.

In this chapter I will not describe the technique of flushing the organ using a special catheter with two balloons, the triple lumen catheter (DBTLC), introduced into the aorta through one of the femoral arteries and the whole technique of determining its best position, filling balloons, and so on. We used this technique for some weeks, but I should inform you that the DBTLC was problematic as in most cases there was bending and/or bad positioning. The abdominal organs, including the kidneys, were not always very well perfused and washed out, so we quickly changed our procurement technique. For over 20 years we have been using for every kind of deceased donation the technique of rapid, massive internal (with a large bore cannula) and external cooling which, briefly speaking, consists of the following steps: opening of the abdominal cavity, aortic cannulation, decompression of the IVC, abdominal organ perfusion with cold preservation solution under pressure and external cooling. I am convinced that the decision to stop using the balloons for multi-organ donation was correct. I also consider that by stopping the DBTLC technique we did the right thing, as evidenced by the very good results of our work, which defend themselves in terms of the quality of the procured and transplanted organs.

## 2.2   Surgical Technique of Kidney Procurement During Multiple Organ Donation from Donation After Brain Death (DBD) and Donation After Circulatory Death (DCD) Donors

### 2.2.1   Introduction

I described the surgical technique of kidney procurement in my previous book, published worldwide by Springer in 2009, entitled "Surgical Technique of Abdominal Organ Procurement, Step-by-step". There I described most important steps of kidney procurement from deceased donors—the so-called "donation after brain death (DBD)" and "donation after circulatory death (DCD)".

In 1995, at a conference in Maastricht (the Netherlands), for the first time in Europe, the definitions of donors after cardiac or circulatory death were officially established on the basis of clinical and legal grounds. This convention has been adopted all over the world and currently classifies donors after cardiac death according to the clinical situation into the following categories [2, 3]:

**A. Uncontrolled categories**:

  I. The donor died at the time of admission—an uncontrolled situation.
  II. Donor died after ineffective cardiopulmonary resuscitation.

**B. Controlled (c-DCD) categories**:

  III.  Donor with severe irreversible brain damage, for donors in whom the brain has been severely damaged, but the donor has not yet met all of the official criteria for brain death. The doctors stop the life-supporting treatment and wait for the heart to stop beating before they start to remove the organs—a controlled situation.

  IV.  Donor with symptoms of brain death who has had sudden cardiac arrest.

  V.  The donor died in hospital after irreversible cardiac arrest because of a euthanasia procedure (category added in 2000).

Donation (donor) after circulatory death (DCD) has become an accepted practice in many countries and remains a focus of intense interest in the transplant community. Controlled DCD (c-DCD) refers to donation from persons whose death has occurred following the decision to withdraw life-sustaining therapies (WLST) which are no longer considered in the best interests of the patient. Countries with DCD activity are: Austria, Belgium, Czech Republic, France, Ireland, Israel, Italy, Latvia, Lithuania, the Netherlands, Norway, Poland, Portugal, Russia, Spain, Sweden, Switzerland and the United Kingdom. Countries planning to start a DCD program are: Bulgaria, Croatia, Denmark, Hungary, Moldova, Romania, Slovak Republic, Slovenia and Turkey. Countries with no present or planned DCD activity are: Armenia, Belarus, Cyprus, Estonia, Finland, Georgia, Germany and Greece. Member states with DCD programs controlled and uncontrolled are: Austria, Belgium, Czech Republic, France, Italy, the Netherlands, Spain and Switzerland. Those with controlled only DCD are: Ireland, Norway, Sweden and the United Kingdom. Those with uncontrolled only DCD are: Israel, Latvia, Lithuania, Poland, Portugal and Russia. DCD is an effective means of expanding the potential donor pool and has a comparable transplantation survival to donation after brain death despite the higher rates of primary non-function and delayed graft function. Countries with successfully implemented DCD programs have achieved this primarily through the establishment of national ethical, professional and legal frameworks to address both public and professional concerns regarding all aspects of the DCD pathway [1–3, 20–22].

At the time of multiorgan retrieval, the kidney is the last organ removed from the abdominal cavity. Please remember that kidneys are located deep in the retroperitoneal space and, especially in obese people, due to the thick layer of fat surrounding them, at the beginning of multiorgan donation, they cannot be practically examined and assessed in terms of their suitability for transplantation. After opening the abdominal cavity, and even during perfusion of the abdominal organs, it is practically impossible to thoroughly inspect the kidneys and comment on their quality, for example, on the presence of infected and uninfected cysts, tumors, anatomical anomalies, quality of perfusion, number of arteries supplying each kidney or the number of renal veins or ureters. In short, each kidney can only be assessed for transplant suitability after it has been procured, inspected just prior to packing (using classic static cold storage—CS) or putting it on the cold pulsatile hypothermic machine perfusion (HMP), and in both methods shipping as quickly as possible to the recipient's hospital [3–22].

Later in this chapter I will describe the most common situations when the kidneys are procured after the pancreas and liver. If the bowels have not been retrieved for transplantation, they are mobilized, their mesentery is closed and cut with a stapler below the uncinate process of the pancreas, and the colon with the small bowel are placed on the donor's thighs outside the abdominal cavity. After the pancreas and liver, or pancreas with the liver ("en-bloc" or after splitting the arterial blood supply in the donor body), are removed, the following organs and structures are found in the abdominal cavity: kidneys, ureters, renal arteries and veins, female uterus and ovaries, urinary bladder, abdominal aorta and IVC, along with iliac arteries and veins. Thanks to the professional surgical abdominal retractor, the operating field remains stable throughout the operation.

Now I will briefly state the most important surgical steps required during multiple abdominal organ procurement, which must take place before kidney retrieval [20–45]:

1. The abdominal cavity and sternum are opened with a median incision from the neck to the pubic bone.
2. The abdominal organs are mobilized.
3. The aorta and the IVC are dissected and cannulated close to their bifurcations, or the aorta only is dissected close to its bifurcation.
4. The whole system before perfusion can be decompressed in two ways:

   a. by almost complete transection of the inferior vena cava (IVC) at the level of the right atrium of the heart (Fig. 2.62) or
   b. by removing the clamp from the drain previously inserted into the IVC's lumen (Figs. 2.1, 2.2, 2.52, 2.63) or
   c. by IVC transection at the level of its bifurcation and putting suction into the IVC's lumen (an emergency situation)

   and then perfused with a cold preservation solution (internal cooling).

5. The external cooling of abdominal organs consists of sterile crushed ice and a chilled Ringer's solution or saline, inserted into the abdominal cavity which, after warming or melting, are replaced regularly.
6. The duodenum is cut off and closed with a stapler on the border between the Treitz ligament and the small intestine and on the border between the stomach and the duodenum at the level of the pyrolus or a little above it.
7. The stomach and esophagus up to the diaphragm are freed very close to their walls from the surrounding tissues along the minor and major curvature of the stomach and esophagus wall up to the diaphragm, the stomach is then moved out of the abdominal cavity to the chest.
8. The small intestine is cut off and closed with a stapler on the level of the Treitz ligament and together with the large intestine moved beyond the abdominal cavity and placed below the pubic bone between the donor's thighs (Figs. 2.1 and 2.2).
9. The left renal vein is cut off from the IVC before liver and pancreas procurement (Figs. 2.3 and 2.4).

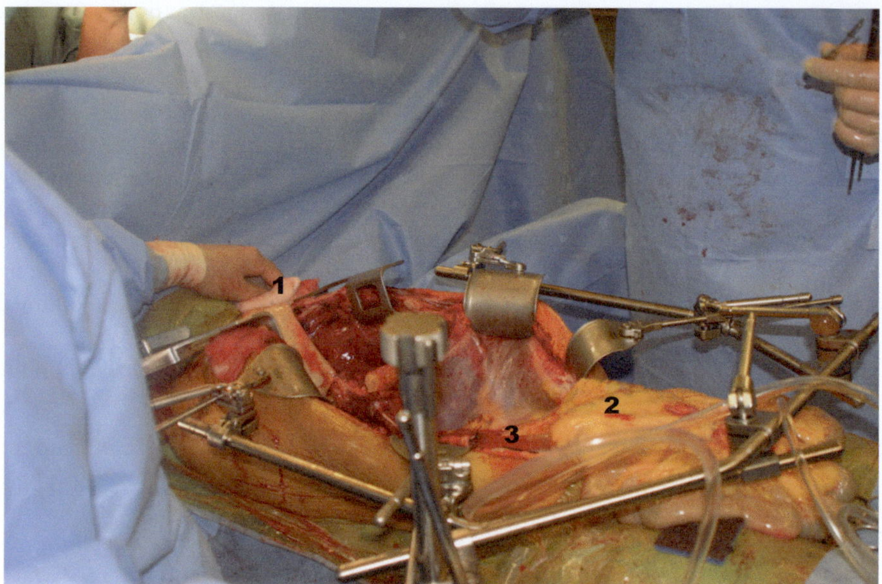

**Fig. 2.1** Multiple organ procurement of the abdominal and thoracic organs. The heart and lungs were retrieved from the chest. The liver and pancreas were moved from the abdomen. 1—The stomach is cut off and closed with a stapler at the pylorus level and moved beyond the abdominal cavity to the chest. 2—The small intestine is cut off and closed with a stapler at the level of the Treitz ligament and together with the large intestine moved beyond the abdominal cavity and placed below the pubic bone between the donor's thighs. 3—The aorta's cannula is placed into the abdominal aorta just above its bifurcation and fixed with a nonabsorbable ligature. In the abdominal cavity there are still kidneys and vessels (tool-kit) for procurement

Regardless of the type of donor (donor with confirmed cerebral death—DBD, or donor after irreversible cardiac arrest—DCD), the kidney as an organ in the case of multiorgan abdominal organ donation is always collected at the end of the procedure, before the vessels (tool-kit). In most cases the tool-kit consists of the iliac vessels (veins and arteries) if they are good quality without atherosclerosis which means that they are suitable for the reconstruction of the vessels of the transplanted organ or vessels of the recipient [17–19].

During organ procurement by DCD all abdominal organs, including the kidney(s), are damaged as a consequence of the effects of ichemia-reperfusion injury (IRI). In order to minimize the damaging effect of IRI, it is critical that cardiopulmonary arrest occurs within a short time (e.g. 2 h). As a result of IRI the retrieved kidney may not work initially after transplantation and dialysis therapy will be required. In such a case the kidney is said to have suffered from delayed graft function (DGF). This occurs in 2% of living related grafts, around 25% in DBD grafts and 50% in DCD grafts. In about 3% of cadaveric grafts the kidney never functions at all and this is called primary non-function [23].

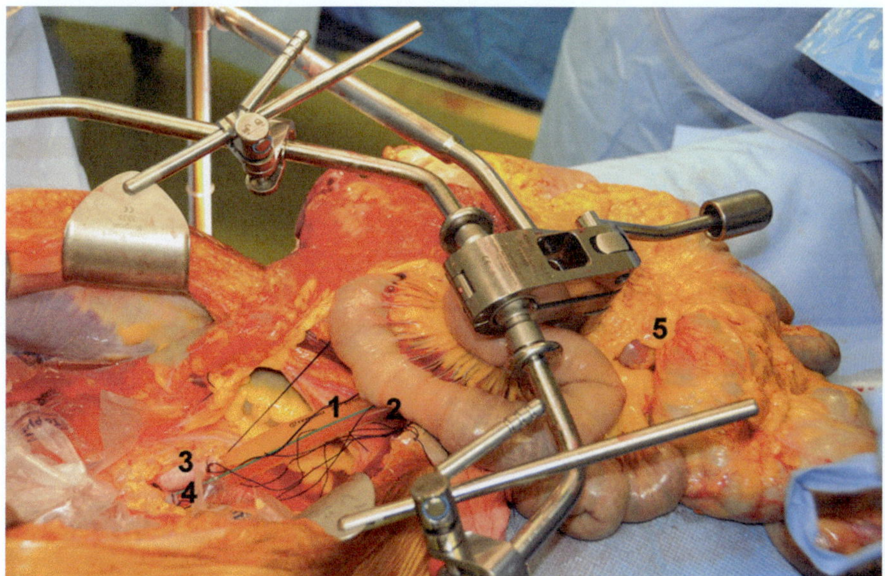

**Fig. 2.2** Multiple abdominal organ procurement. Abdominal aorta just above its bifurcation, cannulated with a large bore aorta's cannula for perfusion (preservation and internal cooling) of abdominal organs. The IVC was cannulated with a chest drain and used for system decompression. 1—Aortic cannula, 2—Chest drain, 3—Thick surgical ligature tied around the aortic wall and around the previously inserted cannula, 4—Chest drain was inserted into the IVC for system decompression, 5—Donor intestines were placed outside the abdomen on the donor's thighs. The next step removes the cannulas from the aorta and the IVC

**Warning! (Left renal vein, retro-aortic left renal vein)**
Even among experienced surgeons, this is very often a subject of serious academic discussion, how the left renal vein should be retrieved: with or without the inferior vena cava patch?

Personally, I agree with the first statement that the left renal vein does not have to be procured with a patch from the IVC, but with one exception—when it runs along the posterior wall of the abdominal aorta. From my experience, I can present arguments that the anastomosis of the left renal vein with the IVC patch is associated with certain inconveniences and is technically more difficult. Here are my arguments: the wall of the IVC is always thicker than that of the renal, common and external iliac vein. The wall of the renal vein itself is generally the same thickness as that of one of the iliac veins, so if both walls are of the same or similar thickness, end-to-side anastomosis should be easier in most cases. The left renal vein should be cut on the left lateral edge of the IVC, especially when the left renal vein runs correctly towards the IVC, along the anterior surface of the abdominal aorta. The left renal vein, cut off just at its entrance into the IVC, is long enough for

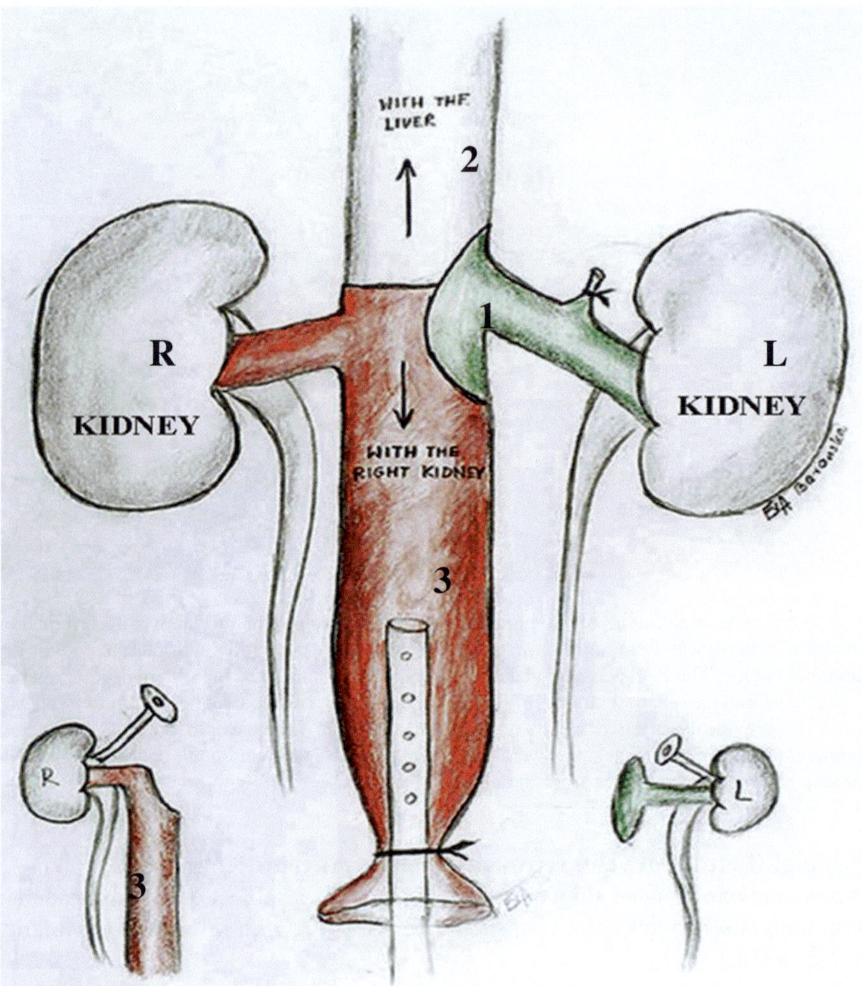


**Fig. 2.3** Splitting of the IVC under the liver between the left and the right kidney and the liver. 1—The green part, the left renal vein, is cut with/without a patch from the IVC, this part has to be given to the left kidney, 2—This white part of the IVC is cut 1–2 cm above the level of the highest ostium of the right renal vein and has to be given to the liver, 3—The red part of the IVC is cut close above the bifurcation of the IVC and has to be given to the right kidney

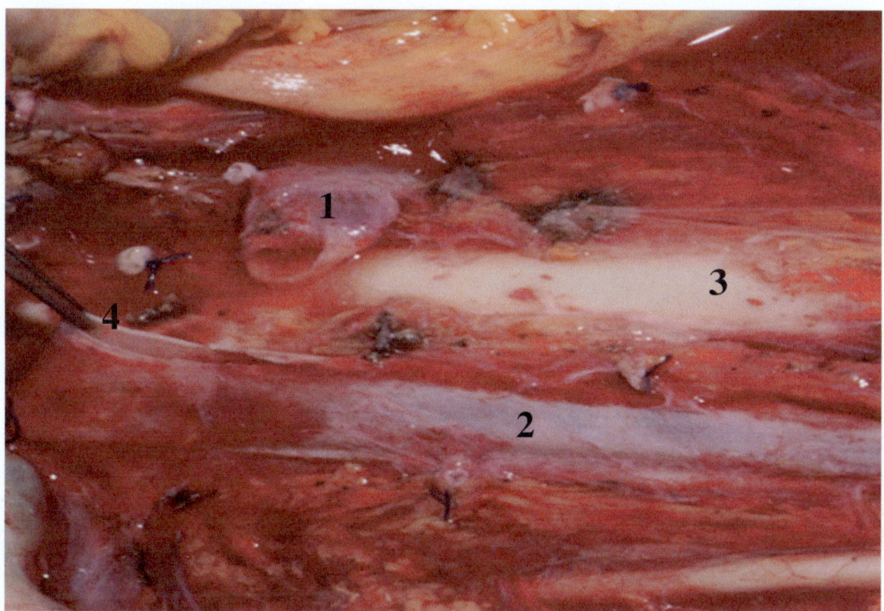

**Fig. 2.4**  The left renal vein is cut off from the IVC, without a patch. 1—Left renal vein, 2—IVC, 3—Abdominal aorta, 4—An opening in the IVC after removal of the left renal vein

transplantation for suturing to iliac vessels on both the right and left side. As is well known, accessory veins may also be present on the left side, so the additional renal vein should be completely preserved and cut off, with or without a patch, but very close to its entrance into IVC.

Each left renal vein running behind the posterior wall of the aorta and entering the IVC should be procured entirely along its length, with or without a patch from the IVC, as close as possible to its entrance into the vena cava, that is right next to its wall. The left renal vein located on the posterior wall of the aorta has usually a very thin wall and a large number of small veins that connect to it. These small veins should be cut off at a sufficient distance from the main renal vein wall during procurement so that they can be ligated or sewn while benching the kidney for transplantation. The retro-aortic renal vein should be prepared very carefully due to its thin wall (Fig. 2.5). Another method of left kidney procurement is to remove the right kidney first. The next step is to mobilize from the retroperitoneal space the posterior surface of this kidney by putting a lot of ice on the anterior and posterior surfaces of this kidney and systematically ligating all venous branches without damaging the main vein wall.

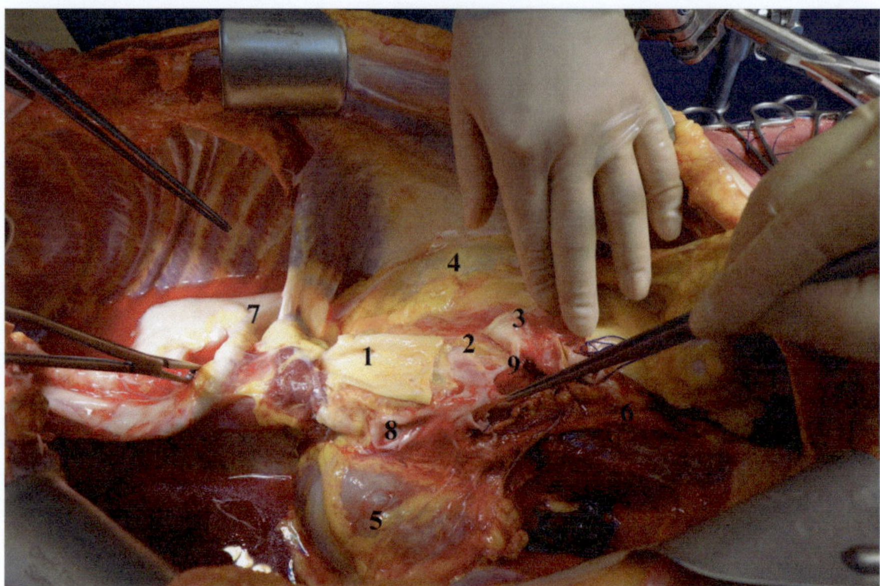

**Fig. 2.5** Left renal vein with retro-aortic course. 1—Abdominal aorta with the visible opening of the left renal artery, 2—Left renal vein with preaortic course, 3—Abdominal aorta cut above the bifurcation to reach and retrieve without damaging the preaortic left renal vein course, 4—Left kidney, 5—Right kidney, 6—Right ureter, 7—Heart, 8—IVC, 9—One of many thin wall branches coming into the left renal vein

### 2.2.2 *Deceased Donor Kidney Procurement Surgical Technique with Separation in the Donor's Body. DBD, DCD—Multiorgan Procurement Surgical Technique in Brief. DBD, DCD—New Kidney-only Procurement Surgical Technique*

#### 2.2.2.1 Differences in Steps Between Multiorgan and "Kidney-only" Procurement

**A. Multiorgan procurement (DBD and DCD donor):**

- Time out with the procurement team(s) and transplant coordinator:

    - DBD before transportation to the operating room (OR).
    - DCD before withdrawal of treatment.

- Mobilization, cannulation, decompression, preservation, internal (perfusion) and external cooling, and if necessary organ splitting.
- First organ retrieved is the small bowel (sometimes), in most cases the liver and pancreas have already been procured for transplantation in bowls filled up with cold preservation solution and ice, the bowels are outside the abdominal cavity, the kidney and great vessels are in the abdomen.
- In the abdomen: kidneys (perfused) and great vessels [24–45].

**B. Kidney-only procurement (DBD and DCD donor):**

- Time out with the procurement team(s) and transplant coordinator:

  - DBD before transportation to the OR
  - DCD before withdrawal of treatment (Insensitive care (IC) or operating theatre (OR)).

- Cannulation, decompression, internal perfusion, cooling and preservation, external cooling, no organ splitting.
- Abdominal part of esophagus, stomach, spleen, pancreas, bowels—"en bloc" outside abdominal cavity—non-perfused and preserved.
- In the abdomen: kidneys and great vessels (perfused, cooled, preserved) and liver not cooled, perfused and preserved (Figs. 2.66 and 2.67).

### 2.2.2.2  Kidney Procurement During Abdominal Multiorgan Procurement from Deceased Donors (DBD and DCD): The Same Surgical Steps in Brief

As I have already mentioned, the kidneys, in the case of multiple abdominal organ retrieval, are always procured at the end of the procedure in the majority of cases after the liver and pancreas and much less often after the small bowel which is usually retrieved as the first organ from the abdomen.

1. After abdominal organ perfusion, cut (perfect external, internal cooling and preservation) with a scalpel the ligature around the aorta and aortic cannula and the ligature around the IVC. Remove the cannula from the aortic lumen. If decompression of the IVC was carried out with the chest tube, cut the ligature and also remove the chest tube from the lumen of the IVC (Figs. 2.6 and 2.7).
2. If you have not already, cut the left renal vein very close to the IVC and mobilize it towards the hilum of the kidney, so that the left renal vein does not contact the anterior wall of the abdominal aorta. The left adrenal vein and the left adrenal gland can be taken together with the kidney, or the left adrenal vein can be cut 3–4 mm off from the renal vein, or the left adrenal vein can be tied. Lift the mobilized left renal vein upwards and place it on the anterior surface of the kidney. The retracted left renal vein is immobilized with a wet swab soaked in cold saline or a Ringer's

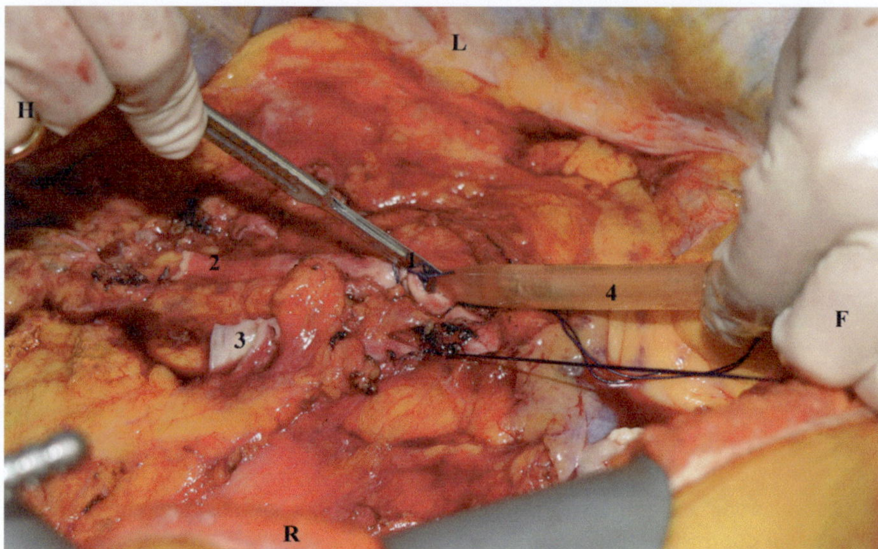

**Fig. 2.6** After removing the chest tube from the IVC, the next stage is to remove the aortic cannula. 1—Cutting, preferably with a scalpel, a thick ligature tied around the wall of the abdominal aorta and around the cannula inserted into its lumen, 2—Abdominal aorta, 3—Cut off IVC above its bifurcation, 4—Cannula inserted into lumen of aorta, H—Towards the head, F—Towards the feet, L—The left side of the patient, R—The right side of the patient

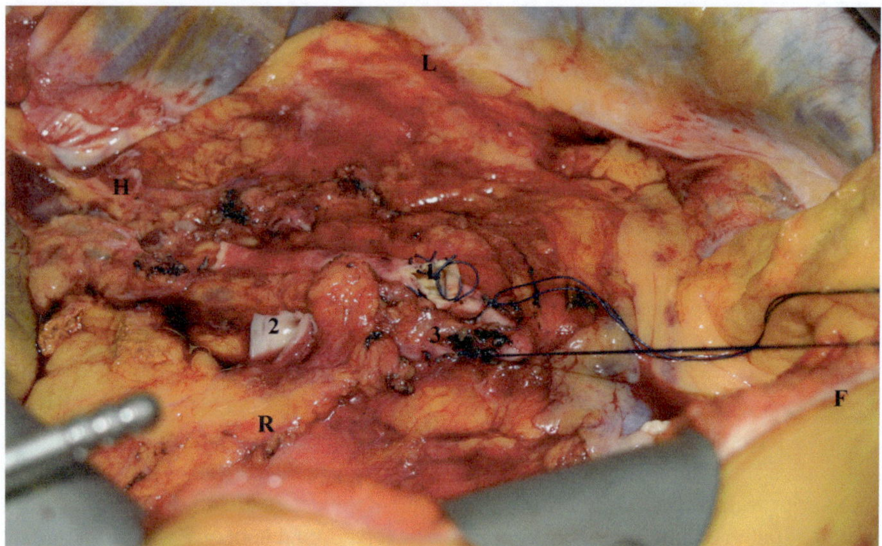

**Fig. 2.7** The cannula was removed from the abdominal aorta, and the chest tube from the IVC. 1—Abdominal aorta, 2—IVC cut off above its bifurcation, 3—IVC just above its bifurcation, H—Towards the head, F—Towards the feet, L—Left side, R—Right side

sterile solution so that the left renal vein does not accidentally fall into the third step of opening the anterior wall of the abdominal aorta.

3. Cut with scissors the medial anterior surface of the abdominal aorta wall along its long axis, from the bifurcation to the ostium of the superior mesenteric artery. A symmetrical cut of the anterior abdominal aorta wall can also be performed in the opposite direction, starting at the ostium of the superior mesenteric artery and ending 1 cm before the bifurcation of the abdominal aorta (Fig. 2.8).

4. After cutting the medial anterior surface of the abdominal aorta wall, check the advancement of atherosclerotic lesions (Fig. 2.9) situated inside the lumen of the abdominal aorta wall and in the ostia of the renal arteries (Fig. 2.10). If there is any doubt about the number of renal arteries ("suspicious" renal artery ostia in the aortic wall), the presence of possible additional renal artery orifices from the aorta can be checked using the following sterile instruments: a special thin metal probe (rounded at both ends) or a thin Fogarty catheter or a thin long silicone tube. After gently placing one of the above-mentioned instruments into the "suspected" lumen (ostium) of one of the extra renal arteries, try to slide very slowly and carefully the instrument into the lumen and slowly move it forward, carefully observing whether it moves towards the hilum or one of the poles of the kidney. If you suspect a renal accessory (a superior or inferior pole artery) or

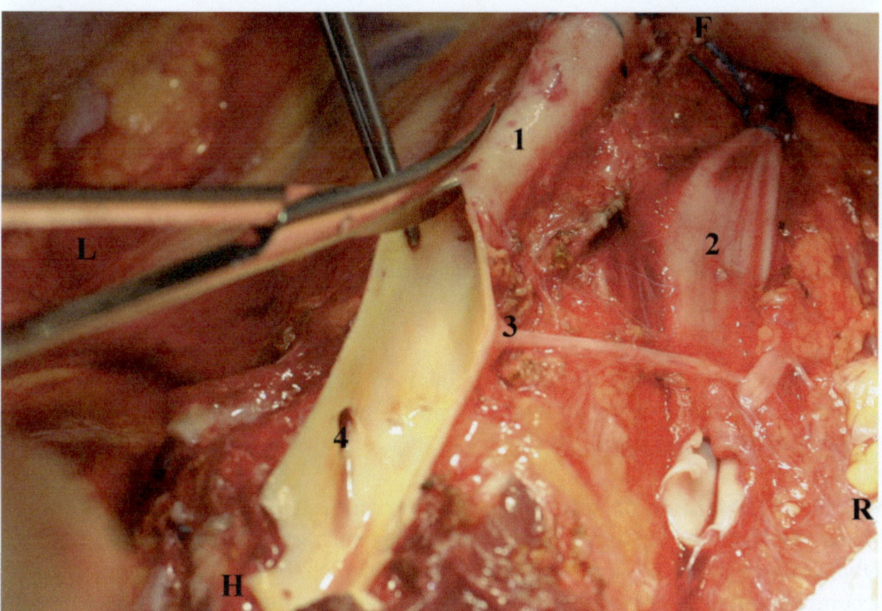

**Fig. 2.8** Abdominal aorta—exactly in the middle of the anterior wall along the long axis of the aorta. The incision was started from the upper mesenteric artery towards the bifurcation of the abdominal aorta (view from the patient's head). 1—The abdominal aorta just above its bifurcation, 2—IVC, 3—Right accessory renal artery, 4—Entry to the aorta of the right renal artery running along the anterior wall of the IVC. H—Towards the head, F—Towards the feet, L—The left side, R—The right side

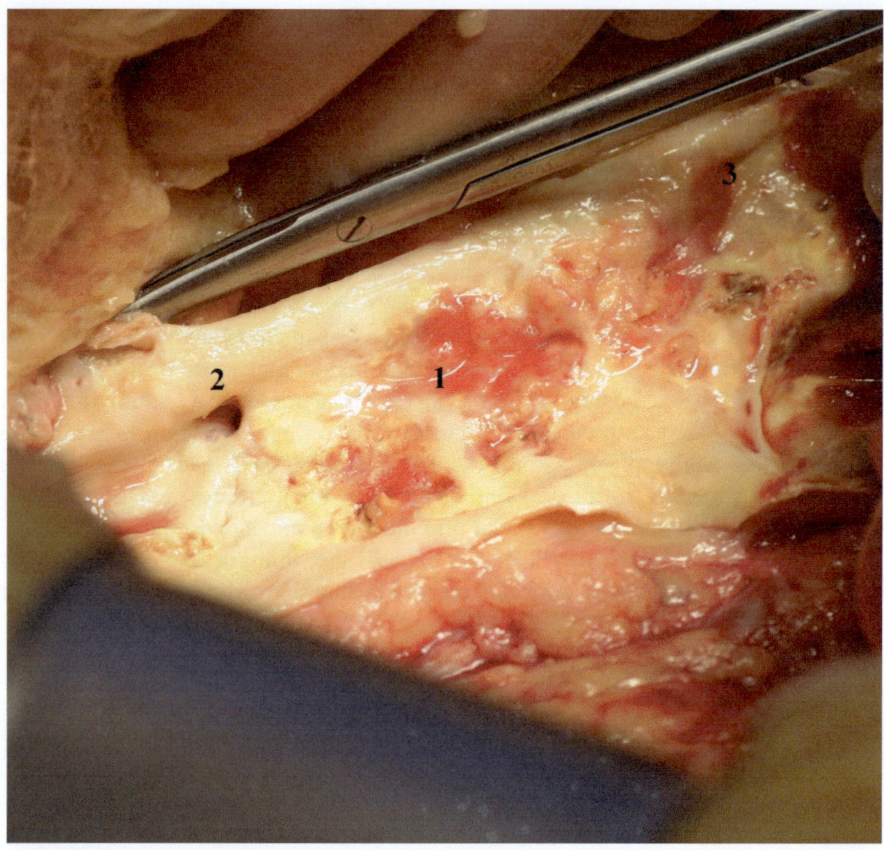

**Fig. 2.9** The anterior inferior wall of the abdominal aorta is cut. 1—Aortic wall with severe atherosclerotic lesions, 2—Ostium of the main renal artery, 3—Atherosclerotic plaque with commencing ulceration

an aberrant renal artery (hilum) examine the ostias of the renal arteries on the left and the right side of the abdominal aorta from the iliac external artery up to the level of the celiac trunk [31].

**Warning! (Definition of accessory and aberrant artery)**
When speaking in anatomical terms, "extra renal artery" may be used with a subclassification of an accessory renal artery which is extra to the main artery accompanying the same direction towards the hilus and entering the kidney through the hilum to supply it, while the aberrant artery supplies the kidney without entering its hilum, thus in most cases supplying the superior and/or inferior pole of the kidney [38–41].

5. Cut the posterior wall of the aorta along its long axis, exactly between the lumbar arteries, so that there are two aortic patches, right and left, extending

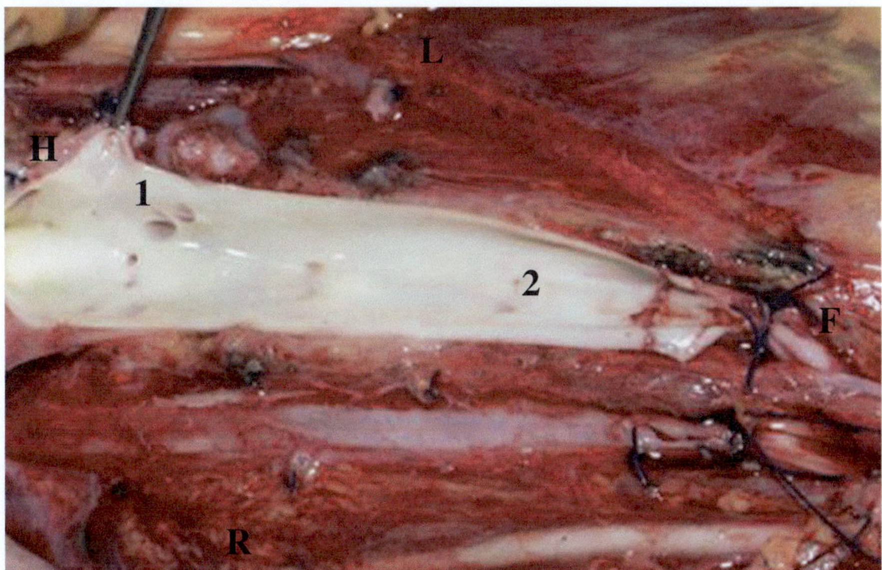


**Fig. 2.10**  1—The orifices of the two left renal arteries from the abdominal aorta. 2—Lumbar arteries, H—Towards the head, F—Towards the feet, L—The left side of the patient, R—The right side

from the aortic bifurcation up to 1 cm above the uppermost ostium of the right or left renal artery. You probably will ask yourself why such a long aorta patch is taken together with the kidneys. The answer is that even if the additional renal artery was not recognized at the time of kidney procurement and packing, procurement with such a long aorta patches provides hope that the patches will contain most or all of the extra renal arteries which are not damaged (Fig. 2.11).

**Warning! (Renal accessory arteries may depart from different places)**

Renal accessory arteries may depart from the abdominal aorta, the celiac trunk, the superior and inferior mesenteric arteries and the iliac arteries. The accessory arteries, especially those running to the hilum and its lower pole, may play an important role in the blood supply to the renal pelvis and ureter [2–5, 31–35]. If you recognize such an artery during retrieval, try to save it with a small patch or cut it off right at the wall of the artery. After the kidney has been retrieved for transplant, immediately before packing, the amount of fat around it should be reduced and the kidney's parenchymal perfusion should be assessed, with particular emphasis on the areas of the kidney supplied by additional (aberrant and/or accessory) renal arteries departing from the aorta or other great arteries in the abdomen. In the case of insufficient perfusion of the entire kidney's parenchyma or its area, the renal artery or extra renal artery or all the renal arteries should be cannulated immediately and perfused with a cold sterile organ preservation fluid with added heparin. The organ preservation solution may be replaced with a sterile cold saline solution or a cold

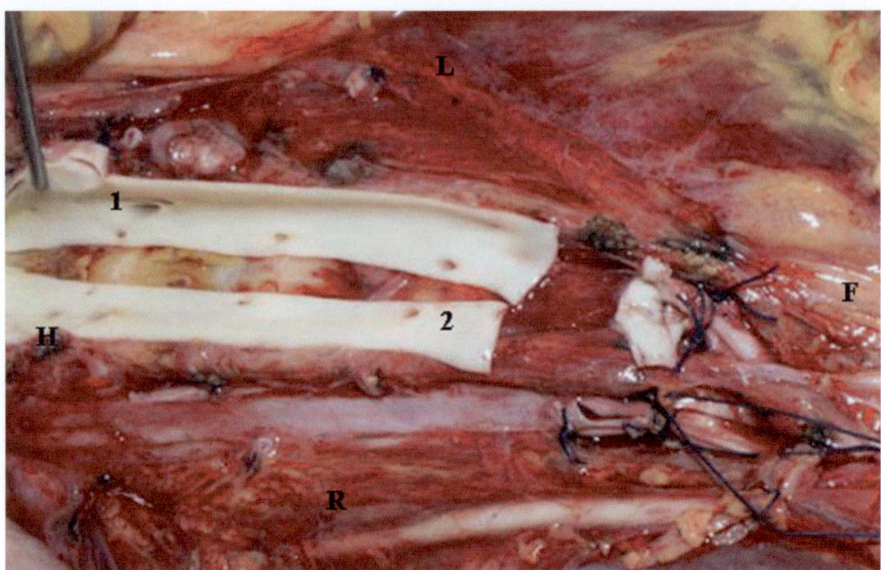

**Fig. 2.11** Abdominal aorta cut off 2 cm above its bifurcation, with its posterior wall cut along the long axis between the lumbar arteries. 1—Aorta orifices of two left kidney arteries, 2—Right aortic patch with the right renal artery and lumbar arteries departing from abdominal aorta, H—Towards the head, F—Towards the feet, L—The left side, R—The right side

Ringer's solution, but it is very important that the solution contains heparin. Additional perfusion always begins with the artery supplying the kidney parenchyma area from which the blood has not been well flushed out. For this purpose, a large syringe with a capacity of 10 or 20 ml, with a thin cannula, Venflon (Becton Dickinson) or a very thin tube attached, may be used, so as not to damage the artery wall and cause its dissection.

**Example:** The right extra renal artery (aberrant artery) from the right common iliac artery to the lower pole (Fig. 2.12) was noticed just prior to procurement and at the beginning of kidney perfusion outside the body (kidney donation from living donor). The celiac trunk before operation did not reveal any extra renal artery. In this case, before the kidney was retrieved the procurement surgeon requested injury avoidance and a long ischemia time and two sets for kidney perfusion by two renal arteries. The preparation requires—besides the two already prepared perfusion systems sets—a special 2 mm thin cannula in order to cannulate and perfuse the small, renal, lower pol artery (always think about the vascularization of the ureter!). After such preparation, cooling and preservation affects the entire kidney simultaneously and not just a part of it. After perfusion through the lower pole and the main renal artery, the differences in color of the lower pole and the remaining renal

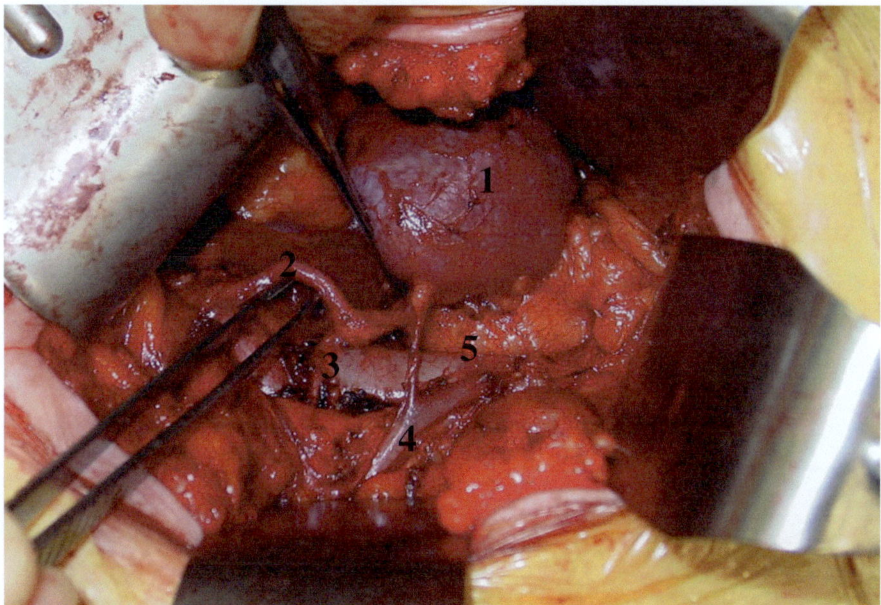

**Fig. 2.12** Renal accessory artery from the right common iliac artery. 1—Right kidney, 2—Right ureter, 3—Additional renal artery deviating from the common iliac artery, 4—Gonadal vein, 5—IVC

parenchyma disappear. Subsequently, the kidney parenchyma was gently palpeted for the presence of tumors. The kidney was considered as normal and suitable for transplantation, after which it was packed in a transport box and then transplanted successfully. In the next chapter I will illustrate the decision making considering a kidney after a multiorgan retrieval where the renal artery has been excised prior to perfusion or arose from the iliac vessels and sent as normal for transplant with a large amount of blood in the part of the kidney supplied by this artery.

6. The IVC should be completely transected near its bifurcation (Fig. 2.13a). If the right renal vein is to be extended with the IVC, there should be no damage to the posterior wall of the right renal vein and the IVC. The lumbar vein should be trimmed to within 2 mm of the IVC wall, has to be cut 2–3 mm from the IVC and can not be torn from the wall during retrieval. Here again I would like to remind you of the right renal vein. Please look again at how thin the posterior wall of the renal vein in particular is. Both walls of the right renal vein are so thin that they are transparent and can easily be damaged (Fig. 2.13b).

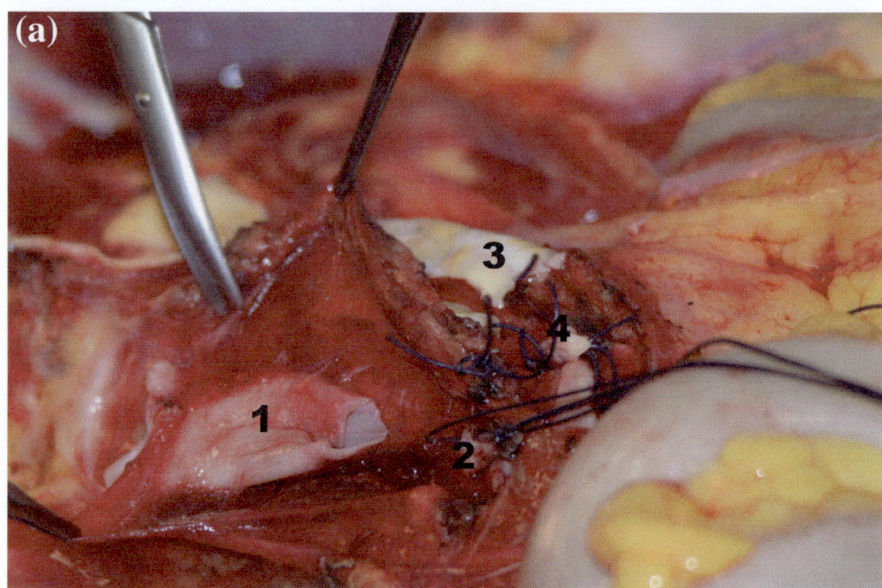

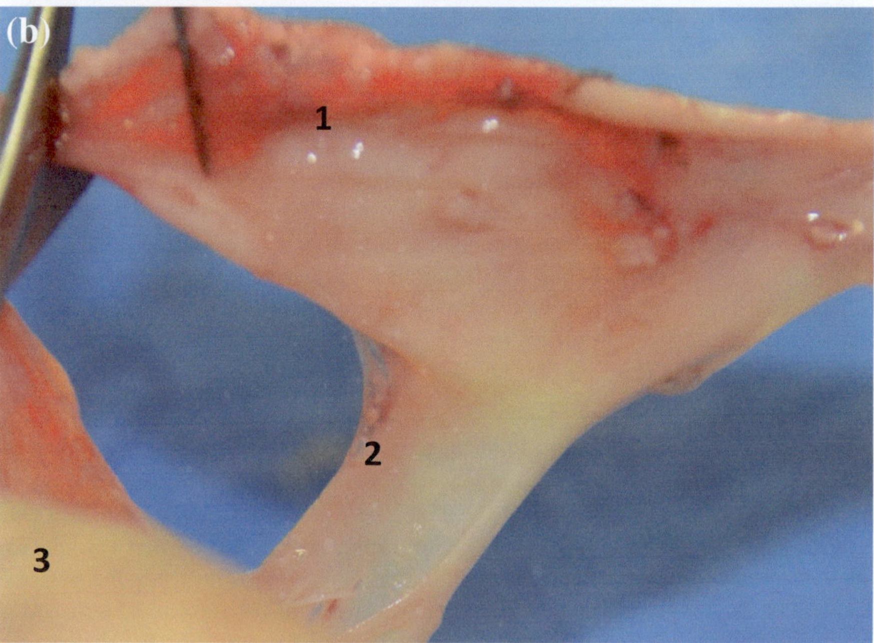

**Fig. 2.13** **(a)** 1—IVC cut above its bifurcation, 2—Bifurcation of the IVC, 3—Left patch of abdominal aorta, including left renal and lumbar arteries, 4—Abdominal aortic bifurcation, **(b)** 1—IVC, 2—Thin and short right renal vein, 3—Kidney hilum

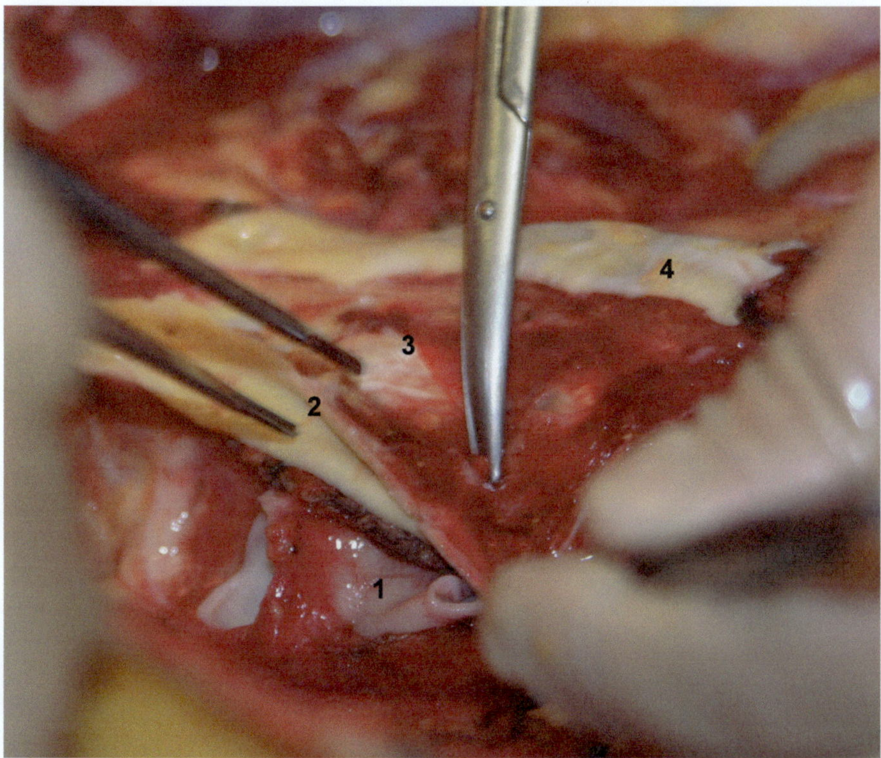

**Fig. 2.14** Using forceps and scissors, mobilize by cutting off the right aorta patch together with the IVC from the anterior longitudinal ligament of the spine as much as possible to the right side. The cuts should be carried out close to the ligament. During cutting be careful not to damage the renal vein, IVC and renal artery. 1—IVC, 2—Right aorta patch, 3—Anterior longitudinal ligament, 4—Left aorta patch

7. Mobilize the right aortic patch along and together with the IVC from the anterior longitudinal ligament of the vertebral column. Carry out the cuts with scissors strictly on the surface of the anterior longitudinal ligament, going to the right (Figs. 2.14 and 2.15) (when cutting, be very careful in order not to damage renal arteries and/or veins). Lumbar veins located on the posterior surface of the IVC should be cut at a considerable distance so that after procurement they are suitable for ligating or suturing.

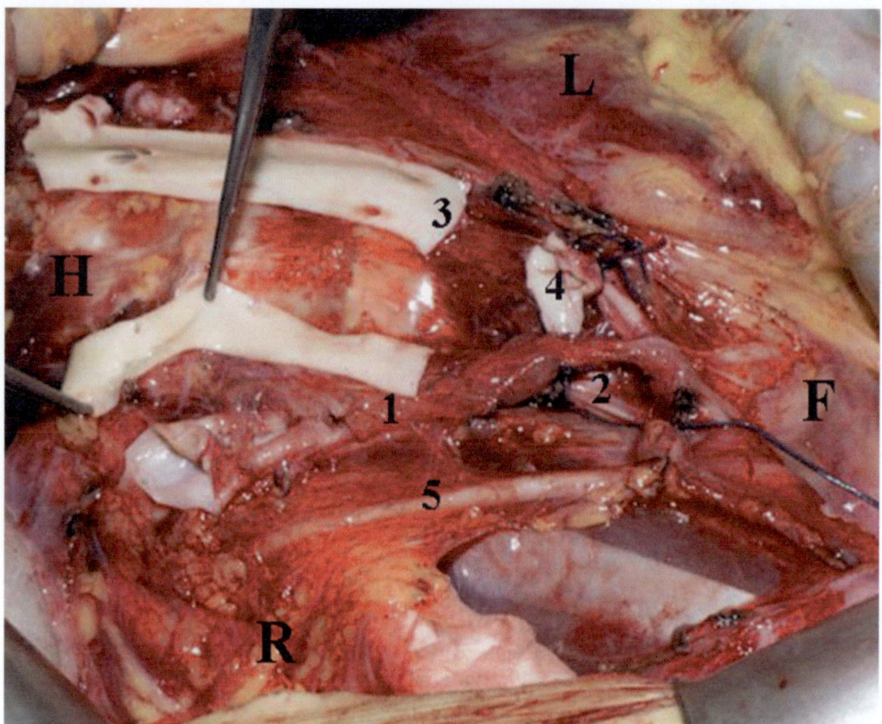

**Fig. 2.15** The abdominal aorta and the IVC were cut just above their bifurcations. The right aortic patch and IVC were cut off with scissors next to the anterior longitudinal ligament maximal to the right side without damaging the renal artery, IVC or right renal vein. 1—IVC, this part after procurement belongs to the right kidney, 2—IVC bifurcation, 3—Left patch of the abdominal aorta, cut off above the bifurcation, 4—Abdominal aortic bifurcation, 5—Localized and dissected right ureter, H—In towards the head, F—Towards the feet, L—Left side, R—Right side

8. Mobilize right kidney from retroperitoneal space. Start from the right side—lateral border and lower pole, posterior surface of the right kidney towards the right side of the column vertebrae. Going down mobilize the right ureter with its surrounding tissue as far as the urinary bladder (Fig. 2.16). The right kidney was mobilized with scissors behind from the retroperitoneal space until the right side of the anterior longitudinal ligament of the vertebral column and then rotated to the left side (Fig. 2.17). As a next step mobilize the upper pole from the retroperitoneal space by cutting the tissues above the upper pole and upper edge of the right aortic patch (Fig. 2.18).

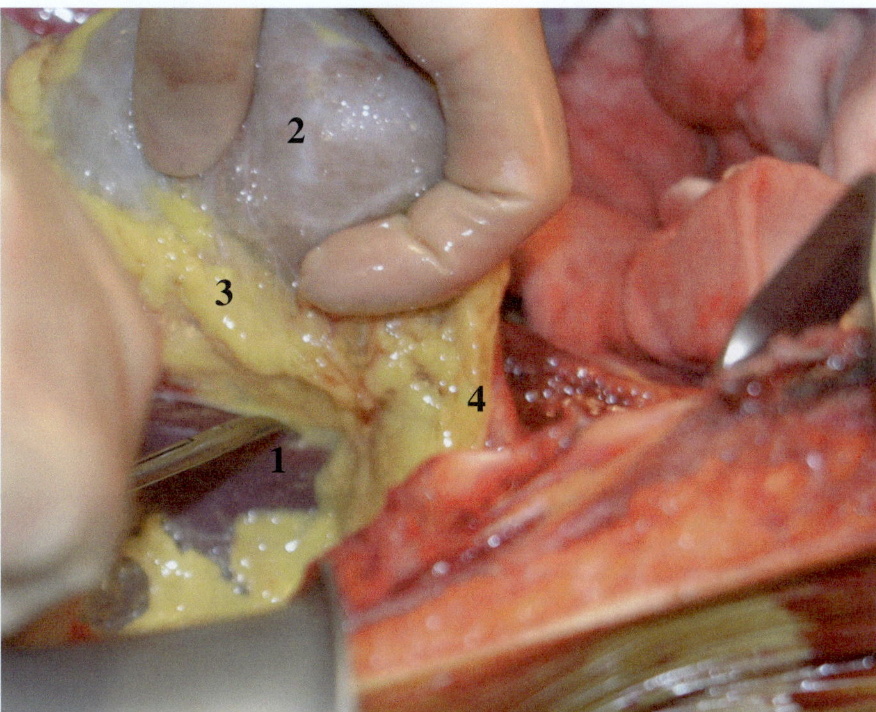

**Fig. 2.16** The posterior surface of the right kidney is completely mobilized from the retroperitoneal space. 1—Cutting with scissors on the right side, including the lateral surface of the vertebral column and anterior longitudinal ligament, 2—Right kidney, 3—Renal pelvis, 4—Right ureter with surrounding tissues

9. The right kidney is fully mobilized from the retroperitoneal space. Hold the kidney in the left hand and gently pull it upwards to reveal tension structures such as the ureter or ureters with the surrounding tissues and running in parallel with the gonadal vessels. This is an excellent opportunity to try to assess the number of ureters. The ureters and vessels mentioned above should be carefully dissected as close to the bladder and then cut with scissors so that they are as long as possible and have enough tissue around to ensure a proper blood supply of the ureter after transplantation (Figs. 2.19 and 2.20).

10. The right kidney, after excision from the abdominal cavity, is handed over to the scrub nurse who, as quickly as possible, places the organ in a sterile right kidney container filled with a cold preservation solution and sterile slush ice. In order not to make a mistake when packing, the sterile container bears the inscription: right kidney.

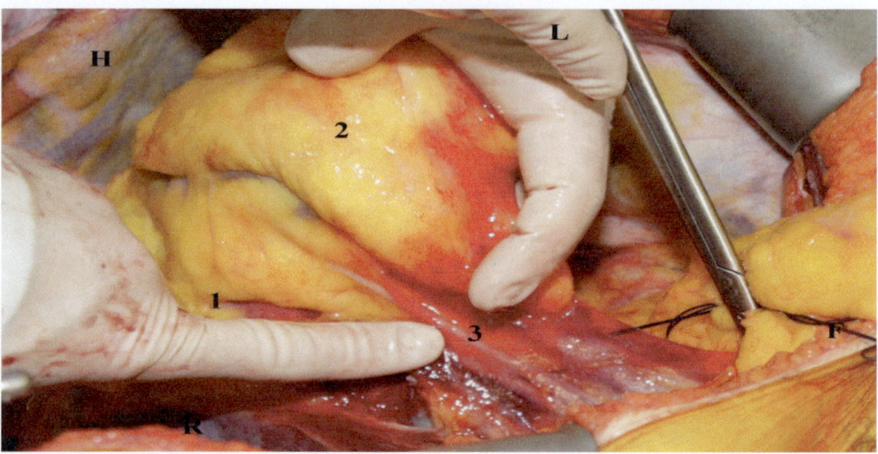

**Fig. 2.17** The posterior surface of the right kidney is completely mobilized from the retroperitoneal space. After mobilizing the vessels, the kidney is mobilized with scissors from above and behind, taking care not to damage the vessels and the ureter. 1—Retroperitoneal space, 2—Kidney with adhering fat mobilized from retroperitoneal space, 3—Right ureter with gonadal vein; the kidney and ureter will be mobilized further towards the bladder, H—Towards the head, F—Towards the feet, L—The left side, R—The right side

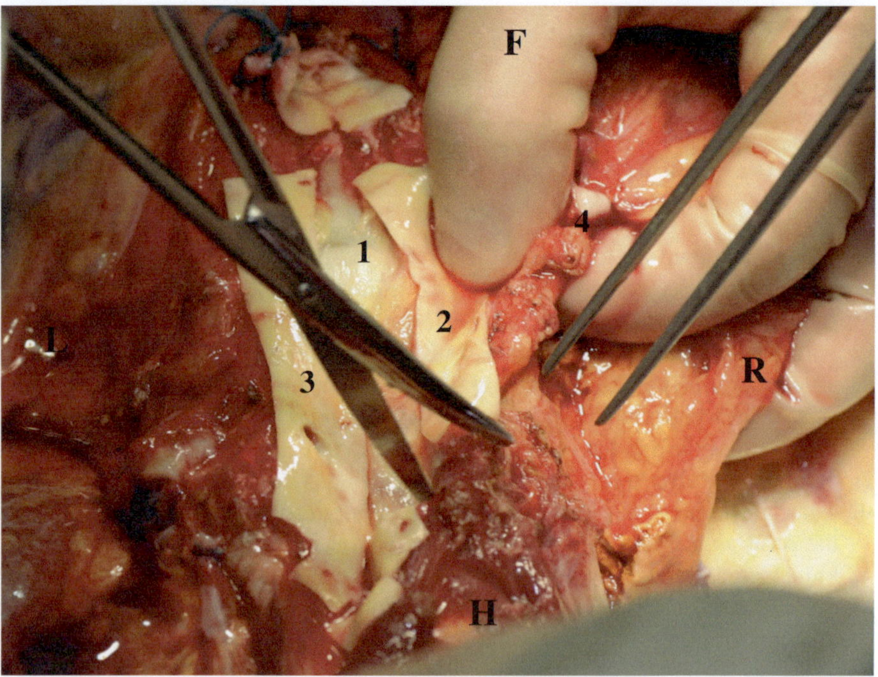

**Fig. 2.18** Mobilization of the upper pole of the right kidney. 1—Anterior longitudinal ligament, 2—Right aortic patch with right renal artery and a tiny bit of the IVC under the thumb, 3—Left aortic patch, 4—A small section of the protruding IVC, H—Towards the head, F—Towards the feet, L—The left side, R—The right side

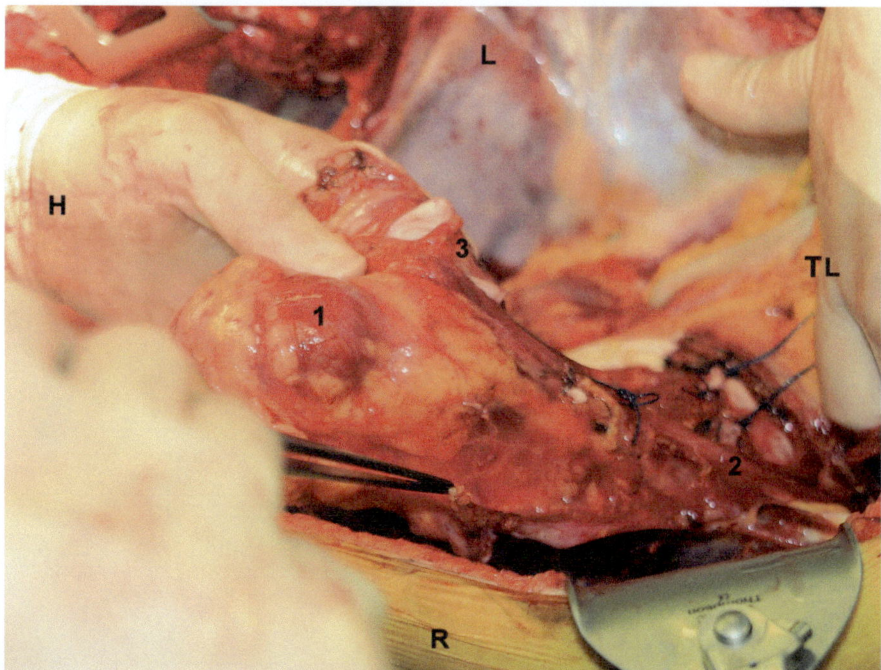

**Fig. 2.19** The right kidney with renal vessels are completely mobilized from the extraperitoneal space. The only non-mobilized element is the ureter and gonadal vein. The ureter together with the gonadal vein will be cut out of the extraperitoneal space with as much tissue as possible by moving the scissors from the apical of the lower kidney pole towards the bladder. 1—Completely mobilized right kidney, 2—Right kidney ureter, 3—IVC, H—Towards the head, TL—Towards the leg, L—Left side, R—Right side

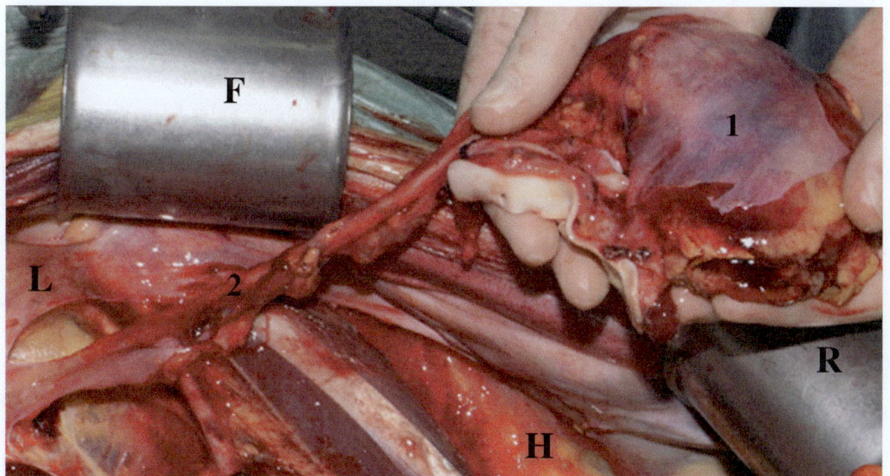

**Fig. 2.20** Completely freed from the retroperitoneal space, the right kidney together with the ureter is mobilized up to the bladder with a large amount of surrounding tissues. 1—Right kidney, 2—Ureter, H—Towards the head, F—Towards the feet, L—Left side, R—Right side

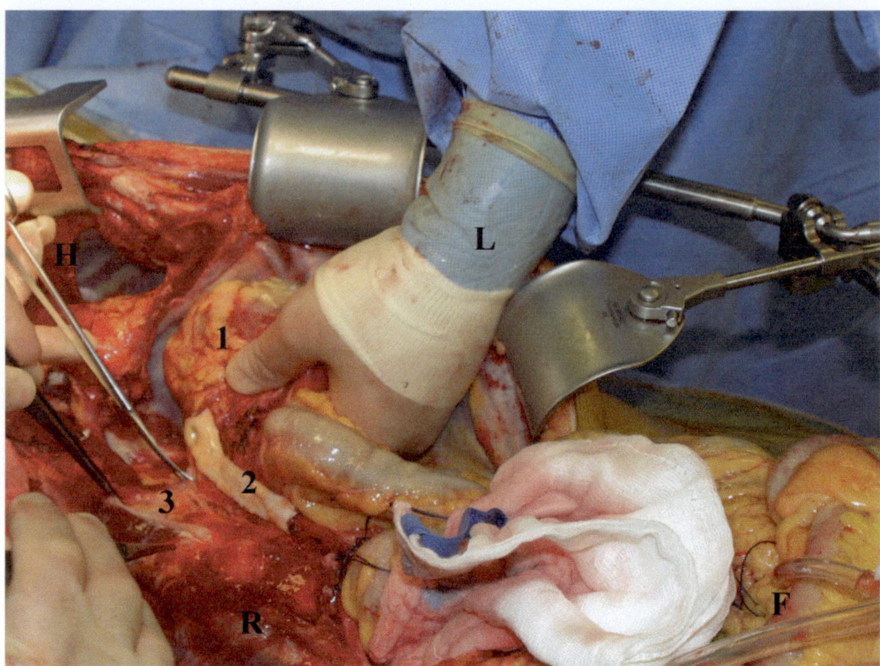

**Fig. 2.21** Left kidney mobilization. First, the left aortic patch and the left renal vein are mobilized with scissors, cutting off all the tissues between the left kidney abdominal aorta patch and the anterior longitudinal ligament of the spine. The next stage is mobilization of the descending and sigmoid colon along the Toldt's line. Then the left kidney is fully mobilized from the retroperitoneal space along with the previously mobilized vessels. The ureter is not yet sufficiently mobilized. 1—Left kidney, 2—Left aortic years, 3—Anterior longitudinal ligament, H—Towards the head, F—Towards the feet, L—Left side, R—Right side

11. Procurement of the left kidney. Cut the aortic patch of the left renal artery very close to the anterior longitudinal ligament of the spine. Pay particular attention to the central and extra-renal arteries and veins (Fig. 2.21).

12. Mobilize the left kidney from the retroperitoneal space. Start from the left side —the lateral border, lower poles, posterior surface of the right kidney to the left side of the column vertebrae. Mobilize the upper pole from the retroperitoneal space by cutting the tissues above the upper pole and upper edge of the left aortic patch. Go down and if it has not been done, cut the peritoneum along the Toldt's line and mobilize from the retroperitoneal space the mesentery of the descending colon and sigmoid together with the left ureter(s) with its surrounding tissues as far as the bladder [24, 31–33].

13. The left kidney is fully mobilized from the retroperitoneal space. Holding the kidney in the left hand and gently pulling it upwards to reveal the tension structures, such as ureter or ureters with surrounding tissues and running in parallel with the gonadal vessel. To easily visualize the ureter(s) and the gonadal vessel in the left retroperitoneal space, the posterior surface of the descending colon mesentery and the sigmoid colon must be freed from the Toldt's line to the left lateral wall of the abdominal aorta and left iliac vessels (Fig. 2.22).

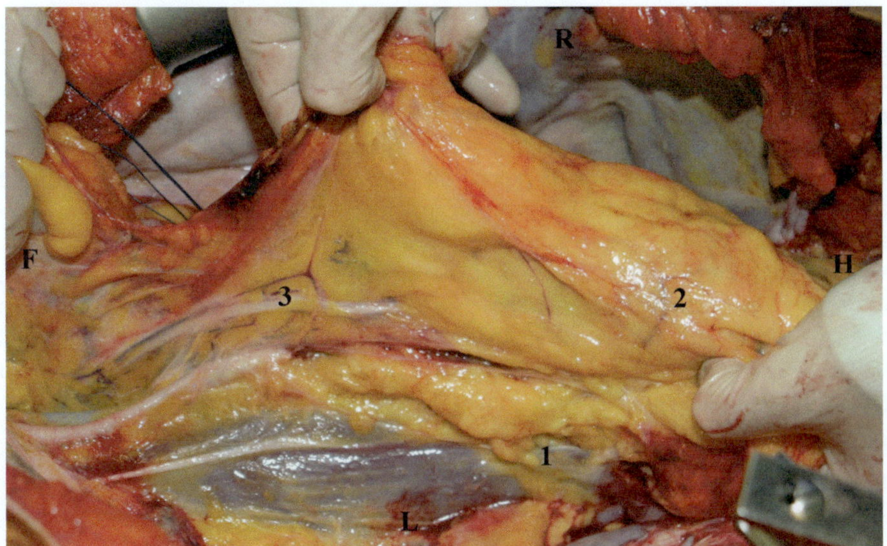

**Fig. 2.22** Left kidney completely mobilized from the retroperitoneal space. In the photo, the left kidney is turned to the right side. 1—Retroperitoneal space on the left side, visible is the major lumbar muscle, 2—Posterior surface of the left kidney covered by fat, 3—Left ureter, H—Towards the head, F—Towards the feet, L—Left side, R—Right side

**Warning! (Finding and recognizing the left ureter is not always easy—tips)**
The best and the easiest way is to identify the left ureter/ureters by performing an incision of the peritoneum along the Toldt' s line and mobilizing the descending colon with sigmoid mesentery up to the left side of the aorta and left iliac vessels. The next step is to gently lift up and turn to the right all the above mentioned structures, so that the posterior surface of the descending colon and sigmoid can be completely visualized. Remember that the left ureter is "glued" to the posterior surface of the descending colon and the sigmoid mesentery and runs along with the testicular or ovarian vein to the urinary bladder. If we are not able to recognize the structures going to the posterior surface of the descending colon and sigmoid mesentery or we are not sure, treat them as with the ureters.

So try to dissect all unidentified structures, preserving as much tissue as possible from the renal pelvis to the urinary bladder. Remember that before organ packing you will have a second chance to identify the ureter or ureters. After kidney procurement and before packing or connecting with the perfusion machine it is always worth examining the lumen of every cut structure (the ureter is star-shaped). If we still cannot recognize the ureter(s) in the cut section, I would recommend placing the kidney in a special sterile container filled with ice and cold preservation solution and perform here one more time a longer and more accurate cut surface inspection, for example by cannulating the lumen of the "suspicious" structure with a thin long tube, which you should very slowly and gently try to move towards the renal pelvis or left renal vein. Another way to identify the ureter after kidney procurement is to insert a thin sterile tube into the lumen of a "suspect" ureter and connect it to a syringe filled with a cold preservative solution or cold saline solution. During the administration of the fluid, carefully and slowly move the cannula towards the renal pelvis. If the ureter is cannulated after the injection of every 5 ml of the cold preservation solution or sterile saline, check the degree of the renal pelvis and ureter distension, or if your catheter is placed into the vein look for the extravasation of the fluid into the surrounding tissues or left renal vein. In the case of significant resistance to fluid injection or to moving the cannula towards the renal pelvis, check whether the ureter is not twisted and how it is physiologically positioned in relation to the procured kidney. If the ureter is twisted, fluid injection should be stopped. In this case, try to unscrew the ureter to allow the fluid and cannula to enter the renal pelvis without any resistance. In every case of ureter resistance close to the renal pelvis, think about uretero-pelvic junction (UPJ) or ureter obstruction [31–33].

14. The left kidney with ureter is fully mobilized, but the ureter, gonadal vessels and surrounding tissues have not yet been cut but dissected up to the urinary bladder (Fig. 2.23).

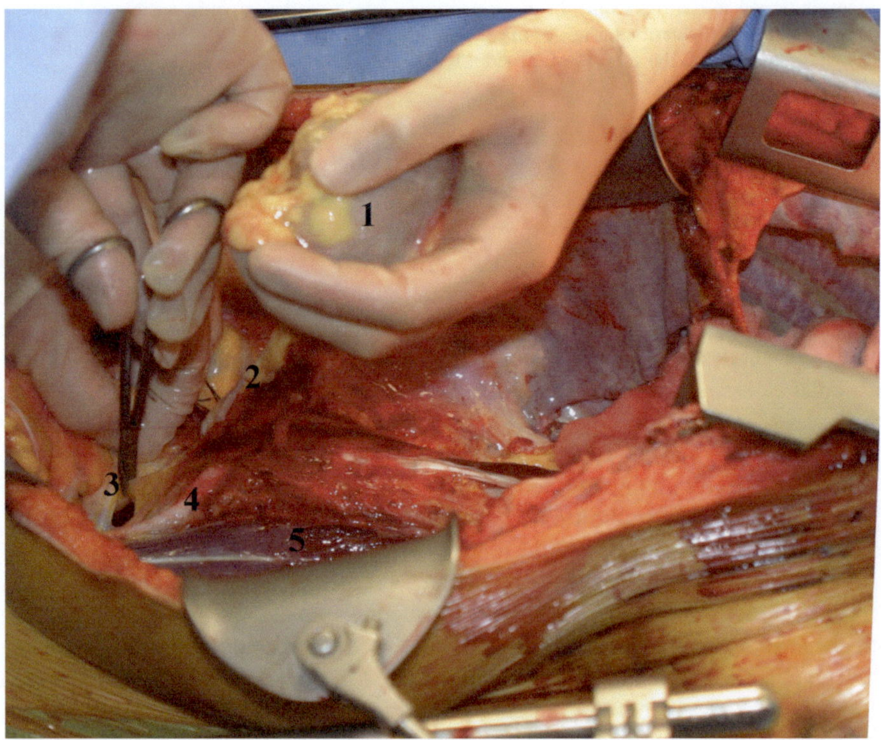

**Fig. 2.23** Left ureter cut right next to the bladder. 1—Retrieved left kidney, 2—Left ureter, 3—Para-vesical area, 4—The left common iliac artery, 5—Major lumbar muscle

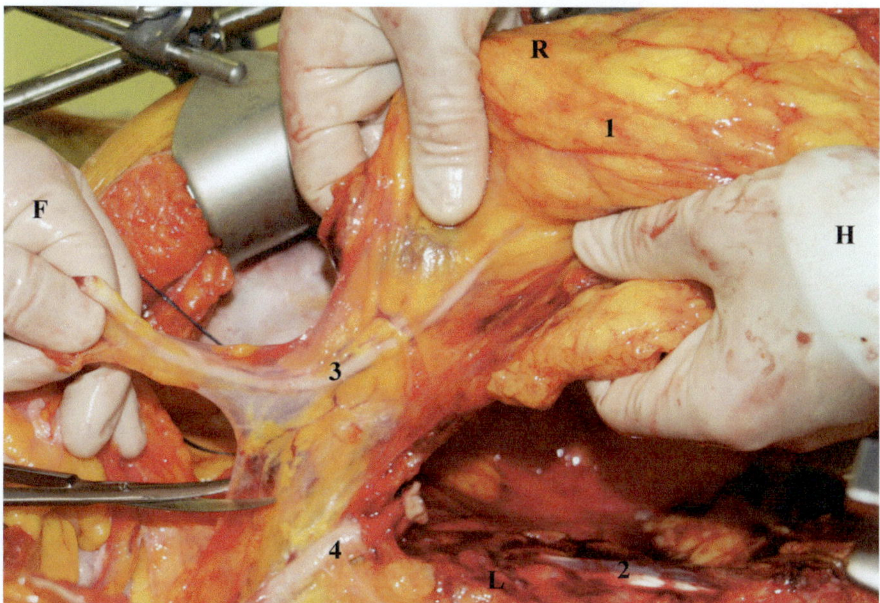

**Fig. 2.24** Completely mobilized left kidney with the ureter cut off close to the bladder. The procurement surgeon tries to retrieve every ureter with as much of the surrounding tissue as possible. 1—Posterior surface of the mobilized left kidney, 2—Retroperitoneal space, 3—Left ureter, 4—Left common iliac artery, H—Towards the head, F—Towards the feet, L—The left side, R—The right side

16. A few centimeters before the urinary bladder, cut off the ureter and hand the procured left kidney over to the scrub nurse who, as quickly as possible, places the organ in a sterile container filled with a cold preservative fluid and sterile slush ice. In order not to make a mistake when packing, the sterile container bears the inscription: left kidney (Figs. 2.24 and 2.25).

**Warning! (To ligate or not ligate ureters?)**

A frequently asked question is whether to ligate or to not ligate, as it may not be necessary to ligate the vesical ureters close to the urinary bladder before cutting them. Personally, during a kidney procurement from a cadaver donor, I don't ligate any ureter, I just cut them 10–15 cm before the urinary bladder. My first argument for not ligating the ureters during procurement from a cadaver donor is that there is a catheter in the urinary bladder which is removed at the end of the organ procurement, so the bladder is already drained out. My second argument is that at the junction of the ureter with the bladder, there are vesicoureteral valves which prevent the return of urine from the urinary bladder to the ureter. Conclusion: if you believe my arguments, it is not necessary to ligate [3].

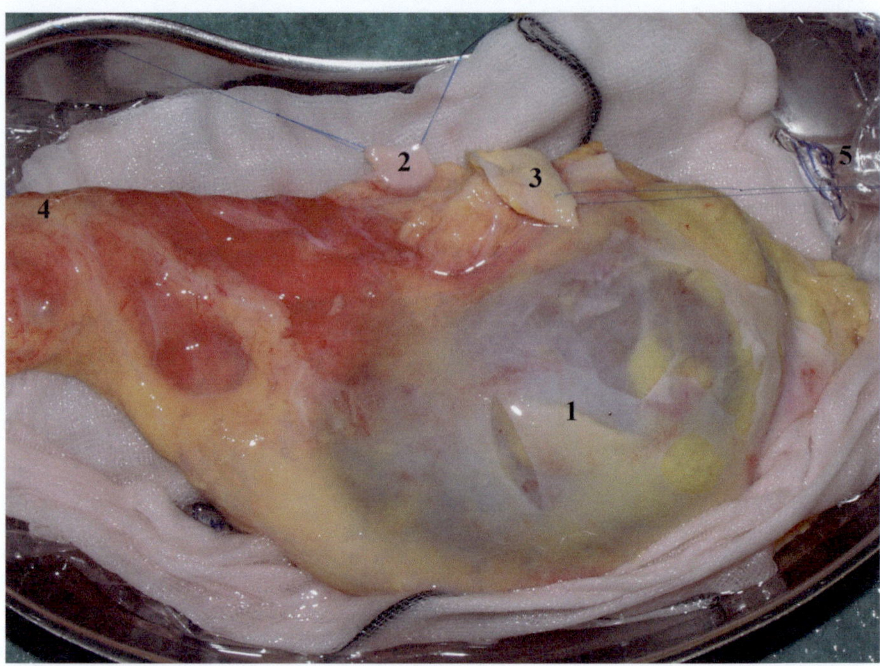

**Fig. 2.25** The left adult kidney is placed in a container filled with a preservation solution and sterile ice after removal. 1—Anterior surface of kidney procured with perirenal fat, 2—Left renal vein, 3—Left renal artery at the aortic patch, 4—Ureter, 5—Sterile ice

**Warning! (Always and everywhere label the right kidney and left kidney)**

When it comes to kidney storage, it is a good idea to have specially labeled containers each time to prevent mistakes (Fig. 2.26). I have learned in the course of many years of practice that most scrub nurses cannot distinguish the right from the left procured kidney outside the body. The kidneys are usually placed in containers marked "right" and "left" in order to avoid confusion during packing. During most donations, the kidneys are packaged by the scrub nurse or put on the perfusion machine by the procurement surgeon, before being thoroughly inspected by the donor surgeon. Inspection of each retrieved kidney for transplantation is mandatory and each retrieved kidney cannot be packaged or put on the machine without being carefully evaluated by the retrieval surgeon.

**Warning! (If possible, always procure the right kidney with the IVC)**

The right kidney, unlike the left one, usually has a shorter vein and a longer artery and more often it has more than one renal vein and should always be procured with the IVC. Some surgeons do not respect this rule. In my opinion, the following situations are an absolute indication for the procurement of the right kidney with the IVC: when the kidney has more than one vein or when the right renal vein is very short; when the recipient is obese with difficult access to the iliac vessels; or the

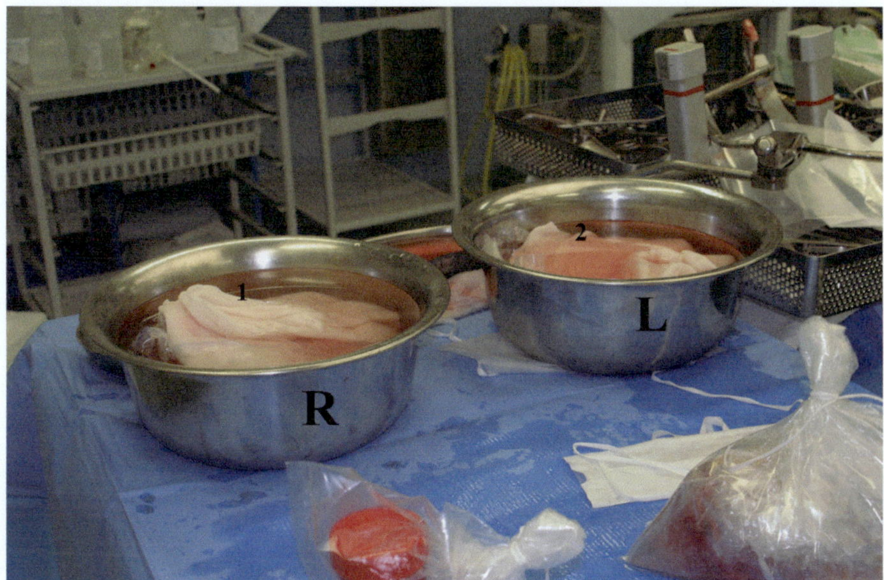



**Fig. 2.26**  Bowels in the operating room of the donor's hospital. The containers are labeled right and left and are used for temporary storage just after the right and left kidney are removed. 1 and 2—Containers filled with sterile ice slush or crushed ice and preservation solution. The bowls have been marked; R—For the right kidney, L—For the left kidney. Each bowl should be labeled to prevent kidney packaging error

transplantation will be very complex (e.g. a second graft on the same side with or without removal of the previous graft). In these cases, elongation of the right renal vein with the IVC can greatly facilitate its transplantation and thus reduce the risks associated with surgery.

17. The procurement surgeon who has procured the kidney(s) should carefully examine each of them before packing (using static cold storage) (Fig. 2.27) or before connecting to hypothermic machine perfusion. The inspection process consists of assessing the number and length of the vessels, the distance between them and whether they were retrieved on an aortic patch, or not, their diameter, assessment of every ostium of the renal arteries arising from the aorta wall, if any—the degree of their damage, the advancement of atherosclerotic changes in the aortic wall, the length of the ureter with its surrounding tissues (Fig. 2.28), an attempt to determine the number of ureters and, if possible, the reduction of fat around the retrieved kidney (Fig. 2.29), but not around the renal hilum, ureter and lower pole. After reducing the fat around the kidney, it's parenchyma should be very carefully inspected and palpated (Fig. 2.30) in order to assess its perfusion, the presence of tumors or cysts, possible surgical or non-surgical damage (due to accident and/or procurement) to the parenchyma, renal pelvis and ureter.

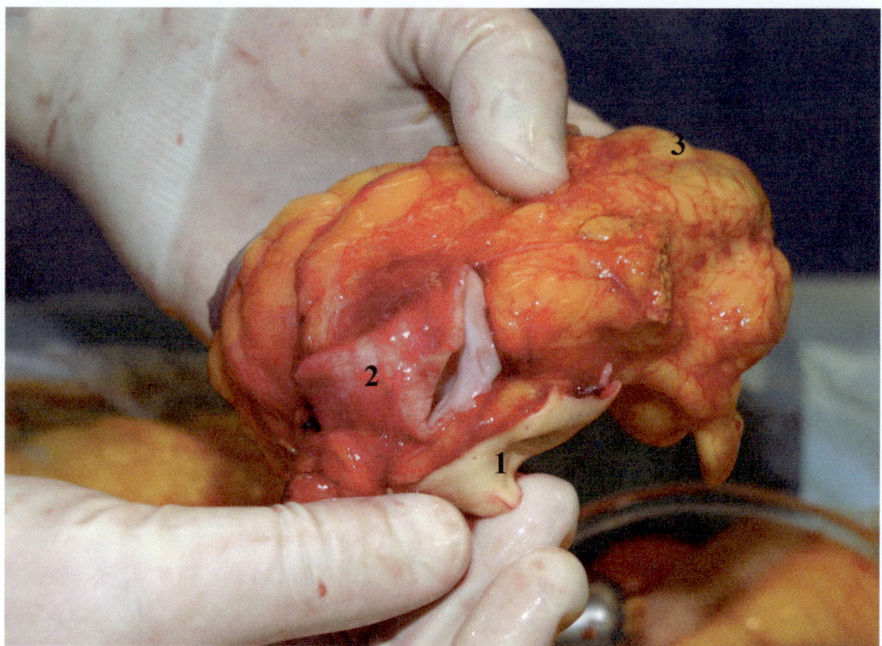

**Fig. 2.27** The right kidney has been procured. Initial assessment of the advancement of atherosclerosis in the patch of the abdominal aorta with careful assessment of the ostium of the renal artery from the aorta. 1—Right renal artery ostium on the aorta patch, 2—IVC retrieved with right renal vein(s), 3—Upper pole of the right kidney

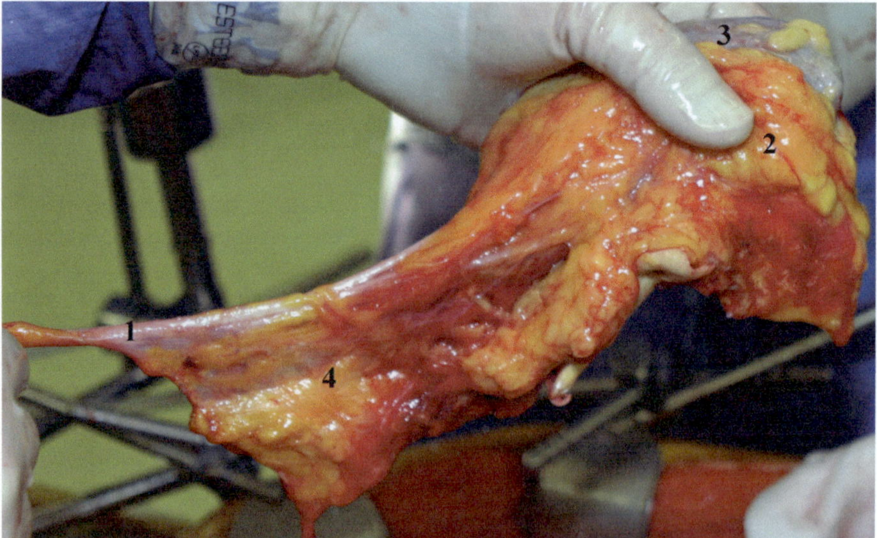

**Fig. 2.28** Assessment of the length and the amount of tissue around the ureter. 1—Ureter, 2—A layer of perirenal fat surrounds left kidney, 3—Left kidney, 4—The tissues surrounding the ureter are taken together with the ureter, giving it a chance to become well supplied with blood. Try to take as many around the ureter as possible, and do not try to reduce their volume or prepare them in the donor hospital

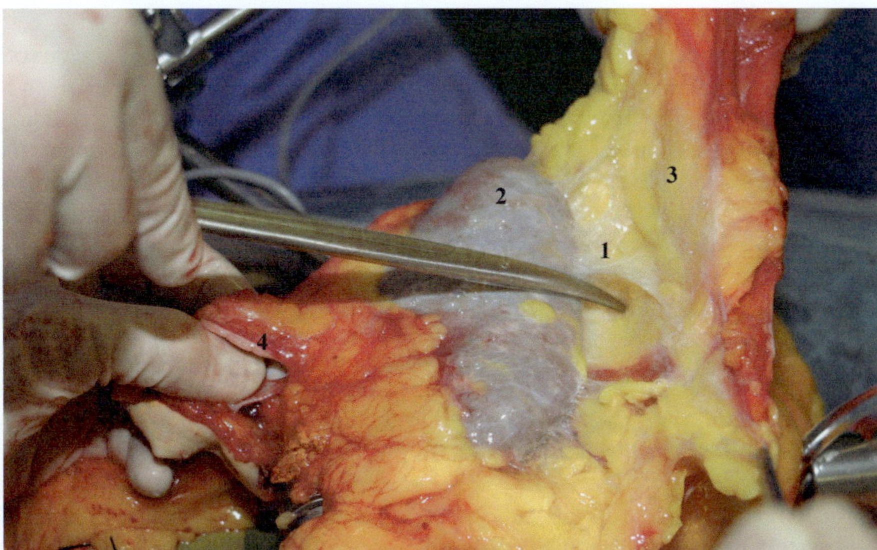

**Fig. 2.29**  Perirenal fat must be reduced around the upper pole, anterior and posterior surfaces, but not around the lower pole and around the hilum. Remember that with excess fat cools from the outside of the kidney may be insufficient, as the fat acts as an insulator. 1—Perirenal fat, 2—Kidney parenchyma without fat upper pole, 3—Perirenal fat released from the anterior surface of the kidney, 4—Kidney hilum with renal vessels

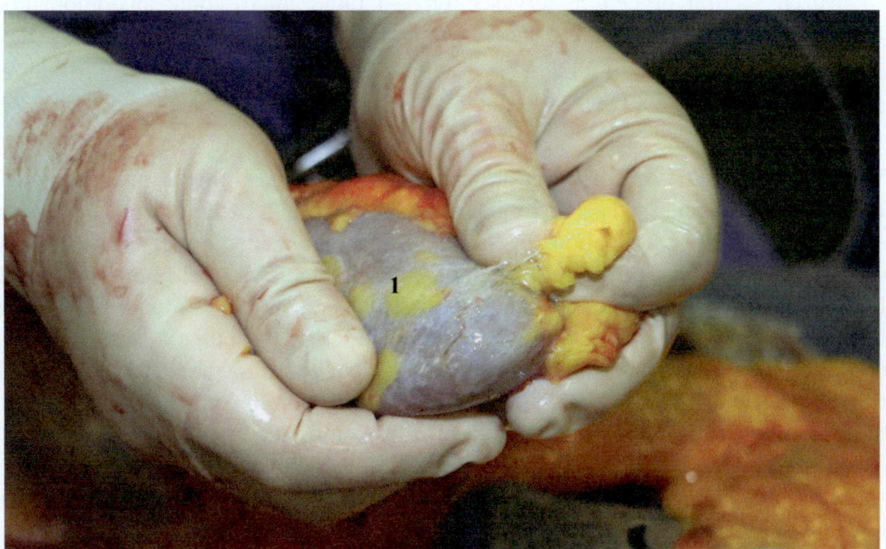

**Fig. 2.30**  The kidney, after a significant amount of renal fat reduction, is gently palpated for the presence of tumors, injuries or pathological fat. 1—Kidney surface with small normal fat islet

**Warning! (Kidney fat reduction is sometimes impossible)**
During the reduction of fat around the procured kidney be very careful and cut out fat that can be easily separated from the kidney capsule and leave the fat ingrown in the kidney capsule. Remember that a large layer of fat around the removed kidney may slow down its cooling process during transport to the recipient's hospital (the fat in this case acts as an insulator). A kidney with a large amount of ingrown perirenal fat may be of considerable size and therefore be suitable for transplantation only to selected recipients who can accommodate such a large kidney in the retroperitoneal space. It is more than advisable at this point to ask the recipient's hospital to clarify this.

18. Check the kidney vessels carefully and in particular the number of veins and arteries. Describe in the kidney quality report not only its suitability for transplantation but also the diameters in the case of multiple vessels and their distances from each other on the aorta patch. Further, it is very important to describe the state of the severity of the atherosclerotic lesions in the wall of the abdominal aorta and in the ostia of the renal arteries departing from the aorta, because they are often affected by atherosclerotic lesions especially in older people. Finally, we evaluate the ureter(s) and here, especially in the case of the left kidney, pay attention to their number. In this case, as already mentioned, the "suspect" ureter can always be cannulated and/or the "suspect" structure can be cannulated and perfused using a thin catheter with a cold preservative solution or examined with a special thin metal probe.

19. If necessary, and there are indications for this, perform a kidney biopsy and a frozen section procedure (cryosection)—a rapid microscopic anatomopathological examination of the specimen. If the pathologist finds something that deviates from the norm, please ask a procurement surgeon to immediately inform the transplant coordinator, the kidney recipient centers and the recipients of the other organs about it [24, 31–33].

**Warning! (Frozen sections, anatomical pathologists, peripheral hospitals)**
In peripheral hospitals it is sometimes impossible to find a pathologist to perform a rapid microscopic examination. In that kind of situation, the collected specimens should be sent to the university hospital of the recipient who is to be transplanted first—thus this will be a heart or lung or liver or pancreas recipient—or to a center that has the greatest experience and can make a quick and accurate diagnosis. In the case when cancer is suspected, inform the transplant coordinators of all the donated organs as soon as possible. If you have a strong suspicion of cancer, try, if possible, to delay all transplant operations until a frozen section procedure result is available. You can send all procured organs to the recipient(s) hospital(s) but write on the shipping box a letter warning that the kidney may be transplanted, like any other donated organ, only after a cancer negative frozen section procedure. After getting the result the transplant coordinator will contact you before getting the result from the frozen section procedure, as using any procured organ for transplantation is forbidden by law.

20. The abdominal organ quality report has to be personally prepared by the procurement surgeon and the transplant coordinator and signed by the surgeon who performed the abdominal organ procurement.

**Warning! (Kidney packing: hypothermic machine perfusion or classic cold storage?)**

After a very detailed assessment of both kidneys, we can allow the scrub nurse to pack organs according to the protocol applicable in the given country. In the Netherlands, this will be a technique of packing organs for transplantation according to the Dutch Transplant Foundation and Eurotransplant protocol, in this case we are illustrating the old method of packing kidneys so called static cold storage (Figs. 2.31, 2.32, 2.33, 2.34, 2.35 and 2.36).

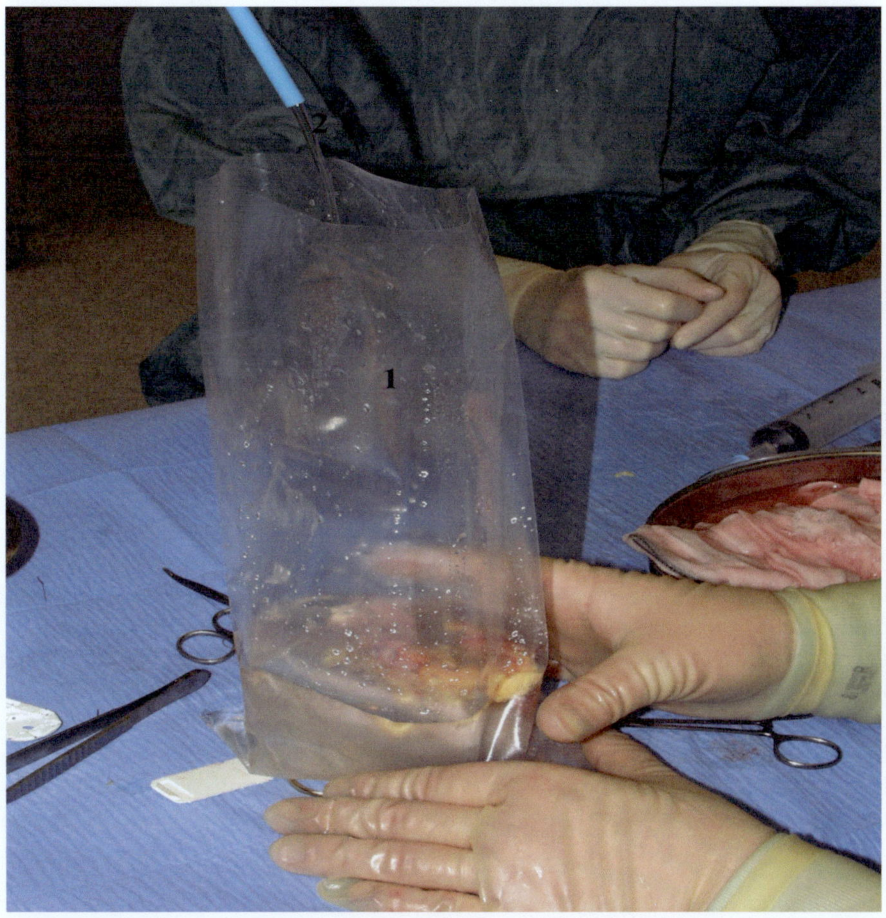

**Fig. 2.31** Packing of procured organs. 1—The removed organ is sterile packed into the first bag which is filled with a cold fresh preservation solution so that the organ is completely covered. The air is removed from the bag before it is tightly tied

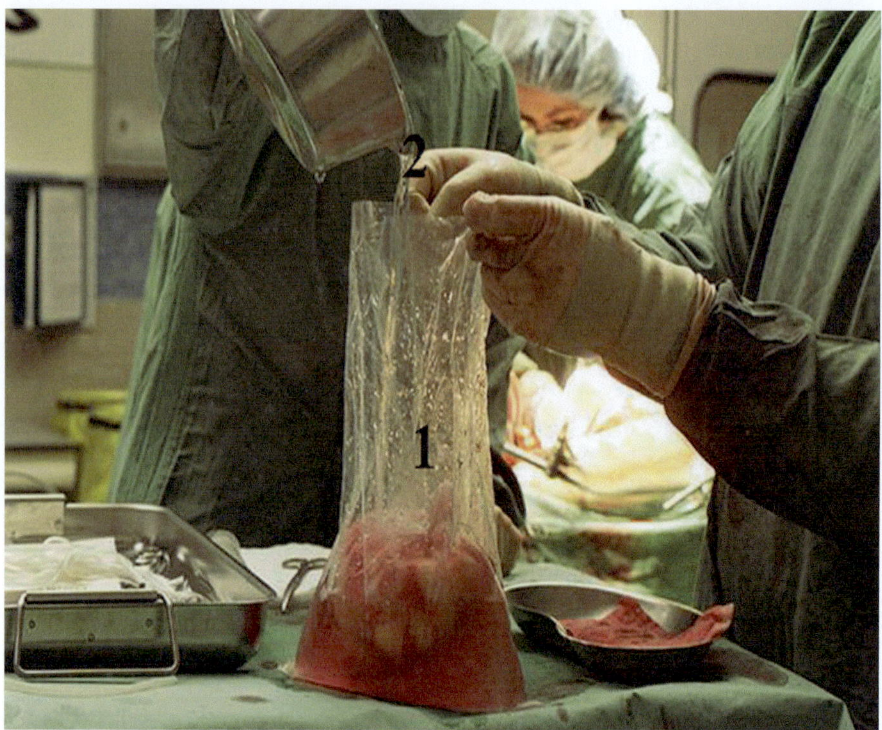


**Fig. 2.32**  1—The first tied bag with the organ removed is inserted into the second larger bag. 2—The second bag is filled with a cold physiological natrium chloride solution or Ringer's solution so that the first organ bag is completely covered with this fluid. The air is removed from the bag and the bag is tightly tied

This is why we use the cold static storage technique in the Netherlands from January 2016: each kidney donated by a deceased donor is connected at the donor hospital to one of the machines in which the kidney is actively cooled and preserved during transport to the recipient hospital. The flow of specially prepared preservation fluid through the organ may be laminar or pulsatile, depending on the type of machine, and the fluid may or may not be saturated with oxygen before entering the donor kidney. Hypothermic machine perfusion (HMP) of the kidney is a long-established alternative to static cold storage. It has been suggested that it is a better method of preservation. Today, as the profile of our deceased donors continues to change in favour of higher risk, lower quality kidneys, we are faced with

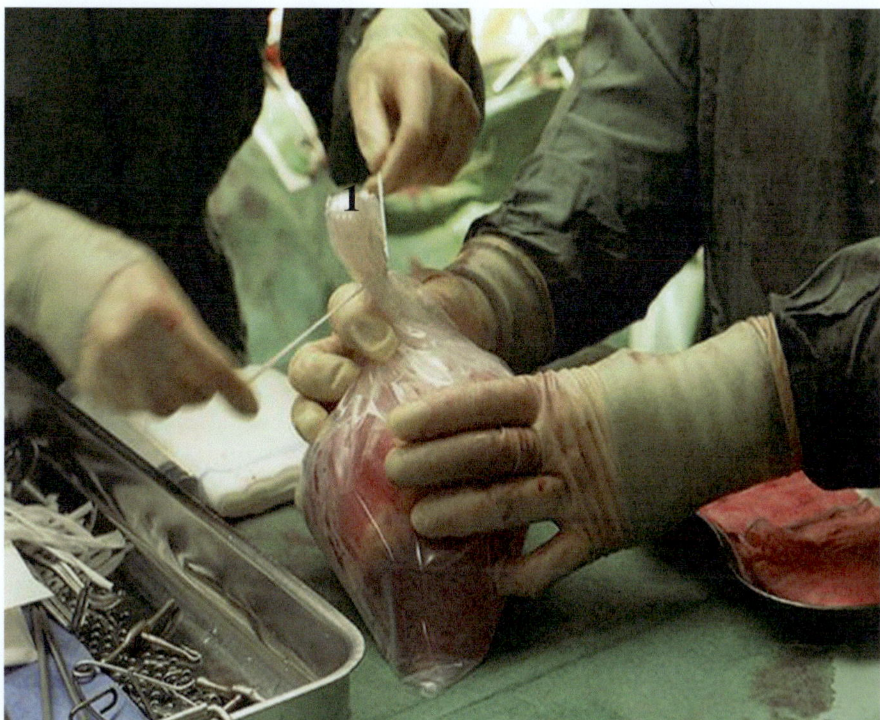


**Fig. 2.33**  1—The third bag does not contain any liquid; it is empty or "dry". Two previously packed bags are placed in the third bag. Air is purged from the last bag which (acts as an insulator) and the bag is tied tightly

the limitation. Interest in HMP as a preservation technique is growing. In addition, HMP also creates a window of opportunity during which the viability and quality of the graft can be assessed prior to transplantation. The kidneys of deceased donors are preserved in cold, hypoxic condition. The provision of oxygen during preservation may improve post-transplant outcomes, particularly for kidneys which are subject to a greater degree of preservation injury. Interest in HMP as a preservation technique is growing. In addition, HMP also creates a window of opportunity during which the viability and quality of the graft can be assessed prior to transplantation. The kidneys of deceased donors are preserved in cold, with provision of

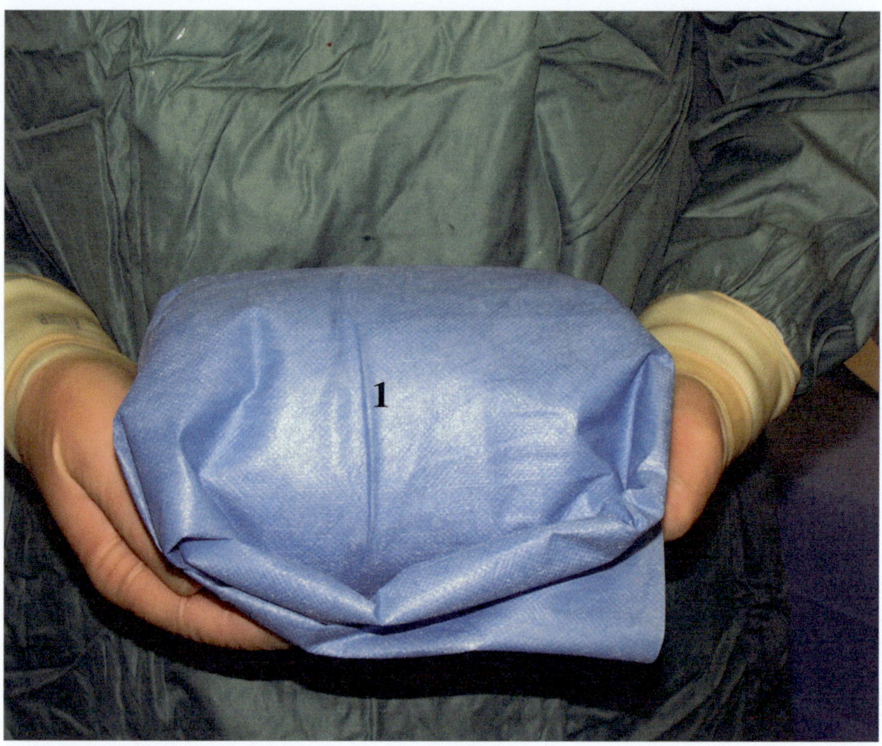

**Fig. 2.34** 1—The retrieved organ, previously packed in three sterile bags, in some centers, before being put into the transport container with ice, has a special napkin wrapped around it

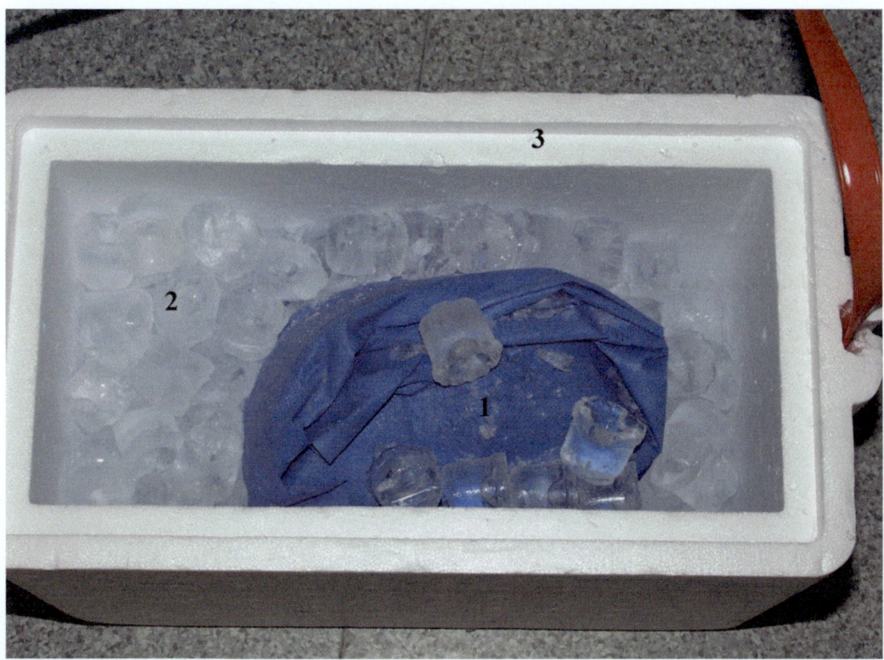


**Fig. 2.35** The removed and packed organ is placed on ice in a special transport box and then completely covered with fresh ice and a napkin. 1—Kidney procured and packed, 2—Ice, 3—Open transport box

oxygen during preservation may improve post-transplant outcomes, particularly for kidneys which are subject to a greater degree of preservation injury. The provision of oxygen during preservation may improve post-transplant outcomes, particularly for kidneys that have suffered greater degrees of ischaemia-reperfusion injury. Hypothermic machine perfusion is able to control the following parameters: temperature, perfusion pressure and biochemical parameters of the perfusion fluid flowing from the renal vein. For this purpose, the machine uses its own electronic circuits connected to a computer that controls the entirety of its operation (Figs. 2.37 and 2.38).

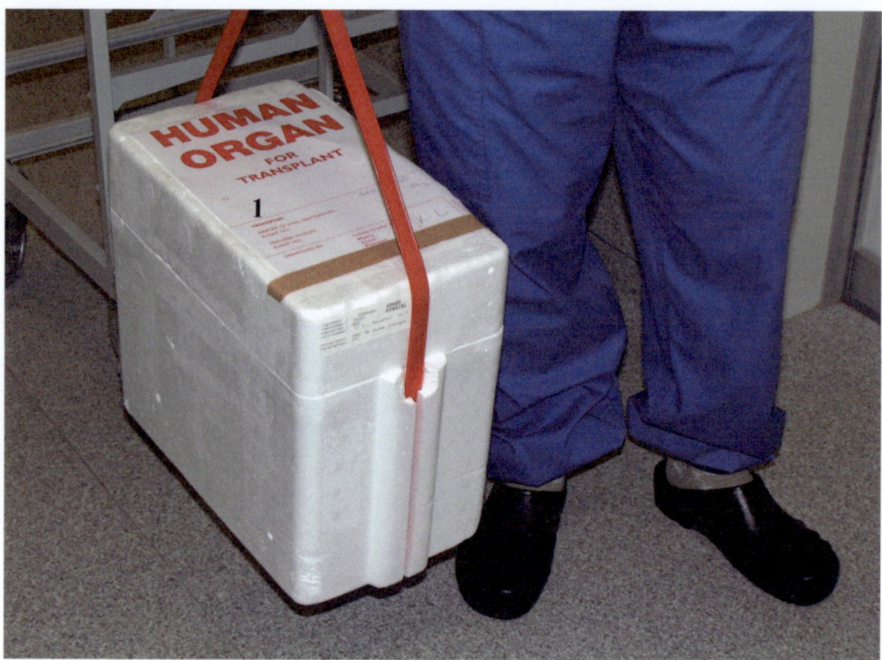

**Fig. 2.36** After filling the transport box with fresh ice, it is sealed, and after affixing all the documents concerning the donor, quality form and the donated organ, the organ can be transported to the recipient's hospital. 1—Professional transport box

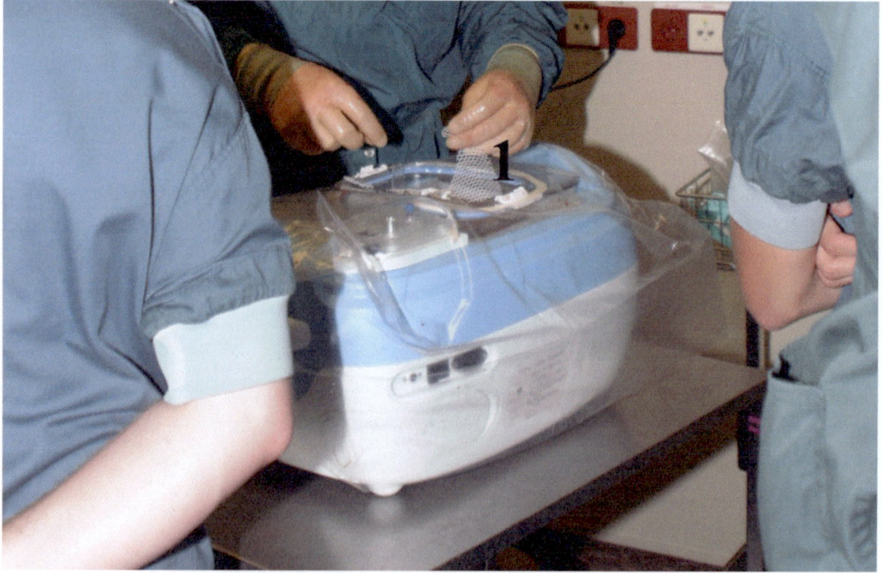

**Fig. 2.37** The kidney is packaged in the LifePort, where it will be continuously perfused with a preservation solution and cooled during transport to the recipient's hospital. 1—LifePort

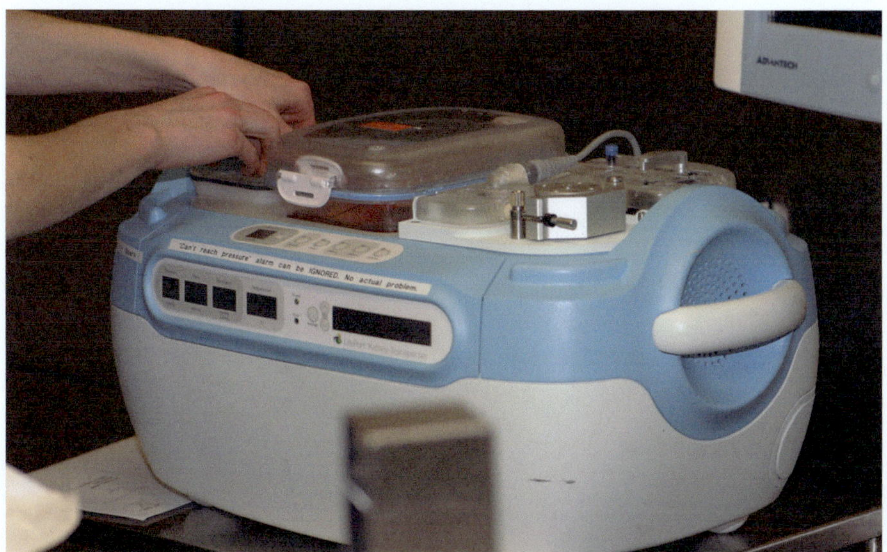

**Fig. 2.38** The kidney is placed and connected to the device which will cool it externally and internally during transport until arrival and/or the start of kidney benching at the recipient's hospital

### 2.2.2.3  Adult and Pediatric Deceases Donor "En Bloc" Kidney Procurement

Introduction: Child Donor Criteria for Kidney Procurement

a. Kidney donor age criteria for DBD: donation of abdominal organs in children:

   – No age limit, from birth onwards (removal by "en bloc" for children up to two years; for older children up to five years, in consultation with the receiving center).

b. Kidney donor age criteria for DCD donation: donation of abdominal organs in children:

   – donor age 5 to ± 75 years.

Steps

1. Mobilize both kidneys from the retroperitoneal space on the right and left side of the abdominal cavity up to the vertebral column.
2. A thick surgical ligature tied around each cannula was cut through the wall of the aorta and inferior vena cava, preferably with a scalpel or scissors. During perfusion of the abdominal organs at the time of procurement, these ligatures allowed the cannulae to be held in the lumen of the aorta and inferior vena cava.

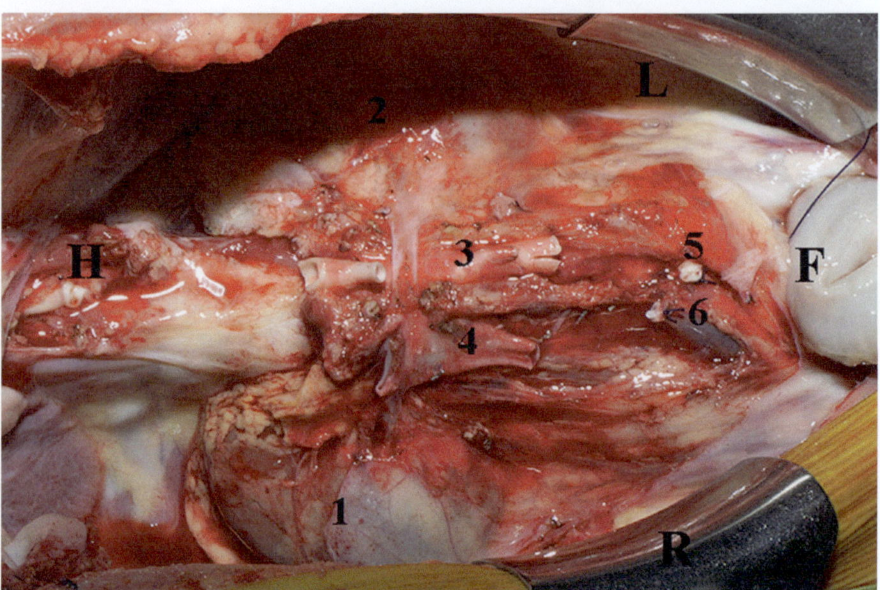


**Fig. 2.39** In this case, the organ donor is a child under the age of five. The liver and pancreas have been removed from the abdominal cavity, and the intestines and stomach moved beyond the abdominal cavity. The abdominal aorta has been cut off between the ostium of the celiac trunk and the superior mesenteric artery and above the aorta's bifurcation. The IVC was cut 1–2 cm above the highest ostium of the right renal vein and above the its bifurcation. 1—Right kidney, 2—Left kidney, 3—Abdominal aorta, 4—IVC, 5—Bifurcation of the abdominal aorta, 6—Bifurcation of the IVC, H—Towards the head, F—Towards the feet, L—Left side, R—Right side

3. Remove the perfusion cannula and thoracic tube if present from the aortic and IVC lumen. Cut crosswise completely the abdominal aorta and the IVC at the level of their bifurcations (Fig. 2.39).
4. Identify and cut both ureters close to the bladder. Use a small mosquito clamp to close the tissue around the end of each ureter. With as much tissue around the ureter as possible, dissect both ureters in the direction of the lower pole and the hilum of each kidney (Fig. 2.40).
5. Grasp the tissues between the wall of the abdominal aorta and/or the IVC with a soft vascular clamp. Gently lift both vessels upwards to reveal the lumbar arteries and veins and the front of the anterior longitudinal ligament of the vertebral column.

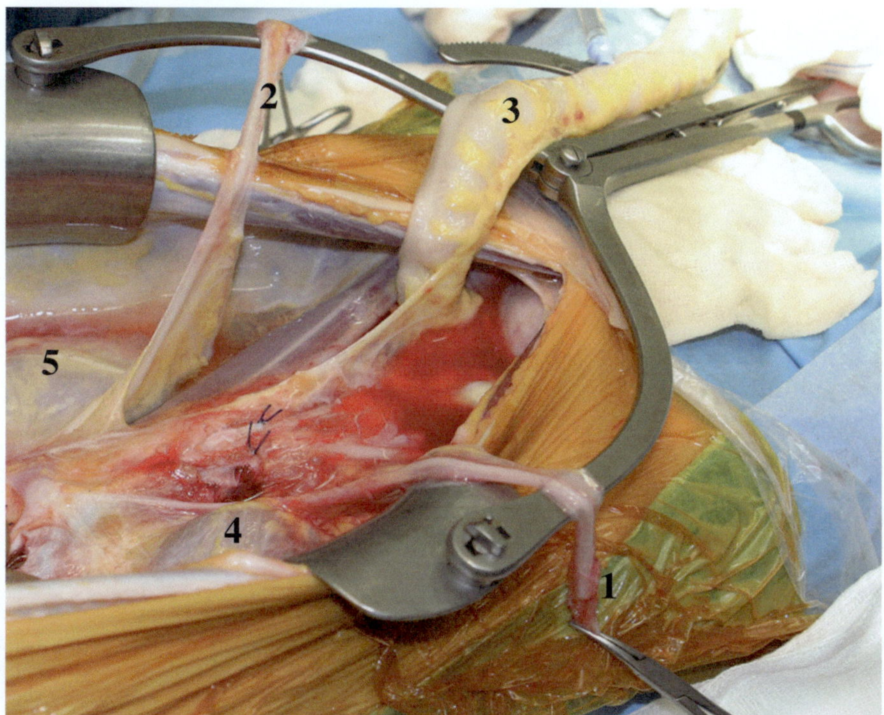



**Fig. 2.40** Mosquito clamps on the surrounding tissues of the ureters. 1—Right ureter, 2—Left ureter, 3—Intestines outside the abdominal cavity (the picture shows a fragment of the large intestine), 4—Right kidney, 5—Left kidney

6. Cut all the tissues with lumbar arteries and veins between the posterior aortic wall and the posterior wall of the IVC and the anterior longitudinal ligament of the vertebral column without damaging the posterior aortic and the IVC wall (Figs. 2.41 and 2.42).
7. Remove both kidneys from the abdominal cavity and transfer them to a sterile container filled with preservation solution or Ringer's lactate or saline with sterile crushed ice. If necessary, the kidneys can now be separated or they can be packed and sent "en bloc" (Fig. 2.43) to the center that is to accept them.

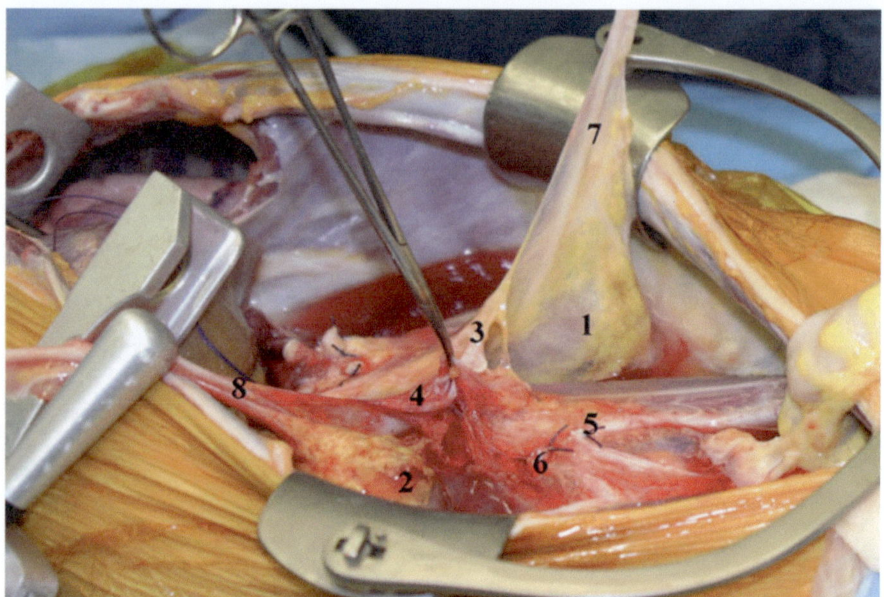

**Fig. 2.41** 1—Left kidney posterior area, 2—Right kidney posterior area of the renal pelvis, 3 and 4—Medial walls of the abdominal aorta and IVC connected together with a small vascular clamp type Mosquito, 5 and 6—Bifurcation region: of the IVC (6) and abdominal aorta (5), 7—Left ureter, 8—Right ureter

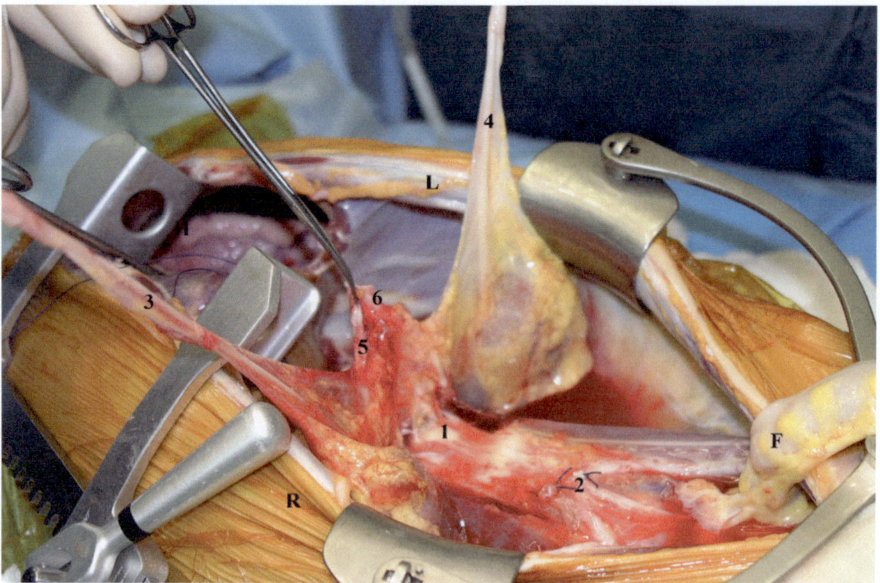

**Fig. 2.42** 1—Anterior longitudinal ligament, 2—Ligated bifurcations of the aorta and IVC, 3—Right ureter, 4—Left ureter, 5—IVC, 6—Abdominal aorta, H—Towards the head, F—Towards the feet, L—Left side, R—Right side

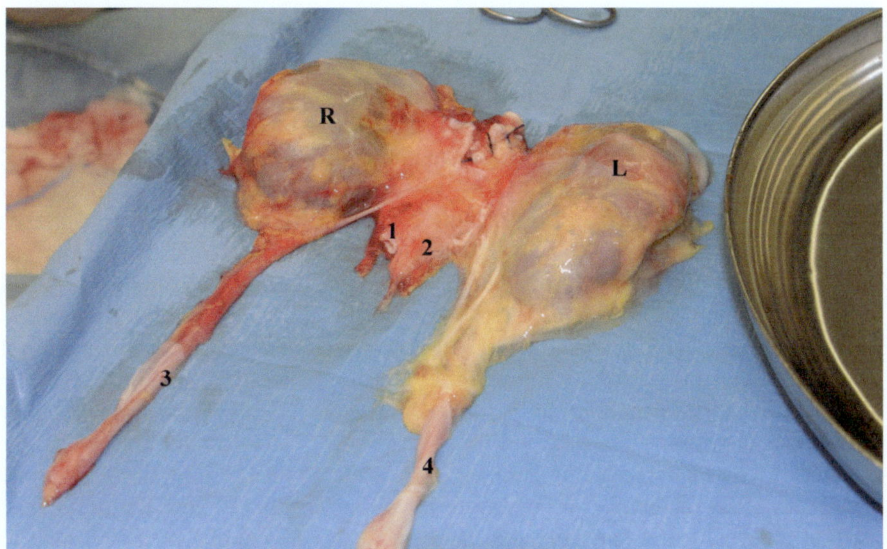

**Fig. 2.43**  Kidneys obtained as "en block" from a donor who is less than 5 years old. R—Right kidney, L—Left kidney, 1—IVC, 2—Abdominal aorta, 3—Right ureter, 4—Left ureter

**Warning! (Kidneys procured "en bloc" sometimes needs vessels)**
We should remember that kidneys procured "en bloc" with the intention of transplanting them, may require additional venous and arterial vessels (tool-kit) for the reconstruction due to various transplant techniques. For this purpose, contact the recipient's hospital on your own or through the transplant coordinator.

### 2.2.2.4  The Surgical Technique used to Separate Kidneys that have been Procured "En Bloc" from a Deceased Donor

Introduction

The surgical technique of separating kidneys procured "en bloc" is generally not different from the technique of separating them in the abdominal cavity, except that "en bloc" takes place outside the donor's body. The kidneys are placed and submerged in a sterile container filled with sterile preservation solution or Ringer's lactate solution or a sterile NaC1 physiological solution and slush ice. Here is a brief description of the entire kidney separation procedure step-by-step.

Surgical Steps

1. Cut off the left renal vein with a patch from the IVC or without a patch close to
   the IVC. Gently separate the renal vein from the anterior wall of the abdominal
   aorta towards the hilum and set it on the kidney front surface. Place the left renal
   vein that has been mobilised in this way on the anterior surface of the kidney
   and stabilise the renal vein by placing a small sterile pad of gauze soaked in
   saline over it.
2. If not already marked, locate the ureters, mark each one by closing a small soft
   vascular clamp on the surrounding tissues at the end in order not to damage it.
3. Invert the donated kidneys 180 degrees so that you can see the posterior wall of
   the aorta and IVC. Make a longitudinal incision to the posterior surface of the
   abdominal aorta, which has to be made along the long axis of the aorta precisely
   between the lumbar arteries.
4. Check the ostia coming out from the aorta's lumen to the right and left kidney
   on both sides of the abdominal aorta. If you are in doubt about the number of
   renal arteries, use a specially designed metal vascular probe or a thin tube to
   examine them.
5. To achieve a complete separation of the kidneys, perform a longitudinal incision
   to the anterior surface of the abdominal aorta.
   The incision has to be made along the long axis of the aorta precisely between
   the ostias of the renal arteries.

**Warning! (Avoid kidney damage and keep it in the physiological position)**
Keep the kidneys during the tissues cutting in the physiological position. Beware of
the ureters and renal vessels at every change of position of the kidney.

6. Before packing the kidneys, perform the following activities to declare each
   kidney suitable or not suitable for transplantation. Reduce the amount of fat
   around each kidney; do not try to remove too much fat in the donor's hospital
   especially around the hilum, lower pole and ureter. After removing excess fat,
   carefully inspect both kidneys for the quality for parenchyma perfusion, the
   presence of tumors, damage, atherosclerosis, thrombosis, and the number of
   renal vessels and ureters. If the perfusion has not been successful, try to flush
   with a preservation solution the less well flushed kidney or the kidney area again
   before packing. At the end of the kidney inspection as a procurement surgeon
   you are going to pass judgment about the suitability of each kidney for transplantation in terms of surgical damage, anatomical anomalies, the number of
   renal arteries, veins and ureters, the severity of atherosclerosis, atherosclerotic
   lesions at, around and above the ostia of the renal arteries, the access severity of
   atherosclerosis or another disease in the renal arteries themselves, the presence
   of tumors in the parenchyma or kidney pelvis, mechanical or surgical damage to
   the kidney (rupture of the parenchyma), the access quality of the kidney parenchyma (cirrhosis, fibrosis), infections, the presence of one or more cysts
   (cystic kidney disease) and ureteral strictures.

**Warning! (Impossible perfusion through the renal arteries)**
If the kidney perfusion through the artery or arteries has failed for one or other reason, you have still one escape in order to save the kidney in the form of retrograde perfusion. The removed kidney may in this case also be perfused under low pressure and cooled through the renal vein with a heparinized cold preservation solution.

**Warning! (Avoid the kidney backtable in the donor's hospital)**
The operating room (OR) in the donor's hospital is not an appropriate place to prepare the kidney for transplantation, but it is the best place for the first general kidney inspection. An attempt to prepare the kidney at the donor's hospital is unnecessary because it lengthens the time of kidney warm ischemia. When attempting to inspect the kidney in the donor's hospital, the surgeon exposes the donated organ to high risk of organ damage due to inadequate conditions in the donor hospital's operating theatre. Lack of adequate lighting and qualified assistance may lead to irreversible accidental technical damage to the kidney and disqualify it for transplantation. Remember that the long inspection of the kidney immediately after its procurement may damage the renal tubular epithelial cells of the kidney which can lead to delayed graft function, acute tubular necrosis or kidney primary non-function. The procured, preserved and cooled kidney is after the procurement still not cold enough on the inside for carrying out a long inspection in the donor's hospital. By prolonging the organ procurement procedure, we can warm the kidney which will cause a growth of metabolism instead of a reduction. A rapid kidney inspection, cold storage packing or connecting with the perfusion machine results in its further cooling and a decrease in its metabolism, and therefore such a procedure is not only good for the kidney, but also for the recipient. Hypothermic machine perfusion means perfusing, preserving and cooling the kidney during transport from the donor to the recipient's hospital, allowing the kidney to survive undamaged and in good condition for preparation (back table) for transplantation and warm ischaemia during transplantation.

**Warning! (If you do not trust the procured kidney perform a biopsy and a frozen section examination)**
If parenchymal disease is suspected, perform a kidney biopsy and a frozen section examination. The test result should be discussed with the anatomic pathologist, transplant coordinator and the recipients centers.

**Warning! (Pediatric donors)**
In donors younger than five years, kidneys should be harvested en bloc, maintaining continuity of the aorta and IVC from their bifurcation to the area 0.4–0.5 cm above the ostia of the renal arteries and veins in the aorta and IVC.

**Warning! (Pediatric kidneys: an important communication)**
When the donor is between two and five years old the technique of procurement of the kidneys (to separate them or not) should be discussed in detail with the center that accepted the kidneys.

**Warning! ("En bloc" surgical technique for kidney retrieval is very often also used in adults)**

The en bloc surgical technique for kidney donation is popular in many centers all over the world. It is also possible to procure kidneys from adult cadaver donors in this way. The adult procured kidneys in the en bloc technique have to be separated in the donor's or recipient's hospital. According to the available literature, kidneys procured en bloc for transplantation are less damaged, which means that the procurement surgeons make fewer technical errors during this procedure [46, 47].

## 2.3  "Kidney-only" Procurement from Deceased Donors; The Surgical Technique

### 2.3.1  Introduction

Although it is perhaps hard to believe, there are situations where the only organs to be procured, due to the age and past diseases of the donor, are the kidneys. Sometimes it does happen that a potential organ donor agrees to donate only one or both kidneys after death by signing an organ donor card during his/her lifetime.

The UK national Transplant Database was analyzed for all cadaveric kidneys donated over a five-year period in the UK. The results are that out of 9014 retrieved kidneys, 96 could not be transplanted because of the severe damage made during the retrieval. Injury was reported in 1726 (19%) kidneys, although by both donor and recipient centers in only 270 (3%). Reported kidney damage was 26% more likely for retrievals of kidneys made only by a renal team as opposed to multiorgan retrieval of 21%; the proportion was lower when a liver team retrieved both liver and kidneys [46].

DCD donations are associated with a significantly increased incidence of procurement related kidney damage especially with regards to ureteric and polar artery injuries. The awareness of this issue should lead to the optimization of procurement techniques to improve the quality of this increasingly important way of kidney transplantation [47].

When only the kidneys are procured, the presence of other organs in the abdominal cavity causes a lack of transparency and stability in the operating field. During kidney-only procurement, the presence of other abdominal organs in the operative field may obscure the view making it difficult to recognize anatomy, hamper good external cooling and proper dissection of important structures. We know from the literature that kidney damage is more frequent whenever kidney alone are procured, especially when they are taken from DCD. The surgical damage caused during kidney-only procurement is the result of various circumstances, such as the failure to properly train the procurement team, the fatigue of the team (e.g. a second or third procurement overnight), insufficient knowledge of the anatomy, unnecessary routines, the rush and even sometimes the takeover by a less experienced team which is often sent with the (false) thought that it is very easy to deal with a kidney-only procurement [28, 29, 46–50].

Finally, I want to recall the French experience in organ retrieval which is performed by urologists involved in the national renal transplantation program. They also have to deal with transplant complications. Arterial lesions were more frequently observed during single-organ procurement in procedures performed by less experienced surgeons, with less than 30 organ procurements with 12% organ injury vs. more than 30 multiorgan procurement procedures with only 3% organ injury. Surgical injuries were more frequently observed during single-organ procurements than during multiorgan procurements: 8.2% versus 3.7% [50].

Surgical damage may affect all of a kidney's elements such as the capsule and parenchyma, the renal vessels and the pelvis and the ureter. A lot of kidney damage can be repaired, but keep in mind that if there are too many and large damages the chance of complications in the recipient will increase and that the graft survival expectancy will get much shorter. Unfortunately, sometimes the damage to the parenchyma of the kidney or the kidney vessels is irreparable—then the kidney will not be transplanted and the person who was supposed to receive the transplant may have lost his/her last chance of being transplanted. Let us remember that by carrying out a successful kidney transplant, we are helping two patients: the one whose kidney has been transplanted and the one for whom a place in a dialysis center has become available.

In this section, I would like to introduce my new surgical technique of kidney-only procurement from deceased donors. This technique allows procurement through a median laparotomy with or without the opening of the sternum. In the case of any organ or vessel removal from the chest or from obese patients, the chest is opened by performing a sternotomy. Some authors state that the higher incidence of delayed graft function (DGF) among kidney-only donors might be explained by their older age; other authors attribute a higher incidence in multi-organ donors to unrecognized warm ichemia during abdominal organ retrieval [28].

The surgical technique I would like to present is not only fast and easy to learn, but it also provides a very stable surgical field and thus protects the kidneys, their vessels, the renal pelvis and ureters as much as possible from any surgical damage and mistakes made by the procurement surgeon. I invented this technique and improved it for two to three years until I found it so simple and easy to learn that it is for me a great satisfaction to describe it and share it with the readers of this book [28–51].

## 2.3.2  Kidney-only Procurement from Donor with Brain Death (DBD) without Sternotomy: A Step-by-step Surgical Technique

### 2.3.2.1  Introduction

Extensive time out with the procurement team(s) and transplant coordinator in a DBD procedure is conducted before donor transportation to the OR. The time out focusses on discussing the relevant patient information, the theater preparation, the transportation from ICU to OR, the placing of the donor on the OR table with a sufficient amount of staff, identification, checking the surgical equipment and explanation of the initial surgical steps.

The donor in the OR is placed on the operating table in a supine position. Most DBD donors are hemodynamically stable and, at the beginning of the abdominal organ procurement, the surgeon can palpate everything and everywhere in the abdomen, such as the arteries' pulsations. The surgeon has more time to dissect the tissues, great vessels, mobilize the organs, recognize anatomical abnormality and peform a thorough inspection of the organs in the abdominal cavity.

### 2.3.2.2  Surgical Steps

1. Disinfect the operating field and cover it with sterile surgical drapes. Disinfect the body surface and cover with sterile incise drapes ("Steri-Drape"). The draping starts from the neck, 2–3 cm above the jugular notch of the sternum and 2 cm below the pubic bone, lateral sides the disposable sterile operating drapes are located along the mid-axillary line (Fig. 2.44).
2. Perform the median laparotomy from the xiphoid process of the sternum to the pubic bone (Fig. 2.45). Ligate and cut round the ligament of the liver (ligamentum teres, or ligamentum teres hepatis) and the liver's falciform ligament. Cut close to the abdominal wall up to the hepatic veins.
3. Install a professional retractor to the operating table and fix it at the level of the donor's pubic bone. Use the attached retractor blades and pull the right abdominal wall to the right and the left wall to the left, and try to obtain the maximum opening of the abdomen.
4. Perform a right medial visceral rotation—the Cattell-Braasch manoeuvre is a technique to mobilise the ascending and 1/3 transverse colon, small bowel, and the extensive Kocher manoeuvre the duodenum, the right part of the pancreas-head and neck up to the right side of the abdominal aorta, celiac trunk and superior mesenteric artery (Fig. 2.46).

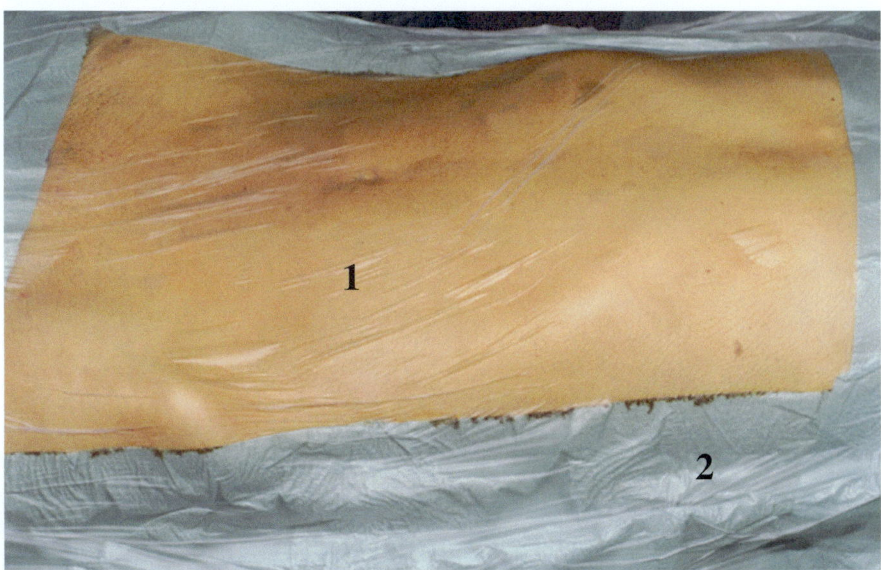

**Fig. 2.44** Disinfected operating field is covered with surgical foil Steri-Drape. The operating field has been covered from the bottom (1–2 cm below the symphysis of the pubic bone, next to the top) 10–15 cm below the jugular notch of the sternum handle and at the end the sides (this is the middle axillary line). 1—Sterile self-adhesive foil Steri-Drape, 2—Sterile drape sticked to sterile surgical draping

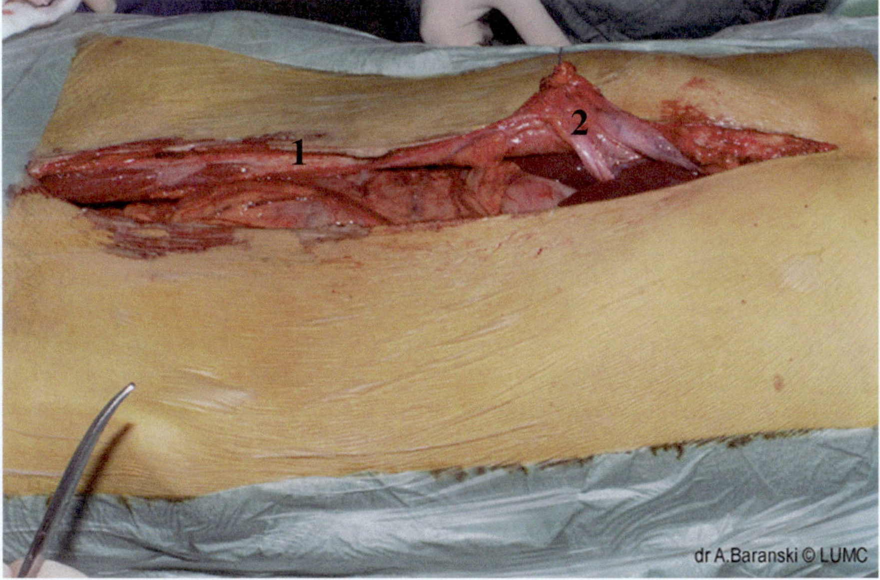

**Fig. 2.45** Median laparotomy. 1—Abdominal wall, 2—Teres ligament before cutting and ligation just above the falciform ligament

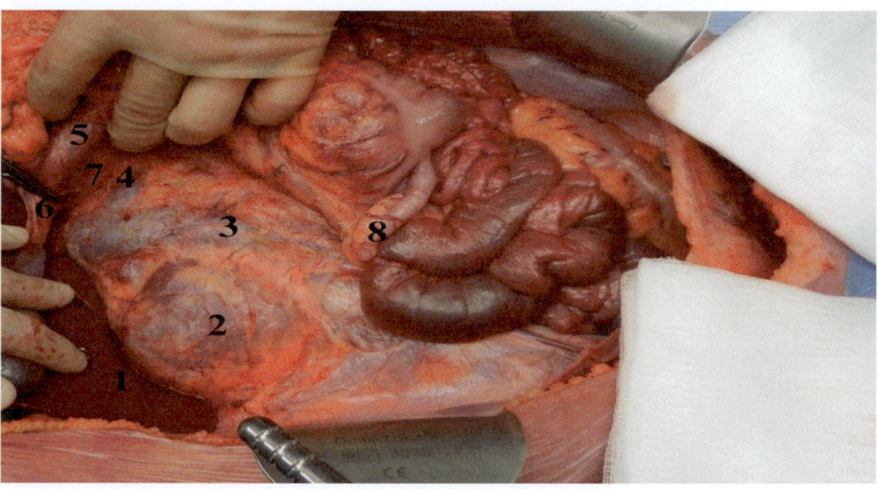

**Fig. 2.46** Right sided medial visceral rotation: the Cattel-Braasch maneuver and additionally the extensive Kocher maneuver. Avascular plane. Extensive mobilization of the duodenum, pancreas head and neck from right side of the abdomen to the abdominal aorta, CT and superior mesenteric artery. 1—Right lobe of the liver, 2—Right kidney, 3—IVC, 4—Left renal vein, 5—Duodenum, 6—Hepato-duodenal ligament, 7—Posterior surface of the pancreatic head, 8—Appendix

5. Dissect the abdominal aorta and IVC, starting from their bifurcations up to the left renal vein or in the opposite direction (watch out for extra renal arteries to the right kidney, which may run on the anterior wall of the IVC) (Fig. 2.47).
6. Place two thick vascular ligatures around the aorta and IVC just above their bifurcations (four ligatures); fix the ends of each ligature outside the abdomen with a small vascular clamp (Fig. 2.48).
7. Localize the CT and SMA and dissect them; free the abdominal aorta wall between the upper edge of the left renal vein and the SMA (Fig. 2.49).
8. Cut the left triangular ligament of the liver and turn the mobilized left lobe to the right side.
9. Cut the hepatogastric ligament (if there is any left accessory hepatic artery present, cut and ligate it) to reach the right and the left crus of the diaphragm, the abdominal aorta and CT under the diaphragm.
10. Use a long right-angled surgical clamp to dissect the tissues with the help of coagulation. Cut the right and left crus of the diaphragm, slowly dissect and visualize the abdominal aorta under the diaphragm. In the second step place a vascular sling or long thick vascular ligature around the abdominal aorta, pin their ends together with a small vascular clamp and place each one of them outside the abdomen (Fig. 2.50) [31–33].

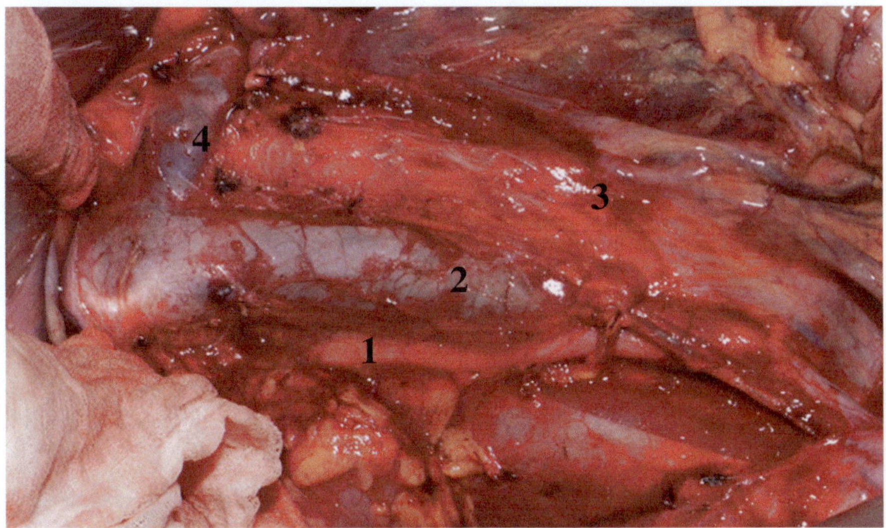

**Fig. 2.47**  The anterior and lateral surfaces of the abdominal aorta and IVC have been dissected from the left renal vein up to their bifurcations. 1—Right ureter, 2—IVC, 3—Abdominal aorta, 4—Left renal vein

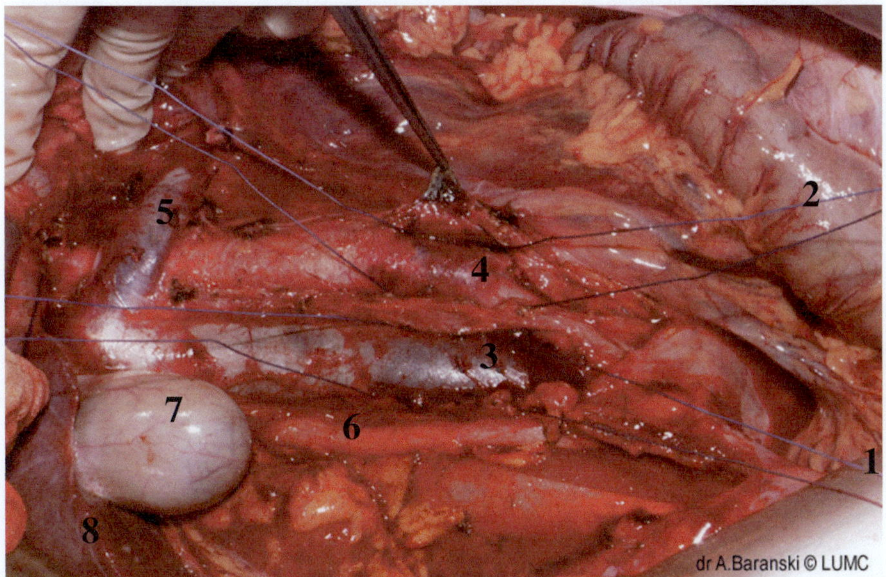


**Fig. 2.48**  Abdominal aorta and IVC have been dissected from the left renal vein up to their iliac vessels; two thick ligatures are placed around the aorta and IVC close to their bifurcations, the ends of each ligature are moved beyond the abdomen and closed with a small vascular clamp. 1—One of the two thick ligatures located around the IVC, 2—One of the two thick ligatures located around the abdominal aorta, 3—IVC, 4—Abdominal aorta, 5—Left renal vein, 6—Right ureter, 7—Gallbladder, 8—Right lobe of the liver

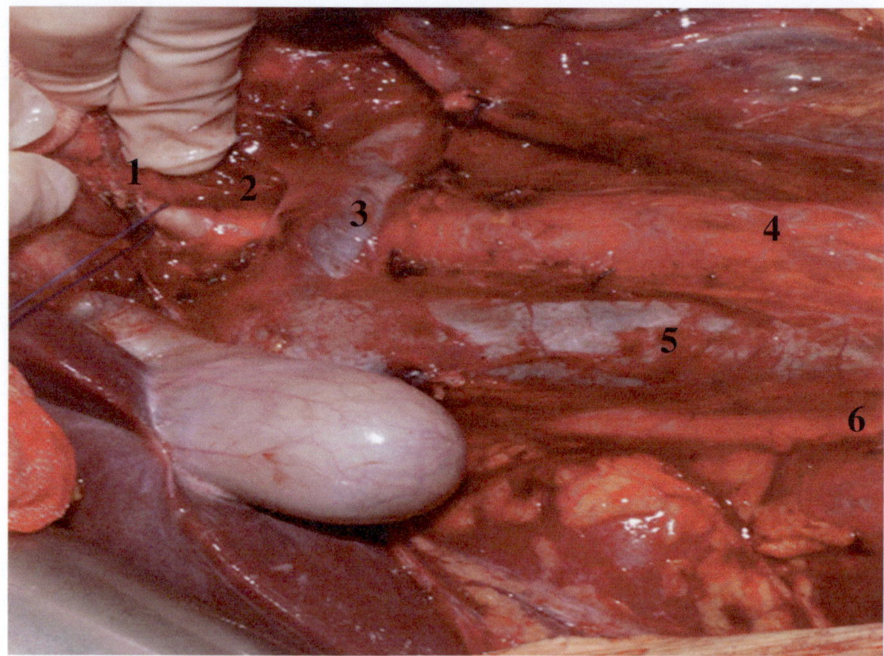

**Fig. 2.49** SMA and abdominal aorta between the left renal vein and the SMA have been dissected. The SMA should be dissected at a distance not further than 1.5 cm from the abdominal aorta. 1—SMA, 2—Abdominal aorta, 3—Left renal vein, 4—Abdominal aorta, 5—IVC, 6—Right ureter

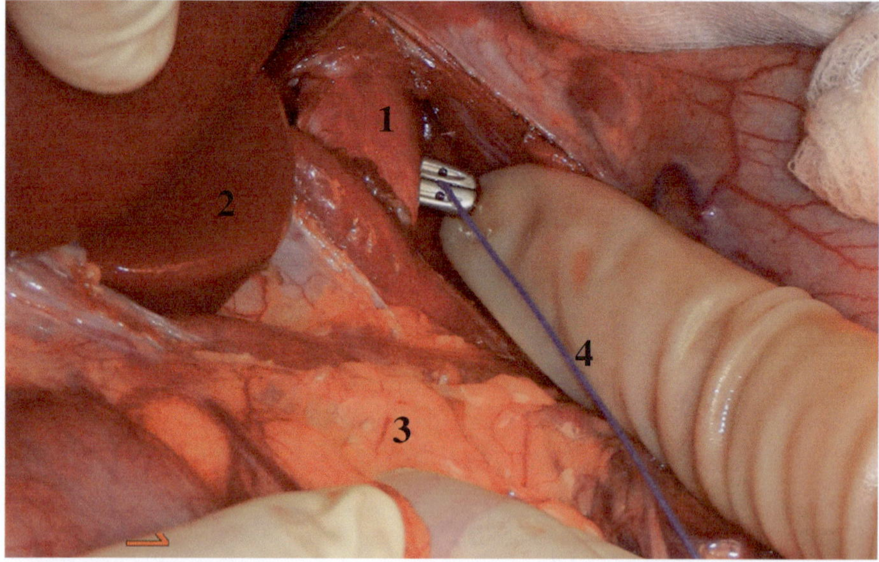

**Fig. 2.50** The right and the left crus of the diaphragm have been cut off. The dissected abdominal aorta lies below the diaphragm. 1—Abdominal aorta below the diaphragm, 2—Caudate lobe of the liver, 3—Pancreas upper edge, 4—A thick ligature or vessel-loop is placed around the abdominal aorta just below the diaphragm

**Warning! (Clamping the thoracic aorta above the left diaphragm without thoracotomy)**

Despite the promises which we may have made to the donor family to not open the chest,remember that sometimes the maximum opening of the abdominal cavity with a long incision and a professional abdominal retractor is not enough to be able to retrieve abdominal organs safely and without any surgical damage. Due to the very small space and bad access to the upper abdomen, the whole procedure may be difficult. Abdominal organ procurement could be especially difficult in obese or very tall and narrow donors, for example when you have to mobilize the left liver lobe in order to free the aorta below the diaphragm. If it is impossible to perform, it should not be done due to the high risk of damage to the abdominal aorta, especially in the donor who has undergone surgery of the subphrenic, thoracic or heart area. Remember that damage to the aorta—such as heavy hemorrhaging and bad organ perfusion—can cause a complete destabilization of the donor. The second method of rapid closure of the abdominal aorta is to cut the diaphragm under the left costal arch, free the lower surface of the left lung from the diaphragm and then lift up and press it against the chest wall with the retractor blade so that you can locate the aorta on the left side of the vertebral column in the left pleural cavity of the chest. The descending aorta can be quickly and efficiently found in the left thoracic cavity and dissected from the surrounding tissue with the fingers or a right-angled surgical clamp and closed with a vascular clamp.

**Warning! (The pericardial sac should be opened last!)**

In my opinion, opening the pericardial sac by cardiac or abdominal surgeons in order to assess the suitability of the heart for transplantation is a mistake at the beginning of multiorgan procurement. Three times in my 30-year career in various countries, excessive and intensive heart inspection by cardiac surgeons has resulted in irreversible donor arrhythmias after which cardiac arrest and reanimation and finally the loss of the heart and in one case also the lungs. That is why I am against the opening of the pericardial sac and the heart examination at the beginning of the multiorgan retrieval. I prefer to carry out a heart inspection after the abdominal organs have been dissected and freed in such a way that in the event of cardiac arrest the abdominal team will be able to save the abdominal organs. On the other hand, whenever a heart inspection was performed after the dissection and preparation of the abdominal organs, not one of the donors from whom I had procured organs had a sudden stop of circulation [31].

11. Ask the anesthesiologist to give intravenous heparin in an amount of 200–300 units/kg/BW for adults and 500 units/kg/BW for children (BW=body weight). Remember that heparin works rapidly but not immediately, which means within 3–5 min after intravenous injection [31].
12. Cannulation of the abdominal aorta. With the first lowest ligature placed around the abdominal aorta, ligate the aorta at the level of its bifurcation. Close the abdominal aorta with your fingers or a vascular clamp 5–10 cm above the first tied ligature. With scissors, transversely (40% of the circumference) cut the

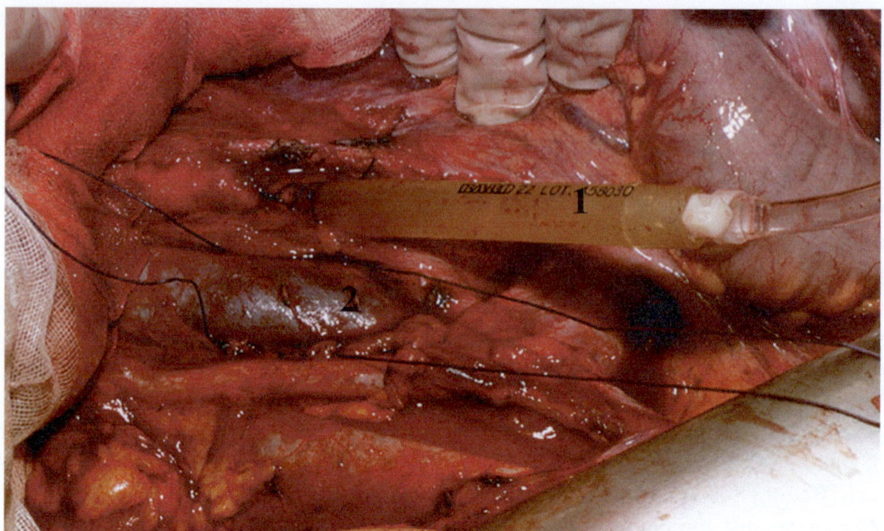


**Fig. 2.51** Aortic cannula inserted into the aorta's lumen and fixed with thick ligatures. 1—The aortic cannula was filled with a cold preservation solution without air bubbles and then inserted into the lumen of the aorta and secured with two thick ligatures. 2—IVC

aorta 2–3 cm above the first ligated ligature and insert the cannula into the aorta's lumen and tie it with a second thick ligature placed around it. With the same ligature fix the aortic cannula in such a way that it does not slip out of the aorta when the clamp is removed and/or the perfusion begins. To fix the properly placed aortic cannula into the lumen of the aorta, we usually use a second upper thick ligature previously ligated around the abdominal aorta and cannula. The entire aortic perfusion system before perfusion is closed by a clamp placed 30–40 cm before connection between the aortic cannula and the connector which joins a reservoir with cold perfusion fluid and heparin with that of the aortic cannula (Fig. 2.51).

**Warning! (How to fix bleeding after aorta cannulation)**
Sometimes after inserting the cannula into the lumen of the abdominal aorta and fixing it, we have a problem with bleeding from the place of insertion into the abdominal aorta or from the place where the aorta is cut, or below the level of its bifurcation. In all cases we are dealing with a leak. The first case you can solve by putting a new ligature around the aorta and the cannula in it and ligating it until the blood leakage between the cannula and the abdominal aorta's wall stops. In the second case, close the lumbar arteries with a metal clip or ligate them. In the third case put a new ligature and ligate it more strongly or put a big clip behind first ligature [31, 32].

**Warning! (Inferior mesenteric artery: to ligate or not to ligate?)**
The question is whether to ligate or not ligate the inferior mesenteric artery (IMA) before aortic cannulation. First of all ligating the IMA has no effect on the

blood supply to the left half of the large intestine and so there is no influence on the procurement process at all. The only indication for a ligation of the IMA is a very short distance between the aorta's bifurcation and the IMS itself. The very short distance may lead to a difficult aortic closing and cannulation and difficulties with aortic cannula fixation, large blood loss, an unstable patient and—as a result—badly perfused and damaged organs [31–33].

13. IVC cannulation. After cannulation of the abdominal aorta, the second large vessel which must be cannulated for decompression of the entire system is the IVC. We use a chest tube for this purpose. With sternotomy the first place of choice for venue decompression of the entire system is the right atrium or the IVC 2–3 cm above the diaphragm. In this case decompression of the IVC in the abdominal cavity is our first choice. As the first step, ligate the IVC with the first lowest ligature at the level of its bifurcation or some millimeters above. When the IVC is closed crosswise with fingers or a vascular clamp, then cut transversely and cannulate with a chest tube. The upper ligature around the IVC is tied on the wall of the IVC and the chest tube. Try to eliminate any degree of blood leakage and treat it as a blood leak from the aorta after its cannulation. The chest tube, once placed in the ICV and fixed, is connected to a drain that takes away the preservation solution mixed with the donor's blood into a special container located under the operating table. Before starting the perfusion, we must first decompress the venue system. For this purpose, we first remove the clamp from the chest tube inserted into the IVC (Fig. 2.52).

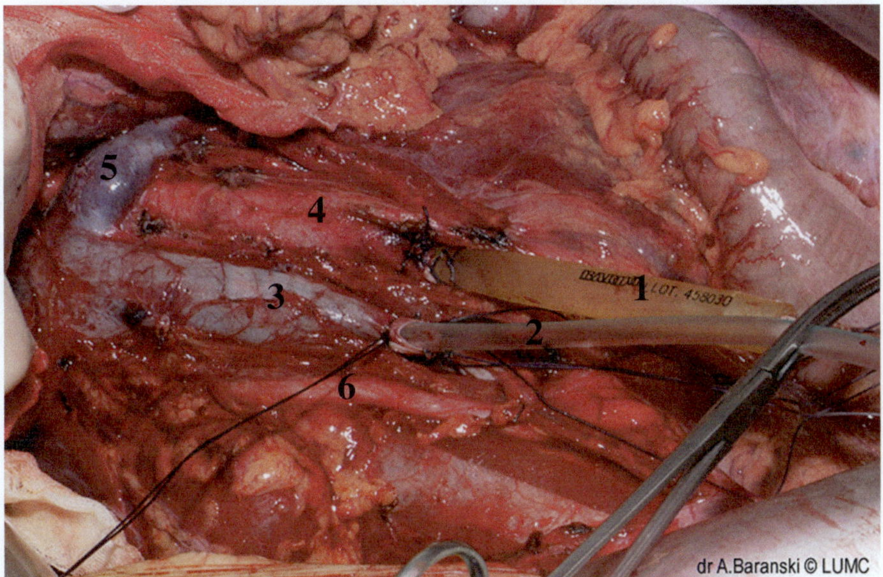


**Fig. 2.52** Cannulation of the IVC with a chest tube. 1—Aortic cannula already placed into the lumen of the abdominal aorta, 2—Chest tube, 3—IVC, 4—Abdominal aorta, 5—Left renal vein, 6—Right ureter

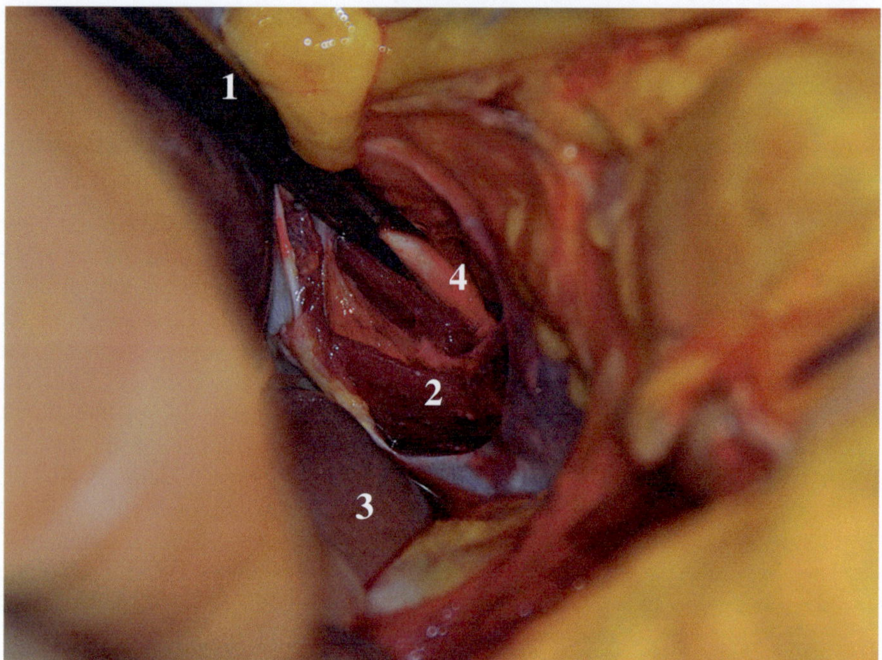

**Fig. 2.53** Below the diaphragm, the abdominal aorta has been closed with a vascular clamp. 1—Vascular clamp, 2—The cut off crura of the diaphragm, 3—Caudate lobe of the liver, 4—Closed abdominal aorta in the subphrenic region

14. Just before beginning or just after the start of perfusion of the abdominal organs, close the abdominal aorta under the diaphragm with a vascular clamp (Fig. 2.53) or ligate it with a thick ligature (Fig. 2.54).
15. First open the clamp that closes the IVC decompression system, then the second clamp that closes the aortic perfusion system and start the internal rinsing and cooling of the abdominal organs. Additionally, the abdominal organs should be cooled externally by systematically adding cold sterile saline or Ringer's solution and sterile ice slush or ice cubes to the abdominal cavity.
16. Cut and close the hepatoduodenal ligament with a vascular stapler or between two vascular clamps (Fig. 2.55).

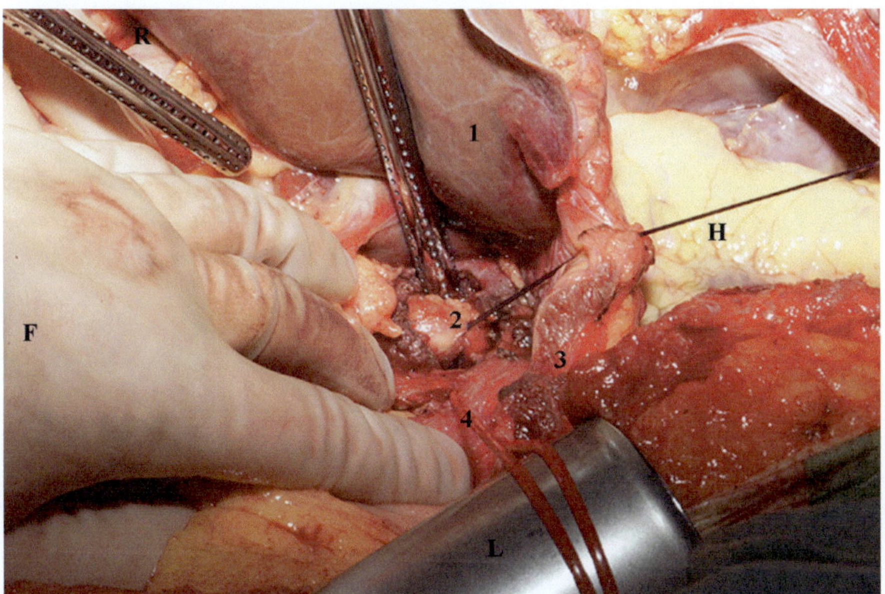

**Fig. 2.54** The aorta was tied with a thick surgical ligature under the diaphragm. 1—Left lobe of the liver, 2—Abdominal aorta below the diaphragm is tied, 3—Left dome of the diaphragm, 4—Esophagus surrounded with a vessel loop, H—Towards the head, F—Towards the feet, L—Left side

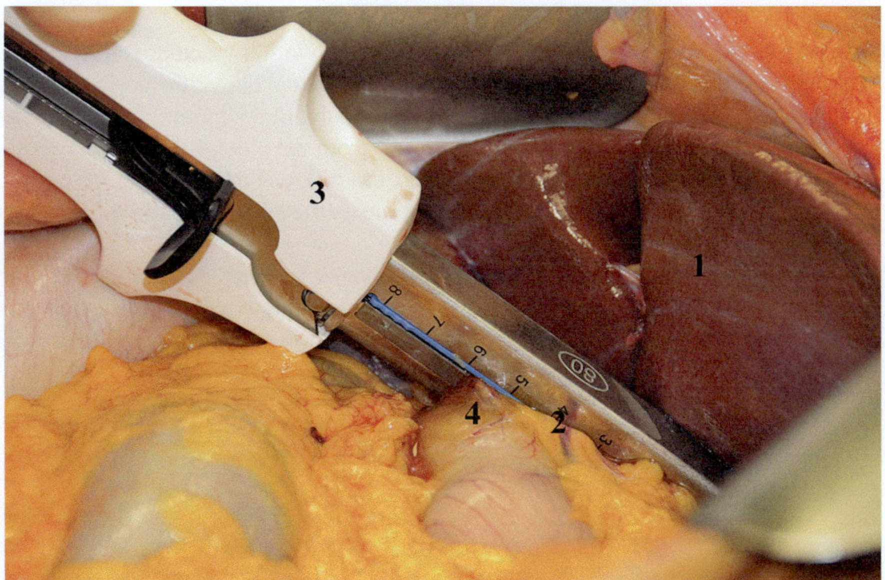

**Fig. 2.55** Cutting and closing with a gastrointestinal stapler (GIA) a hepatoduodenal ligament, which can also be good for this purpose with a vascular cartridge. 1—Left lobe of the liver, 2—Hepato duodenal ligament, 3—Stapler (GIA), 4—Duodenum: pylorus level

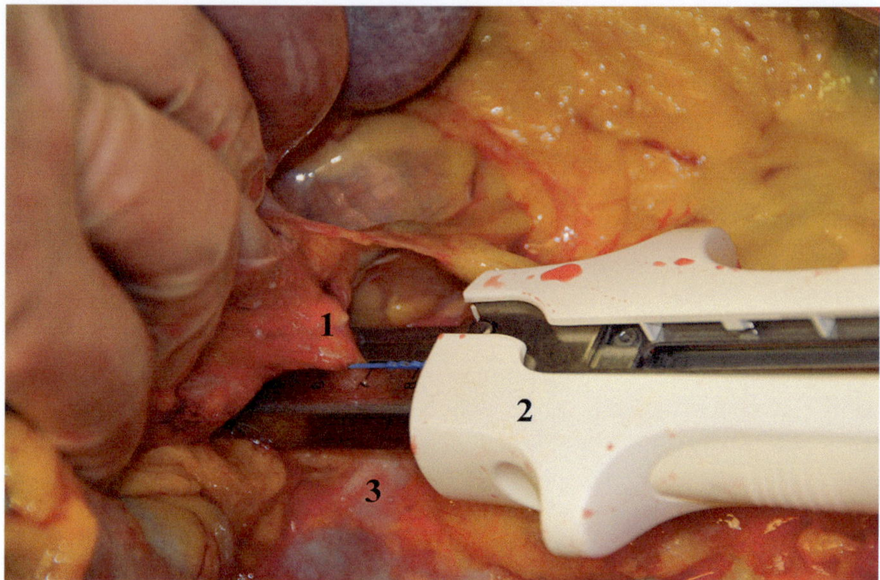

**Fig. 2.56** A vascular or (GIA) stapler or big vascular clamp is placed longitudinally and 5–10 mm above the anterior surface of the abdominal aorta. Be sure of your staple position. Close and cut with a vascular or (GIA) stapler or clamp, the SMA and CT. The stapler or clamp are inserted from below, i.e. from the aortic bifurcation and IVC towards the diaphragm. 1—SMA and CT closed with a stapler. 2—Stapler: GIA (blue cartridge), 3—Left renal vein

17. Close at the same time the SMA and CT and cut with a vascular stapler or use to close a large long clamp; place it parallel and 1 cm above the aorta and then cut the vessels 2 cm above the placed clamp to avoid it slipping. The stapler or clamp is inserted from below, that is to say from the side of the SMA towards the diaphragm. At this point, the CT and the SMA with the celiac plexus are closed and cut, then the only organs that are perfused in the abdominal cavity are the kidneys (Fig. 2.56).

18. Using a big syringe aspirate the gastric contents then replace the gastric tube from the stomach to the esophagus above the diaphragm and cut the esophagus under the diaphragm with a GIA (use a vascular or intestinal catridge or stapler) (Fig. 2.57).

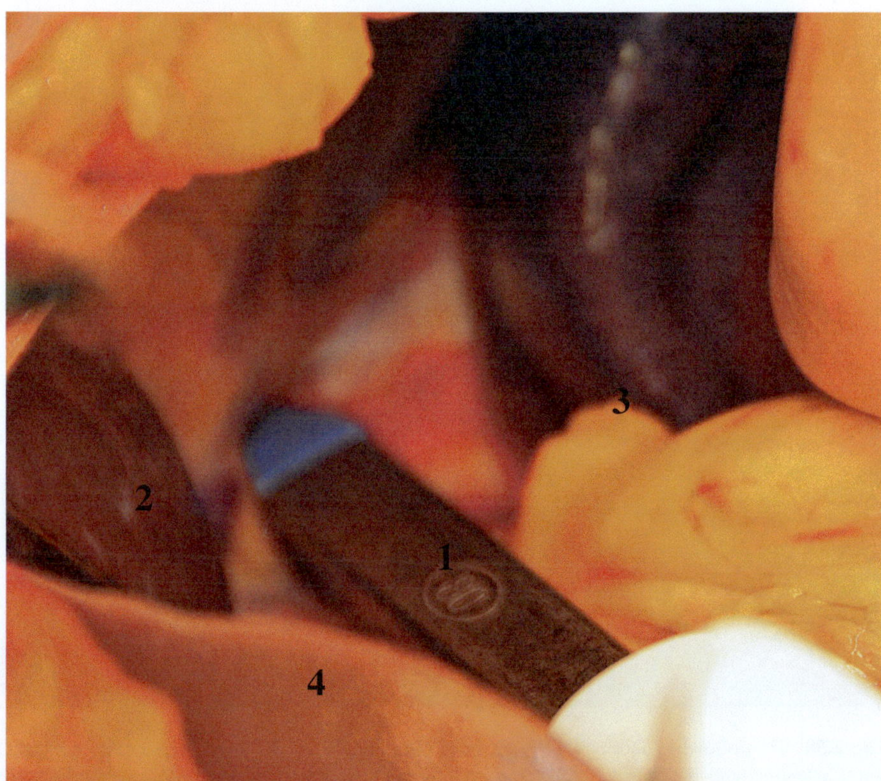

**Fig. 2.57** Move the stomach tube from the stomach to the esophagus. Cut and close the esophagus with a vascular or intestinal staple under the diaphragm. 1—Stapler, 2—Liver left lobe, 3—Spleen, 4—Liver right lobe

19. Mobilize the following abdominal organs with scissors: stomach, duodenum, pancreas, small intestine and large intestine including the descending colon in one bloc. When fully mobilized, move them outside of the abdomen and place them on the donor's thighs. Organs that remain in the abdomen are the kidneys, liver (not perfused) and large vessels (Fig. 2.58).

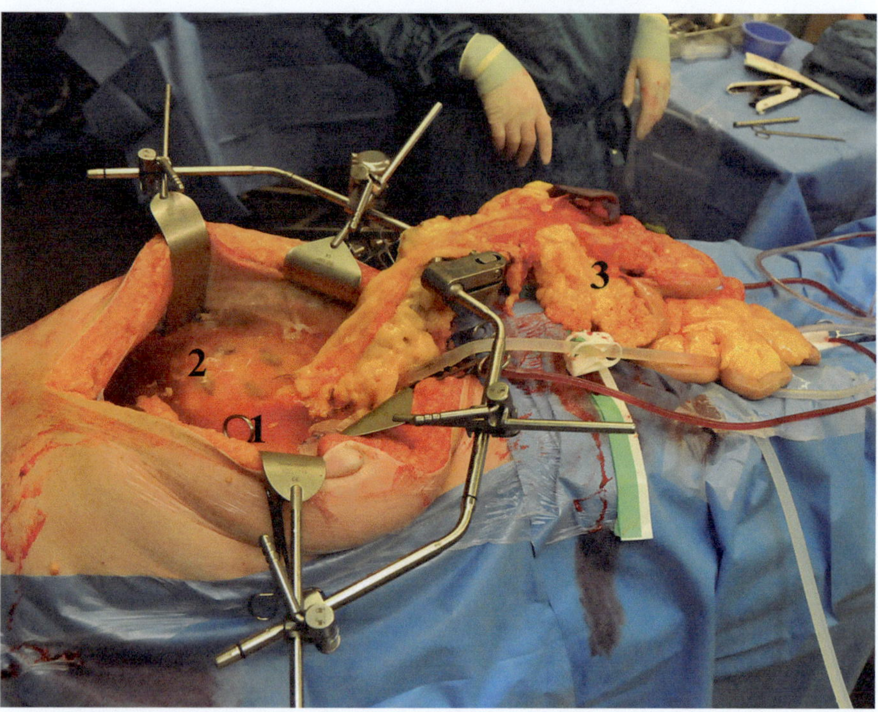

**Fig. 2.58** The following abdominal organs have been mobilised: stomach, duodenum, pancreas, small intestine and ascending, transverse and descending colon. All abdominal organs were mobilised without disruption of the small and large intestines and placed on the thighs of the deceased organ donor. 1—Abdominal aorta under the diaphragm closed with clamp, 2—External cooling of organs with cold sterile solution and sterile ice, 3—Abdominal part of the esophagus, stomach, pancreas, spleen, small and large intestine have been mobilized from the abdominal cavity and placed on the donor's thighs

20. In order to obtain better external cooling, add more cold sterile saline or Ringer's solution into the abdominal cavity and add ice (Figs. 2.59 and 2.60). The liver if necessary is stabilized with one of the blades of a professional abdominal retractor, to facilitate retrieval of the right kidney, push the liver, into the right upper corner of the abdomen together with right diaphragm (Figs. 2.67 and 2.68).

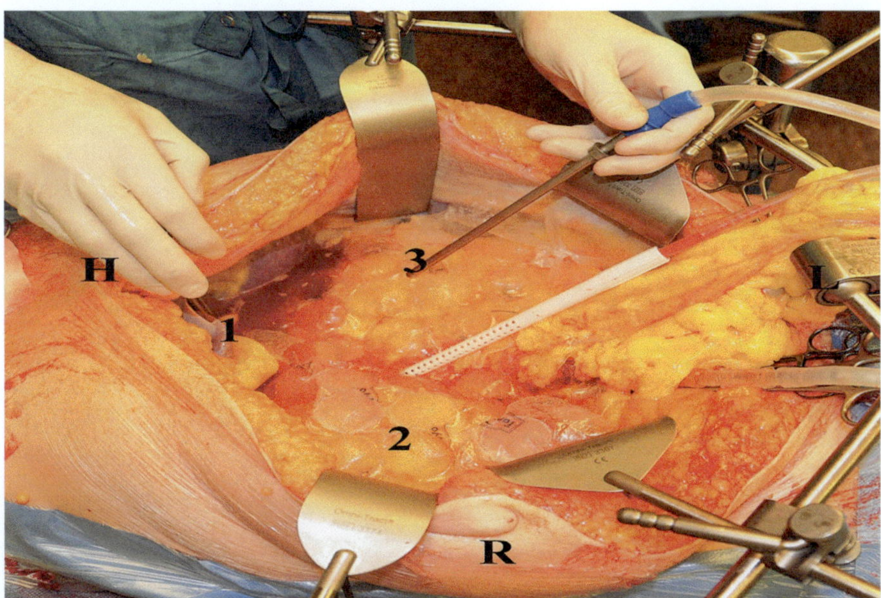



**Fig. 2.59** For better external cooling of the kidneys, during perfusion more cold sterile 0.9% NaCl solution and ice is added in the abdominal cavity. The donor liver which is left in the abdomen is stabilized (pushed up with the blade of the retractor towards the right dome of the diaphragm). 1—Left lobe of liver, 2—External ice cooling right kidney, 3—External ice cooling left kidney, H—Head, L—Towards patient's legs, R—Right side

21. If you retrieve abdominal organs from a very obese donor with a thick layer of fat surrounding the kidneys, you can mobilize their posterior surfaces from the retroperitoneal space and then cover both of their surfaces with sterile ice for the best possible external cooling (Fig. 2.60).
22. The further steps concerning the surgical technique of kidney procurement havebeen described earlier in section 2.2.2).

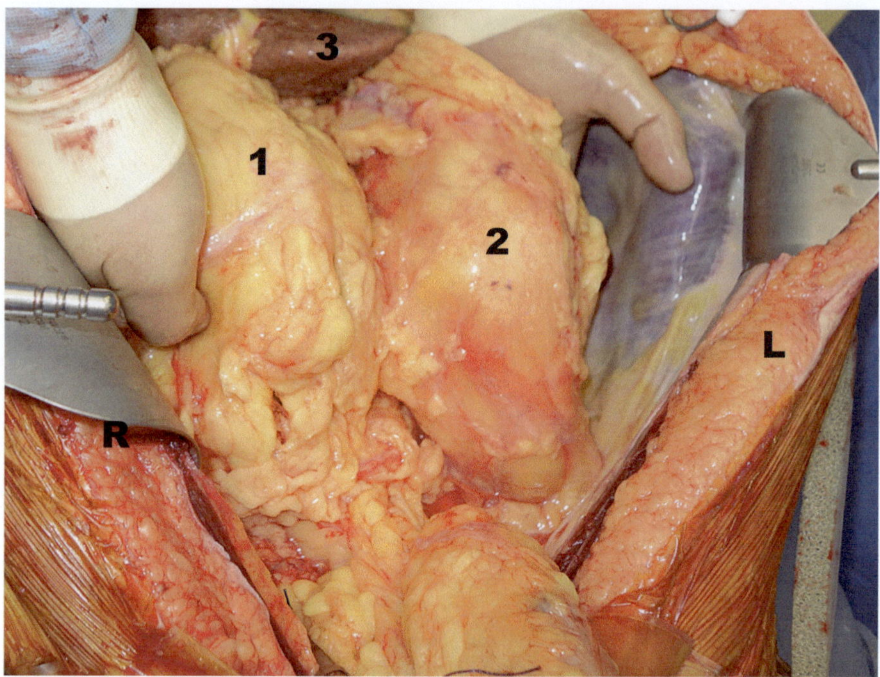

**Fig. 2.60** In the case of a very obese patient and a thick layer of fat surrounding the kidney, I recommend mobilizing the posterior surfaces of both kidneys from the extraperitoneal space to better cool both kidneys by covering their front and back with ice for the best possible external cooling. 1—Right kidney, 2—Left kidney, 3—Left lobe of liver, R—Right side of donor, L—left side of the donor

### 2.3.3  *Kidney-only Procurement from Deceased Donor—with Sternotomy Surgical Technique—brief description*

#### 2.3.3.1  Introduction

Extensive time out with the procurement team(s) and transplant coordinator in DBD procedure is done before transportation to the OR. The time out focuses on discussing relevant patient information, theater preparation, the transportation from ICU to OR, the placing of the donor on the OR table with a sufficient amount of staff, identification, re-intubation, checking of surgical equipment and explanation of the initial surgical steps.

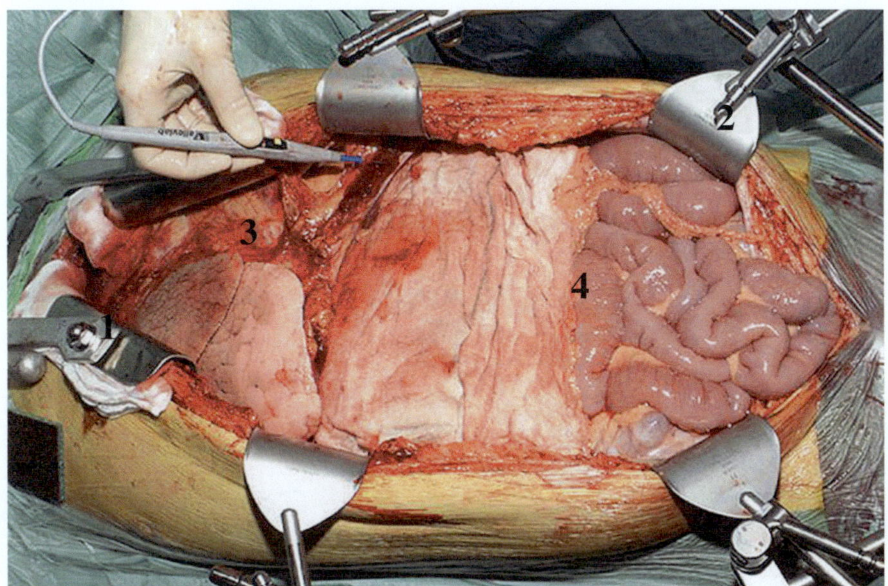

**Fig. 2.61** Midline laparotomy and sternotomy. 1—Professional thoracic retractor, 2—Professional abdominal retractor, 3—Mediastinum, 4—Abdominal cavity—small bowel. Before sternotomy the liver from the abdomen cavity is covered with a large wet gauze

### 2.3.3.2  Surgical Steps

1. Disinfection and draping of the operating field.
2. Perform a midline laparotomy and sternotomy; install a professional abdominal and thoracic retractor (if necessary cut the diaphragm close to the thoracic cavity on both sides) (Fig. 2.61).
3. Perform the Cattel-Braasch maneuver and the Kocher maneuver [2, 33, 34].
4. Ask the anesthetist to administer heparin 25,000–30,000 IU intravenous (I.V.); wait 5 min.
5. Perform cannulation of the abdominal aorta above its bifurcation (Fig. 2.63) as a first choice.
6. Ligate the IVC with one thick ligature at its bifurcation level or just above it.
7. Open the pericardial sac and cut the IVC at the level of the right atrium of the heart or 2–3 cm above the diaphragm. Place good suction in both pleural cavities, but if you have only one, place it in the right thoracic cavity.

**Warnings! (IVC decompression choices)**

- First choice—make a big cut at the level of the right atrium or 2–3 cm above the diaphragm (Fig. 2.62).
- Second choice—ligate the IVC close to the bifurcation, 2–3 cm above the first ligature; place into the IVC lumen a sterile chest tube (20 or 22 F) and fix it (Fig. 2.63).

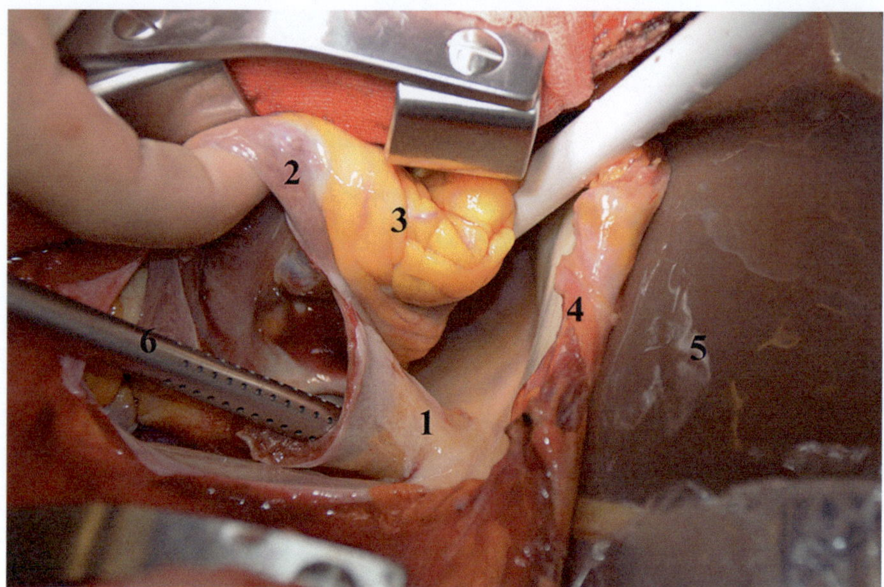

**Fig. 2.62** First choice of system decompressing by opening the IVC at the level of the right atrium. 1—IVC, 2–4 cm above the diaphragm, 2—Right atrium, 3—Heart, 4—Diaphragm, 5—Liver, 6—Poole suction tube located in the IVC. The blood of the donor and preservation solution are drained in the right thoracic cavity

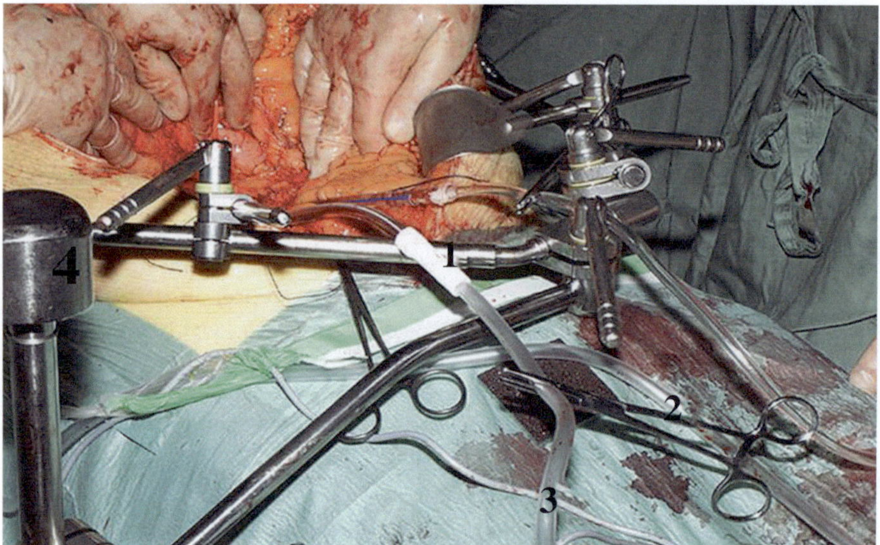

**Fig. 2.63** Cannulated aorta and IVC. Aortic and IVC both cannulae closed with clamps. 1—The chest drain and 2—Aortic drain are closed with clamps; aortic cannula is connected to a bag with a cold preservation solution, 3—The chest drain is placed into a special container located near the operating table, 4—Abdominal retractor

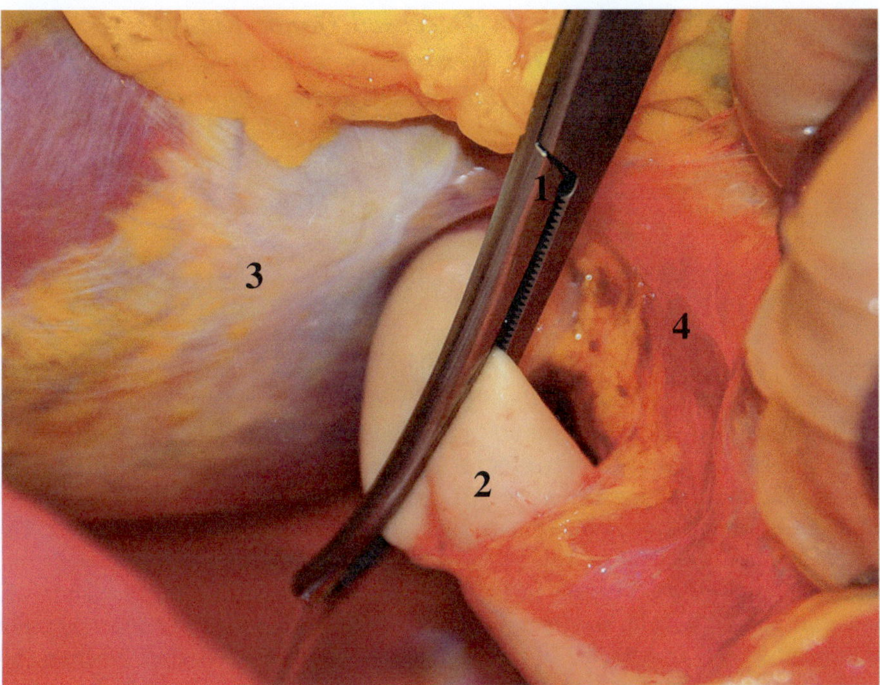

**Fig. 2.64** Closing of the descending aorta close to the diaphragm with vascular clamp in the left thoracic cavity. 1—Vascular clamp, 2—Descending aorta, 3—Left diaphragm, 4—Left side of vertebral column

- Third choice—near and above the IVC bifurcation by cutting and placing an into the lumen of the IVC by surgical suction (unstable or obese organ donors)

  8. Close the thoracic aorta in the left thoracic cavity. After the sternotomy, destroy the left transversus thoracic muscle (attached to the left side of the sternum), this gives you access to the left thoracic cavity. As the next step, if necessary, free the base of the left lung and remove it from the left thoracic cavity and find the descending (thoracic) aorta. This lies on the left side of the vertebral column in the upper part of the posterior mediastinum running on the left side of the spine; free it with your fingers or a right-angled clamp and close it transversally with a vascular clamp (Fig. 2.64).
  9. Start the organ perfusion. The next steps are carried out in the same way and in the same sequence as described in Sect. 2.3.2.

### 2.3.4   Surgical technique for Deceased Donor Kidney Procurement without Sternotomy with direct access to the lumen of the Abdominal Aorta using a large bore cannula

#### 2.3.4.1   Introduction

DCD, previously referred to as donation after cardiac death or non-heart beating organ donation (NHBD), refers to the retrieval of organs for the purpose of transplantation from patients whose death is diagnosed and confirmed using the cardio-respiratory criteria. After an irreversible cardiac arrest, the patient is declared as dead and as a potential organ donor and from that moment the intensive work of the entire team begins to prepare for organ donation. In the UK, an average of 2.7 transplantable organs are retrieved from DCD donors, compared to 3.6 from DBD donors. The biggest contribution of DCD is to kidney transplantation, with 39% of all deceased donor kidney transplants coming from this source in 2019–2020. The lower donation potential of DCD donors is in large part a result of the ischemic injury suffered by solid organs in the time interval between treatment withdrawal and cold perfusion, with the liver and pancreas being particularly vulnerable. For kidney grafts this is reflected in a higher incidence of delayed graft function (requiring a short period of post-implantation renal support), although long term outcomes are similar to DBD grafts. Before treatment withdrawal and donor death the first time of warm ischemia, should be as short as possible and should not exceed 2 h [6–18, 24, 31].

Extensive time out with the procurement team(s) and transplant coordinator in the DCD procedure is done before the withdrawal of treatment. The time out focuses on discussing the relevant patient information, theater preparation, transportation from ICU to OR, the placing of the donor on the OR table with a sufficient number of staff, identification, re-intubation, checking the surgical equipment and explanation of the initial surgical steps.

#### 2.3.4.2   Surgical Steps [24, 31]

1. Rapid disinfection and draping of the operating field.
2. Make with a knife (scalpel) a long midline incision from the sternal notch to the symphysis pubis. On both sides of the navel capture the donor skin with two Backhaus napkin clips and pull them upwards. Now the surgeon can begin to open the abdominal wall, with a scalpel and then with scissors from the xiphoid process of the inferior part of the sternum to the pubic bone.
3. Install a professional abdominal and thoracic retractor (if necessary cut the diaphragm close to the thoracic cavity on both sides). It is very important to create a stable operating field during kidney-only procurement (Fig. 2.61).

4. Replace the bowel to the right side of the abdominal cavity. Ask your assistant to take positions to the right of the donor and the left of the operator. His/her task will be to hold to the right side of the abdomen the intestines until the abdominal aorta is cannulated and the IVC is decompressed.
5. Perform quick cannulation of the abdominal aorta and IVC above its bifurcation (as a first choice).
6. Clamp the abdominal aorta above the CT or under the diaphragm.
7. First decompress the IVC and as a next step start aortic perfusion and external organ cooling.
8. Perform a right medial visceral rotation: the Cattell-Braasch and the extensive Kocher maneuver
9. Cut with a vascular stapler or GIA (white cartridge) the hepatoduodenal ligament or cut it between two vascular clamps.
10. Cut with a stapler or scissors the hepatogastric ligament (if there is a left accessory or aberrant hepatic artery present then cut it), if necessary mobilize the left liver lobe and turn the liver over to the right.
11. Decompress the stomach using the gastric tube and then replace the gastric tube with the upper part of the oesophagus. Cut and close the abdominal portion of the oesophagus using the gastrointestinal or vascular stapler.
12. Close together the SMA and CT with a GIA or vascular stapler or vascular clamp about 1–2 cm above where they arise from the aorta. The stapler or clamp is inserted from below, i.e. from the side of the superior mesenteric artery, towards the diaphragm. At this point, the CT and the SMA together with the surrounding tissues are closed and cut. In the case of a vascular clamp, cut with scissors all the tissues 2 cm above the clamp. At this point, the CT and the SMA with the celiac plexus are closed and cut and then the only organs that are perfused in the abdominal cavity are the great vessels and kidneys.
13. Mobilize with scissors the following abdominal organs: the stomach, duodenum, pancreas, small intestine and large intestine including the descending colon in one block. When fully mobilized, move them outside the abdomen and place them on the donor's thighs. The organs that remain in the abdomen are the large vessel kidneys which are well perfused and cooled and the liver which is not perfused and preserved (Fig. 2.65).
14. In order to obtain a better external cooling, add a cold sterile saline or Ringer's solution into the abdominal cavity and add ice. The operating field is now very stable and transparent (Fig. 2.66). Now we have enough time to check the perfusion quality of both kidneys. In an obese donor, there is a large amount of fat around the kidneys. If possible, try to reduce this fat in the donor's body before packing or putting the kidneys on the perfusion machine. The liver is not perfused but is stabilized with one of the special blades of a professional abdominal retractor, pushing it into the upper right corner of the abdominal cavity, under the right diaphragm.
15. The further steps concerning the surgical technique of kidney procurement have been described earlier (Sect. 2.3.2).

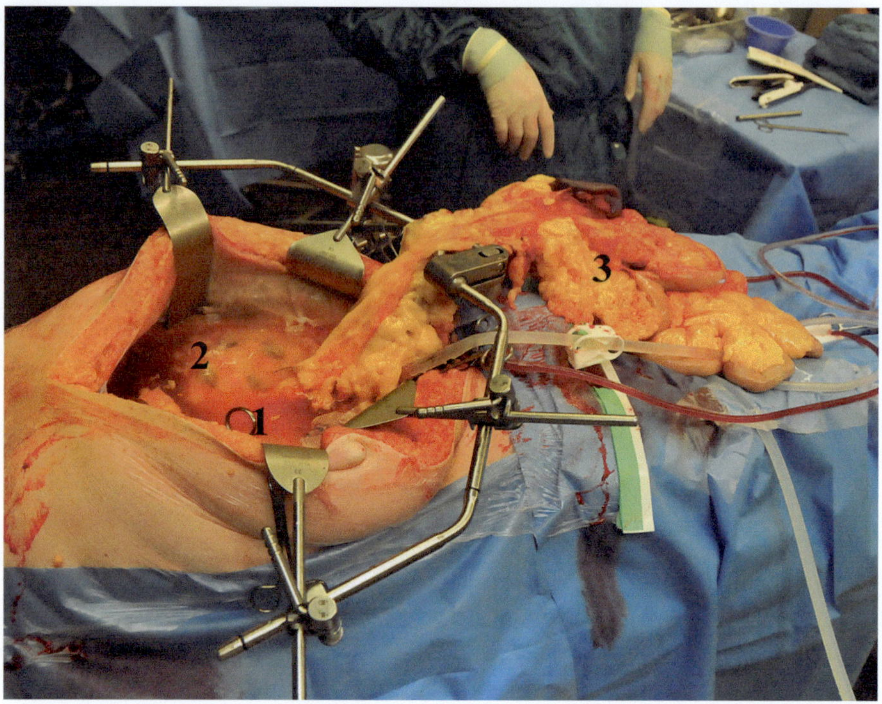

**Fig. 2.65** DCD: kidney-only procurement without opening the chest. Total mobilization of organs from the abdominal cavity: stomach, duodenum, pancreas, small intestine and large intestine including the descendant are mobilized from the abdominal cavity and placed on the donor's thighs. 1—Closing clamp of the abdominal aorta above the celiac trunk, 2—Left kidney, 3—Abdominal organs outside abdominal cavity

**Warning!**

DCD is an operation in which time, experience, speed and precision of movements count. If you are not trained sufficiently and you get stressed easily, remember that it is easy to make mistakes. In this case, be careful when cutting the peritoneum from the right external iliac artery to the bifurcation of the aorta—the right ureter is in your the way and is "waiting for you" not to be damage or cut it at this level.

**Warning! (DCD and heparin doses)**

In a DCD donor, prior administration of heparin is not possible, so it is administered in the organ preservative fluid in the amount of 40–60 thousand international units (IU) in every preservation solution bag. On average, there are 20–30 thousand international units of heparin in each 5 L bag of the preservation solution.

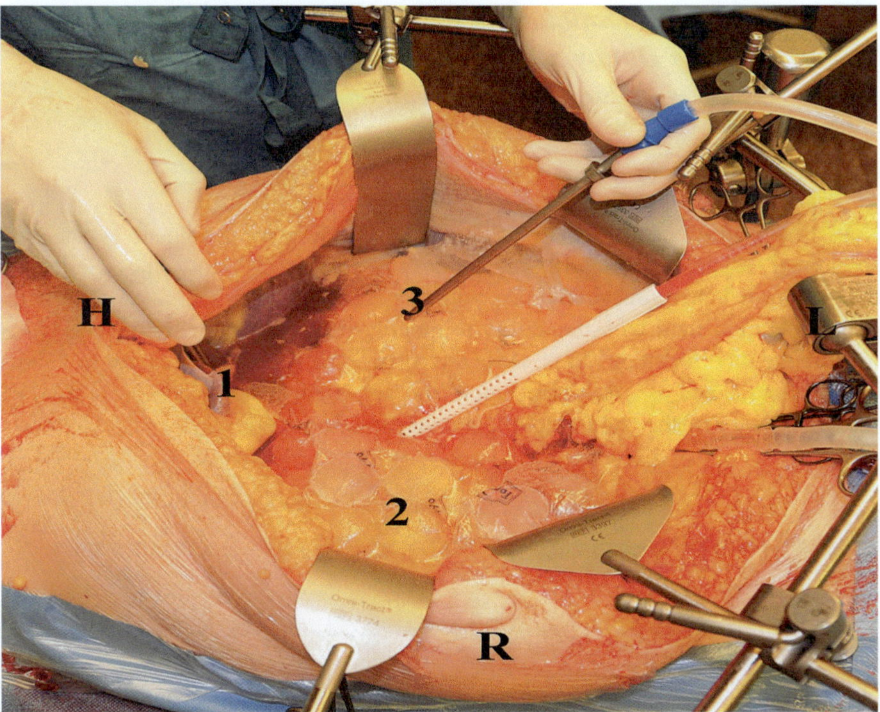

**Fig. 2.66** DCD kidney-only procurement without opening the chest. The operating field is very stable and transparent. Due to the high BMI of the donor and a large amount of perirenal fat, in order to maintain proper external cooling of the kidneys, the latter were mobilized from the retroperitoneal space and covered with cold ice on both sides. 1—Left liver lobe, 2—Right kidney, 3—Left kidney, H—Head, R—Right side, L—Legs

**Warning! (IVC decompression)**
Decompression of the IVC depends always on the situation, according to the previously described methods.

**Warnings! (The hepato duodenal and hepatogastric ligament)**
The fastest way to reach the aorta above the CT is by cutting the hepatoduodenal ligament and hepatogastric ligament with a 60–80–120 mm long vascular stapler or GIA with white cartridge, pushing the liver with one of the blades of a retractor upwards and pulling the pancreas head downwards—this movement gives you very good access to the hepatogastric ligament, the lesser curvature near the right and left crus of the diaphragm and the abdominal aorta above the CT. Now cut the right and left crus of the diaphragm, prepare around the aorta, take it around on the vessel loop above the CT and close it with a vascular clamp. I recommend this method—it is safe, fast and works well, especially in obese donors.

## 2.3.5  Surgical Technique for Kidney-only Procurement from the Donor after Circulatory Death (DCD) with Sternotomy (in Brief)

### 2.3.5.1  Introduction

Now I will briefly describe the technique of kidney procurement as the only abdominal organ, combined with lung retrieval as the only thoracic organ. Performing a laparotomy combined with a sternotomy provides a very clear and stable operating field with the ability to quickly find and cannulate the abdominal aorta above its bifurcation. Next, close the aorta in the left thoracic cavity just above the diaphragm and as a last step before the organ perfusion decompress the IVC above the level of the right diaphragm or right atrium (Fig. 2.67).

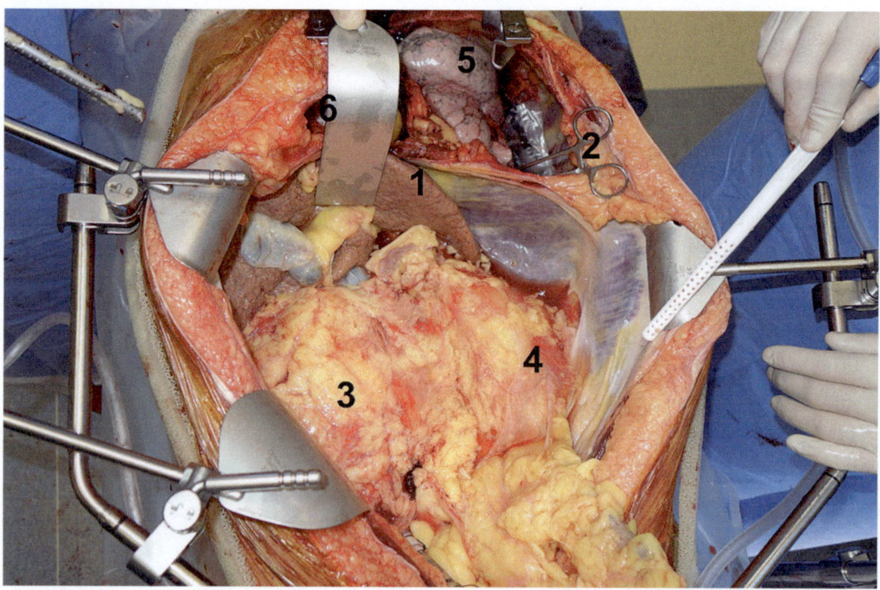

**Fig. 2.67** DCD with chest opening. Laparotomy and sternotomy were performed, which resulted in a clear and stable operating field with the ability to quickly find and close the aorta in the left thoracic cavity and decompress the IVC at the level of the right atrium. 1—Liver pushed by retractor blade up towards right diaphragm, 2—Vascular clamp that closes the thoracic aorta in the left thoracic cavity above the diaphragm, 3—Right kidney, 4—Left kidney, 5—Left lung, 6—Behind the retractor blade is an open pericardial sac with IVC decompression cut

### 2.3.5.2  Operation Steps [24, 31]

1. Rapid disinfection and draping of the operating field.
2. Perform a long midline incision from the sternal notch to the symphysis pubis with a knife (scalpel). With two Backhaus towel forceps, catch the skin on the left and right side of the navel of the donor and pull it upwards. Begin now with opening the abdominal wall with a scalpel and then continue with the scissors to the xiphoid sternum and to the pubic bone.
3. Perform the sternotomy with a pneumatic or Gigli saw (alone or simultaneously with one of the thoracic surgeons).
4. Install an optimal abdominal and thoracic retractor. Cut the diaphragm close to the thoracic cavity up to the midaxillary line on both sides. Slowly open the thoracic retractor to its maximum and reposition the abdominal wall blades to create a stable operating field (Fig. 2.61).
5. Replace the bowel to the right side of the abdominal cavity. Ask your assistant to take his/her position to the right of the donor and to the left of the surgeon. His/her task at this moment is to hold the intestines to the right side of the abdomen until the abdominal aorta is cannulated and the IVC is decompressed (Fig. 2.65).
6. Free the abdominal aorta above its bifurcation, perform a quick cannulation of the abdominal aorta, and ligate the IVC above its bifurcation (as a first choice) —do not start the abdominal organ perfusion yet!
7. After the sternotomy destroy the left transversus thoracic muscle. This gives you access to the left thoracic cavity as the next step is to move the left lung from the left thoracic cavity and pull it up to the right. Now it is easy to find the descending (thoracic) aorta. It lies on the left side of the vertebral column in the upper part of the posterior mediastinum; free it with your fingers or right angled clamp and close it transversally with a vascular clamp (Fig. 2.64).
8. Decompress the IVC by cutting it at the level of the right atrium or above the diaphragm (Fig. 2.63); as a next step start the aortic perfusion and external organ cooling by adding cold sterile saline or Ringer's solution into the abdominal cavity and ice (Fig. 2.68).
9. Perform a right medial visceral rotation—the Cattell-Braasch manoeuvre and the extensive Kocher manoeuvre.
10. Cut the hepatoduodenal ligament with a vascular stapler or GIA with a white cartridge or cut it between two vascular clamps.
11. Cut the hepatogastric ligament with a stapler or scissors (if there is a left accessory or left aberrant hepatic artery present then cut it, but do not ligate it) if the donor is obese and, if it is necessary, mobilize the left liver lobe.
12. Decompress the stomach using the gastric tube. Next, replace the gastric tube higher in the esophagus, cut and close, with a GIA or a vascular stapler, the abdominal part of the esophagus.
13. Close the SMA and CT with a GIA or a vascular stapler or a vascular clamp about 1–2 cm above where they arise from the aorta. The stapler or clamp is inserted from below, that is to say from the side of the SMA, towards the

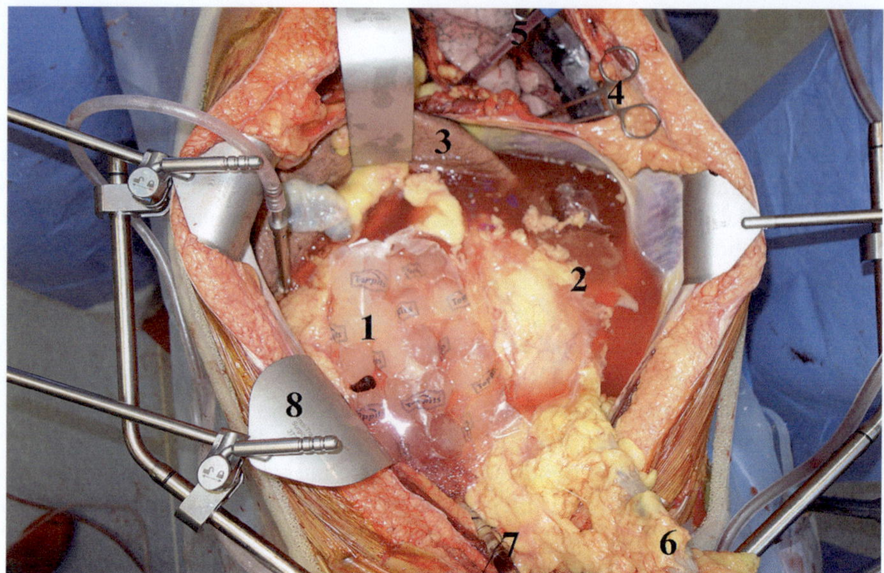

**Fig. 2.68** DCD kidney-only procurement with chest opening. At the Start of perfusion the abdominal organs receive internal and external cooling. 1—External cooling of the abdominal organs using ice and a cold 0.9%NaCl saline solution, 2—Left kidney, 3—Liver, 4—Closed aorta with vascular clamp in the left thoracic cavity, 5—Surgery suction in the left pleural cavity, 6—Mobilized organs of the abdominal cavity mobilized and placed on the donor's thighs, 7—Aortic cannula, 8—Abdominal retractor

diaphragm. In the case of using a vascular clamp, cut with scissors all the tissues and vessels 2 cm above the clamp. Then the only organs that are perfused in the abdominal cavity are kidneys.

14. Mobilize with scissors the following organs from the abdominal cavity: stomach, duodenum, pancreas, small intestine and large intestine including the descending colon. When fully mobilized, move them outside the abdomen and place them on the donor's thighs. The organs that remain in the abdomen are the kidneys which are well perfused and cooled and the liver which is not perfused and preserved (Fig. 2.65).

15. In order to obtain a better external cooling, add a cold sterile saline or Ringer's solution into the abdominal cavity and add ice. The operating field is now very stable and transparent. Now we have enough time to check the quality of the perfusion of both kidneys and, if there is a large amount of fat around the kidneys during perfusion, reduce the fat or put both kidneys in sterile ice bags. The liver, if necessary, is stabilized with one of the special blades of a professional abdominal retractor, pushing it into the upper right corner of the abdominal cavity, under the right diaphragm (Figs. 2.67, 2.68, and 2.69).

16. The further steps concerning the surgical technique of kidney procurement have been described earlier in Sect. 2.2.2.

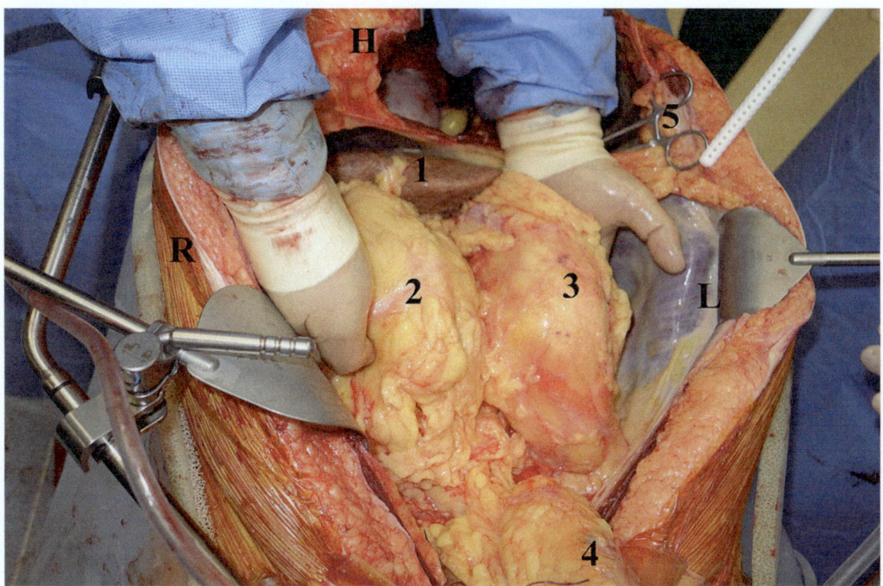


**Fig. 2.69** DCD kidney only. After external and internal cooling and preservation, the fluid from the abdominal cavity was sucked out and the ice removed. The kidneys were the only organs from the abdominal cavity before removal. 1—Liver, 2—Right kidney, 3—Left kidney, 4—Sigmoid colon, 5—Closing aorta in left thoracic cavity, R—Right side, L—Left side, H—Head

**Warnings!**

Keep the temperature in the abdominal cavity as low as possible and extract the organs quickly and carefully. After removal, every organ should be immediately immersed in a special bowl filled up with cold preservation solution with slushed ice, awaiting inspection and bagging/machine connection.

**Comment!**

Retrieving only the kidneys from donors after circulatory death may be more difficult than abdominal multiorgan procurement, especially if the donors are obese and the family or donor agreed to donate only the kidneys or kidney without opening the chest. In the literature techniques of kidney-only retrieval and displacing most of the organs outside the abdominal cavity were described some years ago by me. I hope that the reader will like my surgical technique, which in my opinion is simple, quick, transparent and safe. All surgical techniques described in this chapter by me which we use in the LUMC during an organ procurement deserve to be put into clinical practice, because in my opinion they are fast, the only organs which are being preserved and cooled internally and externally are the kidneys, and the pressure of the preservation solution is less than in the multiorgan procurement procedures. Renal cooling and perfusion is perfectly controlled during retrieval and both the kidneys and ureters can be mobilized from the retroperitoneal space without exposing them to unnecessary loss of preservation solution. Using this method, I procured kidneys successfully dozens of times from DBD and DCD donors. As a rule, I have performed procurement without and with opening the chest using a professional abdominal retractor. The whole operation always took me no more than 90–150 min from skin opening to skin closure. The removed kidneys, their vessels and ureters have never been damaged. Both kidneys were always perfectly flushed and suitable for transplantation. The only inconvenience of the operation is the necessity of cutting the esophagus, but let us not forget that during multiorgan donation we cut the duodenum twice and the trachea once, therefore contamination of the surgical field with kidney-only donation is small and acceptable compared to simultaneous thoracic and abdominal multi-organ procurement. I also taught this method on various hands-on courses dealing with transplant fellows and surgeons with surgical techniques on kidney-only procurement at the following universities: McGill Montreal (Canada), Semmelweis Budapest (Hungary), Tours (France), Leiden (the Netherlands), Padua (Italy), Naples (Italy), St. Petersburg (Russia), Baku (Azerbaijan), Ankara (Turkey) and Ljubljana (Slovenia).

### 2.3.6  *The General Principles of Abdominal Organ Procurement from Donors After Circulatory Death (DCD) and Donors after Brain Death: The Same Steps at Different Time Periods—An Attempt to Undertake the Standardization of Surgical Techniques*

**Remember**: the quality of the procured abdominal organs from the DCD depends on your speed and perfect surgical skills!

**Remember**: first always perfectly learn organ procurement from DBD donors and after that start learning very carefully organ procurement from DCD to avoid big surgical mistakes. Never do it the other way around.

**Introduction**

The general principles for DBD and DCD organ removal are similar. The biggest difference between the procedures is the pace and sequence of steps.

In DBD procedures there is time to perform organ and vessel inspection and dissection before you start cooling, so this is the first priority and difference.

In DCD it is more difficult to identify anatomical structures due to the absence of vessel pulsations creating a higher chance of errors during organ procurement.

In DCD there is an absence of circulation and as a result of donor death leading to the ongoing warm ischemic injury and therefore rapid cannulation and cooling is required to decrease metabolism and preserve abdominal organs.

In DCD procedure the organs are perfused first and examined in detail afterwards. The arterial vascularisation of each organ is asses at the time of organ procurement. If the pancreas and liver procured 'en block' at the time of separation, the arterial vasculature should be divide, if possible, so that both organs can be transplanted. In some cases (anatomical anomalies), it is not possible to separate the arterial vasculature, in which case all the vessels must be donated to the liver and the pancreas if of good quality, can be sent to a centre for isolation of pancreatic islets for scientific research or left in the donor's body. In the case of the kidneys, the vascularisation of the kidneys, both venous and arterial, is assessed at the time of donation (location of the left renal vein and its course in front of or behind the abdominal aorta, the number of renal arteries is assessed after cutting the anterior wall of the aorta). The quality of the parenchyma (presence of tumours and/or cysts) of both kidneys is assess before and after packaging after the early reduction of perinephric fat.

**Procurement Surgery DCD/DBD Differences**

<u>Withdrawal of treatment</u>

DCD—intensive care or anesthetic room or  OR

DBD—OR after decompression and start organ perfusion

<u>Declaring patients death</u>

DCD—the patient's physicians declares death according to the local or international protocol. Location: intensive care or anesthetic room or OR

DBD—day(s) or hours before procurement by specially appointed commission authorized to declare the death of the brain

<u>Transportation</u>

DCD—after death determination and 5 min "no touch" period (different in different countries) the donor is quickly transported to the OR

DBD—the donor is transported to the OR with all the devices which supported his/her life

<u>Time out</u>

Extensive time out with the procurement team(s) and transplant coordinator. DCD —before withdrawal of treatment. DBD before transportation to the OR. The time out focuses on discussing the relevant patient information, theater preparation, transportation from ICU to OR, placing of the donor on the OR table with a sufficient amount of staff, identification, re-intubation, checking of surgical equipment and explanation of the initial surgical steps.

<u>Preparation of operating theater</u>

1. In both procedures of DCD and DBD make sure the OR is ready and everything is in place before the patient arrives

2. In contrast to the DBD procedure, the DCD surgical team has no time to participate in moving the body from bed to the operating table and to place the donor in the required position on the table
3. The DBD surgical team has time to help with moving the donor from the bed to the operating table and to position and scrub him.

Incision
    This is a long midline incision from the sternal notch to the symphysis pubis. DCD—with a knife without hemostasis

DBD—using diathermy saving every drop of blood

Aorta cannulation

Unlike in DBD, where cannulation can be done slowly and meticulously, in DCD the great importance is attached to the speed. For aortic cannulation and perfusion a larger bore single lumen cannula or "double-balloon triple lumen catheter" can be used.

The double-balloon catheter is particularly useful in patients who have had multiple previous abdominal operations and access to the aorta is challenging. If a double-balloon catheter is used, the proximal aorta does not need to be cross-clamped.

Decompression of IVC

The best choices for decompression methods one by one depends on the condition of the donor and whether or not the procurement is done with or without opening the thoracic cavity (DCD or DBD independent).

- First choice—big cut at the level of the right atrium or 2–3 cm above the diaphragm
- Second choice—close to IVC bifurcation with a sterile chest tube (20 or 22 F)
- Third choice—near and above the IVC bifurcation by cutting and placing into the IVC lumen surgical suction (unstable or obese donors).

Organ perfusion: rapid internal and external cooling

Outcomes in recipients of DCD donor organs are very much dependent on rapid cooling to temperatures of less than 5 °C. This should be performed immediately both by internal and external cooling. Aortic cannulation, venous decompression, initiation of perfusion and topical cooling should be done quickly but carefully to avoid unnecessary surgical organ damage.

Starting the procurement surgery

DCD—during the perfusion and cooling of the organ, dissection, examinations and preparations are performed

DBD—precise organ examination; the preparation is finished before the organ perfusion and cooling

In DBD and DCD: donors have the same surgical maneuvers performed, i.e. the Cattel-Braasch maneuver (the right sided visceral rotation) and the extended Kocher maneuver (extended pancreas head mobilization up to the right side of the abdominal aorta), but at a different time. In DBD the maneuvers are performed before the perfusion and in DCD after the perfusion.

In DBD and DCD donors the mobilization of the left liver lobe and turning it to the right in search of the left aberrant hepatic artery in the hepatogastric ligament is performed at the same time.

In DBD and DCD donors, the surgical technique of the abdominal organ procurement is the same after the organ perfusion: the liver and pancreas are retrieved en bloc following by the kidneys and vessels. To save time en bloc liver–pancreas dissection is preferable to in situ dissection, on the condition that a bowl filled with crushed ice and a preservation solution is available for the back table procedure; if not the liver and the pancreas have to be split in situ in the donor's body. Back table perfusion of the liver and/or kidneys is performed when indicated.

The hepatoduodenal ligament dissection in DBD donors is more precise compared to DCD donors.

In DBD and DCD donors there are no differences concerning the surgical technique of kidney procurement. The kidneys can be retrieved individually or en bloc. If the kidneys are being retrieved en bloc, they have to be retrieved with the abdominal aorta and the IVC intact, from the SMA level (including 2–3 mm of the SMA) down to the aortic and IVC bifurcations.

<u>Organ biopsy</u>

In DBD and DCD there is no difference.

The principles with respect to organ biopsy are:

a. Any suspicious lesion in either the chest or abdomen must be biopsied and arrangements made for an urgent frozen section and/or any other tissue sample processing that may be required. Consideration may need to be given to the availability of pathology resources (including the requisite expertise).
b. Biopsy of the liver can be performed either in situ or ex situ.
c. Biopsy of the kidney(s) may also be indicated in donors with risk factors for chronic kidney disease and is best performed on the back table after a comprehensive examination of the cortex has been undertaken. Biopsies for research may also be taken according to national protocols.
d. All biopsies must be appropriately packaged and labeled and the relevant information must be conveyed to the pathology laboratory.

**Be aware** that in DCD procedures the organs are perfused first and palpated later. You then check the quality of the organs, search for malignancies and check the arteries and (aberrant) vessels.

Organ packing

In DBD and DCD there is no difference.

All organs are packed according to the National Standard Operation Procedures. In the Eurotransplant region, organs are triple bagged and immersed in preservation solution surrounding the organs (to protect them from freezing within the ice box); a cold sterile physiological solution is placed in the second bag and the third bag is dry.

Hypothermic machine perfusion is an alternative preservation method for a kidney during transportation from the donor to the recipient's hospital.

Tissue not required/suitable for transplantation

In DBD and DCD there is no difference.

In the Eurotransplant region, any organs or tissues that have been removed and are not required for transplantation, research or pathological examinations should be destroyed at the department of pathology or returned into the donor's body.

Vessels

In DBD and DCD there is no difference.

Vessels have to be packed according to the Standard Operating Procedures for packing, labeling and storage documentation.

The liver and pancreas should each be accompanied by a set of vessels (for example an iliac artery and vein) and if the liver is split, each part should be accompanied by a set of vessels.

The liver requires an arterial graft at least 13 cm long and a vein of 5–10 cm.

The pancreas Y arterial graft needs only to be 5–10 cm (unless the portal vein was cut short).

If the iliac arteries are diseased then the carotid arteries may need to be retrieved.

In the Eurotransplant area vessels cannot be packed in the organ bag and must be packed separately in a specific sterile container. It is the responsibility of the retrieval team to ensure that the appropriate, high quality vessels are sent with the liver, pancreas and small bowel.

Donor body

In the DBD and DCD procedure, standard closure is performed and a dressing applied [2–22].

## 2.4   Surgical Technique for Living Kidney Donation: A Minimally Invasive, Open, Retroperitoneal Approach [51–58]

### 2.4.1   Introduction: Anatomical Basis of This Surgical Technique

The rectus sheath, also called the rectus fascia, is formed by the aponeuroses of the transverse abdominal and the internal and external oblique muscles. It contains the rectus abdominis and pyramidalis muscles. The arrangement of the layers has important variations at different regions of the abdomen. Below the costal margin and above the arcuate line the anterior laminae of the rectus sheath consists of the aponeurosis of the external oblique muscle as well as 50% aponeurosis of the internal oblique muscle; the posterior laminae consists of the aponeurosis of the musculus transversus and 50% aponeurosis of the internal oblique muscle. Below the costal margin and below the arcuate line the aponeuroses of all three muscles (external, internal oblique and transversus) pass in front of the rectus (Figs. 2.70 and 2.71).

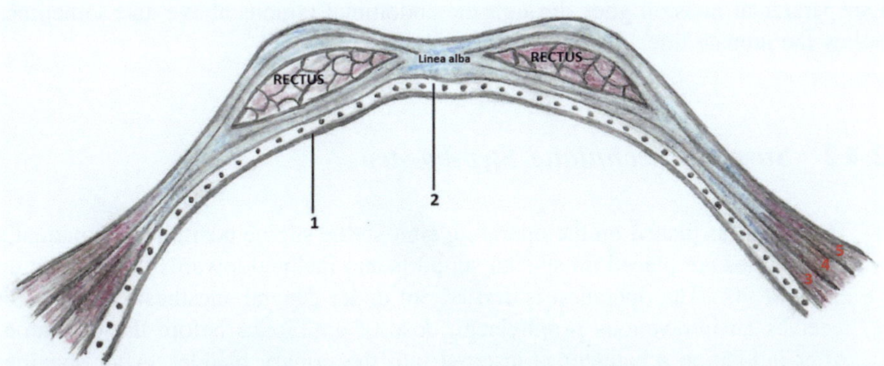


**Fig. 2.70** Above the arcuate line: at the lateral margin of the rectus, the aponeurosis of the internal oblique divides into two lamellae: one of which passes in front of rectus, blending with the aponeurosis of the external oblique as well as the aponeurosis of the anterior half of the internal oblique muscle. The other behind it blends with the aponeurosis of the transvers as well as the posterior half of the internal oblique, and these, joining again at the medical border of the rectus, are inserted into the linea alba. 1—Peritoneum, 2—Transversalis fascia, 3—Transverse muscle, 4—Obliquus internus muscle, 5—Obliquus externus muscle (Drawing drawn by E.A. Baranski)

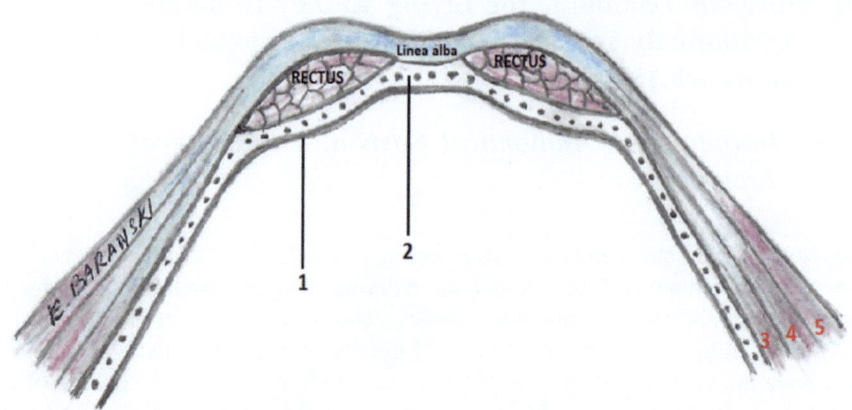



**Fig. 2.71** Below the arcuate line. Below this level, the aponeuroses of all three muscles (including the transversus) pass in front of the rectus. 1—Peritoneum, 2—Transversalis fascia, 3—Transverse muscle, 4—Obliquus internus muscle, 5—Obliquus externus muscle (Drawing drawn by E.A. Baranski)

**Warnings!**

Our pararectal incision goes through the abdominal regions above and sometimes below the arcuate line.

## 2.4.2 Surgical Technique Step-by-step

1. The patient is placed on the operating table in the supine position. The patient's upper limbs are placed on special supports and inclined towards the body at an angle of 90°. The operation is carried out under general anesthesia, the patient receives an intravenous prophylactic dose of antibiotics before the operation. After intubation a catheter is inserted into the urinary bladder. After shaving, disinfection and sterile draping of the surgical field, the surgeon starts the operation.
2. Cut the skin with a scalpel and subcutaneous tissue with diathermy. The incision should be made 5 mm below the costal arch, 1.0–1.5 cm inwards from the lateral side of the abdominal rectus muscle. The length of the incision depends on the patient's height and BMI but on average it ranges from 10 to 15 cm (Fig. 2.72).
3. Free the skin together with the subcutaneous tissue within a radius of about 8–10 cm from the planned incision of the anterior sheath of rectus muscle (Fig. 2.73).

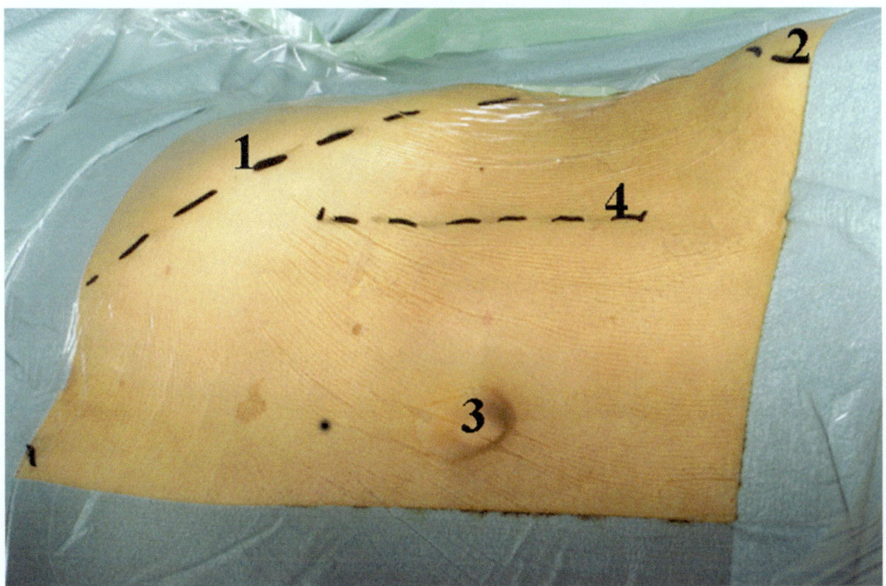

**Fig. 2.72** The incision is done 10 mm below the costal margin, 10–15 mm inwards from the lateral rectus abdominis muscle. 1—Left costal margin, 2—Left anterior superior iliac spine, 3—Umbilicus, 4—Incision line

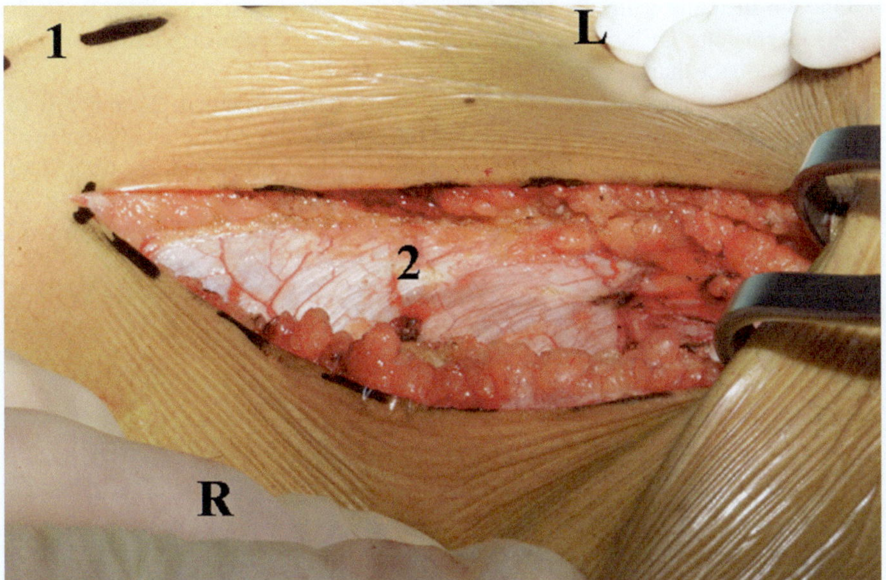

**Fig. 2.73** 1—Left costal margin, 2—Anterior rectus fascia (formed by the aponeuroses of the transverse abdominal and the internal and external oblique muscles). R—Right side, L—Left side

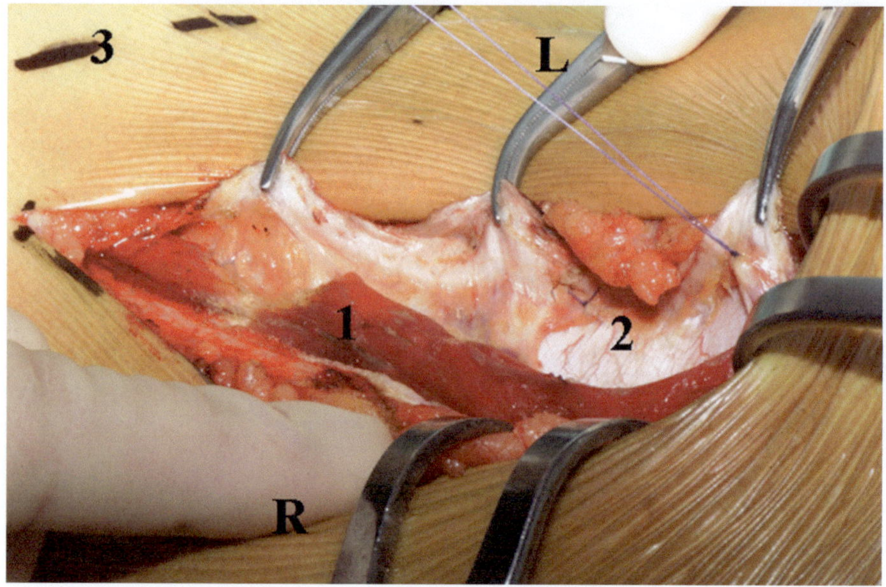

**Fig. 2.74** The anterior rectus fascia was cut 1 cm medially from its lateral edge. 1—The rectus abdominis muscle, 2—The posterior rectus fascia, 3—Marked position of the costal cartilages, R—Right side; L—Left side

4. One cm medially from the lateral edge of the rectus muscle perform vertically 12–15 cm long an incision of the anterior sheath of rectus abdominis muscle (a little longer than a skin incision) (Fig. 2.74).
5. Free the rectus muscle from the anterior and posterior sheath; 1–2 cm below the arcuate line recognize the parietal peritoneum attached to the abdominal wall, and try gently to divide it from the posterior surface of the rectal sheath towards the costal arch (Figs. 2.75 and 2.76).
6. Cut the aponeurosis of the transvers muscle and 50% aponeurosis of the internal oblique muscle towards the costal arch (Fig. 2.77).

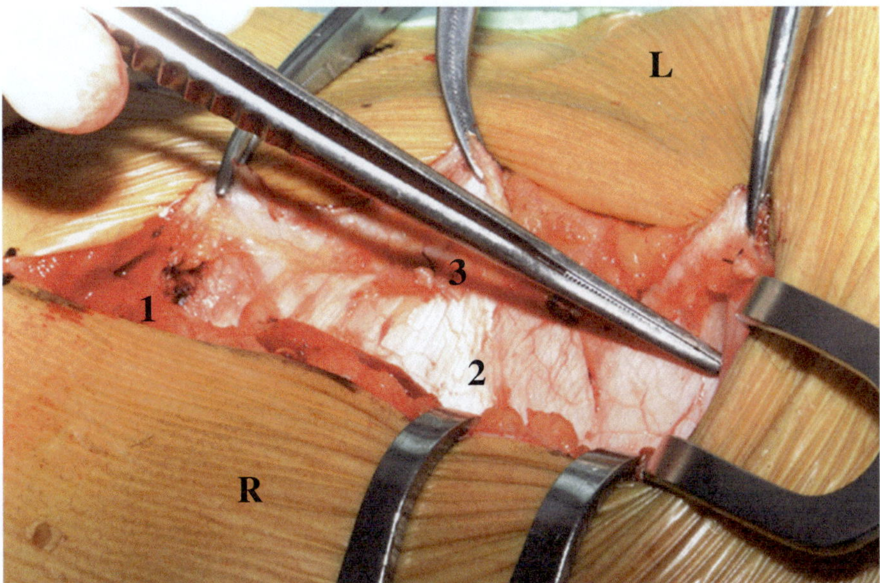

**Fig. 2.75** After incision, release the rectus muscle from the posterior part of the abdominal rectus sheath, coagulate the nerves and ligate the small vessels. 1—The released rectus muscle from its posterior sheath is moved towards the median line in order to reveal its posterior fascia over a distance of about 1–2 cm, 2—The posterior (sheath) part of the rectus muscle capsule, 3—Ligated deep superior epigastric artery perforator, R—Right side, L—Left side

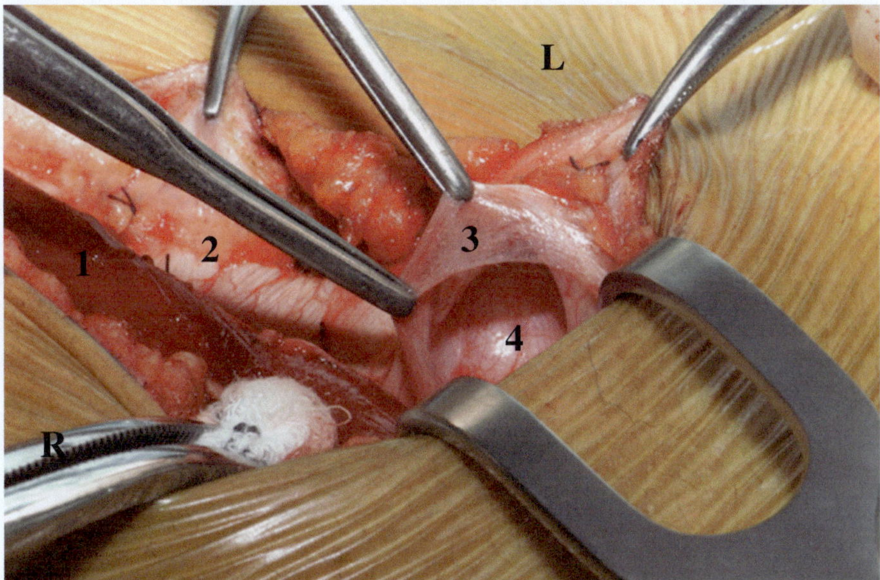

**Fig. 2.76** Cut the posterior rectus sheath lengthwise, starting from the bottom: it is much safer because in the upper part the posterior sheath does not have direct contact with the peritoneum but with the transverse abdominal muscle. 1—Left rectus muscle, 2—Posterior sheath of the rectus muscle, 3—Posterior sheath of the rectus muscle at the level of the arcuate line, detached from the peritoneum with a small gauze swab, 4—Peritoneum, R—Right side, L—Left side

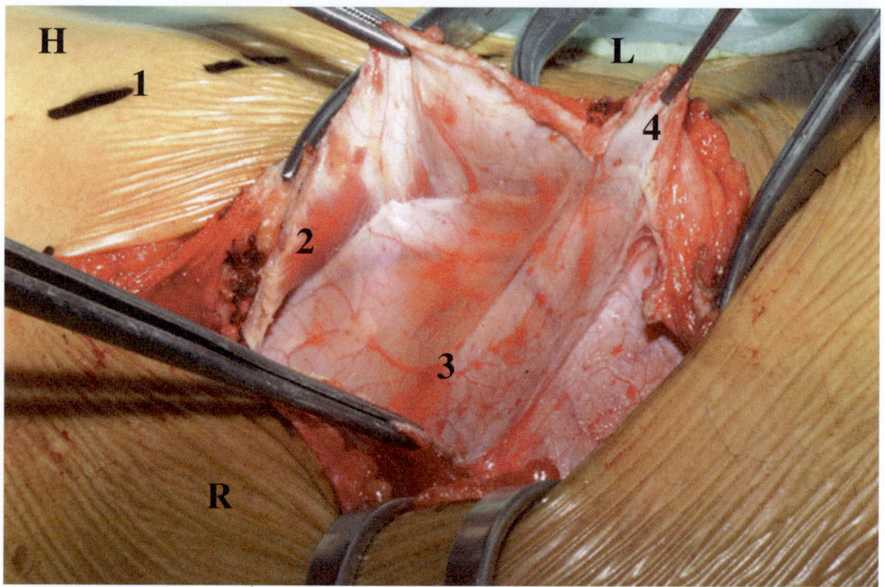


**Fig. 2.77** The peritoneum is gently peeled away from the abdominal wall using an inverted large forceps, and in fact its fixed hinge or small TUPFER with X-ray thread—partially gripped in the jaws of a surgical clamp—as shown in the photo. The peritoneum is detached in the following directions: downwards, laterally, upwards and medially towards the aorta. 1—Left costal margin, 2—Cut transverse abdominal muscle, 3—Peritoneum, 4—Part posterior sheath of the rectal muscle, H—Head, L—Left side, R—Right side

**Warning! (During dissection, try not to damage the peritoneum, located in the subcostal area—it is thin and therefore very susceptible to damage)**

Depending on the size of the transverse abdominal muscle, while detaching the parietal peritoneum, gently move upwards and cut it with an electrocautery on a small curved clamp (for example curved small Mosquito Forceps). Personally, to avoid damage of the parietal peritoneum, I cut the transverse abdominal muscle incompletely and usually I do not cut off the upper part of the muscle located 2–3 cm below the costal arch. At the upper (subcostal) and lateral abdominal regions, the parietal peritoneum is very thin and more prone to tearing. Below the arcuate line and the lower parietal the peritoneum is thicker, stronger and less prone to tearing.

7. Detachment of the parietal peritoneum from the abdominal wall is performed gently with long tissues or a small gauze encased in small Mosquito Forceps. The detachment begins below arcuate laterally, downwards, upwards and medially towards the aorta (Fig. 2.78).

8. After detaching the posterior part of the parietal peritoneum towards the aorta (left side) or IVC (right side) close to the paravertebral line, install a professional abdominal retractor (Fig. 2.79).

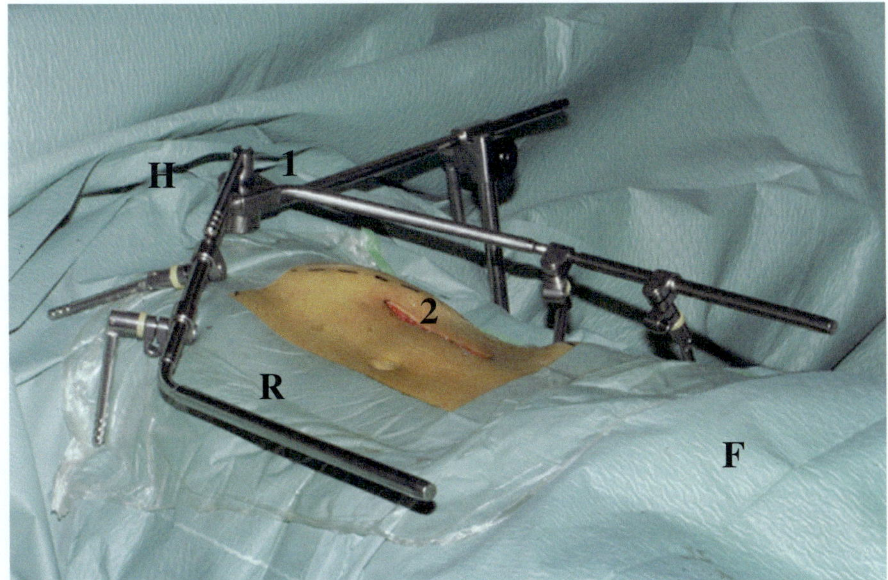



**Fig. 2.78** 1—Optimal installed abdominal retractor, 2—Pararectal incision, H—Head, R—Right side, F—Towards the patient's legs

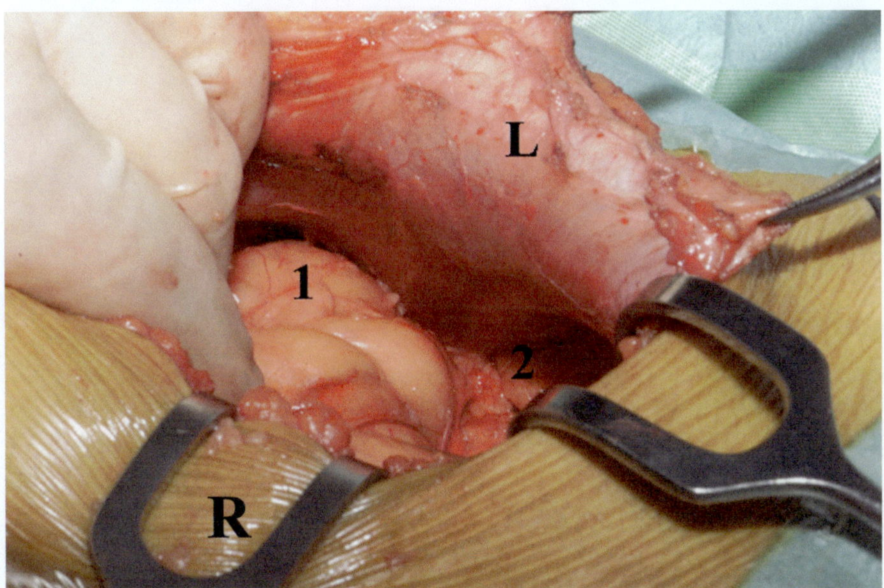



**Fig. 2.79** Using a handle of a large forceps, small gauze swab and a hand, gently peel off the parietal peritoneum from the abdominal wall to the bottom and side, and then, with the help of a long curved vascular clamp, detach the parietal peritoneum from the perirenal fat. 1—Left kidney with perirenal fat, 2—Retroperitoneal space, L—Left side, R—Right side

9. Using as a handle a large forceps (its fixed hinge) and hand, gently detach the parietal peritoneum from the abdominal wall downwards, and then, using a long curved surgical clamp, detach the parietal peritoneum from the perirenal fat. On the left side we detach (free) the parietal peritoneum up to the abdominal aorta and on the right side up to the IVC. On the right side, to visualize the IVC and right renal vein in the subhepatic region, and in order to get very good access to the IVC and right renal artery, we first have to carry out the Kocher maneuver [24, 31, 51–58].

10. Locate the part of the ureter under the renal pelvis and gently mobilize the entire ureter with the surrounding tissues towards the bladder up to below the iliac vessels. As a second step, mobilize the lower part of the kidney (lower pole and renal pelvis) up to the renal vein and carefully dissect the renal vessels (Figs. 2.80 and 2.81).

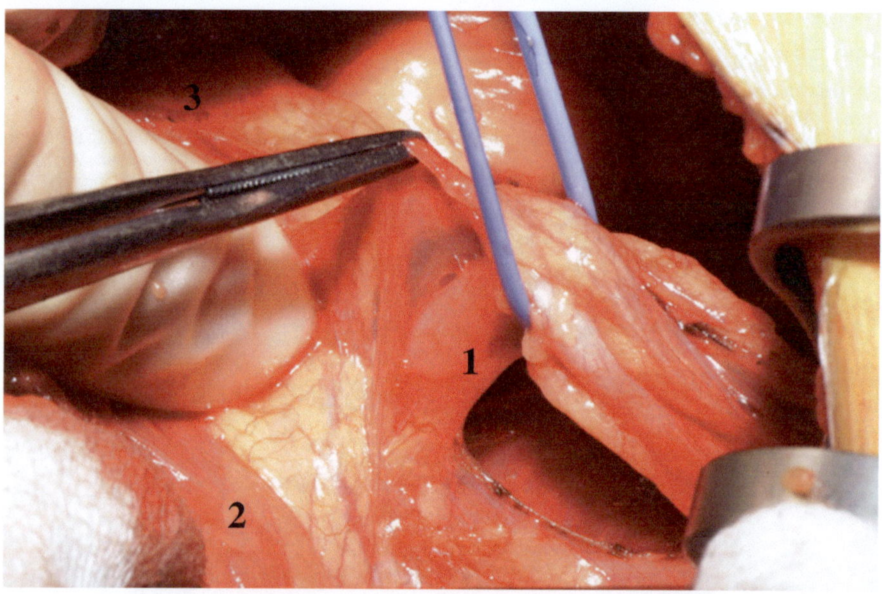

**Fig. 2.80** Location and mobilization of the ureter and renal pelvis up to the renal vessels. 1—Ureter together with gonadal vein and surrounding tissues taken on vascular vessel loop, 2—Peritoneal wall, 3—Perirenal fat

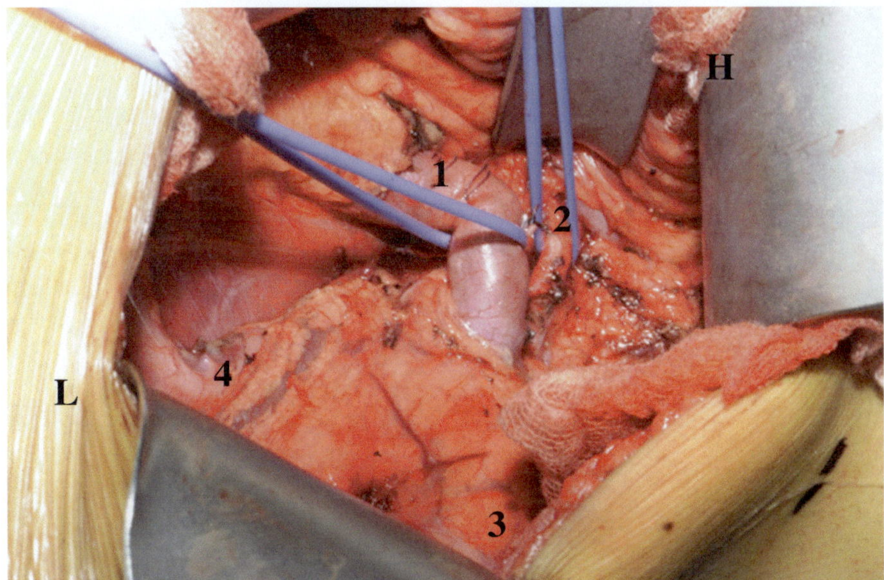

**Fig. 2.81** Left kidney renal vessel dissection—the first one to be prepared is the renal vein, the next one is the renal artery. The adrenal vein is tied up right next to the renal vein, closed right next to the adrenal gland with three clips and divided with scissors. 1—Renal vein, 2—Renal artery, 3—Kidney, 4—Ureter, L—Left side, H—Head

**Warning! (Golden triangle)**

Remember that when preparing the ureter and lower pole of the kidney, the so-called golden triangle (i.e. the arterial blood supply of the ureter) should not be disturbed. Tissues surrounding the ureter contain small vessels which come from the renal artery which is responsible for the arterial blood supply to the ureter. These small vessels are located between the lower and upper pole, renal pelvis and ureter. The idea is to keep the ureter well supplied with blood as long as possible during the kidney procurement for transplantation (Fig. 1.14 and also Sect. 1.5).

11. Using a large angled clamp and diathermy mobilize the kidney entirely from the retroperitoneal space. Reduce as much perirenal fat as possible at the beginning of the procedure. The fat reduction around the kidney will give the kidney more space in the retroperitoneum and more possibilities to change its position during the prepartion of the renal vessels and kidney.
12. First the renal vein is dissected free, then the renal artery (both sides). They are taken apart in the vessel loop. The adrenal vein is ligated close to the renal vein and closed with three clips next to the adrenal gland (left kidney) (Fig. 2.81).
13. The ureter is closed, below the iliac vessels, with two titanium clips and then cut 3–5 mm above the closure (Fig. 2.82).

                                                    

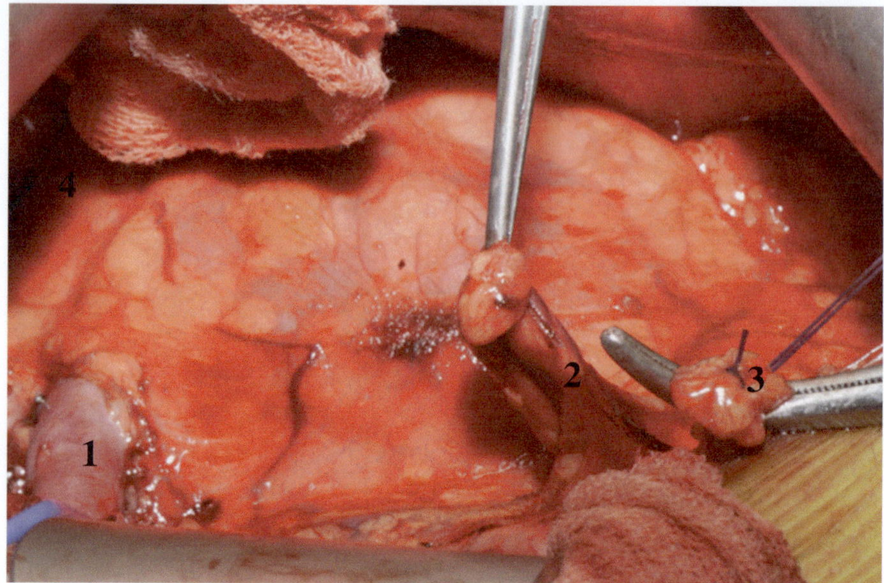

**Fig. 2.82** The ureter is closed, below the iliac vessels with two titanium clips or tied and then cut about 3–5 mm above the closure. 1—Left renal vein, 2—Ureter mobilized and cut, 3—Distal ureter below left iliac vessels, tied, 4—Left kidney

14. The renal artery is closed first (three large tantalum clips are placed one after the other, starting 3 mm from the aortic wall), immediately after that the renal vein is closed with a vascular clamp (Fig. 2.83). The artery is cut first (2–3 mm from the last clip applied) and then the renal vein. Finally, the kidney is removed from the retroperitoneal space and perfused (Fig. 2.84). The kidney preservation consists of an arterial kidney perfusion with cold preservation solution perfusion; the procured kidney is always placed in a bowl submerged with a cold preservation solution and sterile crushed ice (external cooling).

**Warning! (Closing the renal artery. How I do it)**
Closing the renal artery with a clamp and titanium clips is very safe, but requires a lot of experience. Early on as a first technique I ligated the renal artery, then I put a clip on the ligature and beyond. For more than 15 years I have been closing renal arteries with three clips—without any problems for kidney donors.

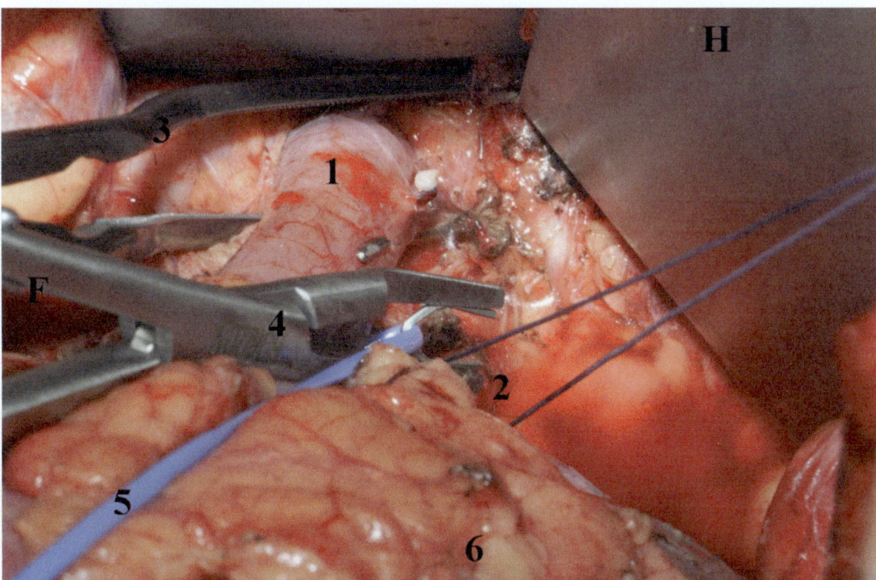

Fig. 2.83   The renal artery is closed first (three titanium large clips are placed one after another starting 3 mm from the aortic wall), immediately afterwards the renal vein is closed with a vascular clamp. 1—Left renal vein, 2—Left renal artery, 3—Vascular clamp closing renal vein, 4—Large clip applier, 5—Vessel loop placed around renal artery, 6—Left kidney, H—Head, F—Towards feet

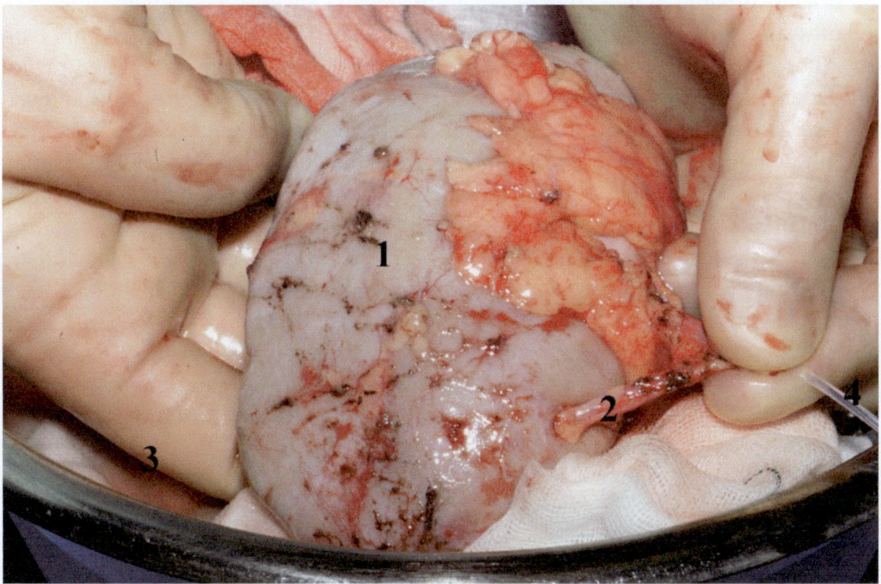

Fig. 2.84   The kidney has been retrieved from the extra-peritoneal space and perfused with a cold preservation solution. 1—Left kidney, 2—Aberrant renal artery, 3—Container with cold saline solution and ice, 4—Soft silicone tube inserted into the upper pole of the renal artery lumen for perfusion on the back table

**For how to safely close the renal arteries with surgical vascular clips, follow the steps below.**

a. In CT, pay attention to the presence of atherosclerotic plaques in the ostium and in the lumen at the beginning of the renal artery.

b. During kidney retrieval, carefully palpate the ostium of the renal artery from the aorta for the atherosclerosis plaque in this place.

c. The renal artery should be closed from the abdominal aorta towards the hilum and the titanium closing clips should be closed beyond the atherosclerotic plaque if the opening of the renal artery is atherosclerotic. Closing the renal artery in the presence of hard plaque in its lumen can lead to the dramatic cutting of the artery and unmanageable hemorrhage. My way of closing the renal artery is that I never close it on the plaque. If the ostium of the renal artery is unchanged, I put the first clip 3 mm from the ostium of the renal artery in the following sequence starting from the aorta towards the renal hilum. The first clip I close only about 80–90%; 1–2 mm further on I put the second clip and close the artery 90–95%; only with the third clip do I gently close the renal artery completely. The artery is cut with scissors 2–3 mm from the last clip. The lumen of the renal vein is sutured with unabsorbable monofilament suture 5/0 from top to bottom and vice versa. The left renal vein, the lumen of which has previously been closed with a suture, is ligated with a 0 ligature made of a soluble material. A stump of right renal vein after placing a clamp on the IVC, the right renal vein is cut off at the level of the IVC wall. The opening in the IVC is sutured by hand two times from top to bottom with the same 5/0 non-absorbable suture, which generally results in very good hemostasis and prevents unnecessary blood loss, while protecting the donor from air embolism.

16. After complete hemostasis, the area of the removed kidney is drained or not, depending on the amount of blood lost and the degree of hemostasis achieved.

17. The wound is sutured with soluble monofilament sutures in layers, in the following order: posterior lamina of the rectus abdominis, anterior lamina, subcutaneous tissue and skin, which is sutured with continuous soluble monofilament intracutaneous suture (Figs. 2.85 and 2.86).

18. After rinsing for blood and cooling, the kidney is packed according to the national packing protocol into three bags and a transport box, where it is signed and ice-covered. The transport box is then closed (Fig. 2.87).

19. A living donor kidney in most cases does not require pre-transplant inspection, but sometimes we need to reconstruct the veins and/or renal arteries. Do this always in a bowl which is submerged in cold preservation solution with added sterile ice (Fig. 2.88) [51–58].

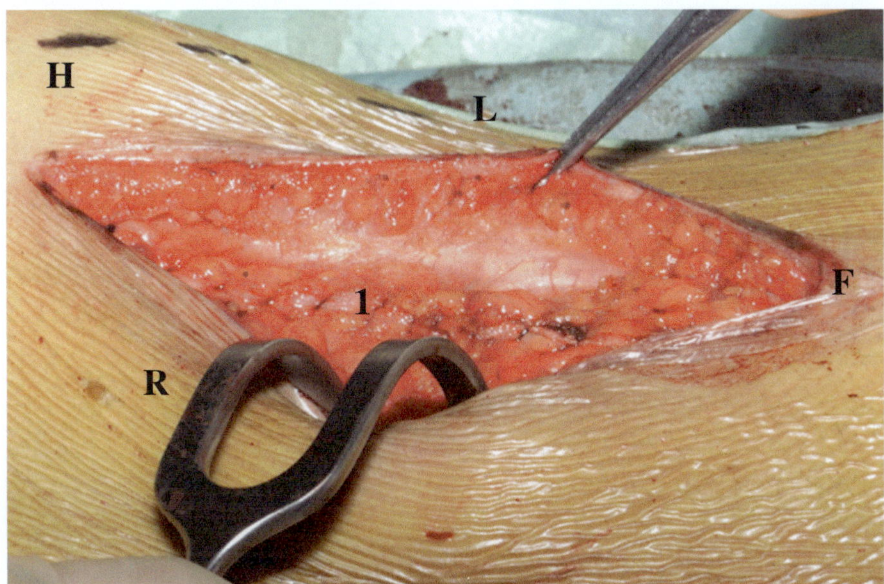


**Fig. 2.85**  The wound is sutured with absorbable monofilament sutures in layers, in the following order: posterior and anterior sheath of the rectus muscle, subcutaneous tissue and skin, which is sutured with continuous absorbable monofilament intracutaneous suture. 1—Sutured subcutaneous tissues, R—Right side, L—Left side, H—Head, F—Feet

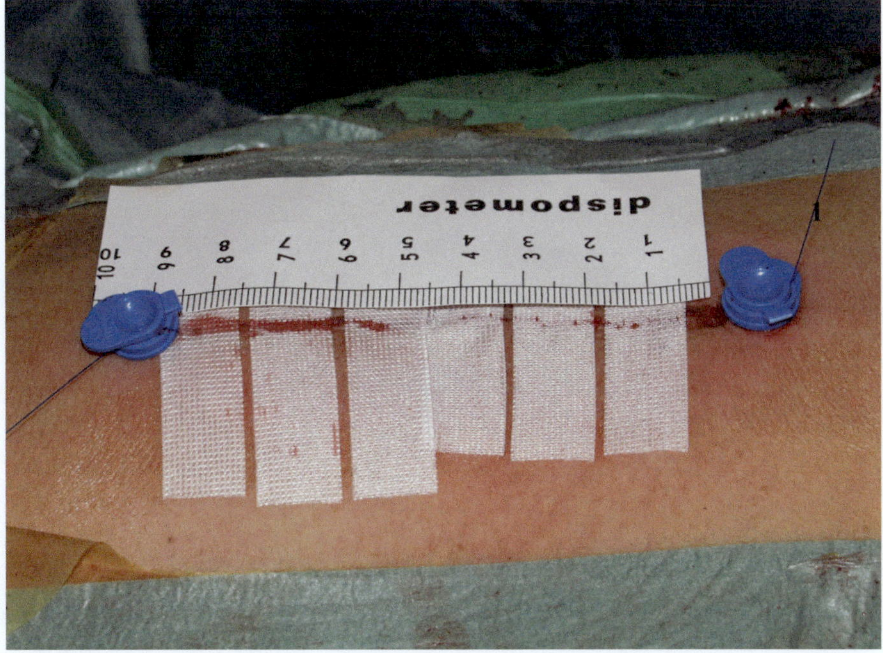


**Fig. 2.86**  1—Completely sutured wound after kidney donation from a living donor, open method, mini-invasive, retroperitoneal

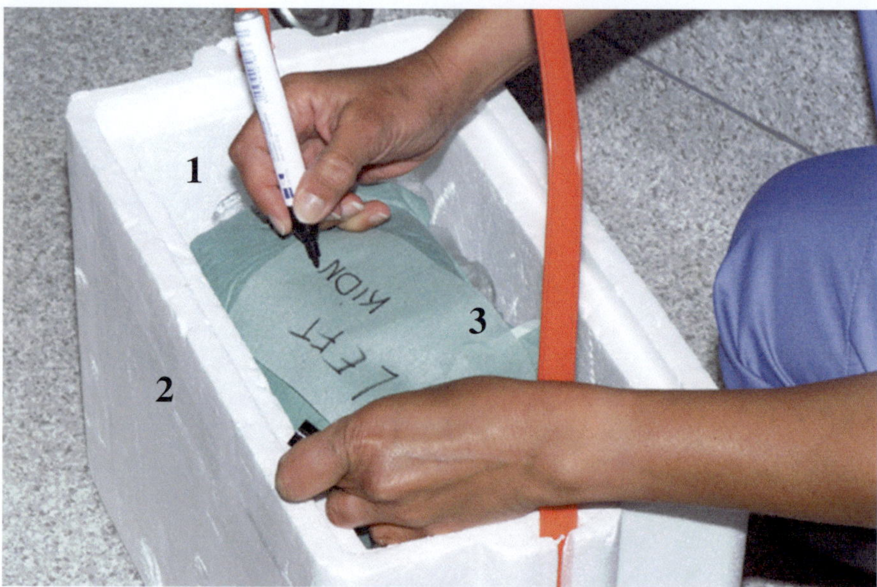

**Fig. 2.87** After kidney retrieval, the kidney is packed according to the national packing protocol into three bags, wrapped, marked and placed on ice in a special transport box. 1—Ice, 2—Transport box, 3—Left kidney packed according protocol

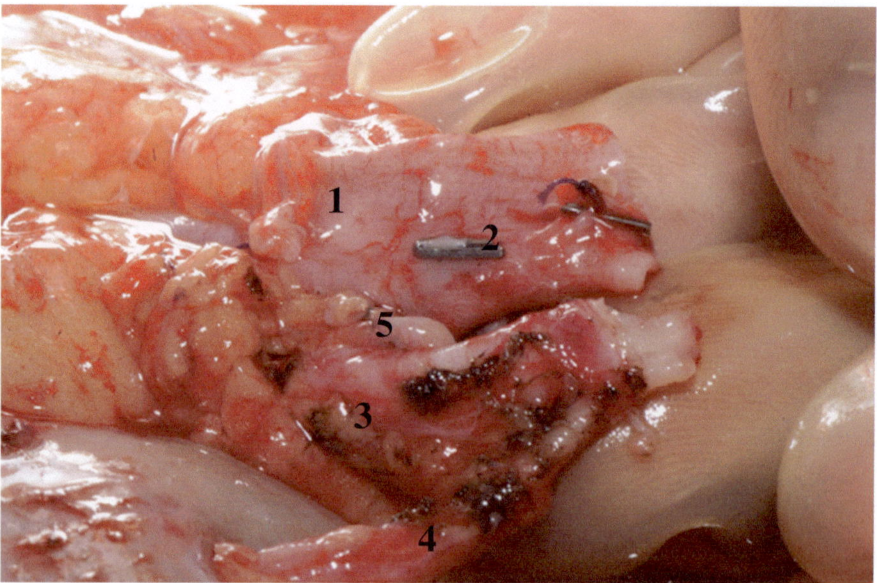

**Fig. 2.88** A kidney procured from a living donor in most cases does not need to be inspected before transplantation, but sometimes we need to reconstruct the renal veins and/or arteries or remove vascular clip(s) to replace them with nonabsorbable ligatures or stitches. 1—Left renal vein, 2—Small vascular clip: before a kidney transplant it is better to remove it and replace it with a safer vascular suture (stitch) or ligate, 3—Main trunk of the renal artery, 4—Aberrant upper pole renal artery, 5—Fat

# References


1. Habets LJM, Helm van dem D, Ramdhani K, Haasnoot A, Vries de APJ, Alwayn IPJ, Baranski AG, Schaapherder AFM, Huurman VAL. Non-muscle splitting MINI donor nephrectomy remains a safe option in the laparoscopic era of live kidney donation. Abstract Bootcongres, Dutch Transplant Foundation. 2021.
2. Thuong M, Ruiz A, Evrard P, Kuiper M, Boffa C, Akhtar MZ, Neuberger J, Ploeg R. New classification of donation after circulatory death donors definitions and terminology. Transpl Int. 2016;29:749–759.
3. Kootstra G, Daemen JHC, Oomen APA. Categories of non-heart-beating donors.Transplant Proc 1995; 27: 2893.
4. Antoine C, Brun F, Tenaillon A, Loty B. Organ procurement and transplantationfrom non heart beating donors. Nephrol. Therap. 2008;4(5):6.
5. Nolan JP, Laver SR, Welch CA, Harrison DA, Gupta V, Rowan K. Outcome following admission to UK intensive care units after cardiac arrest: a secondary analysis of the ICNARC Case Mix Program Database. Anesthesia. 2007;62:1207.
6. Goldberger ZD, Chan PS, Berg RA, et al. Duration of resuscitation efforts and survival after in-hospital cardiac arrest: an observational study. Lancet. 2012;380:1473.
7. Summers DM, Watson CJE, Pettigrew GJ, Johnson RJ, Collett D, NeubergerJM, Andrew Bradley J. Kidney donation after circulatory death (DCD): state of the art. Kidney Int. 2015;88(2):241–249.Kidney donation after circulatory death (DCD): state of the art. Kidney Int. 2015;88(2):241–249.
8. Langhelle A, Tyvold SS, Lexow K, HapnesSA, Sunde K, Steen PA. In-hospital factors associated with improved outcome after out-of-hospital cardiac arrest. A comparison between four regions in Norway. Resuscitation 2003;56:247.10.
9. Shemie SD, Baker AJ, Knoll G, et al. National recommendations for donation after cardiocirculatory death in Canada. Can Med Assoc J. 2006;175:S1.
10. Manara AR, Murphy PG, O'Callaghan G. Donation after circulatory death.Br J Anaesth 2012; 108(Suppl. 1):i108.
11. Sanchez-Fructuoso Al, Marques MPD, Conesa J, et al. Victims of cardiac arrest occurring outside the hospital: a source of transplantable kidneys. Ann Intern Med. 2006;145:157.
12. Detry O, Le Dinh H, Noterdaemer T, et al. Categories of donation after cardiocirculatory death. Transplant Proc. 2012;44:1189.
13. Dominguez-Gil B, Delmonico FL, Shaheen FA, et al. The critical pathway for deceased donation: report able uniformity in the approach to deceased donation. Transpl Int. 2011;24:373.
14. Dominguez-Gil B, Haase-Kromwijk B, Van Leiden H, et al. Current situation of donation after circulatory death in European countries. Transpl Int. 2011;24:676.
15. Sohrabi S, Navarro A, Asher J, et al. Agonal period in potential non-heart-beating donors. Transplant Proc. 2006;38:2629.
16. Bernat JL, D'Alessandro AM, Port FK,et al. Report of a National Conference on donation after cardiac death. Am Journal Transplant 2006; 6: 281.
17. Donation after circulatory death. Report of a Consensus Meeting. Donation after circulatory death steering group. Br Transplant Soc Intensiv Care Soc. http://www.bts.org.uk/transplantation/standards-and-guidelines.
18. Hornby K, Hornby L, Shemie SD. A systematic review of autoresuscitation after cardiac arrest. Crit Care Med. 2010;38:1246.
19. Ausania F, White SA, Pocock P, Manas DM. Kidney damage during organ recovery in donation after circulatory death donors: data from UK national transplant database. Am J Transplant: Off J Am Soc Transplant Am Soc Transpl Surg. 2012;12:932.
20. Smith M, Dominguez-Gil B, Greer DM, Manara AR, Souter MJ. Organ donation after circulatory death: current status and future potential. Intensive Care Med. 2019;45(3):310–21.

21. Manyalich M, Nelson H, Delmonico FL. The need and opportunity for donation after circulatory death worldwide. Curr Opin Organ Transpl. 2018;23(1):136–41.
22. Hosgood, Sarah A, Nicholson, Michael L. The evolution of donation after circulatory death donor kidney repair in the United Kingdom, Curr Opin Organ Transplant. 2018;23(1):130–135.
23. Baker RJ, Watson ChJE. Renal transplantation. Medicine. 2019; 47(10):625–635.
24. Baranski AG, Lam H-D. A modified, rapid and safe technique of kidney only procurement from donors after circulatory and brain death (DCD, DBD). OJOTS. 2016;6:23–8.
25. Starzl TE, Miller C, Broznick B, Makowka L. An improved technique for multiple organ harvesting. Surg, Gynecol & Obstet. 1987;165:343.
26. Starzl TE, Hakala TR, Shaw BW Jr, Hardesty RL, Rosenthal TJ, Griffith BP, et al. A flexible procedure for multiple cadaveric organ procurement. Surg, Gynecol & Obstet. 1984;158:223.
27. Wigmore SJ, Seeney FM, Pleass HC, Praseedom RK, Forsythe JL. Kidney damage during organ retrieval: data from UK national transplant database, vol. 354. Lancet (London, England): Kidney Advisory Group; 1999, p. 1143.
28. Castelo D, Campos L, Moreira P, Furriel F, Parada B, Nunes P, et al. Does multiorgan versus kidney-only cadaveric organ procurement affect graft outcomes? Transpl Proc. 2013;45:1248.
29. Goldsmith PJ, Ridgway DM, Pine JK, Speak G, Newstead C, Lewington AJ, et al. Outcomes following renal transplantation after multiorgan retrieval versus kidney-only retrieval in donation after cardiac death donors. Transpl Proc. 2010;42:3963.
30. Eschwege P, Droupy S, Blanchet P, Hammoudi Y, Laassou K, Hadj AE, et al. Surgical injuries occurring during kidney procurement performed by a renal transplantation team. Transpl Proc. 2002;34:844.
31. Baranski AG. Surgical technique of abdominal organ procurement. Springer; 2009, ISBN: 9781848002500.
32. Baranski AG, Kramer WLM. Chirurgische technieken voor het uitnemen van de abdominale organen bij pediatrische donoren. Handboek Kindertraumatologie. Bohn Stafleu van Loghum. 2019, Chap. 20, pp. 215–233(in Dutch), ISBN: 9789036818698.
33. Baranski AG, Lam H-D, Braat AE. The dorsal pancreatic artery in pancreas procurement and transplantation: anatomical considerations and potential implications. Clin Transplant. 2016;30:1360–1364.
34. Shaffer D, Lewis WD, Jenkins RL, Monaco AP. Combined liver and whole pancreas procurement in donors with a replaced right hepatic artery. Surg Gynecol Obstet. 1992;175:204–7.
35. Ville de Goyet J de, Hausleithner V, Malaise J, et al. Liver procurement without in situ portal perfusion: a safe procedure for more flexible multiple organ harvesting. Transplantation. 1994;57:1328–32.
36. de Ville de Goyet J, Reding R, Hausleithner V et al. Standardized quick en bloc technique for procurement of cadaveric liver grafts for pediatric liver transplantation. Transplant Int. 1995;8:280–285.
37. Squifflet JP. A quick technique for en bloc liver and pancreas procurement Transp. Int. 1995;9:520–1.
38. Imagawa DK, Olthoff KM, Yersiz H, et al. Rapid en bloc technique for pancreas-liver procurement. Improved early liver function. Transplantation. 1996;61:1605–9.
39. Hirshberg A, Mattox KL. The crash laparotomy. The top knife the art & craft of trauma surgery. Castle Hill Barns, Harley, Shrewsbury Harely: Publishing Ltd; 2005. p. 53–70.
40. Cattel R, Braasch J. A technique for the exposure of the third and fourth portion of the duodenum. Surg Gynecol Obstet. 1960;11:379.
41. Nghiem DD. Rapid exenteration for multiorgan harvesting: a new technique for the unstable donor. Transplant Proc. 1996;28:256–7.
42. Abu-Elmagd K, Fung J, Bueno J, et al. Logistics and technique for procurement of intestinal, pancreatic, and hepatic grafts from the same donor. Ann Surg. 2000;232:680–7.
43. Pinna AD, Dodson FS, Smith CV et al. Rapid en bloc technique for liver and pancreas procurement. Transplant Proc. 1997;29:647–.

44. Jan D, Renz JF. Donor selection and procurement of multivisceral and isolated intestinal allografts. Curr Opin Organ Transplant. 2005;10:136–47.

45. Molmenti EE, Molmenti P, Molmenti H, et al. Cannulation of the aorta in organ donors with infrarenal. Pathologies, Digestieve Diseases and Science. 2001;46(11):2457–245.

46. Wigmore SJ, Seeney FM, Pleass HC, Praseedom RK, Forsythe JL. Kidney damage during organ retrieval: data from uk national transplant database, vol. 354. Lancet (London, England): Kidney Advisory Group, p. 1143.

47. Ausania F, White SA, Pocock P, Manas DM. Kidney damage during organ recovery in donation after circulatory death donors: data from UK National Transplant Database. Am J Transplant. 2012;12(4):932–6. https://doi.org/10.1111/j.1600-6143.2011.03882.x Epub 2012 Jan 6 PMID: 22225959.

48. Salaman J.R., Clarke A.G., Crosby D.L The management of kidney transplants damaged during their removal from the donor. Br. J. Urol. 1974; 46: 173–177.

49. Signori S, Boggi U, Vistoli F, et al. Regional procurement team for abdominal organs. Transplant Proc. 2004;36(3):435–6.

50. Eschwege P, Droupy S, Blanchet P, Hammoudi Y, Laassou K, Hadj AE, et al. Surgical injuries occurring during kidney procurement performed by a renal transplantation team. Transpl Proc. 2001;34:844.

51. Habets LJM, Van der Helm D, Ramdhani K, Haasnoot A, Dam R APJ, de Vries Braat AE, Dubbeld J, Lam HD Nijboer WN, De Vries DK, Alwayn IPJ, Baranski AG, Schaapherder AFM, Huurman VAL. The non-muscle splitting mini-open donor nephrectomy is a safe alternative in the laparoscopic era of live kidney donation. Abstract sent for Botcongers of Dutch Transplant Foundation in 2021.

52. Subramanian T, Dageforde LA, Vachharajani N, Wellen J, Doyle MBM, Lin Y, Khan A, Senter-Zapata M, Chapman W, Shenoy S. Mini-incision versus hand-assisted laparoscopic donor nephrectomy in living-donor kidney transplantation: a retrospective cohort study. Int J Surg. 2018;53:339–44.

53. Ratner LE, Ciseck LJ, Moore RG, Cigarroa FG, Kaufman HS, Kavoussi LR. Laparoscopic live donor nephrectomy. Transplantation. 1995;60:1047–9.

54. Kok NFM, Alwayn IPJ, Lind MY, Tran KTC, Weimar W, IJzermans JNM. Donor nephrectomy: mini-incision muscle-splitting open approach versus laparoscopy. Transplantation. 2006;81:881–887.

55. W.R. Halgrimson, J. Campsen, M.S. Mandell, M.A. Kelly, I. Kam, M.A. Zimmerman; Donor complications following laparoscopic compared to hand-assisted living donor nephrectomy: an analysis of the literature. J. Transplant. 2010;2010:825689.

56. Yadav K, Aggarwal S, Guleria S, Kumar R. Comparative study of laparoscopic and mini-incision open donor nephrectomy: have we heard the last word in the debate? Clin Transplant. 2016;30:328–34.

57. Neipp M., Jackobs S., Becker T. i wsp. Living donor nephrectomy: flank incision versus anterior vertical mini-incision. Transplantation. 2004; 78: 1356–1361.

58. Yang SL, Harkaway R, Badosa F, et al. Minimal incision living donor nephrectomy: improvement in patient outcome. Urology. 2002;59:673–7.

# Further Reading

59. Manuals hypothermic machine perfusions : LifePort Kidney Transporter 1.1 Operator's Manual. https://4fetz713plu53drexe2d10ht-wpengine.netdna-ssl.com/wp-content/uploads/2020/10/755-00002-Rev-P-LKT101-Operators-Manual.pdf.

60. Kidney assist—stark medical empower the healer. https://www.starkmed.com.au/pages/kidney-assist-organ-perfusion-system.

61. Bridge to Life: https://bridgetolife.eu/wp-content/uploads/english-4088-eu-belzer-mps-ifu-070820.pdf.

62. Damji S, Callaghan CJ, Loukopoulos I, et al. Utilisation of small paediatric donor kidneys for transplantation. Pediatr Nephrol. 2019;34:1717–26. https://doi.org/10.1007/s00467-018-4073-5.
63. Baranski AG, Kramer WLM. Chirurgische technieken voor het uitnemen van de abdominale organen bij pediatrische donoren. Handboek Kindertraumatologie. Bohn Stafleu van Loghum. 2019, Chap. 20, page 215–233 (in Dutch), ISBN—9789036818698.
64. Baranski AG. Surgical technique of Abdominal Organ Procurement, Springer 2009, ISBN—9781848002500.
65. Baranski AG, Lam H-D. A Modified, rapid and safe technique of kidney only procurement from donors after circulatory and brain death (DCD, DBD). OJOTS. 2016; 6:23–28.

# Chapter 3
# Kidney Transport, Inspection and Preparation for Transplantation

## 3.1 Introduction: Some Definitions

Currently, the literature often uses terms that I have mentioned, such as bench surgery, inspection, preparation and back table. I wanted to find a phrase or English phrases which, despite the fact that they are often used in the literature, will correspond most closely to the stage in which the procured, sent and transplanted kidney is prepared for transplantation. Here I have cited parts of the definitions that most relate to the preparation of organs prior to the transplantation. I have taken all definitions from the Free Dictionary by Farlex and the Cambridge and Oxford Dictionary [1, 2].

**Bench surgery** is performed on an organ that has been removed from the body and repaired at the site, after which it is reimplanted back into the body. This is also called ex vivo surgery.

**Inspection** is the act of looking at something carefully to check its quality or condition, or to scrutinize, or to make an official visit to a building or organization to check that everything is correct and legal.

**Preparation** means "a substance especially prepared" for the things that you do or the time that you spend preparing for something. Preparations are made to prevent hemorrhage after reperfusion of the donor organ. The vascular anatomy is assessed and reconstructed prior to the implantation of the donor organ.

**Back table procedure/preparation** is an operation performed on an organ that has been removed from a patient before it is replaced; or it is defined as preparing the donor organ following procurement and prior to transplantation into the recipient. The back table is used to remove excess donor tissue and adequately prepare the allograft for implantation.

Following these definitions we may say that the preparation of the kidney before transplant is as follows: inspection, preparation, back table procedure and

© The Author(s), under exclusive license to Springer Nature Switzerland AG 2023

A. Baranski, *Kidney Transplantation*,

https://doi.org/10.1007/978-3-030-75886-8_3

preparation. Bench surgery is more suited to describe the repair procedures of the same organs performed outside the human body, which are implanted in the same place after repair. The organ donor and recipient are the same person [1–4].

## 3.2  Shipping a Kidney from the Donor to the Recipient's Hospital

The transport of each procured organ from the donor's to the recipient's hospital must be organized professionally and safely. The transplant coordinator is responsible for organizing and coordinating the transport of the procured organs to centers that have accepted these organs. If the transport is prolonged for one reason or another, the coordinator, in consultation with the recipient's hospital and the police, obtains a permit to transport the organs to the recipient's hospital by ambulance with high speed and flashing warning lights and sirens. In order to ensure that the organ(s) reach their destination safely, the transplant coordinator should choose the means of transport that will provide the fastest and safest delivery of the organ to the accepting (recipient) center. Well-organized transport reduces the time of total organ ischemia time, which in turn affects the length of the patient's stay in the hospital and the patient's and organ's survival. The most common means of transport is an ambulance that is well-marked for this purpose.

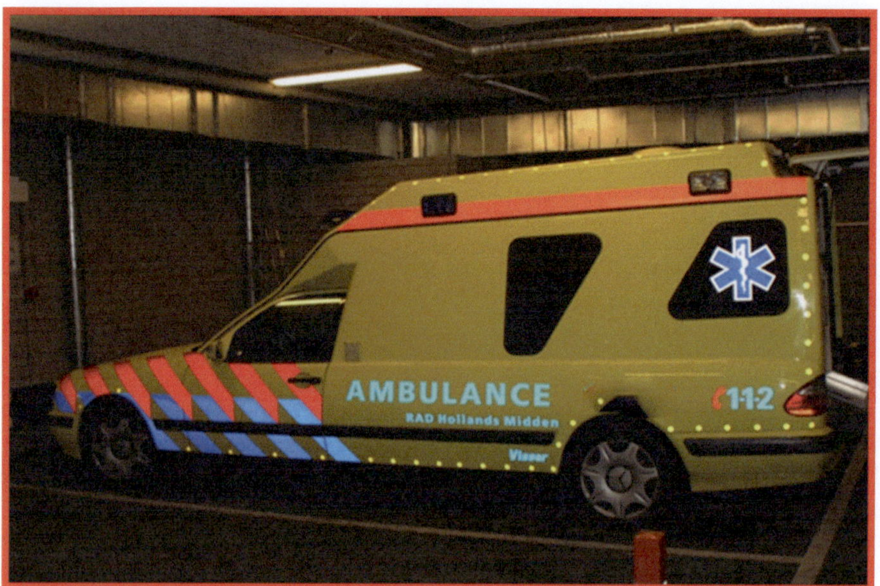


**Fig. 3.1** A well-marked and safe ambulance is the most common means of transport used to convey collected organs to the hospital of the recipient

Other modes of transport, such as helicopters, airplanes and ships, are rarely and only under extreme circumstances used (Fig. 3.1).

During the organ transportation the hospital should be informed of the means of transport, how long it will take, where and when the organ will be deposited in the hospital and who will be the first to be informed of the arrival of the organ [3, 4].

In hospitals where one or more organs are transplanted, there should be a designated area where the retrieved organ(s) is(are) left under constant specialist care. In all organ transplant hospitals in the Netherlands, in order to avoid unnecessary mistakes, a protocol for the delivery of an organ to the recipient's hospital has been developed. I will briefly describe this system. The organ for the transplantation is initially handed over to the hospital security by the ambulance driver. The hospital security notifies the transplant surgeon, the nephrologist and the staff of the immunological laboratory. The immunology technician goes to the hospital security and takes the transport container with the kidney to the laboratory where the parameters of the donor and recipient are first checked. Depending on the situation, the staff of the immunological laboratory will remove the spleen and/or the lymph nodes, serum and/or blood of the donor from the transport container—if the recipient is highly immunized or otherwise indicated, a crossmatch is performed prior to transplantation. The immunology laboratory personnel are trained and responsible for maintaining complete sterility while opening the organ transport box. In the immunology laboratory, after carrying out the necessary steps to remove certain materials, the transport container is closed again and with the kidney is then transported to the permanent storage place at the transplant department. The hospital security officer, the on-duty nephrologist or other qualified personnel notify the time of the organ's arrival at the place of permanent storage. If a cross-match must be performed, the result is notified to the on-call transplant surgeon and nephrologist. After the organ arrives in the transport box at the permanent storage place, specially trained nurses for these purposes open it and check the amount of ice and the condition of the kidney packing (Fig. 3.2). If there is any fluid leakage from any of the bags, the transplant surgeon is immediately informed. The surgeon transports the kidney to the operating room, where it is immediately inspected and sterile repacked into new bags according to the national protocol for packing organs intended for transplant. If the bags in which the organ is packed are intact, preservation solution for bacterial examination is taken from the first bag in which the organ is stored. The newly sterile packed kidney is placed in a new transport container—the old one is wet and therefore non-sterile and usually for some days unusable. If nothing leaks and the packaging is dry, the transport box with the kidney is opened in order to add ice in it, so as to maintain the proper storage conditions for the organ. At the same time, nephrologists, anesthesiologists, scrub nurses and operating theater staff prepare the operating room for the organ inspection and later for the transplantation [5].

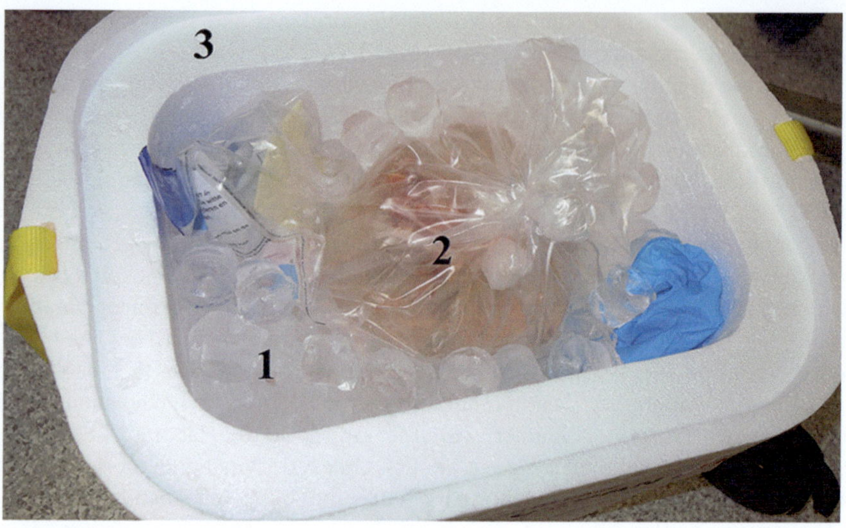



**Fig. 3.2** At a separate location in the transplantology ward, the transport box is opened upon arrival. Specially trained personnel check the amount of ice and the state of packaging of the organ, with particular attention paid to the leakage of any liquid from the last bag. 1—Ice, 2—Kidney packed in three bags, 3—Transport box

## 3.3   Kidney Transport to the Operating Room

After the kidney arrives at the recipient hospital, and if the crossmatch if necessary is performed (if mixing a very small amount of the patient's serum with a very small amount of the potential donor's white cells is negative) or does not need to be performed, the surgeon and the operating theater agree on the time of kidney inspection and preparation, the necessary instruments and the type of preservation fluid that will be used during the preparation (including the same preservation solution in which the kidney was preserved at the time of procurement). The surgeon and/or a transplant fellow or someone from the hospital security picks the kidney up from the permanent storage area for delivery to the operating theater [3–5].

## 3.4   Preparation of the Operating Room for Kidney Inspection Before Transplantation: Necessary Surgical Tools and Materials

After the kidney has been delivered to the operating room, the surgeon reads the organ quality rapport filled in by the procurement surgeon in the donor's hospital. The organ quality report forms the most important information on the donation process filled in by the procurement surgeon who informs the surgeon in the recipient's hospital about: general and clinical donor data; most recent medication and biochemistry; organ preservation (time of administration and given units of heparin, time to start cold perfusion of abdominal organs and portal vein, type of preservation solution, volume of preservation solution, time of first ischemia); anatomy of procured organ; organ quality; anatomical abnormalities such as one that is abnormal in size or location, or has abnormal morphology (color, size, form, consistency); number of renal arteries, veins, ureters and their morphological variations, degree of atherosclerosis in the renal arteries and the abdominal aorta wall; time of nephrectomy; type of perfusion solution; surgical injuries to the kidney (damage to the capsule, kidney parenchyma, kidney vessels or renal pelvis, ureter/ureters), presence of kidney cysts (what is their size), quality of kidney parenchyma; perfusion and preservation in general, in this regard assessment of organ quality and their suitability for transplantation. The kidney inspection takes place before kidney preparation for transplantation. Both procedures, just like the transplant itself, take place in the operating room under sterile conditions. The surgeon and the assistant prepare themselves for the kidney inspection and preparation. They both dress sterile and, after having prepared the operating room, alone or together with a scrub nurse or student or fellow, they begin the kidney

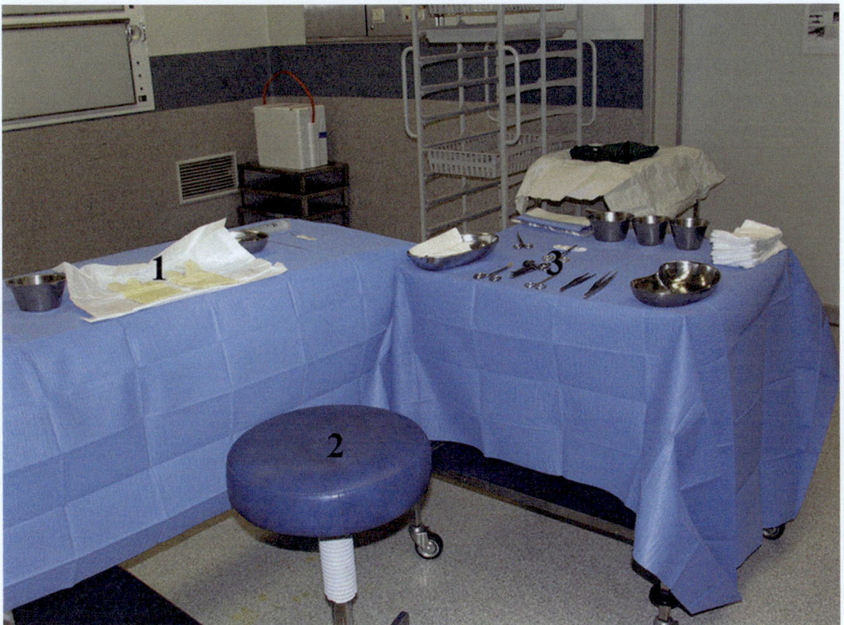


**Fig. 3.3** Operating room prepared for kidney inspection. One or both of the tables are covered with sterile napkins before the inspection. The kidney inspection is done sitting down. 1—Sterile surgical gloves, 2—Foot-adjustable surgical chair, 3—Surgical instruments necessary for kidney inspection

inspection and if the kidney is suitable for transplantation they will begin kidney preparation.

The operating tables and the surgical stools are covered with sterile drapes. Inspection and preparation of the kidney is done in a sitting position on specially adapted surgical stools with the possibility of foot adjustment of the surgeon's seat height. The necessary surgical instruments, gases, swabs, a container(s) or bowl(s) in which the kidney will be inspected and prepared, ice, fresh and cold organ preservation solution, syringes, drains and other objects necessary for kidney inspection will be stored on the table; the preservation solution in the transport box on ice or in refrigerator under conditions of full sterility (Figs. 3.3 and 3.4).

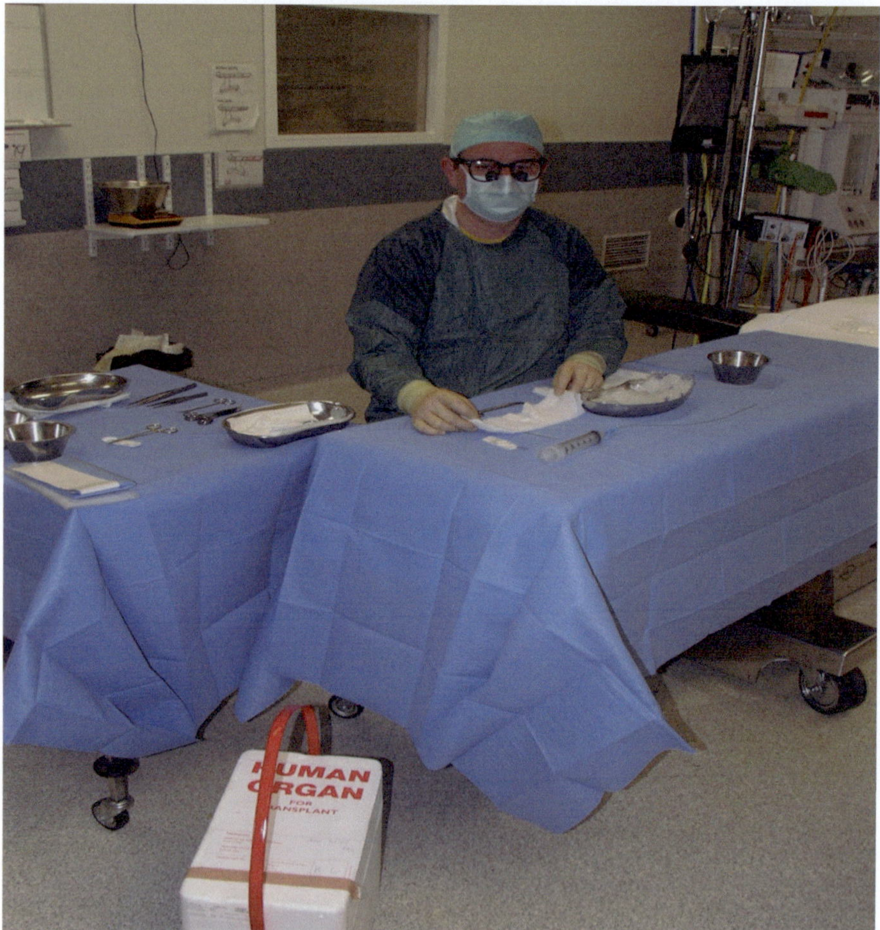


**Fig. 3.4** Kidney inspection in a sitting position. Therefore, to be fully comfortable, the surgeon and assistant need suitable chairs with a foot-adjustable seat height during the inspection and tables without leg bars. In conditions of full sterility, the necessary surgical instruments, gauze, small and suitable bowls (containers), ice, syringes, tubes, and other things necessary for kidney inspection are placed on the table

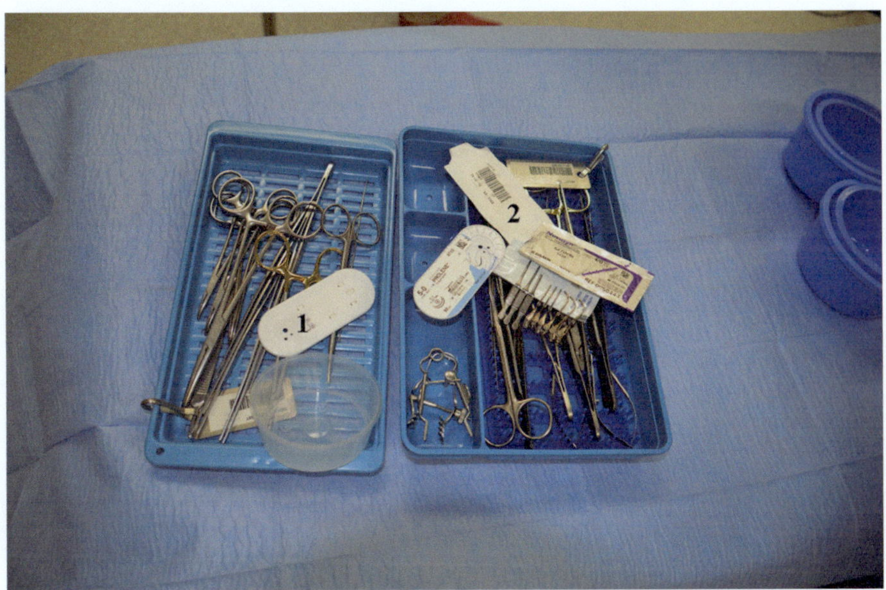

**Fig. 3.5**  Surgical instruments necessary for kidney inspection. 1—Basic set, used for basic kidney inspections not requiring vascular reconstruction, 2—Microsurgical instruments set used for microsurgical vascular reconstruction

Depending on the complexity of the kidney inspection, there is always a normal set available and a set of sterile microsurgical instruments on hand (Fig. 3.5) in case there is a need for complex reconstruction. All microsurgical reconstructive procedures are firstly intended to repair damaged renal vessels and ureters at the time of preparation on specially adapted sterile surgical tables—in such a way that the kidney can be transplanted with the lowest possible risk for its recipient. Secondly, all microsurgical reconstructive procedures are intend to reduce the number of vascular anastomosis in the recipient's body to a minimum—which means a minimum time of warm ischemia of the kidney during transplantation. In the

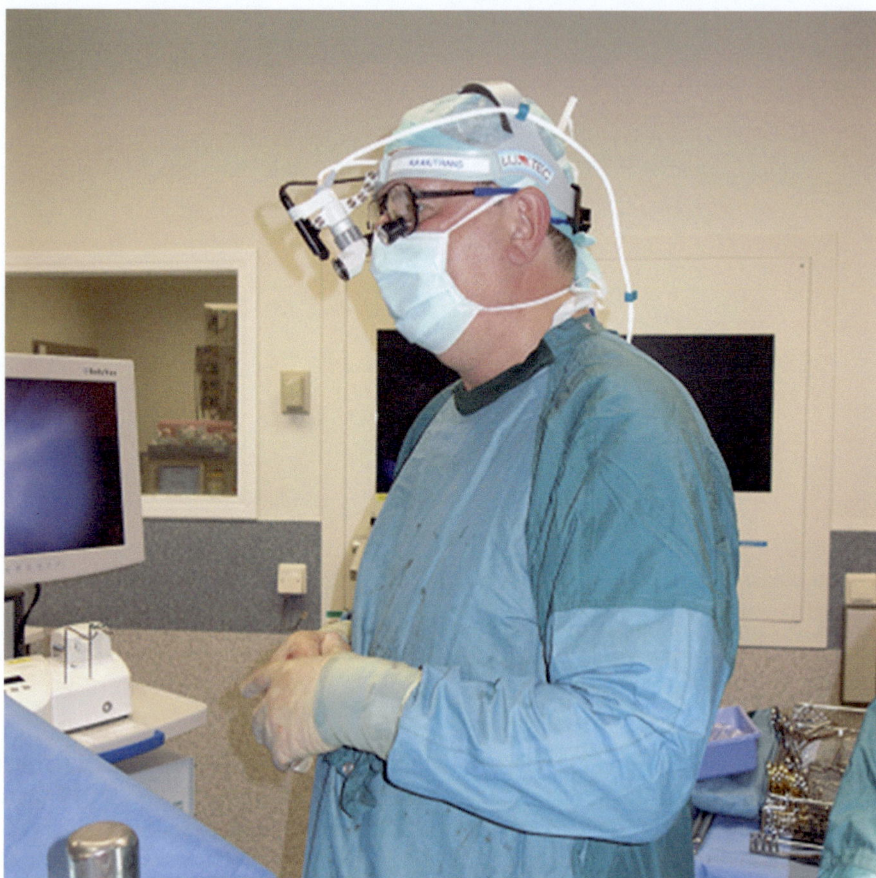

**Fig. 3.6** In the operating room, an essential and indispensable tool of a transplant surgeon must be a good quality surgical magnifying glasses with a magnification of at least 2.5 times, providing high comfort in preparing the kidney for transplantation

operating room, a necessary and indispensable tool of the transplant surgeon is good quality surgical magnifying glasses, magnifying at least 2.5 times, giving comfort and precision during the inspection (Fig. 3.6). Light in the operating room is always a topic of discussion: there are centers that do not use operating lamps during the inspection and preparation, in some centers the use of operating lamps is even strictly prohibited which is explained by the fact that during the inspection and preparation the lamps heat the organ. We and other centers use headlamps with cold light, which does not cause heating of the organ (Fig. 3.7).

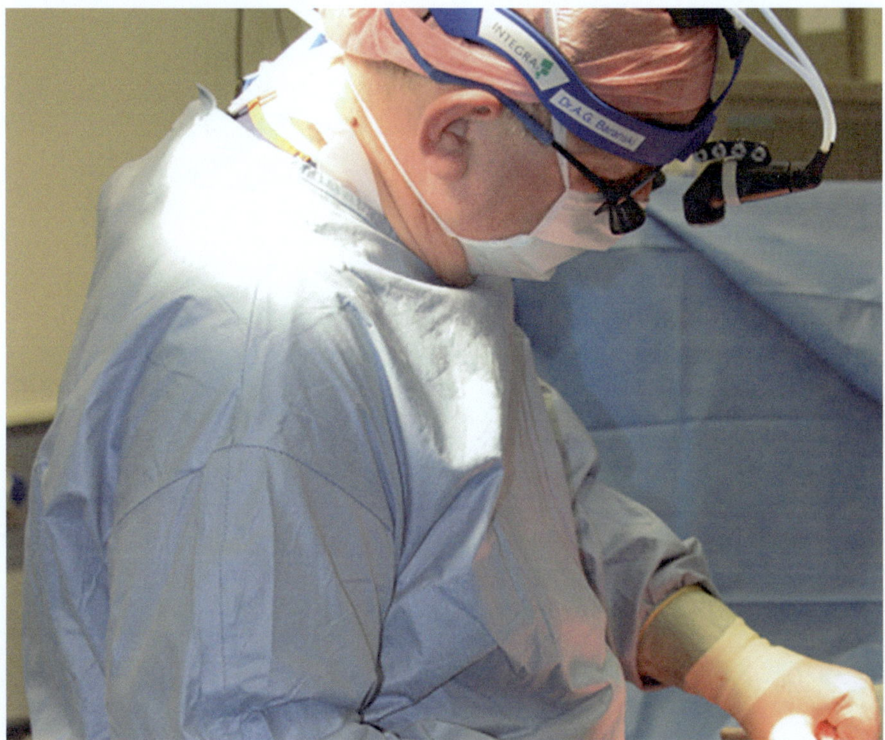

**Fig. 3.7** The surgical headlamp provides an independent light source. It is ideal for inspection of any organ especially if it generates cold light

## 3.5   Removing the Kidney from the Transport Box and the Bags (Unpacking Procedure)

On a specially adapted trolly, the organ transport box with a kidney is brought into the operating room (Fig. 3.8). The trained scrub nurse or the circulating nurse opens the organ transport box and removes the packed kidney. Taken from the transport box, the kidney, packed in three bags, is placed on the top of the operating trolley.

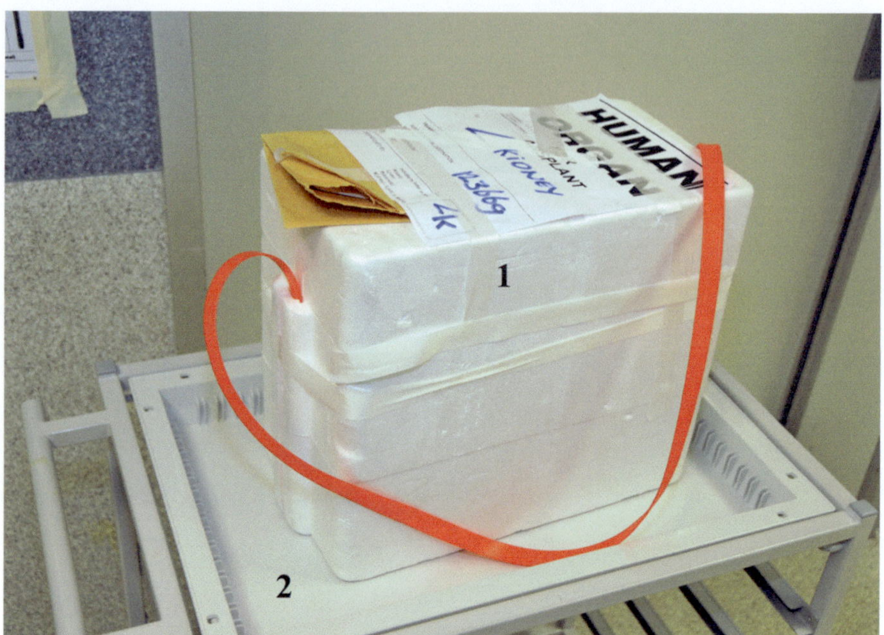



**Fig. 3.8** On a special table, a transport box with a kidney is brought into the operating room. 1—Transport box, 2—Operating theater transport table with movable shelves and moving wheels

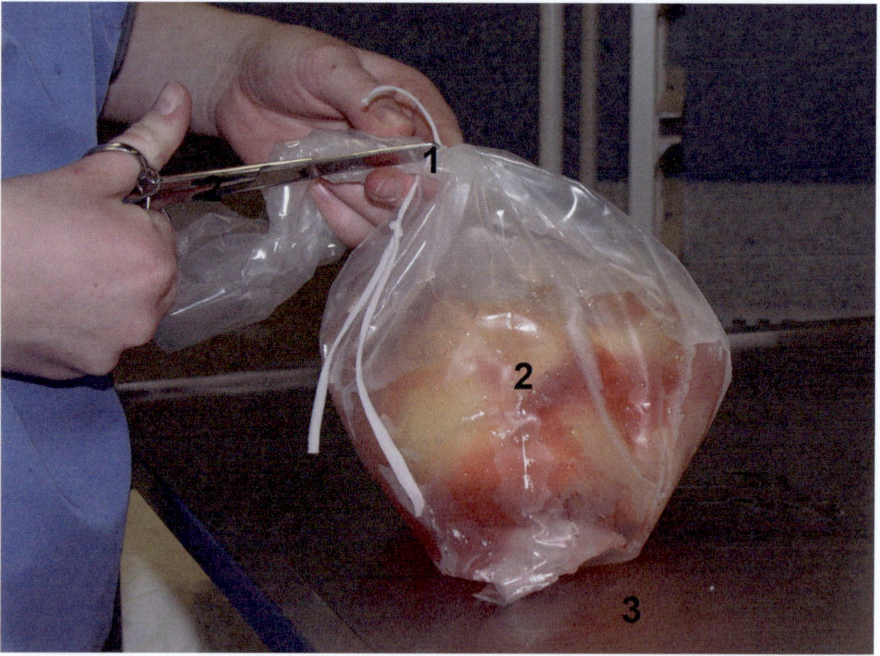



**Fig. 3.9** The nurse takes a kidney packed in three transport bags from the transport box. 1—Cutting the ribbon closing the third bag with scissors, 2—The third bag; the outside of the bag is non-sterile, and the inside is sterile from the bottom to the point where the ribbon is tied. 3—Top of the operating trolley

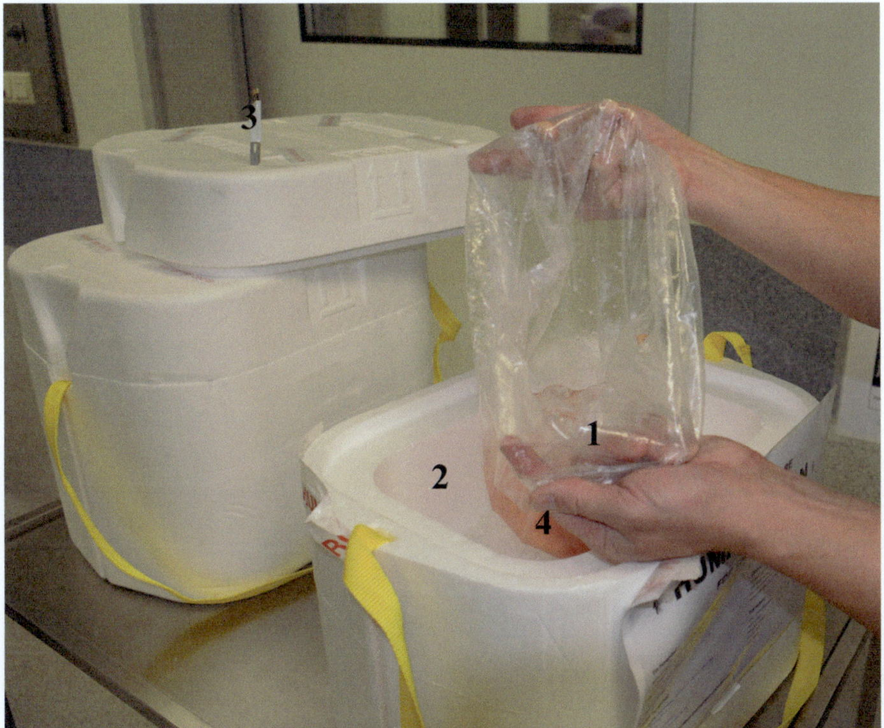

**Fig. 3.10**  The trained scrub nurse or the circulating nurse rolls the edges of the bag outwards in such a way as to retain the sterile inner side of the third bag, the so-called "dry" side not containing any liquid. 1—Third "dry" bag, 2—Transport box, 3—Scalpel placed into the transport box cover in case it is necessary to cut the ribbon (ligature), 4—Kidney removed: empty third bag

In order to sterilely remove a kidney packed in three bags the operating room nurse has to perform the following steps.

1. Cut off the closing ribbon of the first outer bag—this bag is not sterile from the outside (Fig. 3.9) and curl the edges of the first non-sterile bag on the outside so that the inner side of the bag remains sterile (Fig. 3.10).

**Warning! (Watch out for the kidney, don't drop it)**
When taking the packed kidney from the scrub nurse and removing it from the bags, you must be very careful that the kidney does not fall out of the bag on the sterile surgical table or on the unsterile floor of the operating room.

2. To maintain complete sterility, take the second sterile bag which is filled with cold Ringer solution or 0.9% NaCl solution and place it in a bowl filled with ice (Fig. 3.11).

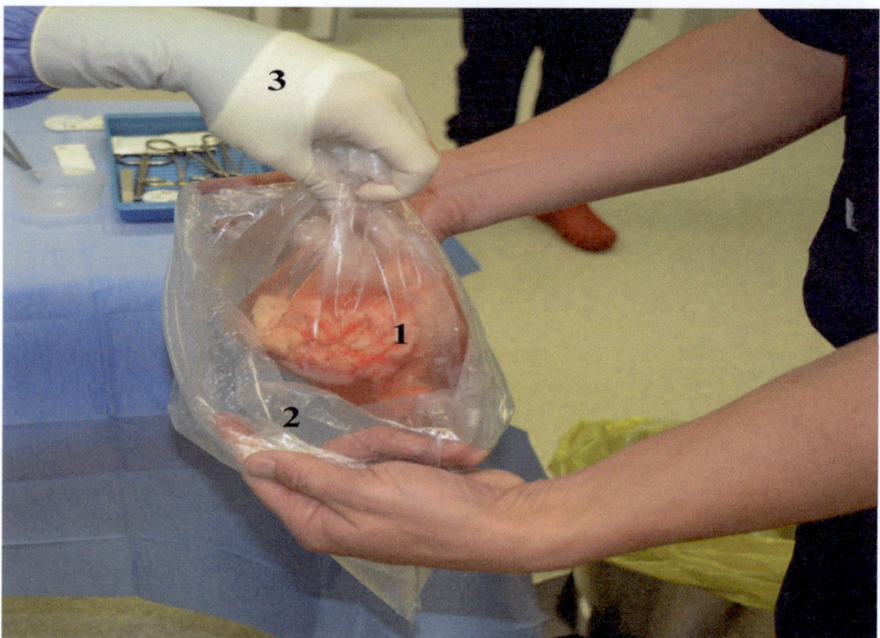

Fig. 3.11 The second dry bag is rolled outside to ensure the internal sterility of the bag. The surgeon dressed sterilely takes the kidney, which is packed in the first bag. 1—Kidney packed in first bag, 2—The walls of the second bag have been turned outwards, 3—A surgeon taking the kidney sterilely packed in the first bag which contains preservation solution

3. Cut the tape which closes the second bag with scissors or cut the bag off beneath the tape's knot (Fig. 3.12). After removing the second bag, the kidney is then only packed in the first bag which is filled with preservation solution. The second bag (with the sterile solution) is thrown away into the trashcan which is located close to the surgeon who is inspecting and preparing the kidney for transplantation (Fig. 3.13).
4. The first bag, in which the kidney is completely submerged in the preservation solution, is opened by the surgeon in the same way as the previous two bags. The first step to be done after opening the first bag is to take into a syringe 5–10 ml of the preservation solution (a sample) for bacteriological examinations (Fig. 3.14) [3–5].

**Warning! (Always perform bacterial examination of the preservation solution)**

The kidney preservation solution taken from the first bag should be immediately examined for microorganisms and sown on special seedbeds for the presence of bacteria, yeast-shaped fungus (candida) and fungi. Early detection of pathogenic microorganisms in the preservation solution gives a greater chance of starting

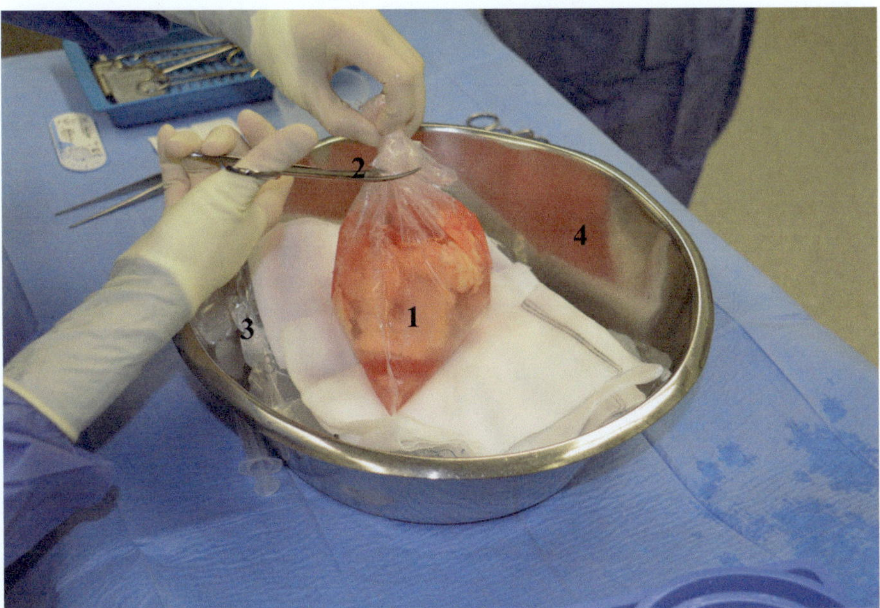

**Fig. 3.12** The surgeon uses sterile scissors to cut off the ribbon that closes the first sterile bag from the outside, in which there is preservation solution and in which the procured kidney is immersed. 1—First bag with inside procured kidney, 2—The bag is cut from the outside with scissors: try not to damage the kidney when opening the bag, 3—Sterile ice, 4—Sterile bowl designed for organ inspection

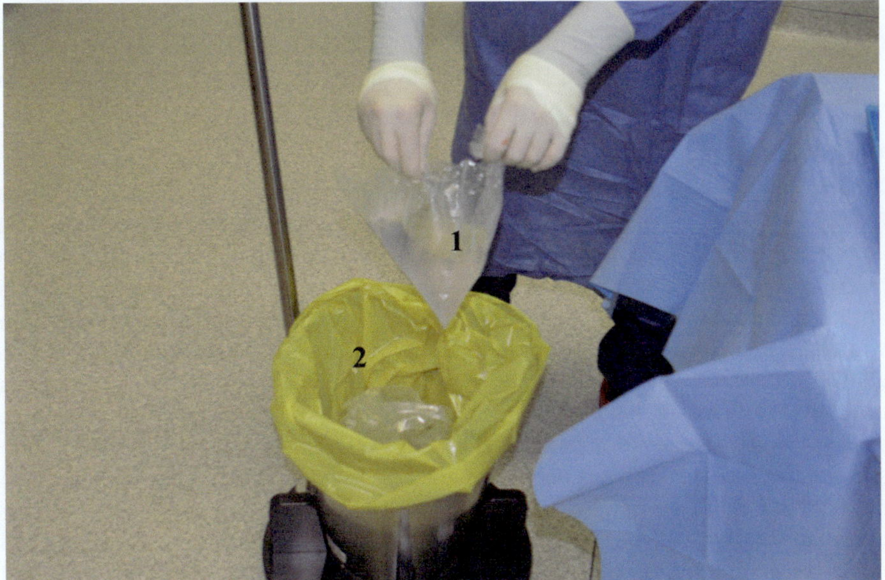

**Fig. 3.13** 1—A second bag from the outside with physiological NaCl solution is thrown by the surgeon into the waste bag or handed over to the scrub or circulating nurse, 2—Waste bag

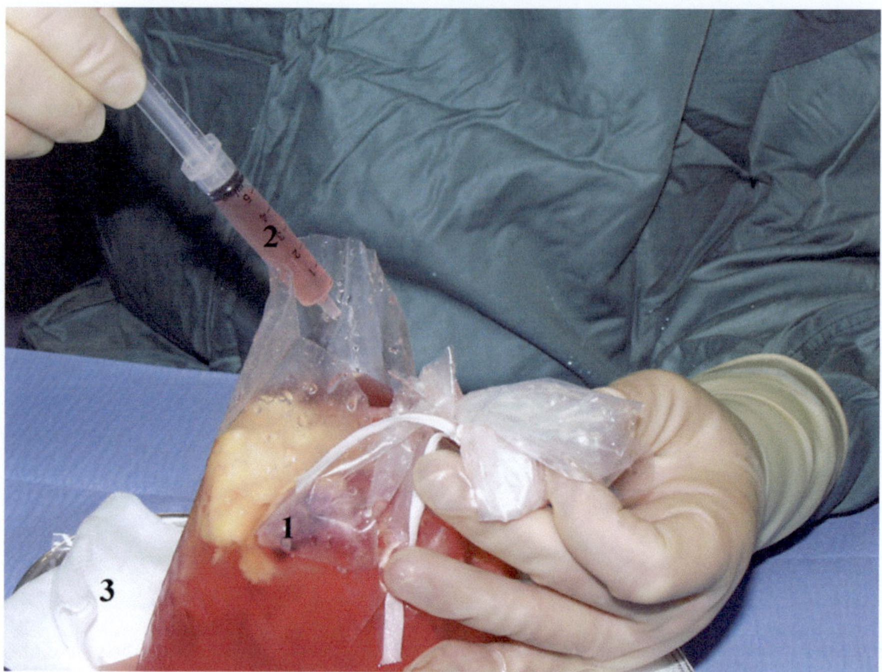

Fig. 3.14 The first step after opening the bag in which the kidney is stored is to take a syringe of approximately 5 ml of preservation solution for culture. 1—Transport bag contain kidney immersed in preservation solution, 2—A syringe filled with preservation solution, 3—Bowl and gauze in which the kidney inspection will be performed

targeted treatment quickly and thus preventing infection or worse complications, such as septic hemorrhage, usually leading to organ loss, lower limb loss and from time to time even loss of life by the transplant recipient.

**Warning! (Mixing preservation solutions?)**

If necessary, the amount of preservation solution necessary for the inspection of the kidney is always supplemented by the scrub nurse, so that the kidney is at least almost completely or completely submerged in it throughout the inspection and preparation. Some centers prefer to use the same or other preservation solution during inspection. In our center we are allowed to perform the kidney inspection whileit is immersed in the preservation solution from the first bag. We are also allowed to mix two of the same preservation solutions during the organ inspection or to use an other cold fresh organ preservation solution; for example, if we receive an organ for transplantation from outside the Netherlands and a preservation fluid such as Celsior or IGL-1 has been used for preservation, and we do not have such preservation fluids at our hospital. Still, we have to prepare the kidney for the transplant, so we use our preservative fluid. Especially during cold storage and organ inspection, kidney must be flush with cold UW solution, which is stored until transplantation. It has to be said here that after 25 years of such practice, we have never observed any side effects of such an exchange or mixing up of the preserving fluids in the form of a delayed function of the organ or its original lack of function.

**Warning! (For organ flushing always use a fresh preservation solution)**
It is not permitted to use the preservation solution from the first bag (donor's hospital), or to mix the old and fresh preservation solutions for flushing the organ through vessels to wash out the rest of the blood or to check vessel permeability. The explanation for this is the presence of fat particles in the transport preservation solution, which can lead to fat micro-embolisms during the flushing of the organs through the vessels or during the flushing of the vessels themselves which may cause a malfunction or non-function of the procured organ after transplantation. Using a very sophisticated filter for the old preservation solution from the first transport bag is more expensive than using a new fresh and cold preservation solution.

5. After collecting the sample for bacteriological examination, the rest of the preservation solution is poured into a sterile dish with ice at its bottom. The ice is covered with a thin layer of wet gauze to prevent the kidney being injured due to freezing during the inspection and preparation (Fig. 3.15).

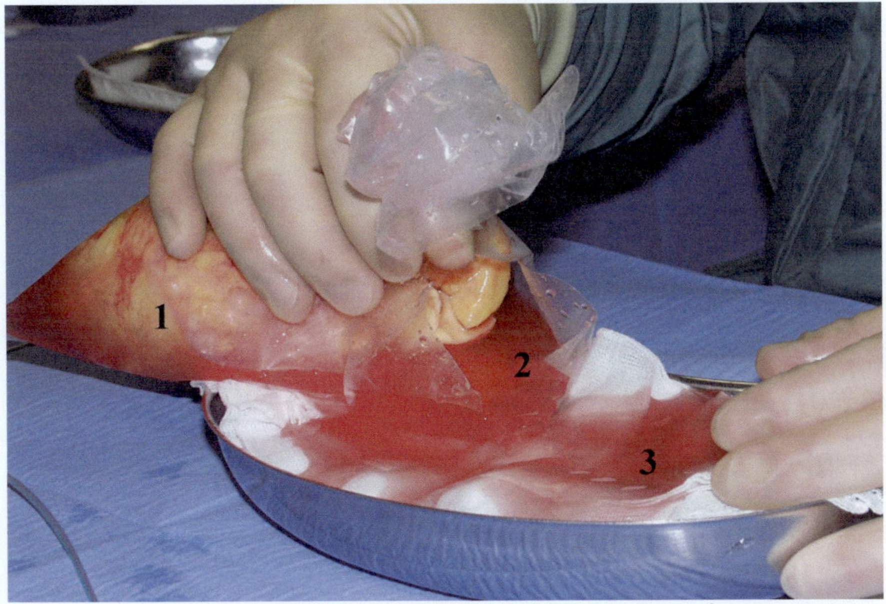


**Fig. 3.15** Some or all of the preservation solution is poured into an bowl with ice for kidney inspection. 1—Bag with kidney and preservation solution, 2—Preservation solution, 3—Bowl with sterile ice at the bottom and a small peice of gauze to prevent frostbite in the kidney

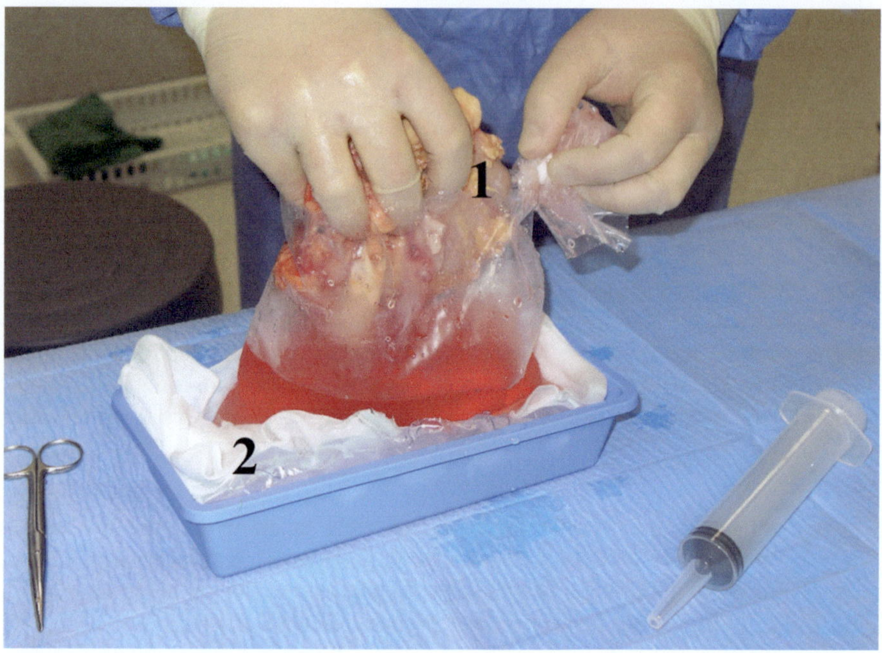

**Fig. 3.16** Carefully, so that the kidney does not fall on the floor of the operating room, take it out of the bag and put it on the gauze in a bowl filled with ice and a cooled preservation solution, in which the kidney will be inspected. 1—Kidney, 2—Container for kidney inspection with sterile ice at the bottom and a small gauze to prevent frostbite

6. Carefully, so that it does not fall on the floor of the operating room, remove the kidney from the bag and put it on the gauze in a container filled with ice and cooled preservation solution, in which the inspection will be performed (Fig. 3.16).
7. If necessary, pour the rest of the preservative fluid from the bag into the container where the kidney inspection will take place. One of the surgeons gives the first bag to the scrub nurse or throws it in the trash bin (Fig. 3.17) [6].

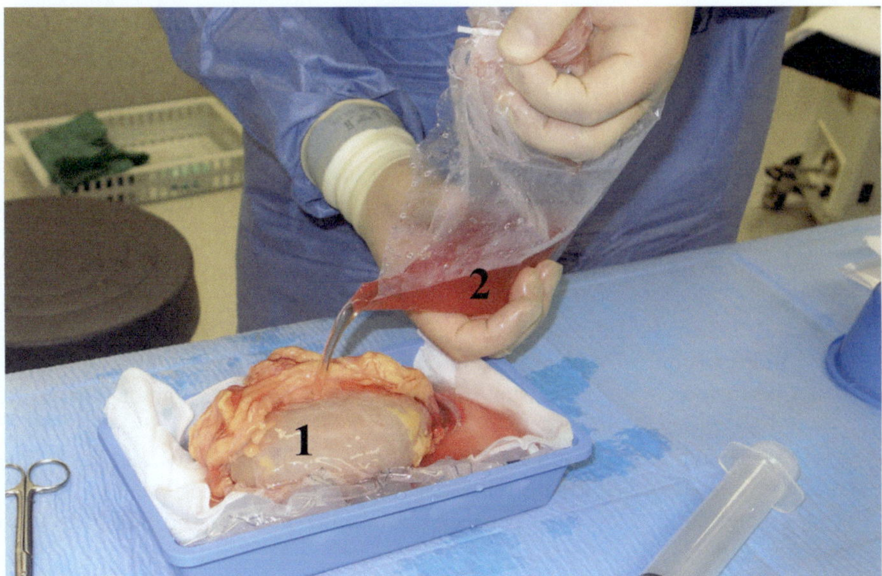

**Fig. 3.17** If necessary, pour the rest of the preservation solution from the bag into a container for kidney inspection. 1—Kidney is placed on gauze and ice and sterile container, 2—Pour the preservation solution into the kidney inspection container

## 3.6   Kidney Removal from the Transport Device for Continuous Hypothermic Kidney Perfusion

### 3.6.1   Introduction

The first perfusion system, built by Truman, was used in 1968 by Belzer to perfuse the kidney taken from the deceased donor. Modern kidney perfusion systems allow us to monitor the following parameters during transport: pressure (systolic and diastolic pressure in the kidney), flow rate of the perfusate through the kidney, vascular resistance within the kidney, temperature, infusion time and battery life. Currently, several portable systems are available on the market. The procured kidney and the renal artery are connected to the continuous perfusion machine and continuously cooled and perfused during transportation to the recipient's hospital. The kidney's recipient is less likely to have a delayed graft function after transplantation and the need for dialysis after the transplant. In particular, this treatment very often applies to kidneys that are taken from donors after cardiac death especially those DCD donors with a long first warm ischaemia time lasting more than an hour.

### 3.6.2  *Steps for Removing the Kidney from the Hypothermic Machine Perfusion: The LifePort Kidney Transporter of Organ Recovery Systems [4, 5, 7]*

1. Move the LifePort Kidney Transporter into the operating room. Movement of this type of equipment is very easy: it has an excellent driving system and a handle to maneuver it (Figs. 3.18 and 3.19).
2. Unlatch and remove the LifePort Kidney Transporter cover (Figs. 3.20 and 3.21).
3. Carefully place the LifePort Kidney Transporter disposable sterile drape onto the LifePort Kidney Transporter, lining up the drape gasket and the well of the outer perfusion circuit lid. Ensure the arrow on the orientation guide is pointing toward the pump deck.
4. Unfold the sterile drape in the following order: right, left, front and back. The drape gasket should fit securely into the well of the outer perfusion circuit lid.
5. Unlock and remove the inner perfusion circuit lid. Place the lid facedown onto the sterile field.

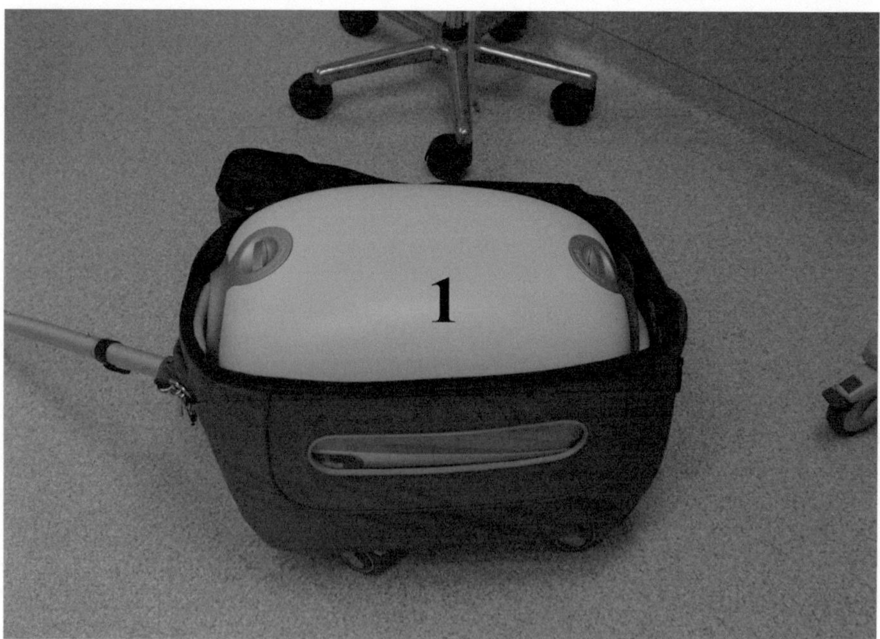


**Fig. 3.18** One of the portable kidney hypothermic perfusion systems delivered to the operating room. It has excellent handling properties and a handle for pulling. The whole device is protected from damages from the outside by a specially designed container. 1—The cover of the device

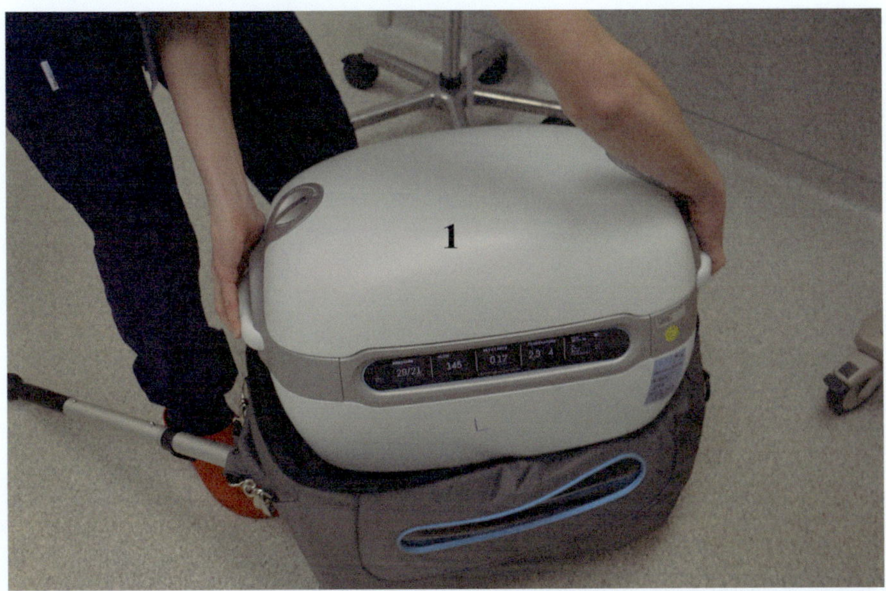

**Fig. 3.19** Hypothermic continuous perfusion device—the kidney transport container. 1: Device cover

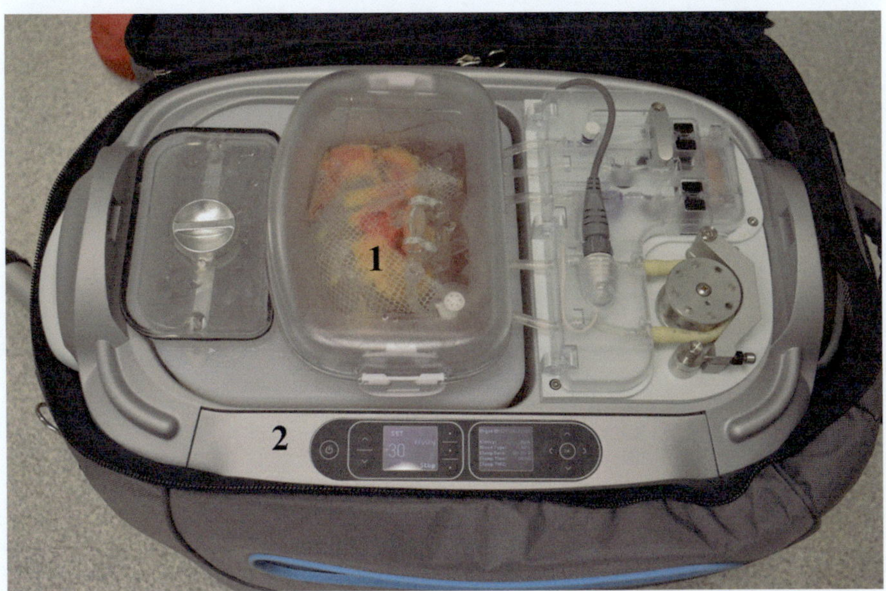

**Fig. 3.20** The cover of the hypothermic continuous kidney perfusion device is removed in the operating room. 1—Sterile kidney perfusion and cooling chamber, 2—Control panel

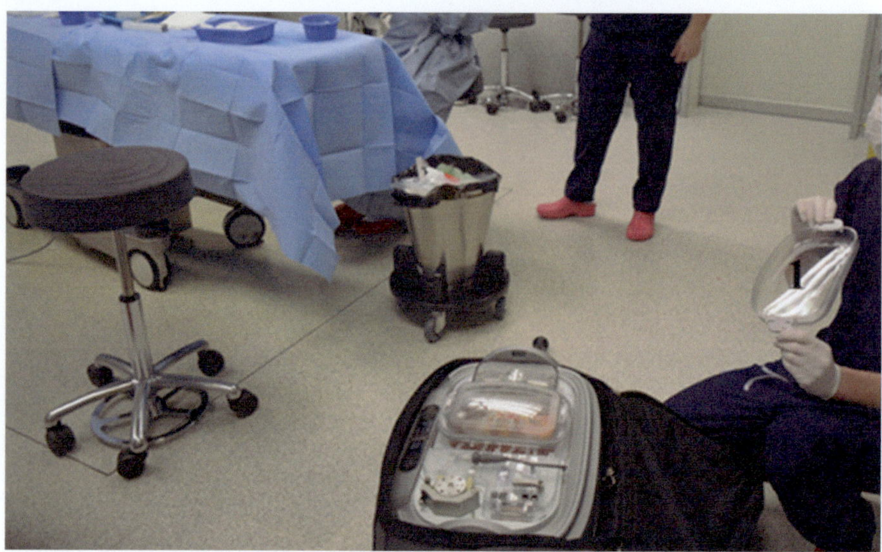

**Fig. 3.21** Removal of the first cover of the kidney perfusion and cooling chamber. 1—First cover

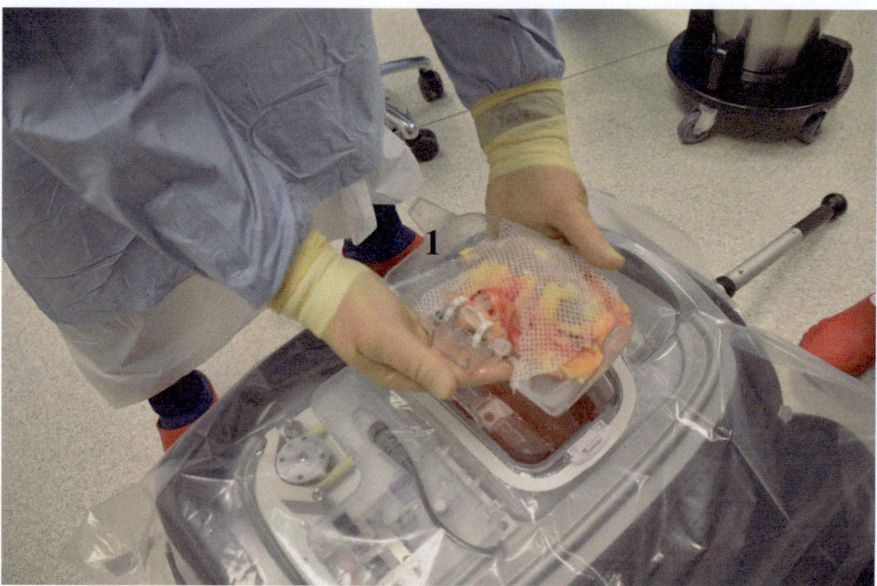

**Fig. 3.22** Covering the kidney perfusion and cooling chamber with a sterile foil allowing the sterile opening of the second cover, which closes the sterile chamber. The disconnected kidney from the perfusion pump is removed from the chamber onto a special platter where it is fixed with mesh. 1—Kidney fixed with mesh so that it does not shift during transport

6. Press the STOP button.
7. Unscrew or cut the infusion line.
8. Carry the kidney cradle, with the cannulated kidney, to your organ inspection table (Fig. 3.22).
9. Unhook the mesh which immobilized the kidney (Fig. 3.23).

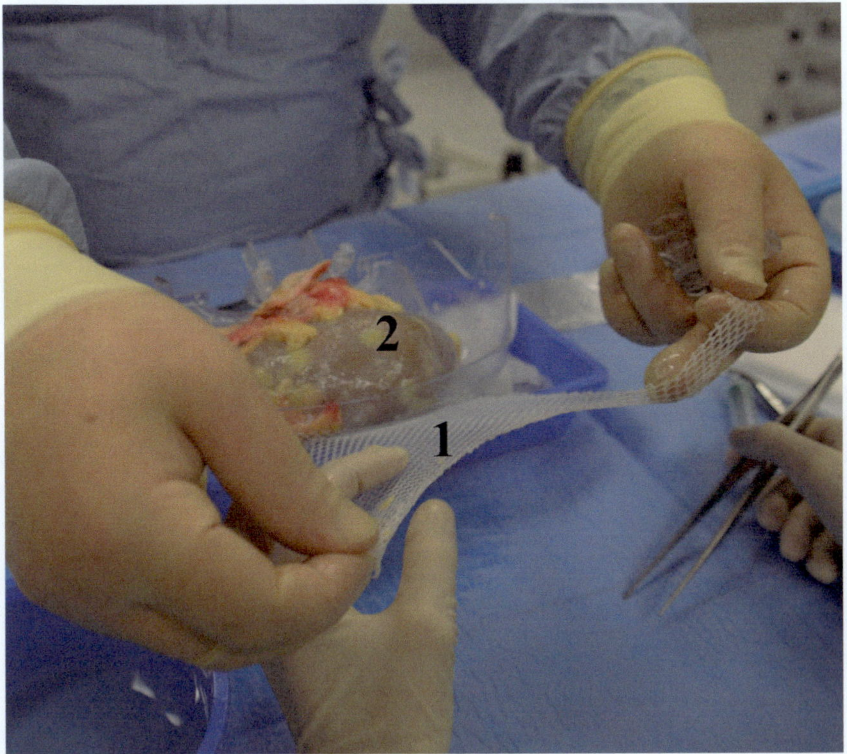

**Fig. 3.23** Transfer of kidney from device platter to inspection container. Release of the renal artery and the kidney itself from the mesh. 1—Special mesh holding the kidney during transport, 2—Kidney

10. Unpin the mesh and remove the renal artery connector.
11. Put the kidney in its own container on ice and submerge in cold preservation solution and start kidney inspection (Fig. 3.24) [7].

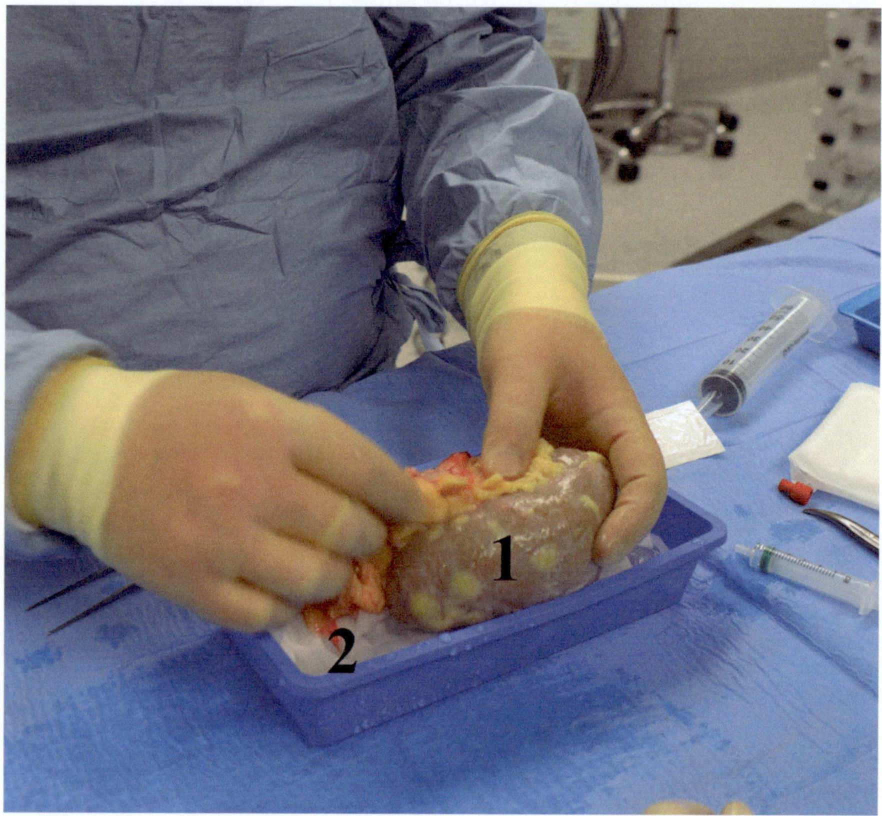

**Fig. 3.24** Placing the kidney in a container filled with ice and fresh preservation solution for inspection. 1—Kidney, 2—Container with ice, a small gauze and cooled preservation solution

## 3.7  General Rules for Kidney Inspection

1. The kidney is placed in a sterile container or bowl with ice which at the bottom is covered by a gauze and cold preservation solution or ice slush. If you are inspecting the left kidney, you have to position it in a way that the first vessel from above is the left renal vein and the ureter(s) faces the right hand of the surgeon and that the aorta patch with the ostia of the renal arteries are in front of him or her (Fig. 3.25).

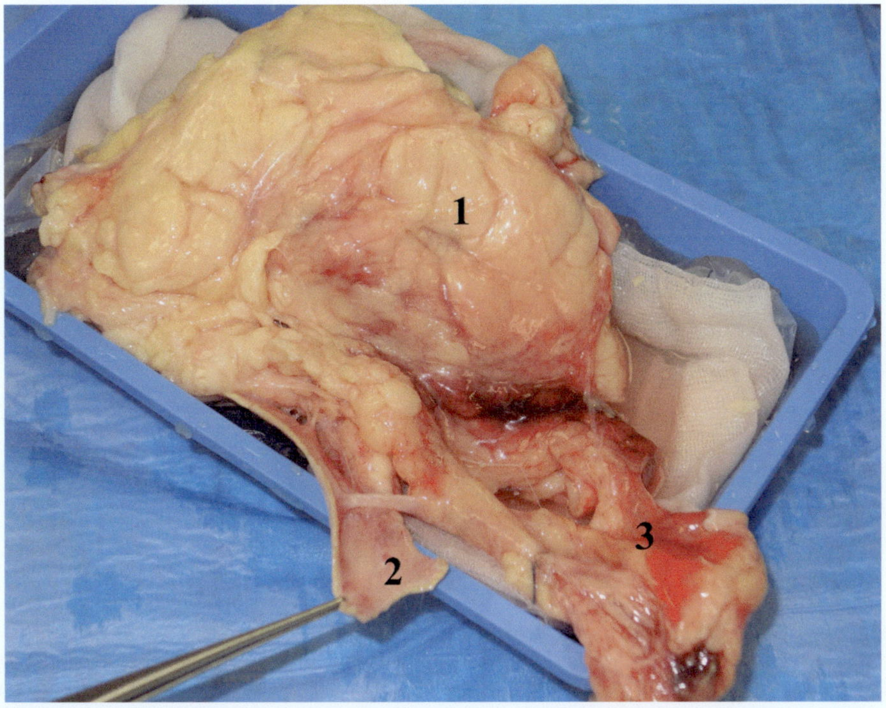

**Fig. 3.25** The left kidney is placed in a container filled with preservation solution and a small wet gauze is placed on sterile ice. 1—Kidney: with this amount of fat, palpating the kidney may be difficult, 2—Patch from abdominal aorta, 3—Tissues around ureter

2. In the case of the **right** kidney, place it in the bowl in such a way that the first vessel from above is the right renal vein and the inferior vena cava (IVC) with the ingoing right renal vein or veins and the ureter(s) facing the left side or left hand of the surgeon; the ostias of the renal artery(-ies) face the surgeon (Fig. 3.26).

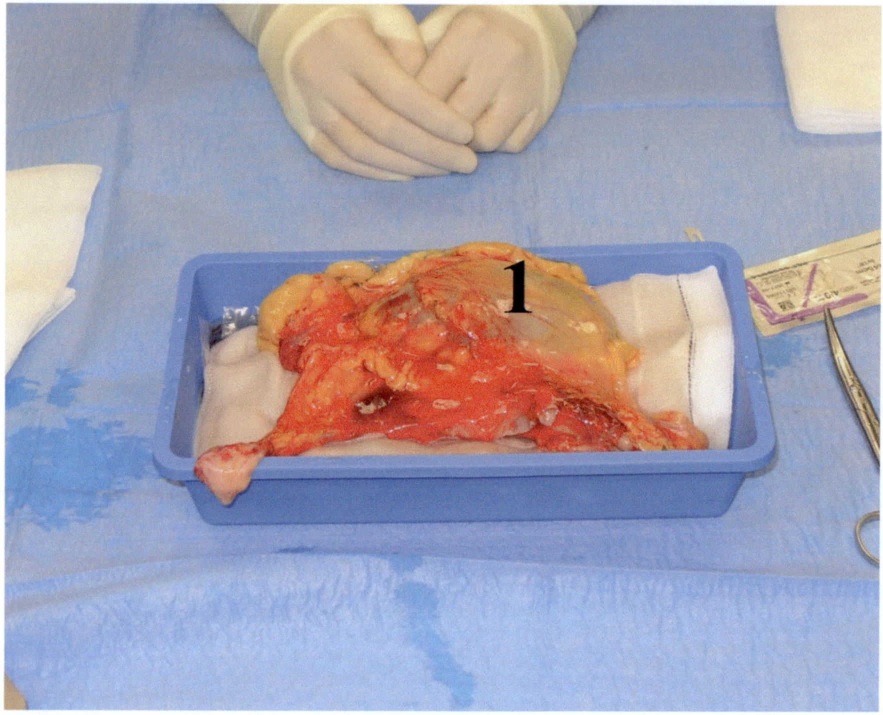

**Fig. 3.26** The right kidney. The right ureter faces the surgeon's left hand. The first vessel from the top is the right renal vein or the right renal vein attached to the IVC. In this case, the amount of fat is minimal and the kidney parenchyma shows through a thin layer of perirenal fat. 1—Right kidney

3. Kidney examination: inspection.

- evaluation of the amount of fat around the kidney and the possibility of reducing it (Fig. 3.27);
- the quality and diameter of visible renal vessels (Fig. 3.28);

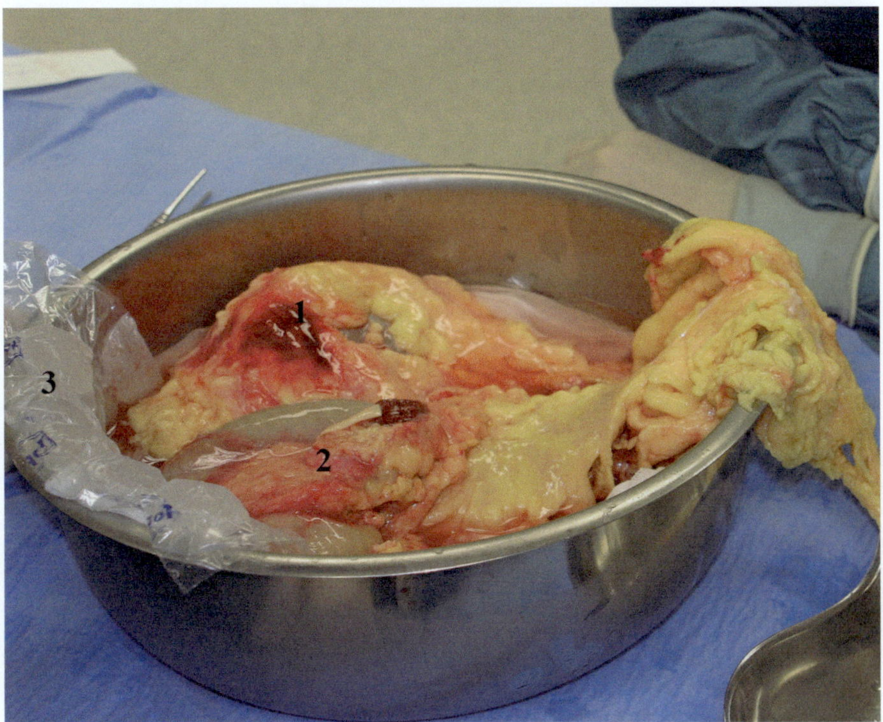


**Fig. 3.27** A donor with a very high BMI. There is a very high amount of fat around the kidney and pancreas. If I ask you where is the kidney and where is the pancreas? I think that many of you would struggle to answer. 1—Kidney, 2—Pancreas, 3—Sterile ice

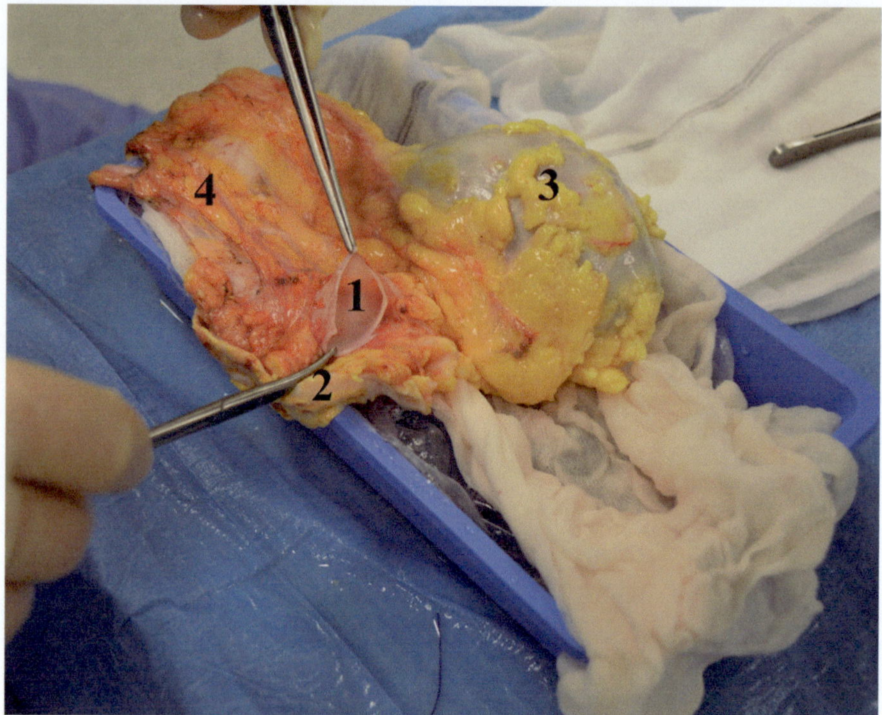

**Fig. 3.28** Visible ostia of two renal veins of the retrieved right kidney. 1—IVC lumen, 2—Aortic patch with severe atherosclerosis, 3—Kidney, 4—Ureter

- advancement of atherosclerosis lesions in the abdominal aortic wall (Fig. 3.29);
- the presence of the hematomas (Fig. 3.30);
- visible damage to the capsule and kidney parenchyma (Fig. 3.31);

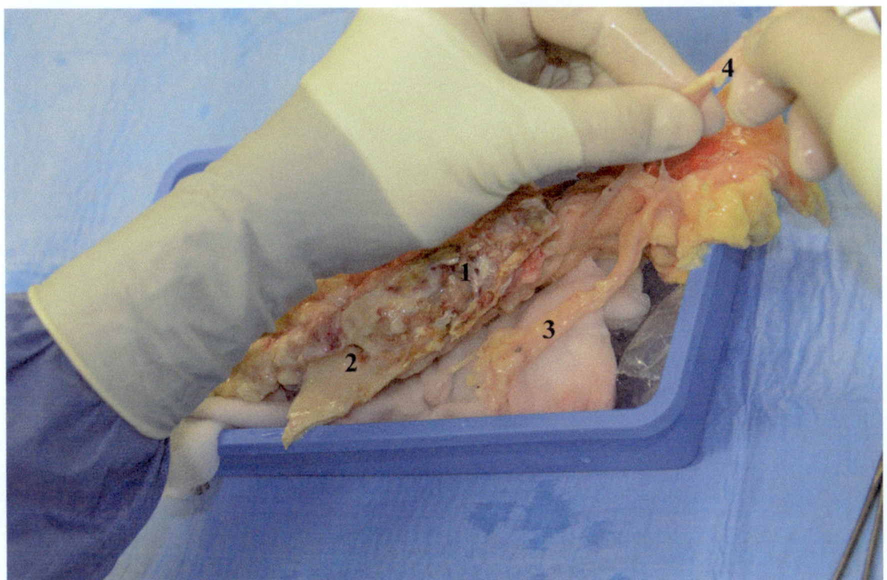

**Fig. 3.29** Very advanced atherosclerotic lesions are visible in the center of the abdominal aorta wall. 1—Patch taken from the abdominal aorta, 2—Ostium of the left renal artery, 3—Ureter, 4—Searching with small silicone tube for a second ureter

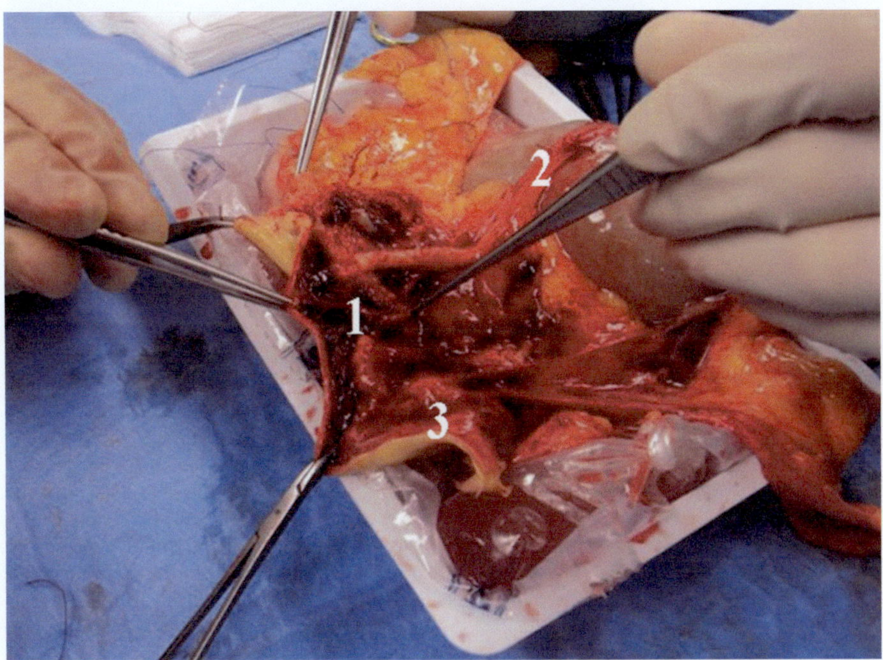

**Fig. 3.30** Damage to the abdominal aorta and the onset of the renal artery during a traffic accident. Massive bleeding into the extraperitoneal space. 1—Hematoma, 2—Freed left renal vein lying on the surface of the kidney, 3—Aortic patch. Massive hematoma reaching into the hilum of the procured kidney; kidney badly washed out of the blood. An attempt was made to flush the kidney through the renal arteries with cold preservation solution, though this gave great resistance. This kidney was not transplanted

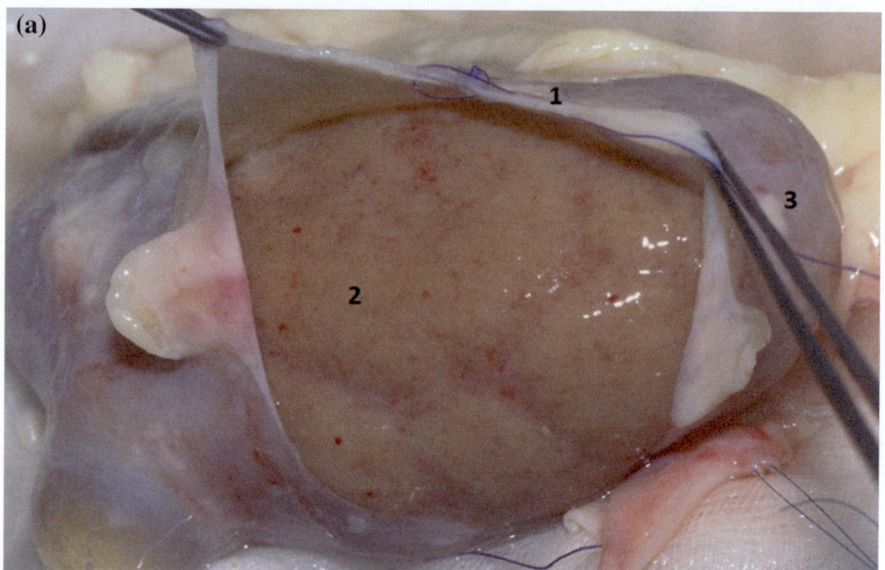

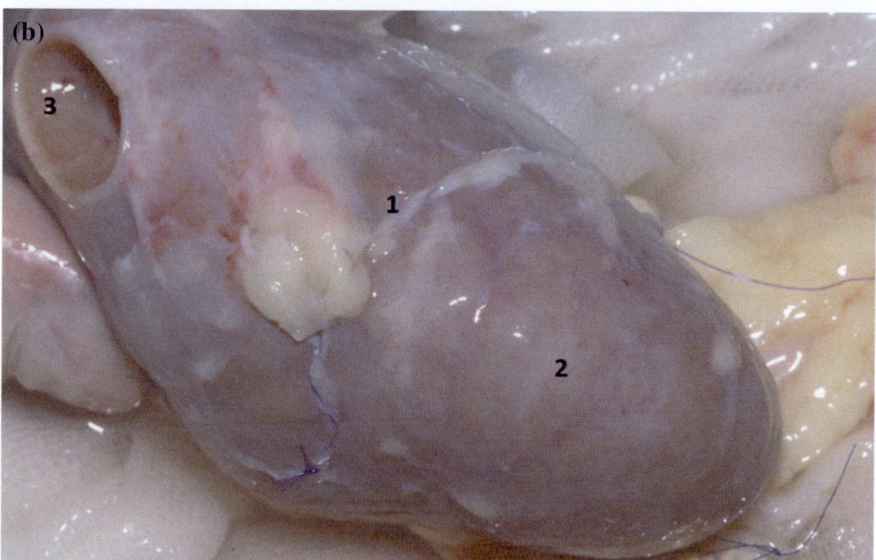

**Fig. 3.31** (**a**) Kidney procurement: damage to kidney capsule. 1—Tear kidney capsule, 2—Decapsulated kidney parenchyma, 3—Kidney upper pole. (**b**) Kidney procurement: damage to kidney capsule. 1—Repaired tear to the kidney capsule absorbable monofilament: 4/0, 2—Decapsulated kidney parenchyma, 3—Renal cyst. (**c**) Kidney procurement: damage to the parenchyma and kidney capsule. 1—Kidney parenchyma, 2—Kidney capsule

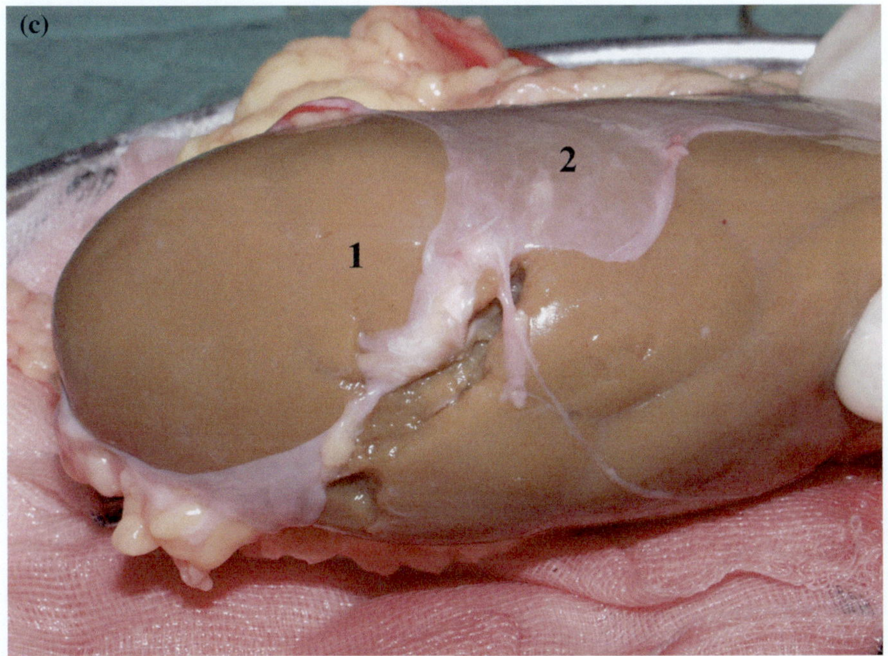

Fig. 3.31 (continued)

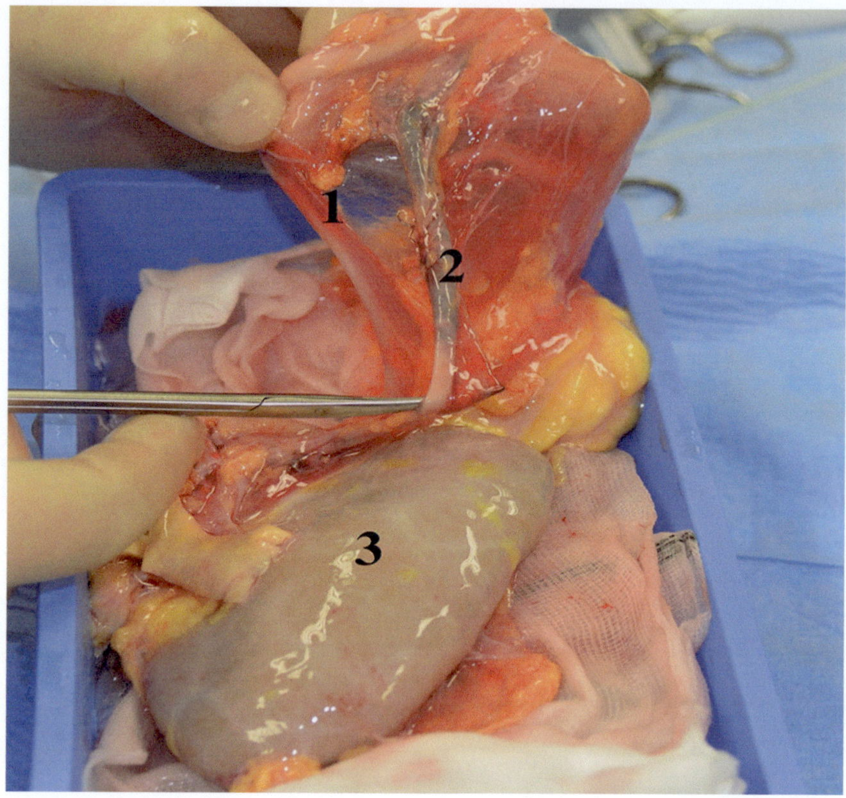

**Fig. 3.32** 1—Left ureter, 2—Partially thrombosed left gonadal vein, 3—Kidney parenchyma

- the number of injuries to the ureter(s) (Fig. 3.32);
- visible tumor of the kidney parenchyma (Fig. 3.33);
- visible kidney tumor excised and submitted for examination; kidney parenchyma sutured after tumor excision; renal artery aneurysm (Fig. 3.33a, b).
- gonadal vein and renal artery thrombosis (Figs. 3.32 and 3.34).

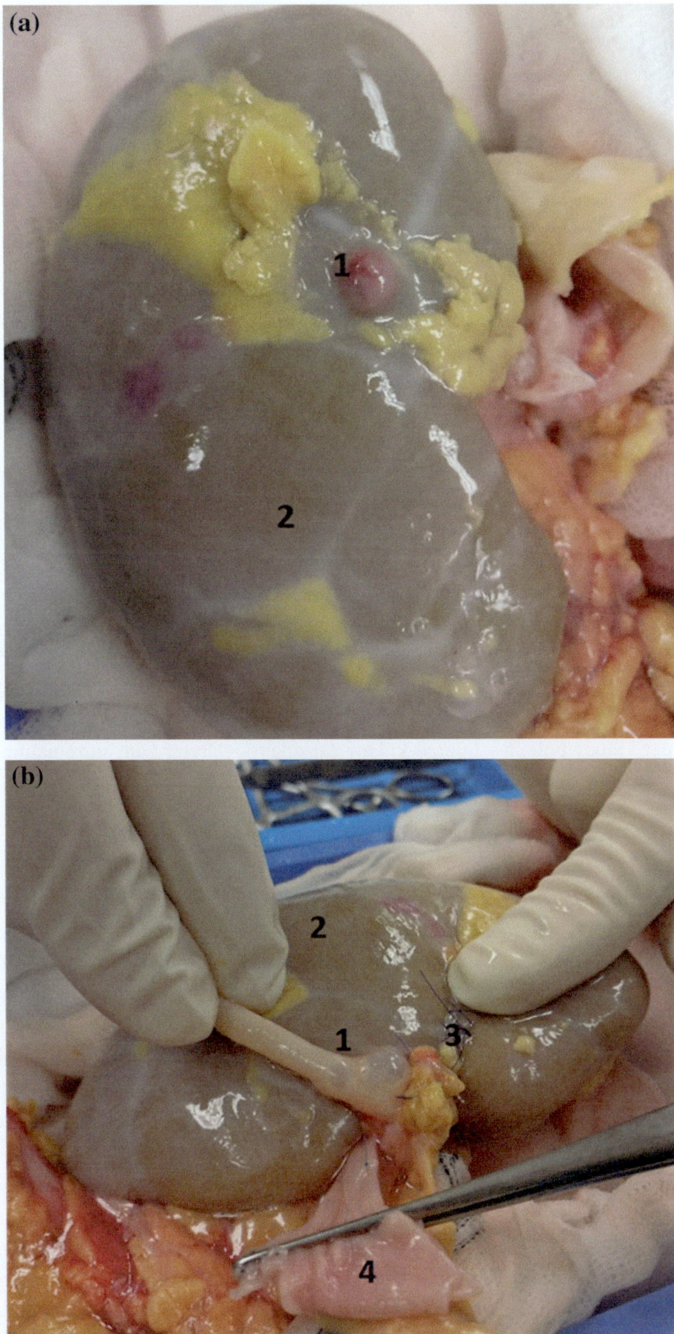

**Fig. 3.33** **(a)** Evident kidney tumor. Biopsies and a quick pathological examination were performed. Test result: cancer. The kidney was disqualified from transplantation. 1—Kidney tumor: in this case we found the kidney cancer, 2—Kidney parenchyma. **(b)**Visible kidney tumor excised and submitted for intraoperative fresh frozen section pathological examination; kidney parenchyma sutured after tumor excision; renal artery aneurysm. 1—Renal artery aneurysm, 2—Renal parenchyma, 3—Kidney parenchyma sutured after excision, 4—Renal vein

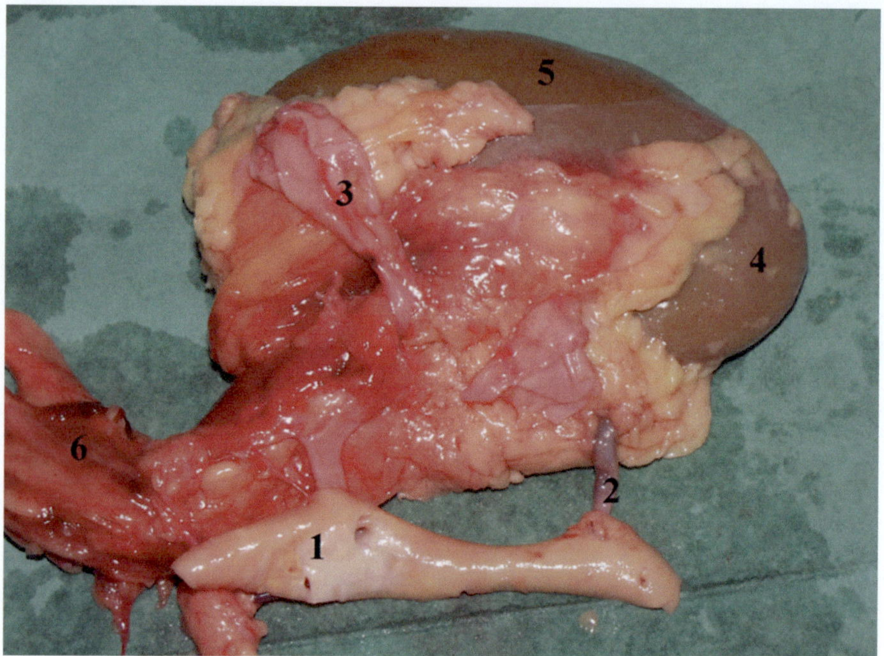

**Fig. 3.34** Damaged parenchyma and capsule; thrombosed renal artery bringing blood to the upper pole. 1—Aortic patch, 2—Thrombosed aberrant superior (upper) pole renal artery, 3—Right renal vein, 4—Upper kidney pole, 5—Injured kidney capsule, 6—Ureter with surrounding tissues

**Warning! (Perirenal fat: what to do and how to reduce it)**

The amount of fat around the kidney depends on the BMI of the donor. Perirenal fat in older and obese people is often ingrown into the capsule and parenchyma of the kidney. At the donor's hospital, the donor surgeon can try to reduce the fat layer located on the kidney to allow it to cool properly during transport to the recipient's hospital. If in the donor's hospital reduction of perirenal fat is for many reasons impossible, the fat should not be removed in a hurry by force. The donor surgeon together with the transplant coordinator are responsible for the notification of the recipient center that fat reduction has failed. The donor surgeon through the transplant coordinator (TC) should ask the recipient center if they would like to accept a kidney without fat reduction and thus with fat around it. This is a very important message, because if the kidney is large in size and is additionally surrounded by ingrown fat, it will probably be not cooled efficiently enough during transportation (static cold storage). A kidney with fat around it can be large in size and volume. In some cases it may exceed the capacity of the recipient's retroperitoneal space—for example when the recipient is a small adult or small child. In such a case it should be remembered that if the amount of fat cannot be significantly reduced, the kidney may not be accepted and transplanted. Depending on the time and distance of transport of the kidney to the recipient's hospital, because of the need to properly cool the organ due to the thick layer of fat, it is possible to consider adding ice cubes to the second bag in order to better cool the kidney. The best solution is to put the kidney before transportation to the recipient's hospital on the hypothermic oxygenated or not oxygenated perfusion machine which will perform internal cooling with a cold preservation solution through the renal artery. Do not forget that a thick layer of fat around the procured kidney acts as an excellent insulator and that without the additional ice in the second bag (static cold storage) or continued internal cooling with a cold preservation solution after a long period or distance of travel, the kidney could be inappropriately cooled [6, 8, 9].

4. Personally I look in detail at the kidney, using two very delicate surgical forceps with which I slowly carry out a preliminary inspection of the renal vessels in terms of their number and location. I estimate the severity of atherosclerosis of the abdominal aortic wall and the intensity of atherosclerotic lesions at the site of arising of the renal artery towards the renal hilum. I check the number of ureters and vessels; in case of doubt, any structure similar to the ureter or vessel, if it has lumen, will be examined with a fine vascular probe or cannulated with very thin cannula and flushed with a cold preservation solution (Fig. 3.35). With a vascular probe from the side of the abdominal aortic wall, I cannulate the ostia of the renal arteries from the abdominal aorta patch towards the hilum of the kidney—thus we check the number and course of renal arteries and distance between them (Fig. 3.36).

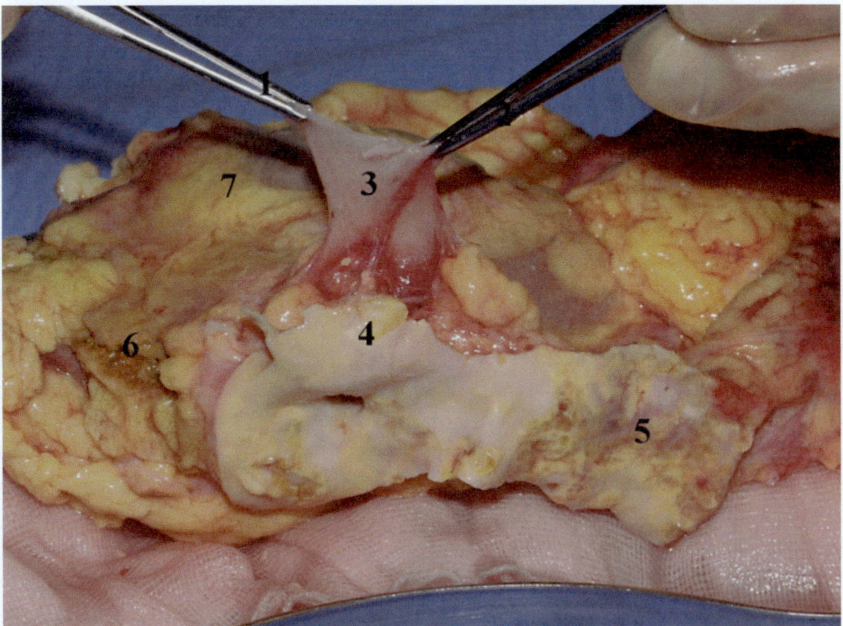

**Fig. 3.35** 1 and 2—Forceps, 3—Left renal vein, 4—Aortic patch in the center ostium of the left renal artery, 5—Distal abdominal aorta wall with advanced atherosclerotic changes, 6—Left adrenal gland, 7—Left kidney

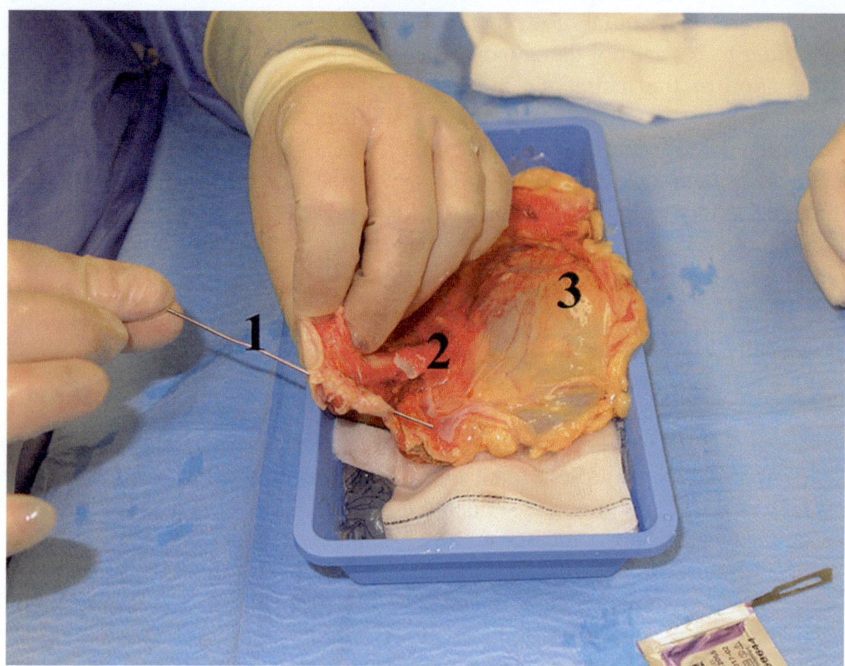


**Fig. 3.36** 1—Special vascular probe with which from the inside of the abdominal aorta we cannulate the "suspicious" artery ostium of the abdominal aorta wall. In this way we check during inspection the number of renal arteries. 1—Vascular probe, 2—Renal vein, 3—Kidney

5. If the perirenal fat does not stick to the kidney capsule it is necessary to remove it from the parenchyma surface but not from the hilum and its surroundings (Fig. 3.37).

**Warning! (Perirenal fat)**

The removal of the perirenal fat should be done very carefully and should cover the whole surface of the kidney except the kidney hilum, the renal pelvis, the ureter(s) and the medial part of the lower kidney's pole. Fat removal is usually done with scissors. I start removing the fat from the back of the kidney and finish 1–2 cm before the kidney hilum. Very carefully I palpate the fat around the ureter, vessels and fat in the kidney hilum—if it is hard and it resembles cartilage, I take a biopsy from it for an intra-operative consultation by the pathologist, a frozen section procedure, for example a liposarcoma, or the presence of atypical cells which could turn into a malignant tumor a few years after a kidney transplant. In my 30 years of career the anatomopathologist confirmed my cancer (liposarcoma) suspicions only in three cases and found atypical cells in more than ten cases. The kidneys in which cancer and/or the atypical cells were found were not transplanted.

We have two types of kidney fat: fat that can be easily removed from the kidney capsule; and ingrown fat that cannot be easily removed. If such a kidney with

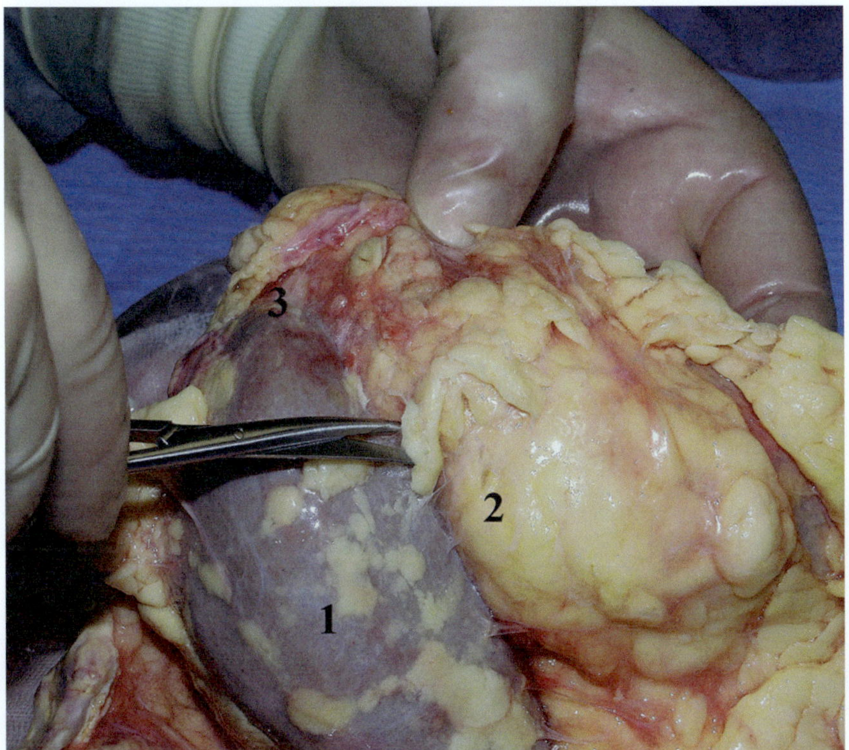

**Fig. 3.37** Fat reduction in the recipient's hospital. 1—Kidney, 2—Perirenal fat, 3—Upper pole of the kidney

ingrown fat is suitable for transplantation, it is necessary to try to reduce it as much as possible up to the kidney capsule (Fig. 3.38).

When removing fat, remember the extra renal arteries, which do not penetrate the kidney through the renal hilum. These arteries can be easily damaged during fat removal and are usually difficult to reconstruct later. The more fat is removed, the lower the risk of necrosis, the better the position of the kidney and the better its cooling during inspection, storage and the transplantation process itself.

6. Palpation of the kidney and ureter for tumors and cysts (Figs. 3.39 and 3.40). Kidney tumors and any suspected ones should be immediately verified by performing a kidney biopsy. When it comes to kidney cysts (Fig. 3.41), there are always questions: whether the contents of the cyst are clear or not and whether each kidney cyst should be opened or not.

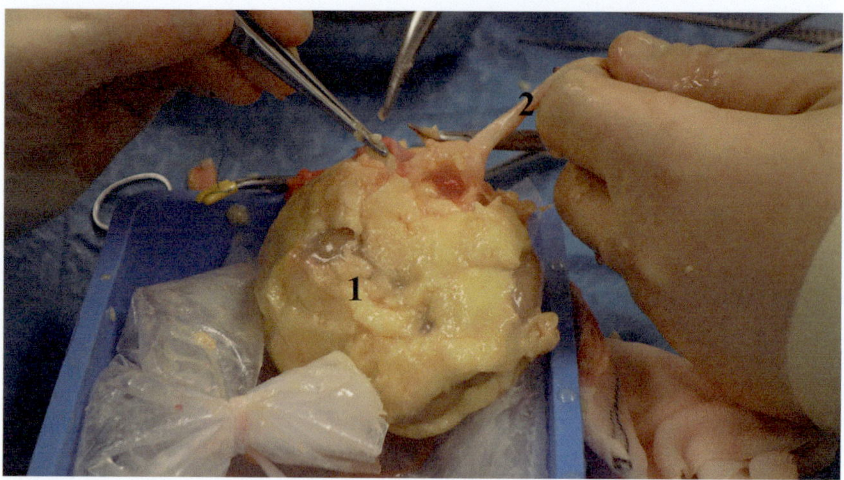

**Fig. 3.38** Maximum reduction of perirenal fat which has grown deeply into the kidney parenchyma. Visible areas without the kidney capsule when we have been trying to remove the fat. 1—Kidney, 2—Renal artery

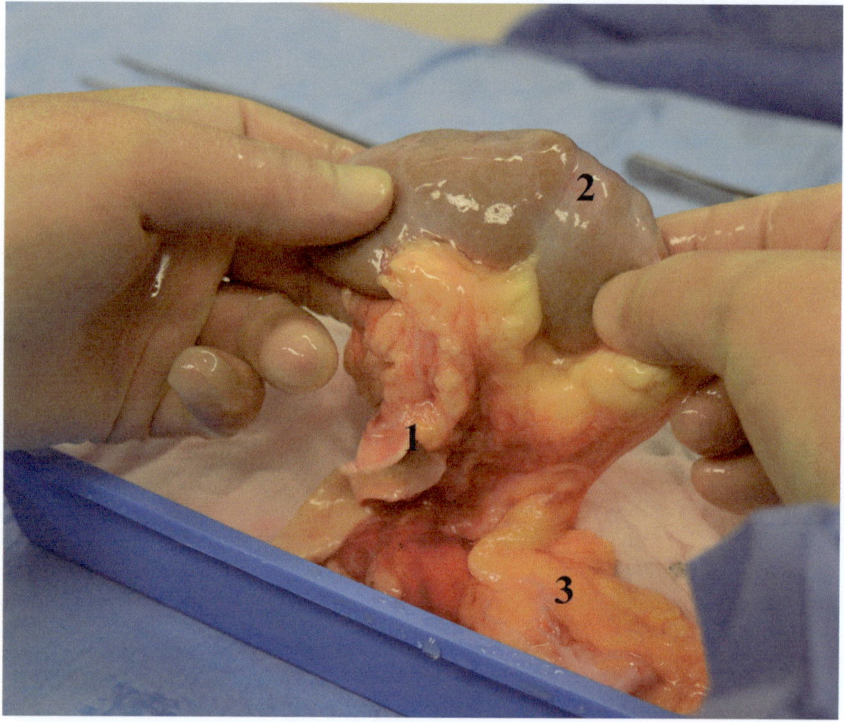

**Fig. 3.39** Palpating the kidney parenchyma for tumors; the picture shows normal kidney. 1—Renal artery, 2—Kidney, 3—Ureter

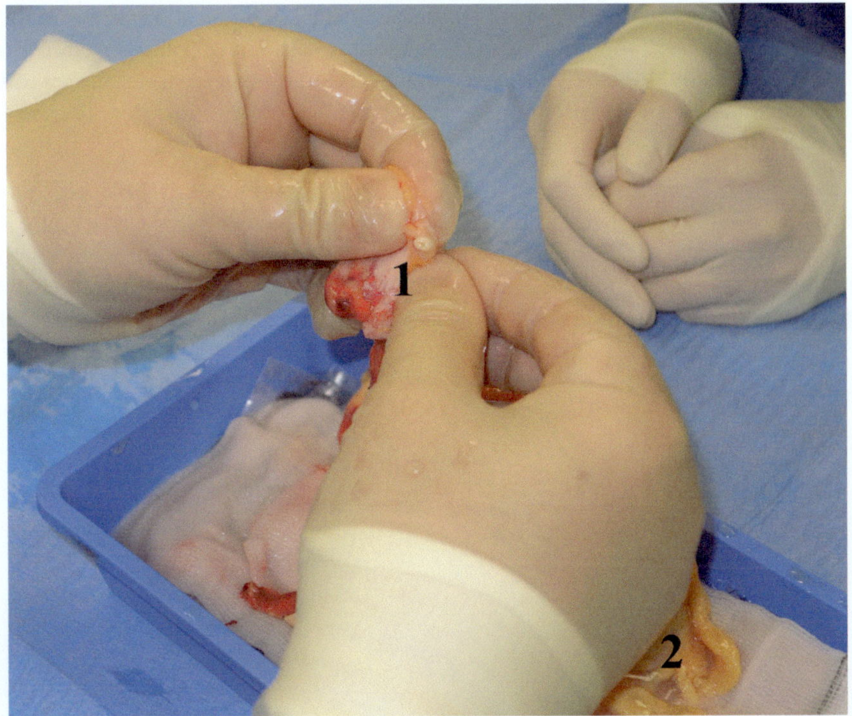

**Fig. 3.40** Palpating the ureter to look for tumors and other abnormalities. 1—Ureter, 2—Kidney

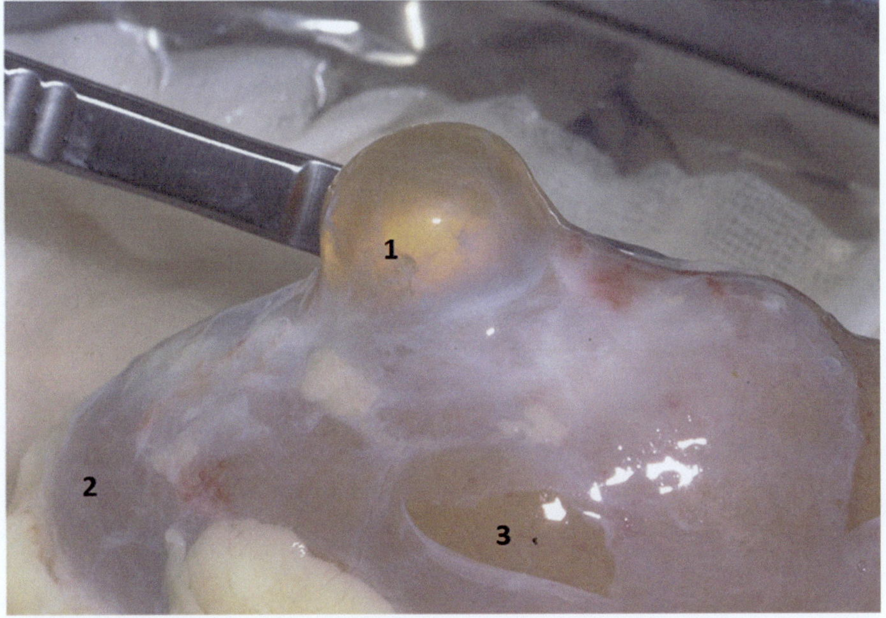

**Fig. 3.41** Retrieved kidney with cyst, most probably Bosniak I. 1—Renal cyst, 2—Kidney parenchyma, 3—Tear in renal capsule

(a) It has been more than 30 years since the Bosniak classification of cystic renal masses was first proposed. This CT-based classification was introduced in 1986 and originally divided cystic renal masses into one of four classes after exclusion of infectious, inflammatory and vascular etiologies (Fig. 3.42) [10–16].

Bosniak 1: Benign simple renal cyst requiring no follow-up. These lesions do not contain septa, calcification or any solid component. Simple cysts account for 80–85% of all space-occupying lesions in the kidneys. Although the etiology of simple cysts is unclear, the age distribution indicates that they are acquired lesions. Pathologic studies have shown that cysts start as dilatations or diverticula of the

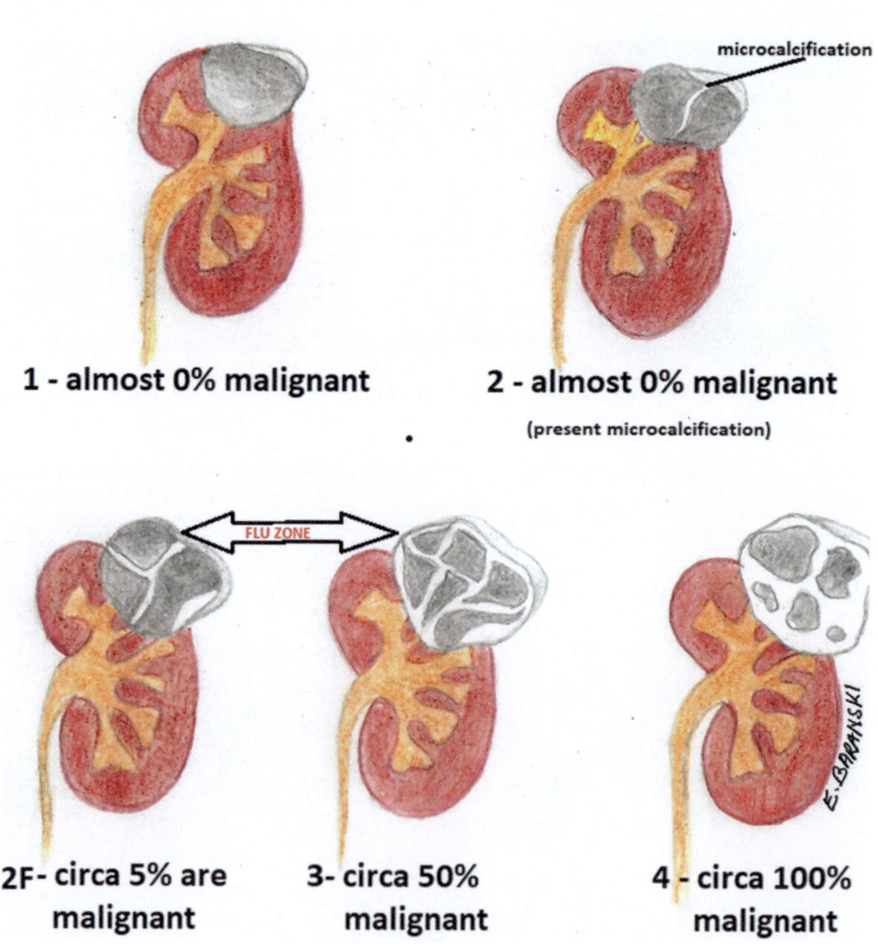


**Fig. 3.42** Bosniak classification system of renal cystic masses

tubules in the nephron and they are thought to arise from focal infarcts or inflammation [1–5, 7].

Bosniak 2: Benign renal cyst requiring no follow-up. A few thin <1 mm septa or thin calcifications (thickness not measurable), non-enhancing high-attenuation (due to proteinaceous or hemorrhagic contents) renal lesions <3 cm; these lesions are generally well marginated; work-up: none; percentage malignant: ~0%. Like category 1 lesions, category 2 lesions have no malignant potential and therefore require no further imaging. However, unlike category 1 lesions, category 2 lesions may contain a few hairline thin septa, fine calcification, or short-segment slightly thickened calcification within the wall or septa. Uniformly high attenuation cysts measuring <3 cm are also included in this category [10–16].

Bosniak 2F: cystic renal mass. The large majority of Bosniak 2F masses are benign. When malignant, nearly all are indolent. Generally, Bosniak 2F masses are followed by imaging at 6 months and 12 months, then annually for a total of five years to assess for morphologic change. Hyperdense cyst >3 cm diameter, mostly intrarenal (less than 25% of wall visible); no enhancement. Percentage malignant about 5%, lesions may contain multiple hairline thin septa or smooth, minimally thickened wall or septa, which may contain calcification that may be thick and nodular [10–16].

Bosniak 3: cystic renal mass. Bosniak 3 masses have an intermediate probability of being malignant. If not already obtained, consider urology consultation. Thick, nodular multiple septa or wall with measurable enhancement, treatment/work-up: partial nephrectomy or radiofrequency ablation in elderly or poor surgical candidates; percentage malignant about 55%; lesions demonstrate enhancing, thickened, irregular, or smooth walls or septa and require surgical removal due to their high potential for malignancy [10–16].

Bosniak 4: cystic renal mass. The large majority of Bosniak 4 masses are a malignant solid mass with a large cystic or a necrotic component treatment: partial or total nephrectomy, percentage malignant about 100%, lesions typically contain enhancing soft-tissue components adjacent to, but independent of, the wall or septum [10–16].

**Warnings! (Danger with many thick enhancing septa)**
The Bosniak classification asserts (for example) that masses with many or thick enhancing septa are associated with a higher probability of malignancy than masses with few or thin septa, but the manner in which this is true is unknown. Although there is no size threshold that separates benign from malignant masses nor indolent from aggressive cancers, size may be an important factor when considering surveillance of cystic renal masses.

Size and growth rate are not included in the update proposal. Small masses may be malignant and large ones benign; however, the smaller the mass, the more likely it is to be benign.

The classification does not distinguish clinically significant aggressive cancers from indolent cancers unlikely to affect a patient's lifespan.

Simple renal cysts are a common finding in the normal population older than 50 years of where their incidence is 25–40%. There are many reports on the use of cadaveric kidneys with cysts. On the long term follow-up, they are found to provide adequate renal function until there is graft failure due to the growth of the cysts or due to some other reasons. If the donor has a simple renal cyst, cyst growth is relatively slow, especially if the donor age is older than 50 years. Renal cysts are a common routine imaging finding, and autopsy studies suggest that more than half of patients of 50 years of age and older have at least one renal cyst. Although most cysts never cause symptoms, some cause pain, collecting system compression, hematuria, hypertension and secondary infection.

There are obvious advantages of transplantation over dialysis even if we are using kidneys with cysts. Reports of the use of cadaveric kidneys with cysts have clearly shown that the growth of these cysts is slow. The long-term graft and patient survival data for recipients having a graft with a cyst are not available at present. Once they are available, I will be able to further assess the feasibility of using such kidneys for transplantation.

If during the kidney inspection there is a cyst which has an irregular thick wall or turbid/hemorrhagic content, perform a frozen section biopsy of the wall of the cyst and/or a biochemical evaluation of the fluid—even when in doubt a biopsy should be advocated. When in the kidney from the cadaver donor the cysts appear complex (Bosniak type 3 to 4), it is necessary to perform frozen section biopsies in order to

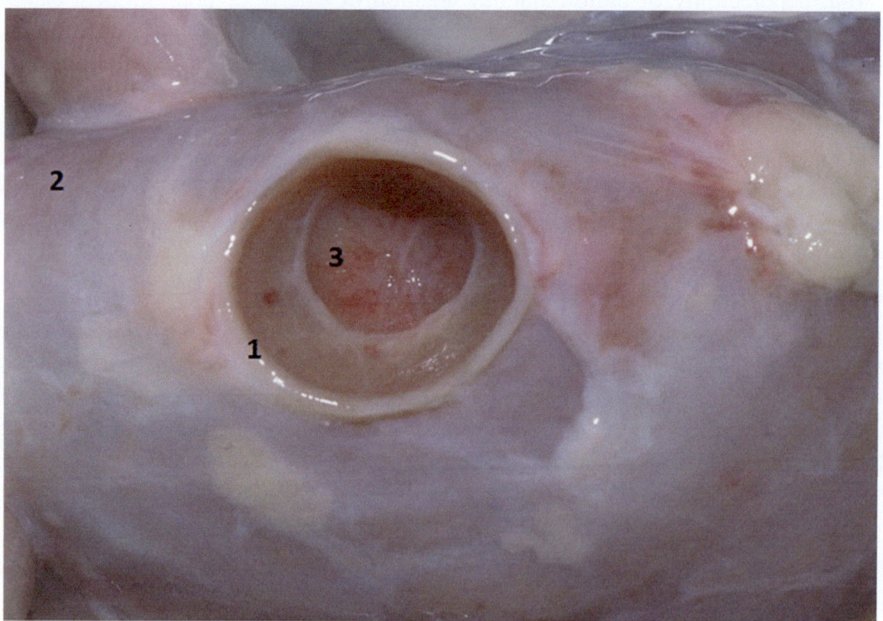

Fig. 3.43  The cyst wall is resected and sent to pathology for frozen section. 1—Margin of the cyst will be, after reperfusion, cauterized with an Argon Beamer or electrocoagulation, 2—Normal kidney parenchyma, 3—Bottom of the cyst. The cyst is then destroyed and deroofed

confirm malignancy (Fig. 3.42). In this case, there should be no doubt that the cyst's wall and/or the fluid inside it should be examined for cancer by the Department of Pathology. The literature encourages us to support the use of kidneys with a cyst if the donor is elderly and there are only a few small cysts (<5 mm in diameter). The decision to use such kidneys should be made in consultation with both donor and recipient, depending on the availability of other donors.

From cysts which have a thick irregular wall and have a diameter larger than 2–3 cm, the fluid has to be aspirated and sent to cytology. The cyst's wall has to be resected by the surgeon and sent for pathology examination (Fig. 3.43). The remaining wall of the cyst has to be visually inspected and if any are present, suspected tissues have to be resected and sent for frozen section. Then the cavity of the cyst is coagulated using an Argon Beamer of electro-diathermy. The cavity of the cyst is packed with Surgicel (Ethicon—oxidized regenerated cellulose) and—if necessary and depending on its position—fixed with glue or absorbable sutures [10–16].

## (b)  Urinomas

Ureteral obstructions with calyceal rupture and trauma (blunt, penetrating, or iatrogenic) are the most common causes of urinomas. Blunt or penetrating trauma can cause perinephric urinomas by two mechanisms—direct disruption of the pelvis or collecting system or by degeneration of nonviable tissue. These urinomas are often perinephric, but can also occur in a subcapsular location. This review will discuss the diagnosis, classification and treatment of renal cysts and urinomas. When urinomas arise spontaneously, the likely cause varies with the patient's age. Blunt or penetrating trauma can cause perinephric urinomas by two mechanisms—direct disruption of the pelvis or collecting system or by degeneration of nonviable tissue. These urinomas are often perinephric, but can also occur in a subcapsular location [16].

Several times, during preparation of the kidney, a cyst started to grow and became even bigger and sometimes even more tensed than the renal pelvis when I started to check the ureter and renal pelvis by administering cold preservative fluid into the ureter and renal pelvis with a soft, thin drain.

If there is a small connection between the cyst and the renal pelvis and the cystic wall or the parenchyma of the kidney is of a good quality, the connection should be closed and the kidney transplanted. After suturing the connection between the renal cyst and the renal pelvis, I repeat one more time the test of permeability by administering a cold saline solution into the pelvis. The lack of leakage of fluid into the lumen of the cyst allows for the next step consisting of filling the cyst cavity (for example with one of the absorbable hemostatic agents) and then closing the renal parenchyma above the connection with a few stitches. The tightness of the repaired connection between the calyx of the renal pelvis and the cyst must be checked again by administering sterile, cold preservation solution through the ureter into the renal pelvis [16].

Remember that a transplanted kidney has a high chance of developing urine leakage from the renal pelvis after surgery. In order to try to treat the kidney conservatively after transplantation, drain the area around the transplanted kidney with at least two large surgical drains. If it is impossible to repair the connection (and thus there is still a leakage), the kidney should be disqualified and proposed to other transplant centers. If no center wants to accept such a kidney, the kidney is—of course in accordance with the donor's family—used for research or burned in our Department of Anatomy [10–16].

## 3.7.1  *Step-by-Step Preparation of the Left Kidney for Transplantation*

### 3.7.1.1  Introduction

The left renal vein is more than three times longer than the right one (about 7.0–7.5 cm). Due to its relatively long course across the abdomen, the left vein receives several tributaries from other organs including the left ovary/testicle, left suprarenal gland and left portion of the diaphragm. The tributaries of the left vein include: left gonadal vein, left inferior phrenic vein, left adrenal vein and capsular veins of the left kidney. The left gonadal and left adrenal vein play a role during left vein preparation. Occasionally, there can be two left renal veins present. When this happens, one runs anterior and the other posterior to the aorta forming the 'renal collar'. The vein that runs posterior to the aorta is also referred to as the retro-aortic left renal vein (Fig. 1.12).

### 3.7.1.2  Kidney Position and Left Renal Vein Preparation in Steps

After reducing the perirenal fat and detailed general inspection, we can conclude that the kidney is suitable for transplantation and the next step will be its detailed preparation in such a way that, after transplantation, blood loss after reperfusion is as small as possible [17–19].

### Steps

1. The kidney is placed in a sterile bowel or dish filled with ice and preservation solution in such a position that the left renal vein is the first vessel from above, the ureter is to the right, the renal artery is on the aortic patch behind the left renal vein, the ostium of the renal artery and the left renal vein are located in front of the surgeon (Fig. 3.44).

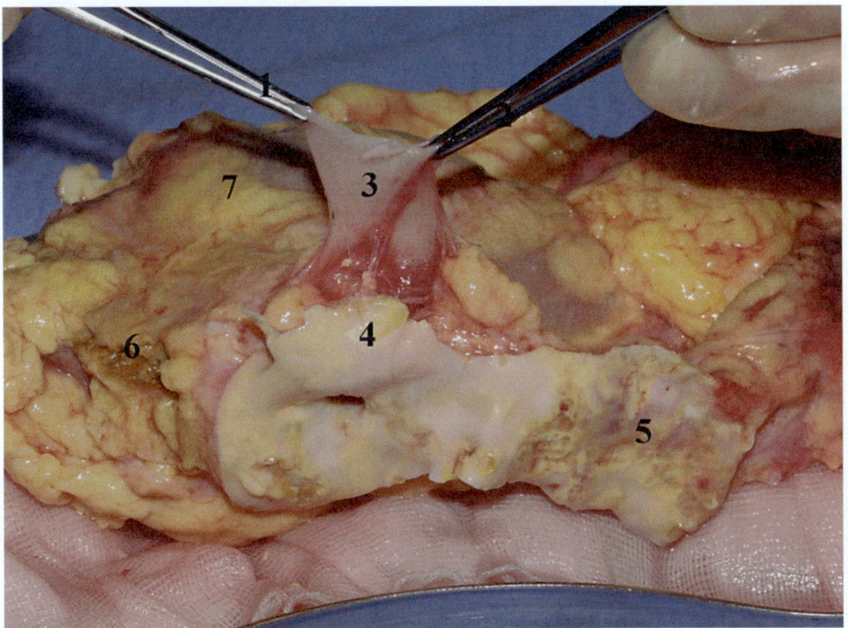

**Fig. 3.44** Put the left renal vein very gently into two vascular forceps and try to look into the lumen of the renal vein. 1 and 2—Vascular forceps, 3—Left renal vein, 4—Aortic patch below with orifice of the left renal artery, 5—Atherosclerotic changes, 6—Left adrenal gland, 7—Kidney parenchyma with perirenal fat tissue

2. Inside the lumen of the renal vein, at the mouth of its entrance into the lower main vein, using a nonabsorbable 5/0 or 6/0 monofilament suture, we put on two "orientation" or "stay sutures". The puncture made by the needle includes a small part of the patch taken from the IVC and inner surface of the left renal vein wall (Fig. 3.45). Tie this suture at a distance of 2–3 cm from the renal vein. So tied the "stay suture" is easier to remove, without damaging its wall. At the end of the "stay suture" we put on a special small vascular clam, the jaws of which have been covered with a plastic or rubber band to prevent direct damage to the suture. A second orientation stay suture is placed on the opposite side of the vein (Fig. 3.46). Orientation sutures are used to tighten the renal vein during the time of its preparation and to keep the vein in its physiological position (Fig. 3.47). An alternative to orientation or stay sutures is a clamp on the patch of the IVC or small soft vascular clamps on the left renal vein wall (Fig. 3.48).

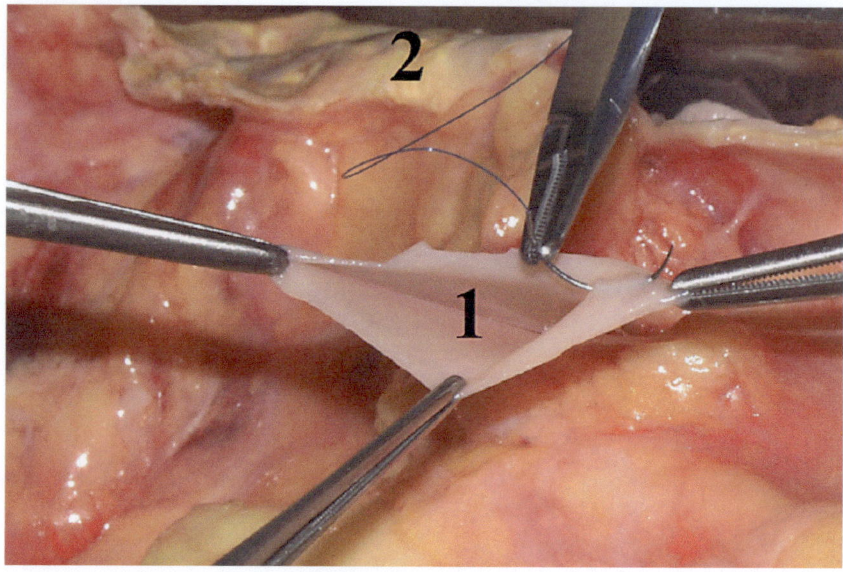

**Fig. 3.45** With the help of forceps the left renal vein has been put in a physiological position. After gentle lumen opening of the left renal vein we put from inside the first "stay suture" (nonabsorbable monofilament 5/0 or 6/0). 1—Left renal vein light, 2—Renal artery with aorta patch

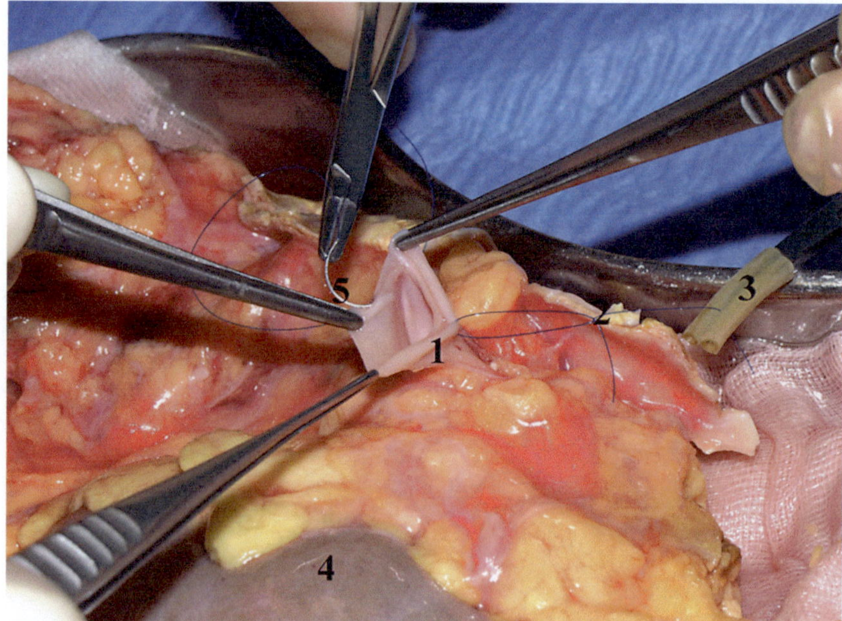

**Fig. 3.46** Fitting from inside a second stay suture. 1—Left renal vein, 2—First top corner stay suture tied about 3 cm from the wall of the left renal vein, 3—Special vascular clamp whose jaws are covered with rubber, in order not to damage the suture during kidney inspection, 4—Kidney parenchyma, 5—Bottom corner stay suture

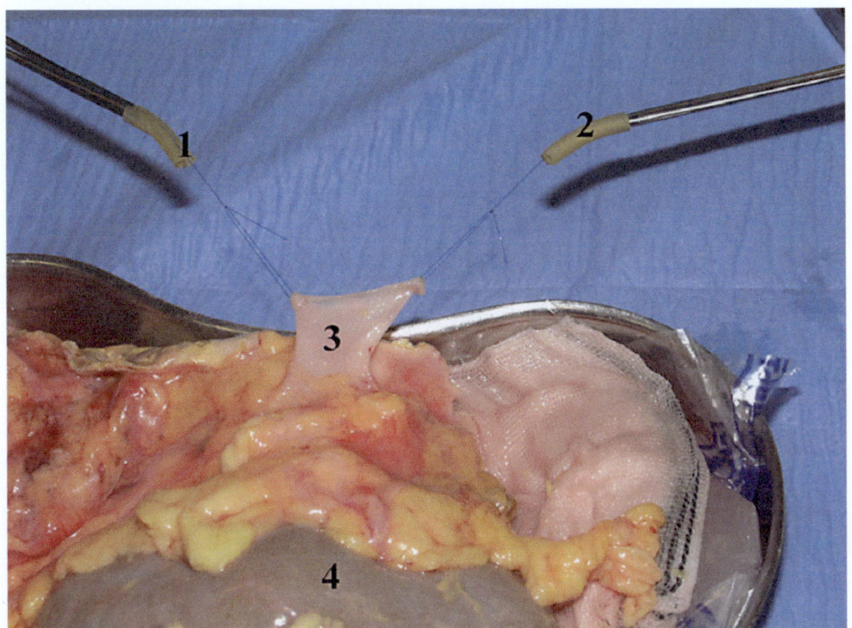

**Fig. 3.47**  Correctly inserted directional stitches (stay sutures) tied at some distance from the wall of the left renal vein, fastened with special small vascular clamps, the jaws of which have been covered with special sterile rubber tubes in order to protect the suture from cutting. 1 and 2—Stay stitches held by vascular clamps with covered jaws, 3—Left renal vein, 4—Kidney parenchyma

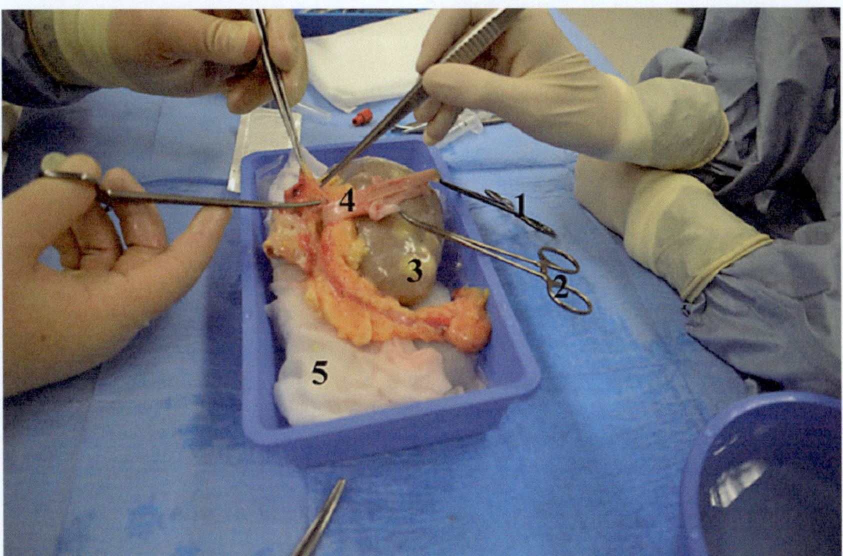

**Fig. 3.48**  An alternative to the stay sutures is the fastening of small soft vascular clamps on the edges of the patch from the IVC to create a top and bottom corner and anterior and posterior wall of the renal vein. 1 and 2—Small vascular clamps, 3—Kidney parenchyma, 4—Renal vein, 5—Sterile ice small wet gauze immersed in cold preservation solution

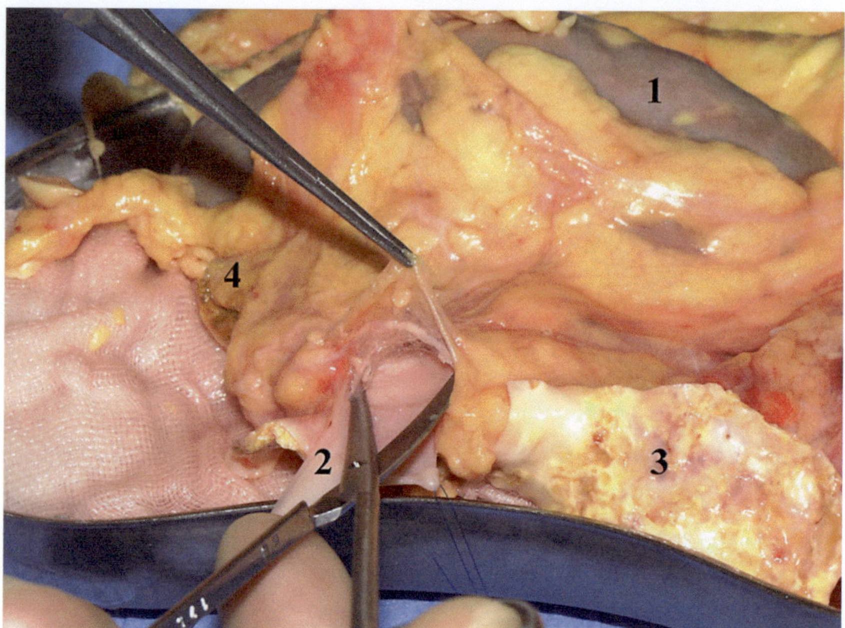

**Fig. 3.49**  The surgeon, holding forceps in his left hand and small preparation scissors in his right hand, grabs the fat tissue located above the anterior surface of the left renal vein and then gently lifts them up. Now with gentle horizontal movements of the preparation scissors, separate the fat tissue from the anterior surface of the renal vein starting from ostium of the left renal vein. Preparation of the anterior surface is continued towards the renal hilum. 1—Kidney, 2—Left renal vein, 3—Aortic patch, 4—Left adrenal gland

3. After stretching the left renal vein, the surgeon who is holding the forceps in one hand and the dissecting scissors in his other hand, grabs and gently lifts the fatty tissue situated on the anterior surface of the left renal vein with forceps. Then, with gentle horizontal movements of the preparation scissors, the surgeon separates the fat from the anterior surface of the left renal vein, starting from its venous opening into the IVC or its lumen. The preparation of the anterior surface of the left renal vein continues towards the hilum (Fig. 3.49).

4. After separating the first few centimeters of fat, from the anterior surface of the renal vein, preparation scissors are placed vertically, continuing to lift up the prepared fat with forceps. The separated fat is cut in the middle and along the long axis of the renal vein. The separation and cut of fat with scissors should be finished 2.5–3 cm from the renal hilum (Fig. 3.50).

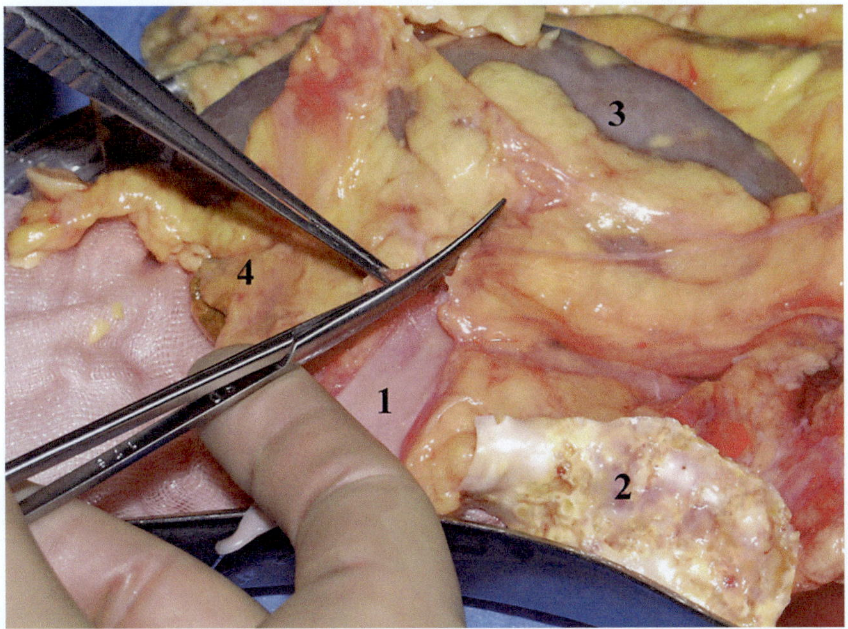

**Fig. 3.50** After separating the first few centimeters of fat tissue, invert the preparation scissors vertically, while still lifting the prepared fat tissues of the anterior surface of the left renal vein with the forceps upwards. Cut the prepared fat and tissues in the middle and along the long axis of the renal vein. Cutting the fat and tissues with scissors should end approximately 2.5–3.0 cm from the hilum of the kidney. 1—Left renal vein, 2—Aortic patch, 3—Kidney, 4—Left adrenal gland

5. In most cases the accessory renal arteries and the branches of the main renal artery may run along the anterior upper surface of the renal vein—the earliest branching occurs at a depth of about 2.0–2.5 cm from the kidney hilum. During the inspection be therefore focused and watch out. Take small steps and try to recognize and locate them quickly and do not damage them. After the dissection is completed, the anterior surface of the left renal vein must be exposed along with the adrenal and ovarian/testicular veins from which the blood flows into it (Fig. 3.51).

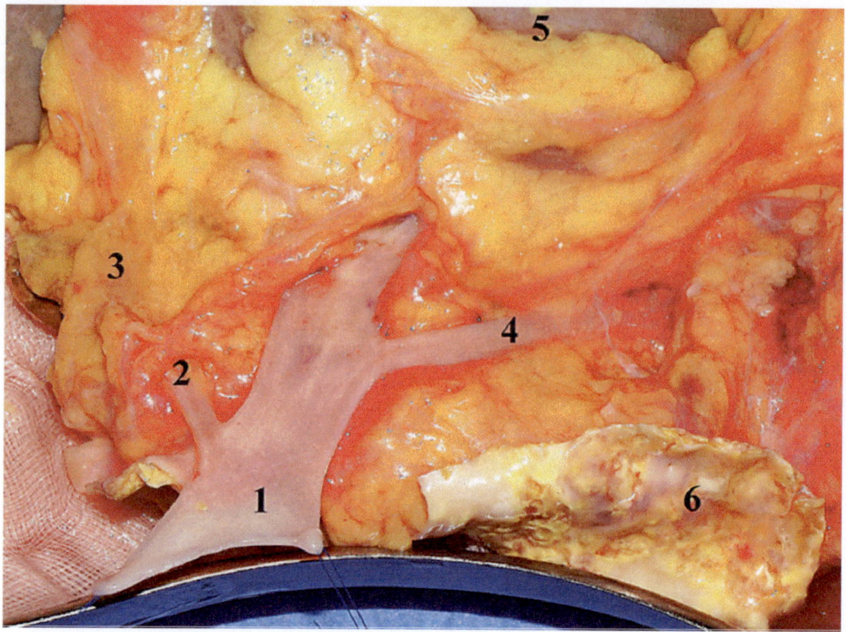

Fig. 3.51 After completion of the preparation, the anterior surface of the left renal vein is completely exposed. 1—Left renal vein, 2—Left adrenal vein, 3—Left adrenal gland, 4—Gonadal vein, 5—Kidney, 6—Aortic patch

6. Now the only thing left to do is to dissect the posterior wall of the left renal vein: to do this, ask the assistant to gently grasp both vascular clamps and lift them equally gently upwards, thus slightly straining the left renal vein. After the fat is dissected from the posterior surface of the left renal vein, the lumbar vein begins to become visible (in approximately 30% of the population). It is also possible that the lumbar vein escapes into the left renal vein on its posterior surface, but this happens less frequently. If the recognition of the branch of the renal vein is difficult, we should use a thin metal vascular probe (Fig. 3.52) to identify and distinguish the retroperitoneal branch escaping into the left renal vein from the early branch of the renal vein leading blood from the kidney to the IVC. The adrenal, testicular/ovarian, lumbar and veins other than the renal veins or their branches should be carefully ligated or sutured with a non-absorbable vascular suture (Fig. 3.53).

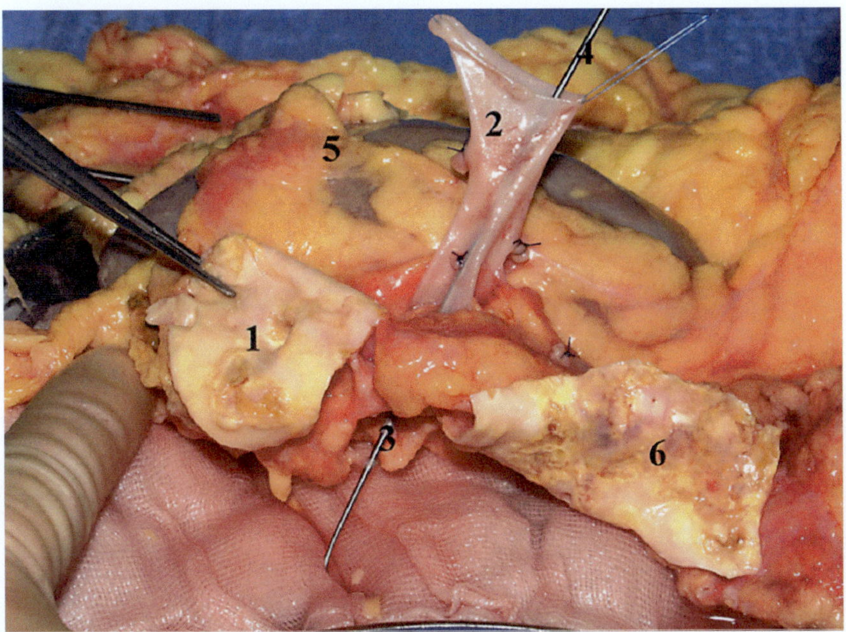

**Fig. 3.52**  During fat tissue removing from the posterior surface of the left renal vein, the lumbar veins drain the blood into the renal vein and in about 30% of cases to the left renal vein on its posterior surface. If recognizing the course of the lumbar vein becomes difficult, you should use a metal vascular probe. 1—Aortic patch with left renal artery ostium, 2—Left renal vein with a metal probe inside the lumbar vein, 3—Vascular probe outside—opening in the lumbar vein, 4—Vascular probe in the middle of the renal vein, 5—Kidney, 6—Rest of the aortic wall

7. The removed fat from the anterior and posterior surface of the left renal vein is ligated and cut 2.5–3.0 cm from the kidney's hilum (Fig. 3.54). Ligate the fat in the area of the anterior side of the renal hilium (more than 2.5–3.0 cm) and ligate all the lymphatic vessels. In this way we can prevent the formation of lymphocele which can arise due to the unclosed lymphatic vessels of the transplanted kidney. After reducing the fat, the renal vein is placed on the anterior surface of the left kidney. The next step of kidney benching will be the preparation of the renal artery (Fig. 3.55).

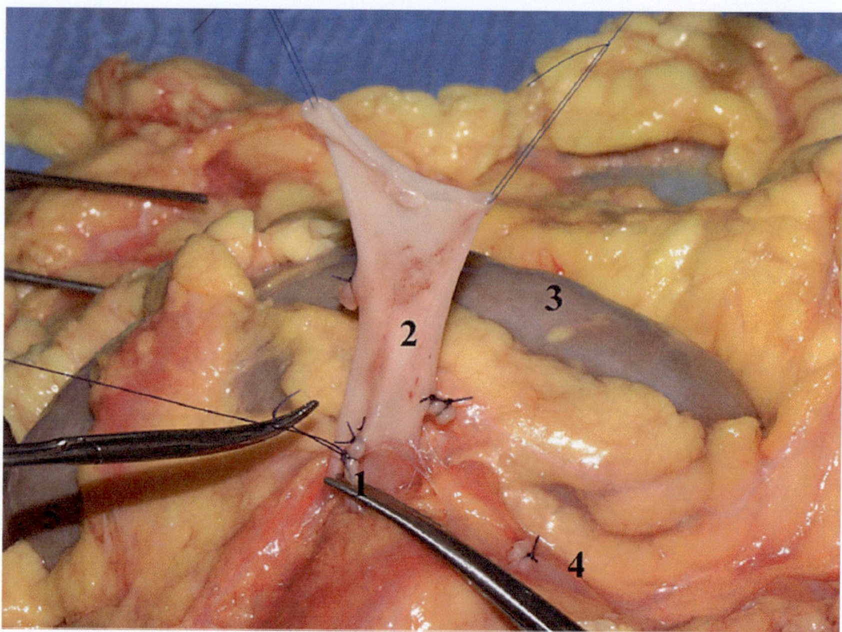

**Fig. 3.53** Lumbar vein tied on the posterior wall of the left renal vein. 1—Lumbar vein ligated and cut off, 2—Left renal vein, 3—Kidney, 4—Gonadal vein ligated and cut off

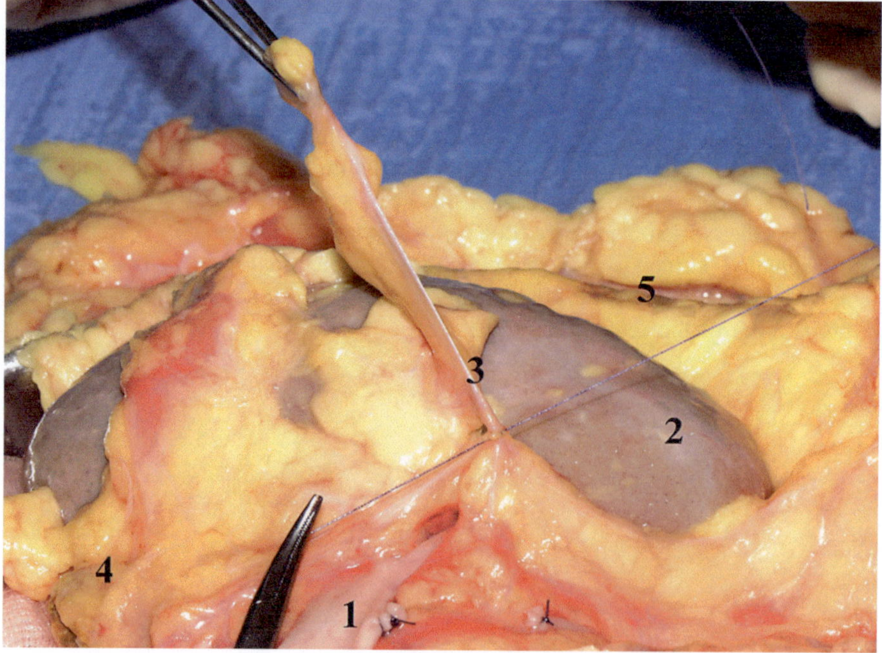

**Fig. 3.54** Excess of prepared fat tissue in the kidney hilum area. The fat tissue and lymphatic vessels are ligated 2.5–3.0 cm from the kidney hilum and cut off. 1—Left kidney vein, 2—Lower pole, 3—Excessive amount of fat, 4—Left adrenal gland, 5—Freed perirenal fat

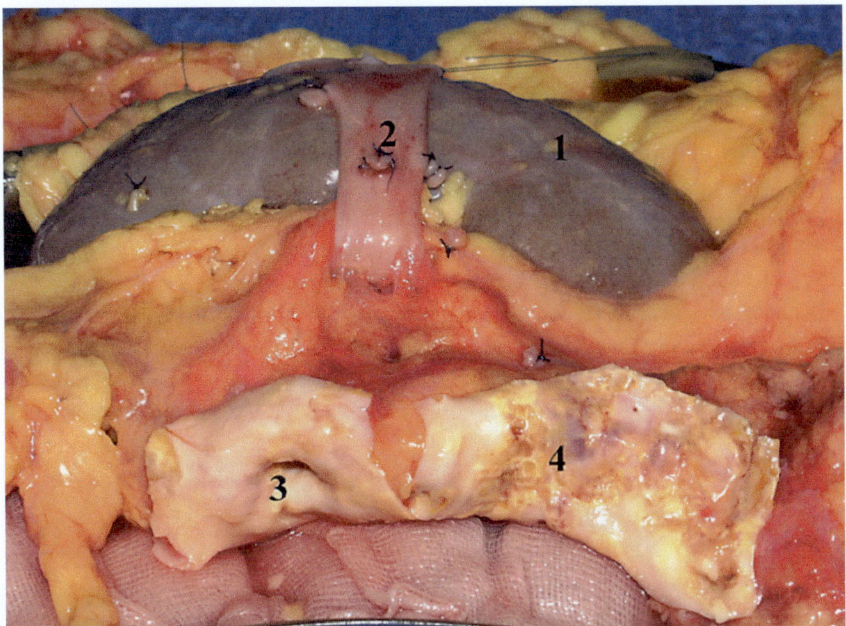

**Fig. 3.55** The limit for the reduction of excess perirenal fat tissue runs between the surface of the kidney parenchyma and its hilum. After reducing the amount of fat, the prepared left renal vein is put on the kidney surface and we proceed to the preparation of the renal artery. 1—Kidney, 2—Left renal vein prepared and placed on the upper surface of the kidney, 3—Aortic patch with ostium of the left renal artery, 4—Rest of the aortic wall

## Warnings! (Early branching, multiple arteries)

The additional renal arteries and their very early divided branches which are essential for blood supply to the kidney and ureter, can run along the anterior upper surface of the renal vein. Be therefore focused and try to prepare in small steps. In most cases the early branching of the renal artery begins 2.0–2.5 cm before the renal hilum and thus by tying the lymphatic vessels at a distance of more than 2.5–3.0 cm from the renal hilum we try to prevent damage to the branches of the previously early divided renal artery. Be very careful and predictive during the preparation and use surgical magnification loops and a cold light source (LED) to not heat up the procured kidney during the inspection.

### 3.7.1.3   General Rules for the Preparation of the Artery Before Any Vascular Anastomosis, Regardless of Its Thickness and Severity of Arteriosclerosis

A.  reduce as much adventitia as possible;

B.  dissect vessels from surrounding tissues with very gentle handling;

C.  reduce adventitia from the edge of each vessel (in most cases it hangs and obstructs the lumen of the vessel, is very thrombogenic and should be removed);

D.  irrigate each vessel lumen with heparinized physiological saline solution;

E.  if necessary, perform very gently mechanical dilatation of the artery or vein;

F.  if necessary, perform chemical dilatation (papaverine 40 mg in 100 ml 0.9% NaCl or Verapamil-based on Taha AY–21, and personal experience in the King Faisal Specialist Hospital & Research Centre, Riyadh, Saudi Arabia).

### 3.7.1.4   Preparation of the Left Renal Artery in Steps

1.  Before starting preparation of the renal artery, we once again inspect the aortic patch for the presence of additional renal arteries. The number of arteries observed on the aortic patch is compared with the number of arteries described in the donor report-organ quality form by the procurement surgeon. For this purpose, it is best to use a vascular probe which allows us to trace the course of additional renal arteries up to the renal hilum and/or poles of the kidney. If the

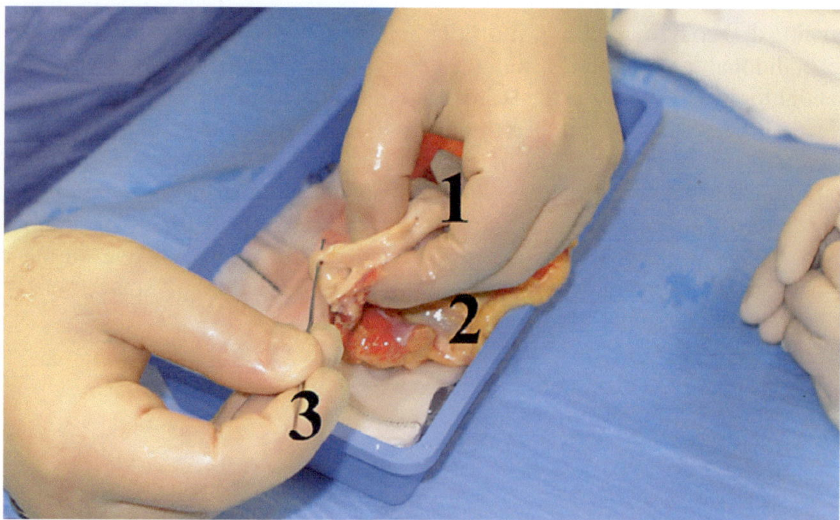


**Fig. 3.56** Before the preparation of the renal artery, we check the number of additional renal arteries arising from the abdominal aorta wall. 1—Aortic patch, 2—Kidney, 3—A special thin vascular metal probe with a finished thin head: use to recognize the course of aberrant and/or accessory renal arteries from the aortic patch

probe is too thick to determine the path and location of the renal arteries, a thin cannula can be used. Very careful, gentle and slow inspection of the renal arteries can prevent them from being damaged (Fig. 3.56).

2. The preparation of the renal artery is similar to that of the renal vein. For this purpose, we put two "stay" or orientation sutures on the aortic wall 1–2 cm to the left and right side of the ostium of the main renal artery, using a non-absorbable monofilament 5/0 or 6/0 suture. The suture that was pierced through the aortic wall is tied 2–3 cm away. On the sutures tied in this way on both sides of the artery's ostium, we place separately small vascular clamps, the jaws of which have been secured with plastic to prevent the suture from cutting. Two "stay" sutures are used to lift and tighten the renal artery during its preparation. The advantage of the use of stay sutures is that they prevent damage to the aorta patch or the ostium of the renal artery. Keep the stay sutures in a physiological position during the transplation to prevent the twisting of the renal vein and artery during the vascular anastomosis (Fig. 3.57).

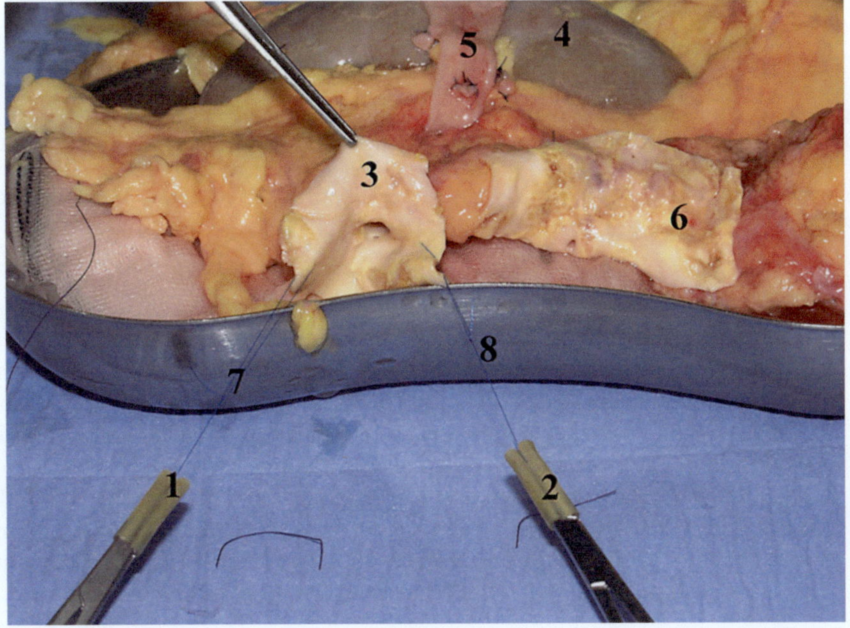

**Fig. 3.57**  Preparation for safe dissection of the renal artery. Two stay sutures over the aortic patch in a safe distance from the opening of the renal artery to the aorta. 1 and 2—Small vascular clamps fastened at the directional sutures. Small clamps jaws are covered with rubber so as not to damage the thin stay sutures, 3—Aortic patch with the ostium of the renal artery, 4—Kidney, 5—Renal vein, 6—Cut off unnecessary severe arteriosclerotic parts of the aortic patch, 7 and 8—Superior and inferior stay sutures are tied at a distance of 2–3 cm from the wall of the abdominal aorta; during the inspection the sutures can keep the renal artery under tension in a physiological position to prevent renal artery damage

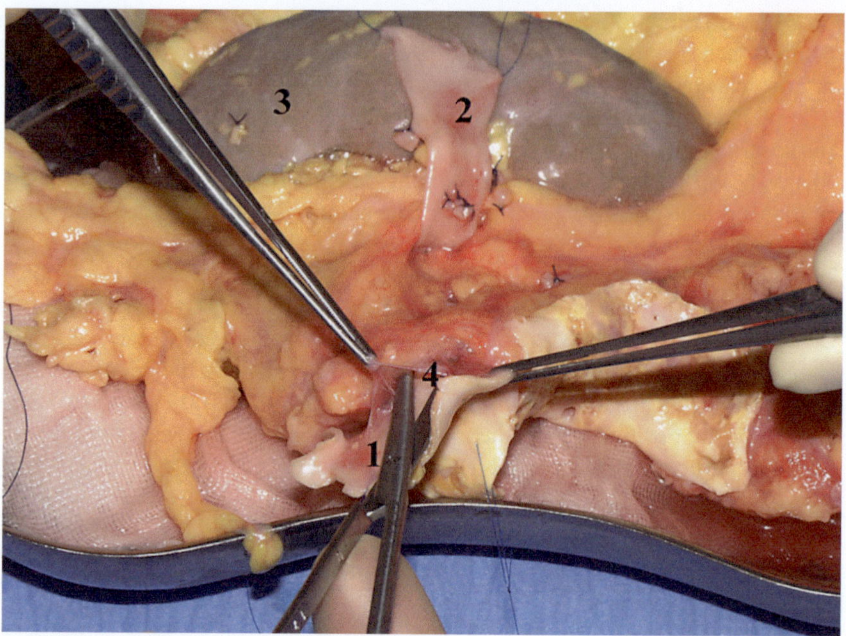

**Fig. 3.58** Preparation of the aortic patch and the beginning of the renal artery. The surgeon performs very gentle horizontal movements of the blades of the preparation scissors to separate the fat tissue from the upper surface of the renal artery. We start preparing the renal artery from its abdominal aorta patch. 1—Aortic patch, 2—Left renal vein, 3—Kidney parenchyma, 4—Renal artery

3.  After a slight stretching of the left renal artery by use of stay sutures by an assistant, the surgeon holds the forceps in one hand and the dissecting scissors in the other. With the forceps he or she grabs and lifts the fat above the renal artery up and then with a very gentle horizontal movement of the blades of the scissors attempts to separate the fat from the anterior surface of the renal artery from its opening to the aorta towards the hilum (Fig. 3.58).
4.  Turn the preparation scissors and position them vertically and continue to lift the separated fat with the forceps, which we cut in the middle and along the long axis of the artery, from its ostium towards the renal hilum. The vertical cutting with the scissors should end 2.5–3.0 cm from the renal hilum (Fig. 3.59).

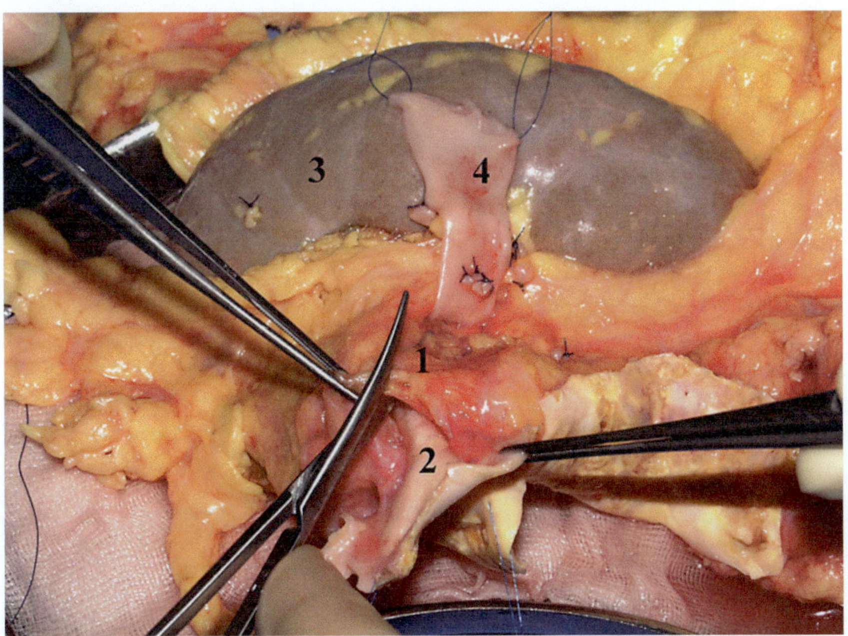

**Fig. 3.59** Turn the preparation scissors vertical, still lifting the fat tissue adjacent to the anterior side of the renal artery with forceps and separate the adipose tissue upwards. Cut the fat tissue along the long axis of the renal artery in the middle, from the aorta patch towards the kidney hilum. When cutting the fat tissue with scissors you should end approximately 2.5–3.0 cm from the hilum of the kidney. 1—With forceps raised the fat tissue covers the anterior surface of the renal artery, 2—Renal artery, 3—Kidney parenchyma, 4—Renal vein placed on the kidney

**Warning! (When inspecting the arteries, beware of the veins and vice versa)**
The additional renal veins and branches of the very early divided essential renal veins may run on the anterior surface of the renal artery. Perform the preparation carefully (using surgical magnification loupes and good, preferably cold, light), think about the veins, try to recognize them quickly, locate them and try not to damage them.

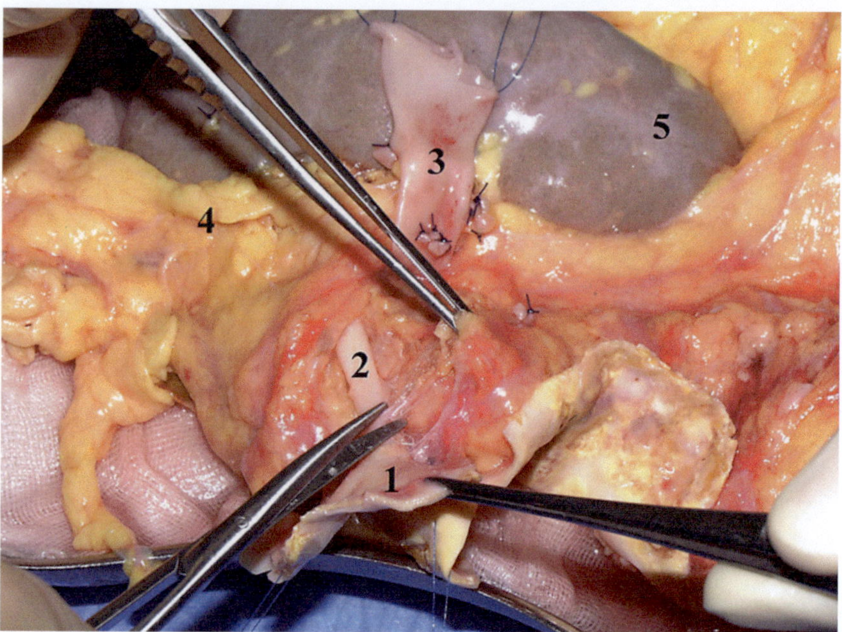

**Fig. 3.60** The anterior superior and inferior surface of the left renal artery should be prepared with departing arteries: the most permanent artery is the lower adrenal artery towards the upper pole. 1—Aortic patch, 2—Renal artery, 3—Renal vein, 4—Left adrenal gland, 5: Kidney—lower pole

5. The anterior surface of the left renal artery should be dissected with a small arterial branch arising from it: the inferior adrenal artery has the most consistent course (Fig. 3.60). Preparation of the early division of the renal artery must be completed 2.5–3.0 cm before the hilum of the kidney. Be very careful and perform the preparation very carefully—remember that the renal artery may subdivide at any level (Fig. 3.62).

**Warning! (Problem with identifying renal artery arteries)**

If you have a problem identifying the small branches of the main trunk of the renal artery or small aberrant or accessory renal arteries (for instance in the left kidney), remember that the artery going from the renal artery upwards to the upper pole of the kidney is usually the lower adrenal artery (and has to be ligated) (Fig. 3.61). A small branch of the main trunk of the renal artery close to the renal hilum going towards the lower pole of the kidney is most likely a ureteral artery. This artery plays a very important role in the blood supply to the renal pelvis and the ureter. In

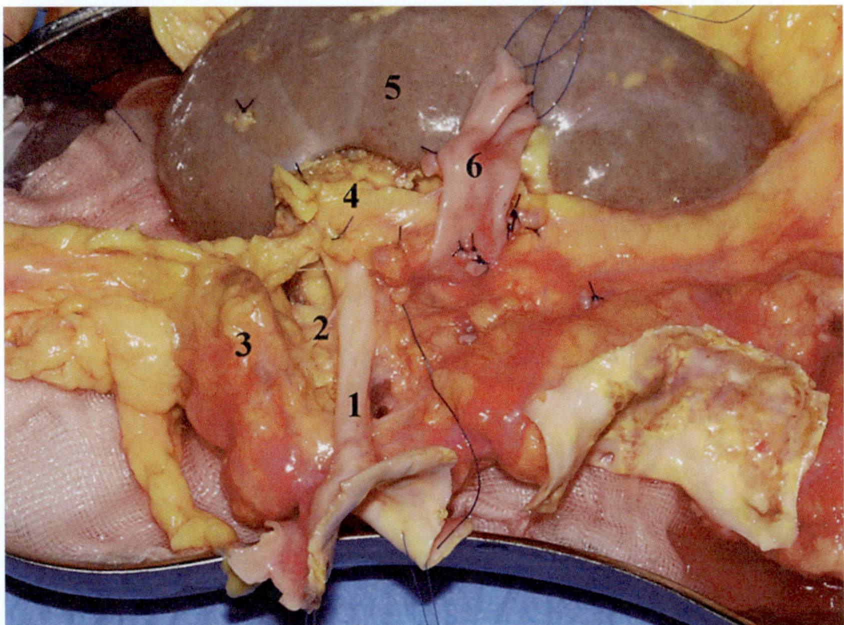

**Fig. 3.61** Preparation of the renal artery must be completed approximately 2–3 cm before the hilum. During preparation, think about the possibility of dividing the renal artery at each level. 1—Renal artery, 2—Lower adrenal artery, 3—Left adrenal gland, 4—Tied fat tissues: preparation of the renal artery completed about 2.5–3.0 cm from the renal hilum. 5—Kidney parenchyma, 6—Right renal vein

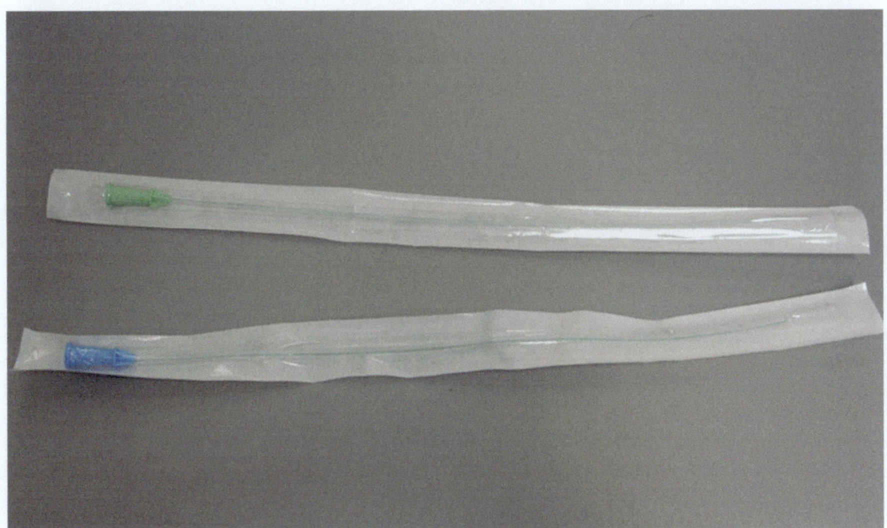

**Fig. 3.62** Thin silicone catheters, which can be used not only to identify the vessels but also to check their tightness after kidney preparation for transplantation

order to find and recognize all small branches of the main trunk renal artery and the small aberrant and accessory arteries and to regard them as small but very important branches during kidney inspection, you must first have knowledge of the anatomy and have thin cannulas, thin vascular probes (Fig. 3.62) and ultimately very thin Fogarty catheters at your disposal in the operating room.

6. The assistant lifts the renal vein and slightly pulls down the renal artery so you can very gently dissect fat and other tissues from the lateral posterior surfaces of the renal artery with scissors. Pay special attention to the proper identification of its branches that sometimes appear as a result of its early division, which is directly involved in the vascularization of the renal parenchyma. We finish the preparation of the posterior wall of the renal artery, 2.5–3.0 cm from the hilum (Fig. 3.63).

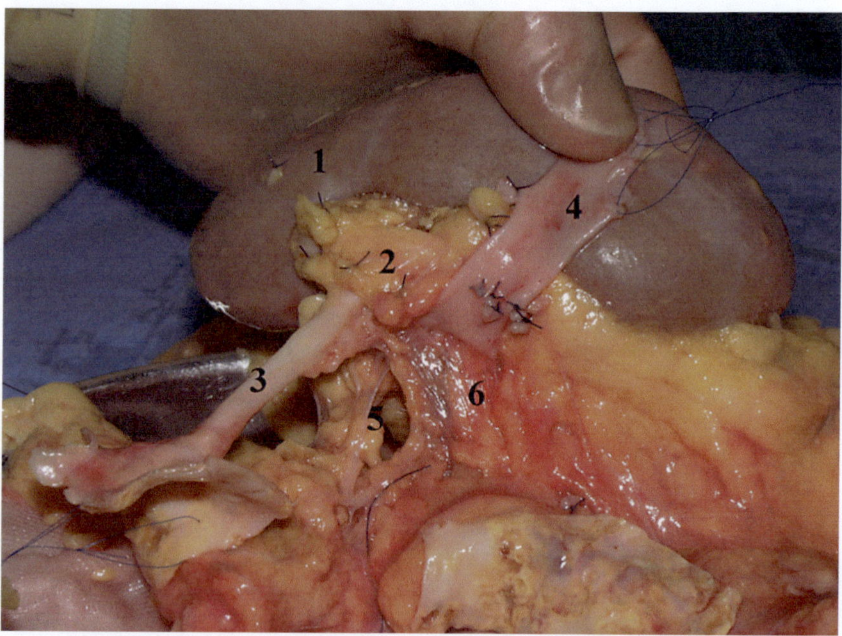

**Fig. 3.63** After the assistant lifts the renal vein and slightly pulls down the renal artery, fat tissue is dissected from the posterior surface of the renal artery. We finish the posterior wall of the renal artery preparation 2.5–3.0 cm from the hilum. Pay special attention to the correct diagnosis of early branches of the renal artery directly flowing into the renal parenchyma. 1—Kidney, 2—Kidney hilum, 3—Renal artery, 4—Renal vein, 5 and 6—Fat tissue close to the kidney's hilum with lymphatic vessels

7. Place the prepared artery on the anterior surface of the kidney and start reducing the excess fat in the area of its upper pole. Small amounts of fat along with the lymphatic vessels are ligated 2.5–3.0 cm from the hilum with 4/0 soluble surgical ligatures from the upper pole of the kidney towards the ureter (Fig. 3.64).
8. Fat preparation around the kidney's lower pole must be performed very carefully due to the blood supply to the ureter. Try to save the "golden triangle"—i.e. the optimal arterial blood supply of every procured kidney—during the preparation (Fig. 3.65).

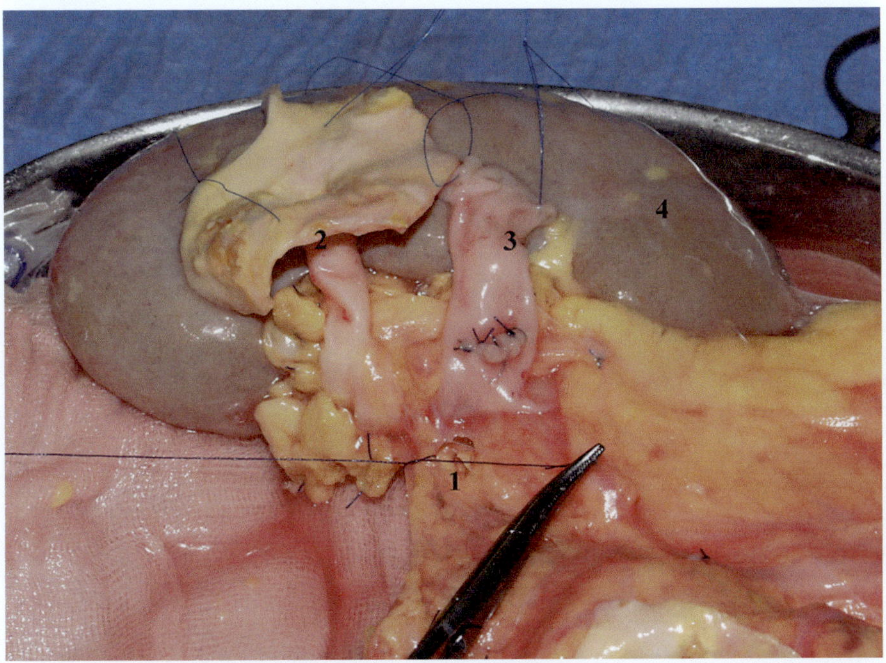

**Fig. 3.64** Place the prepared renal artery on the anterior surface of the kidney and start to reduce the excess fat in the kidney's hilum towards the ureter. Fat tissue and lymphatic vessels are ligated 2.5–3.0 cm from the kidney hilum with absorbable sutures 4/0. 1—Lymphatic vessel and fat tissue ligation, 2—Renal artery, 3—Renal vein, 4—Kidney

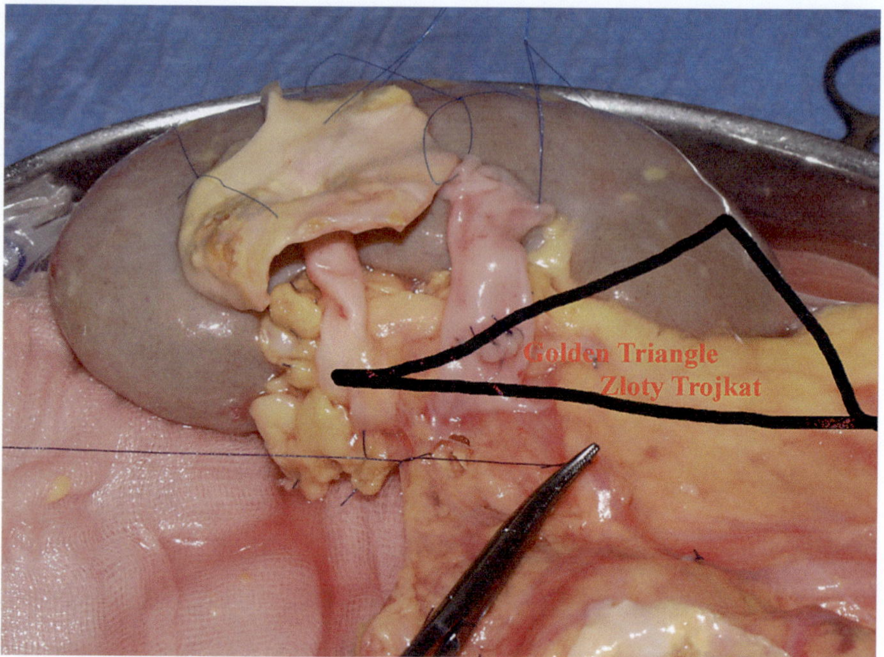


**Fig. 3.65** Preparation of fat tissue around the lower part of the hilum and the lower pole must be done very carefully due to the blood supply to the ureter. Here is the "golden triangle" that forms the lower pole, renal vessels and the ureter with uretero-pelvic fat tissue together with the small vessels that carry blood to the ureter

### 3.7.1.5  Kidneys with Multiple Renal Arteries

Introduction

Generally the management of multiple renal arteries (MRA) is technically demanding. According to certain authors, cadaver kidney procurement with an en bloc technique has helped to significantly decrease accidental injury to polar arteries. In addition back table repair of arterial injuries and bench reconstruction of multiple arteries have helped to significantly expand the pool of cadaver and living donor renal grafts. Technical difficulties with a renal arterial anastomosis can lead to the infarction of the graft segment, infection, calyceal fistula or ureter necrosis. These issues lead to an increased number of complications, increased morbidity and a higher rate of graft loss. Lower polar arteries must be precisely anastomozed as their occlusion can cause ischemia, infarction and urological complications, such as calyces or ureter necrosis with bad healing and at the end fistulas may result. Results of renal artery reconstruction improved with the introduction of extracorporeal microsurgical repair of arterial injuries. Bench reconstruction or back table of MRA have become commonplace in the major kidney transplant centers all over the world.

## MRA: Most Common Techniques for Back Table Reconstruction

Several techniques for back table reconstruction of MRA have been described: the smaller artery usually is anastomozed in end to side fashion to the main trunk of the renal artery; if for example two arteries from the same kidney have the same size—common ostium—side to side anastomosis in this case should be done. Another major known technique to implant MRA is performed by using the external iliac artery with end to side anastomosis, using the internal iliac artery and inferior epigastric artery for end to end anastomosis. Rossi et al. [8] used a Teflon patch to perform end to side with patch multiple artery anastomosis. Back table work when repairing and reconstructing might prolong the cold ischemia time which does not affect renal function if it is adequately perfused and cooled. The presence of an aortic patch does not have an impact on graft outcome or on the rate of complication. Kidney grafts with a single artery can be anastomozed either end to end to the hypogastric or end to side to the external iliac artery with equal results. Panwar et al. [20] similarly showed that the five-year graft survival for end to side anastomosis was markedly lower at 40% compared to 70% for the side to side (common ostium) group and 90% for the direct anastomosis group. Separate implantation of a smaller artery in an external or internal iliac artery runs the risk of prolonging the warm ischemia time (WIR) potentially leading to worse graft outcomes, although sequential anastomosis of the smaller artery with the inferior epigastric artery is another good option described earlier by Panwar et al. The inferior epigastric artery may not always be available due to atherosclerosis or an insufficient diameter relative to the accessory renal artery. The smaller renal artery may also be prone to thrombosis or stenosis. Panwar et al. [20] believe that pantaloon anastomosis (common ostium) overcomes the above complications of its alternative options while providing a larger diameter channel thus reducing the risk of stenosis. Panwar et al. [20] routinely dilate both arteries using vascular dilators during bench dissection. This widens the smaller artery and may help in performing side to side anastomosis. Although their follow-up is short, none of the patients in the pantaloon group developed arterial thrombosis or graft loss and there were no re-explorations in the group. In their conclusion you can read that pantaloon anastomosis is feasible in renal grafts with double renal arteries with significant luminal discrepancy and offers the advantage of a lower warm ischemia time in the recipient compared to separate implantation techniques [40].

Li et al. [21] evaluated arterial blood supply using methylene blue (MB) perfusion, and accessory arteries supplying less than 10% of the total MB perfusion volume were ligated. The other cases were assessed using a conventional method in which arteries with diameters less than 2 mm were ligated. The back-table surgical time, Doppler ultrasonography index, renal function and complications were compared between the two groups. No differences in the Doppler ultrasonography index or postoperative complications were noted. The conclusion is that MB perfusion provides an easy and effective method to make decisions regarding arterial ligation and helps to preserve renal function without increasing the number of complications after transplantation [21].

Kidneys with MRA should therefore be implanted using the technique that not only fits best in a particular situation, but also that is the most comfortable for the individual transplant surgeon [22–34]. Example multiple artery reconstructions have been performed by the author (Figs. 3.129, 3.131, 3.134, 3.136, 3.138 and 3.139).

### 3.7.1.6   Preparation of the Ureter in Steps

1. The localization of the ureter is usually not difficult: it shows through the tissues, is whiter and, even with little experience, it is usually easy to recognize. However, sometimes it is not easy to recognize—especially in obese patients— but you can help yourself by using surgical loupes. When trying to identify the ureter, remember that its lumen is in the shape of a star. Another tip for finding and identifying the ureter is to cannulate it with a soft thin sterile tube and inject sterile cold physiologic saline or Ringer's solution, or preservation fluid into its lumen. The slow enlargement of the renal pelvis will provide the evidence that we are dealing with the ureter.
2. The next step in the preparation of the ureter is to reduce the amount of fat tissue around it. The reduction of fat can be done from the bottom to the top or vice versa. Remember that the arterial supply of the ureter depends only on the ureter's small arterial branch departing from the renal artery, so the amount of tissues around the ureter, going from the renal recess to its end, should decrease. The previously cut off ovarian or testicular vein, if it is not very much associated with the ureter, should be removed and its branches around the ureter ligated with a thin (e.g. 4/0 or 5/0) absorbable suture (Figs. 3.66, 3.67 and 3.68 show a kidney after vessel and ureter preparation and fat reduction) [22].

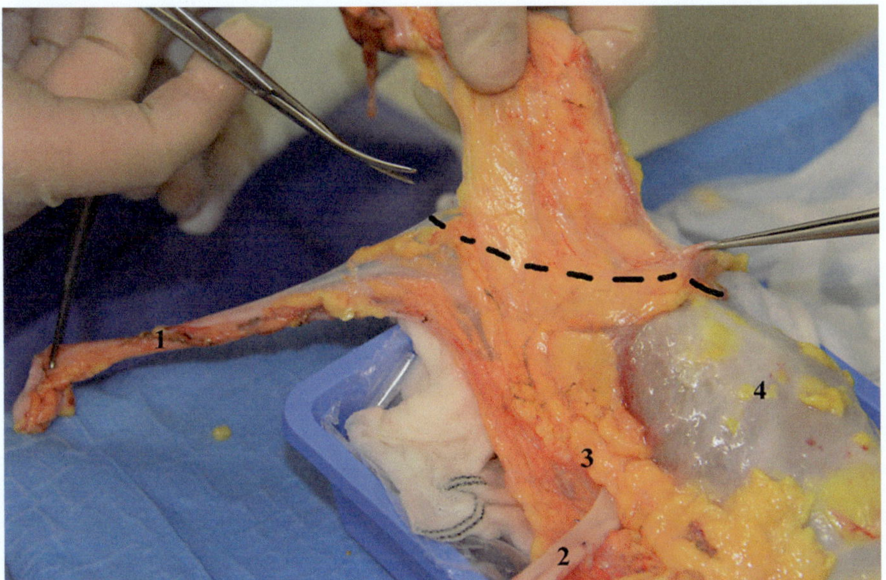

**Fig. 3.66** The next step is to reduce the amount of fat tissue in the ureter area, which can be done from the bottom up or vice versa. Remember that the arterial supply of the ureter depends only on the ureter's small arterial branch departing from the renal artery, so the amount of tissues around the ureter from the renal recess to its end should be reduced. 1—Ureter, 2—Renal vein, 3—Surrounding the renal hilum (small artery to the ureter), 4—Kidney parenchyma and the black dotted line shows the border of fat tissue cutting in the area of the hilum and lower pole of the kidney, preserving the golden triangle and providing good ureteral perfusion

**Warning! (Be careful to save the golden triangle)**

Distal ureteral ischemia and necrosis secondary to compromised blood supply is thought to be the main culprit for early ureteral complications in most patients in the absence of technical difficulties during the transplant operation. In contrast to the native ureters, which derive their blood supply via both renal arteries and pelvic collaterals, the transplanted ureter depends solely on the blood supplied by the branch of the renal artery that traverse in peri-ureteric tissues. This area, also known as the golden triangle (Fig. 3.65), contains important arterial branches, such as the lower polar artery, which supplies the distal ureter. In order to prevent disastrous urinary complications, it is important to preserve the peri-ureteral connective tissue.

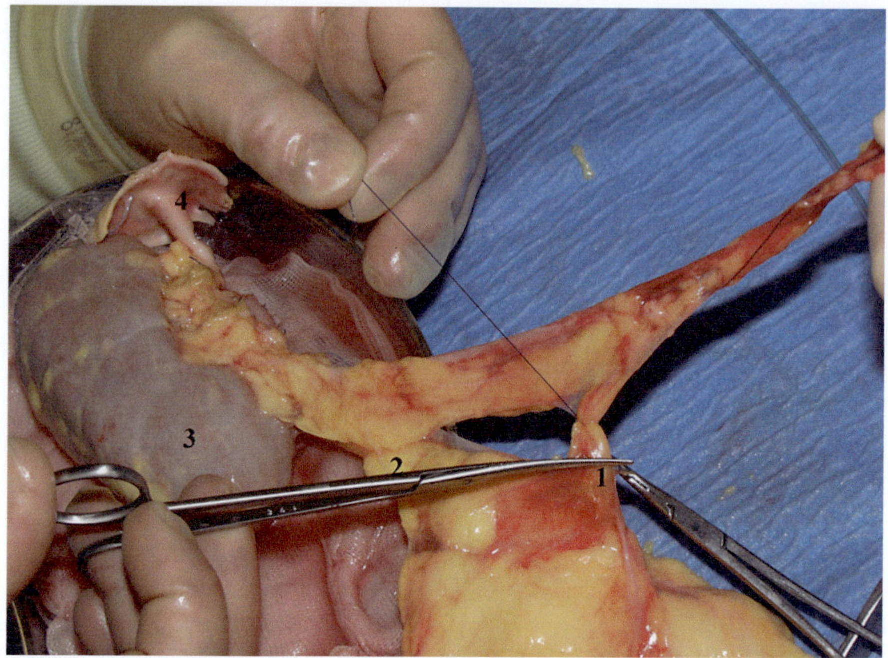

**Fig. 3.67** Remember that the arterial supply of the ureter depends only on the ureteral small arterial branch departing from the renal artery, so the amount of fat tissues around the lower part of the renal hilum and the ureter going from the kidney hilum to its end must be reduced to avoid ischemia. 1—Fat tissue reduction around the ureter, 2—Ureteral fat tissue, 3—Kidney parenchyma, 4—Renal artery

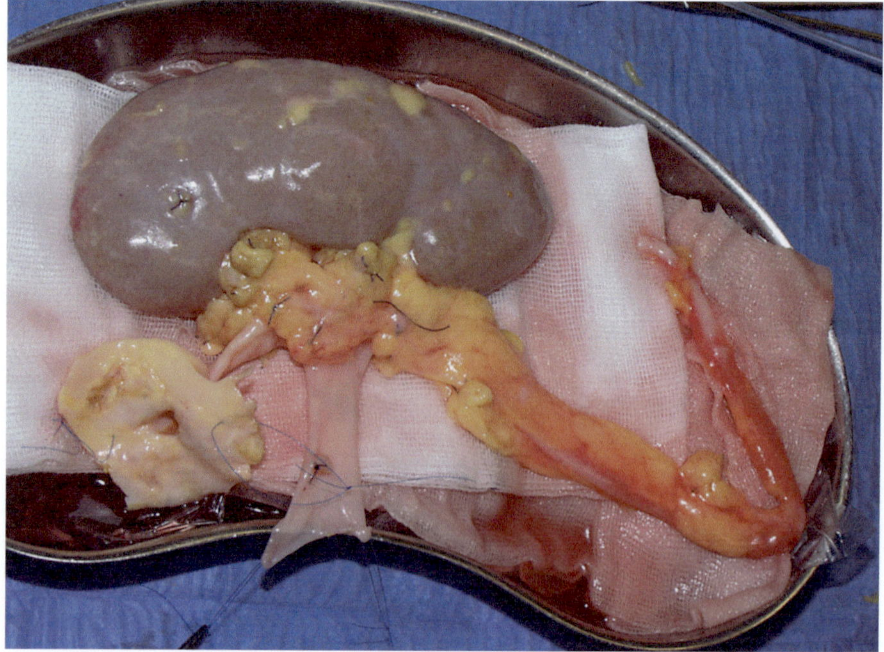

**Fig. 3.68** Kidney after inspection prepared for packing and transplantation

### 3.7.2  Testing of Renal Vascular Tightness and Renal Parenchyma Perfusion Quality: Detection of Mechanical Damage or Stenosis to the Renal Mediastinum and Ureter

#### 3.7.2.1  Testing the Renal Artery and Vein Separately

The surgeon asks the scrub nurse to pour into sterile bowls located on the preparation table a fresh cold preservation solution or to prepare an infusion set with a bag of cold preservative solution suspended on a drip stand (I do not recommend this because the perfusion solution heats up quickly) (Fig. 3.69). After filling the sterile bowls with cold, sterile perfusion solution, fill a 50 ml syringe with it and connect it to a thin sterile catheter. In the next step, remove excess air from the

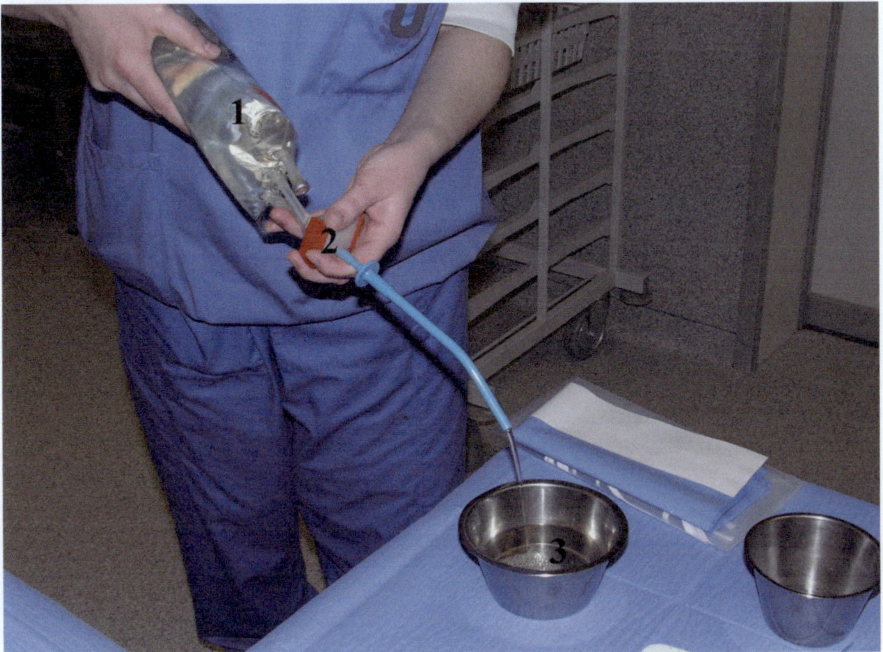

**Fig. 3.69** The surgeon preparing the kidney asks one of the scrub nurses to pour into a sterile container located on the preparation table a cold, fresh preservation solution. 1—Chilled preservation solution taken straight from the fridge, 2—Filter, 3—Fresh cold preservation solution poured into the sterile small bowls

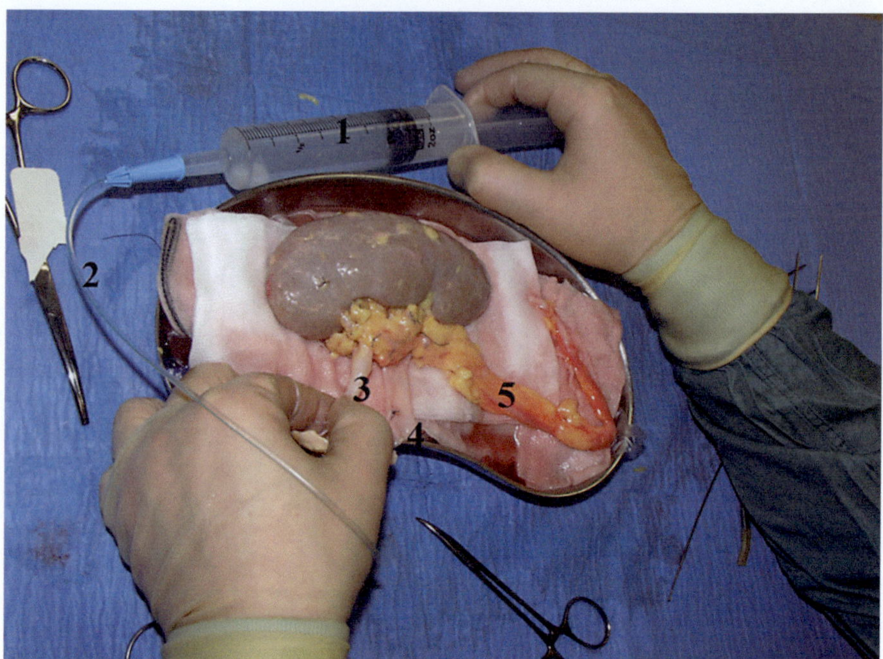

**Fig. 3.70** Prepared kidney. Testing the integrity of the vessels and ureter after preparing (benching) the kidney for transplantation. 1—Syringe, 2—Silicone tube, 3—Renal artery cannulated with silicone tube, 4—Renal vein, 5—Ureter

entire system. Very gently insert the catheter into the lumen of the renal artery, not further than halfway along the length, and very slowly close the lumen of the renal artery around the drain with your fingers. During injection into the lumen of the renal artery, avoid solution leakage between the inserted catheter and the artery lumen (Fig. 3.70). Pay attention to solution leaks from the holes in the artery wall and/or small branches. If out of small openings or cut off branches of the vessels fluid emerges, these should be tied or sutured, depending on the lumen diameter, with a 6/0 or 7/0 non-absorbable suture (Fig. 3.71 and 3.72).

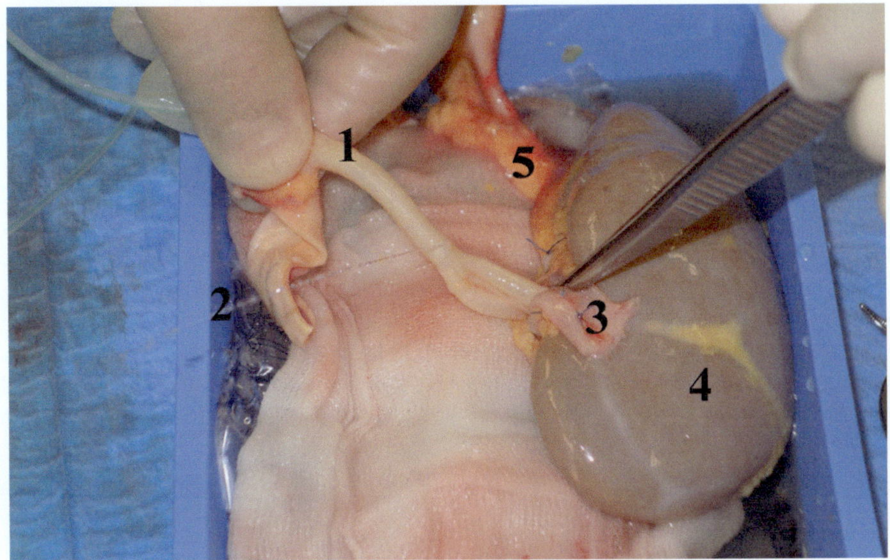

**Fig. 3.71**  1—Renal artery, 2—Leakage of preservation solution from the wall of the renal artery as a result of a small arterial branch being torn out at the time of kidney procurement, 3—Kidney hilum, 4—Kidney parenchyma, 5—Ureter

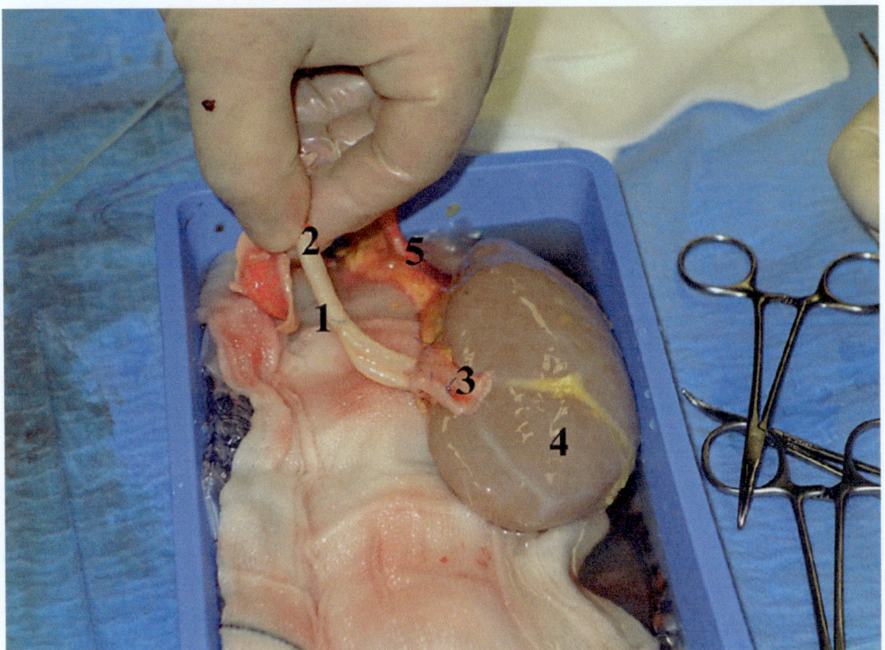

**Fig. 3.72**  Leakage of preservation solution from the wall of the renal artery was sutured. 1—Place of leakage: the leakage area was closed with a 7/0 non-absorbable suture, 2—Renal artery, 3—Renal vein, 4—Kidney, 5—Ureter

**Warning! (When there is reduced blood loss—test the vessels!)**
In the same way you can test the renal vein wall for leaks.


### 3.7.2.2  Quality of Parenchyma Rinsing

When flushing the kidney through the renal artery, pay close attention to the color of the fluid coming out of the renal vein. If the color is bloody, this indicates that the kidney was not rinsed well for blood and preserved. In this case, continue flushing until a pale pink or clear preservation solution begins to flow out of the renal vein (Fig. 3.73). As you can see in the figure the kidney during organ procurement was flushed through the main artery, but its lower pole, unfortunately, has not discolored and you can still see blood in it (Fig. 3.74). In the case shown here we need to try to locate the additional renal artery responsible for the lower kidney's arterial blood supply or damage at the level of the renal hilum to one of the renal artery branches

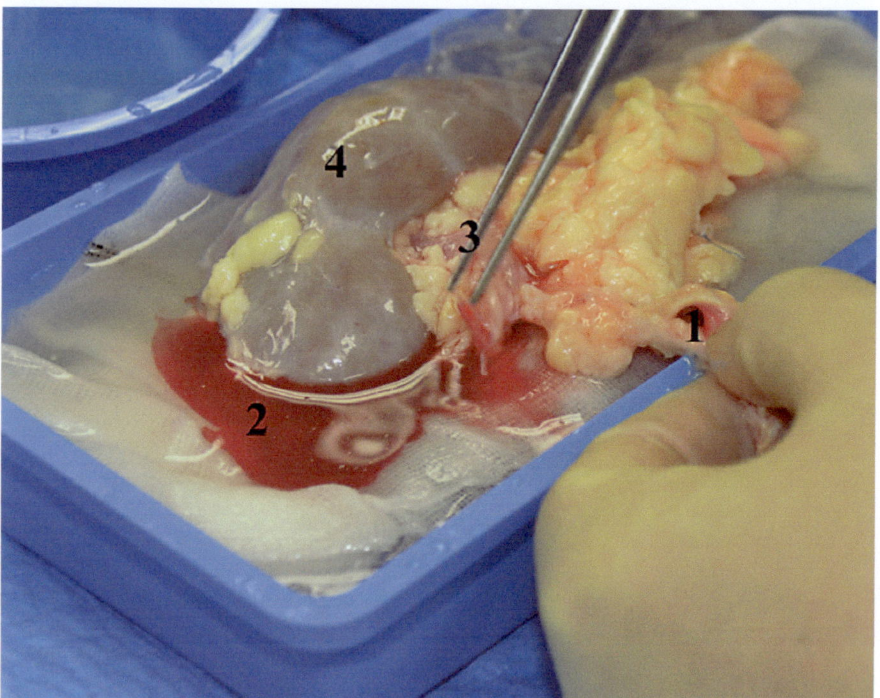


**Fig. 3.73**  Badly flushed lower pole kidney: after slow rinsing of the renal artery blood comes out of the renal vein. 1—Renal artery, 2—Blood coming out of the renal vein, 3—Renal vein, 4—Kidney

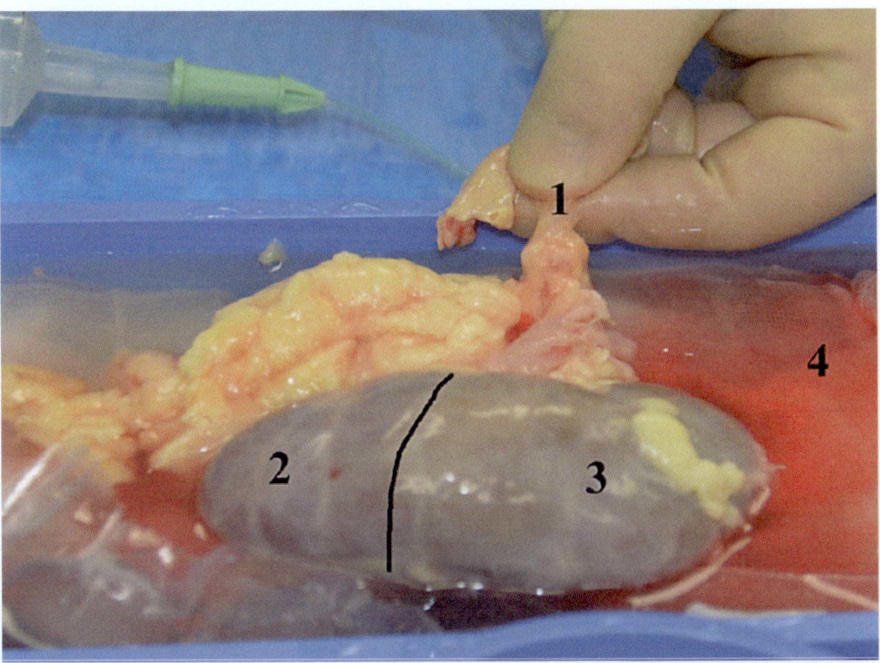

**Fig. 3.74** 1—Washing out kidney through the renal artery: unfortunately the lower pole of the kidney has not discolored and still contains blood. 1—Kidney artery, 2—Lower pole, 3—Upper pole of the kidney, 4—Blood coming out of the renal vein

from the main trunk of the renal artery responsible for vascularization of the lower pole of the kidney. After a thorough inspection of the kidney, the renal hilum was intact. The only logical explanation for this seems to be the presence of an aberrant renal artery not identified at the time of organ procurement, for example arising from the iliac vessels or from the abdominal aorta close to its bifurcation. Indeed, after a thorough inspection of the fat, we found an aberrant left renal artery to the lower pole (Fig. 3.75).

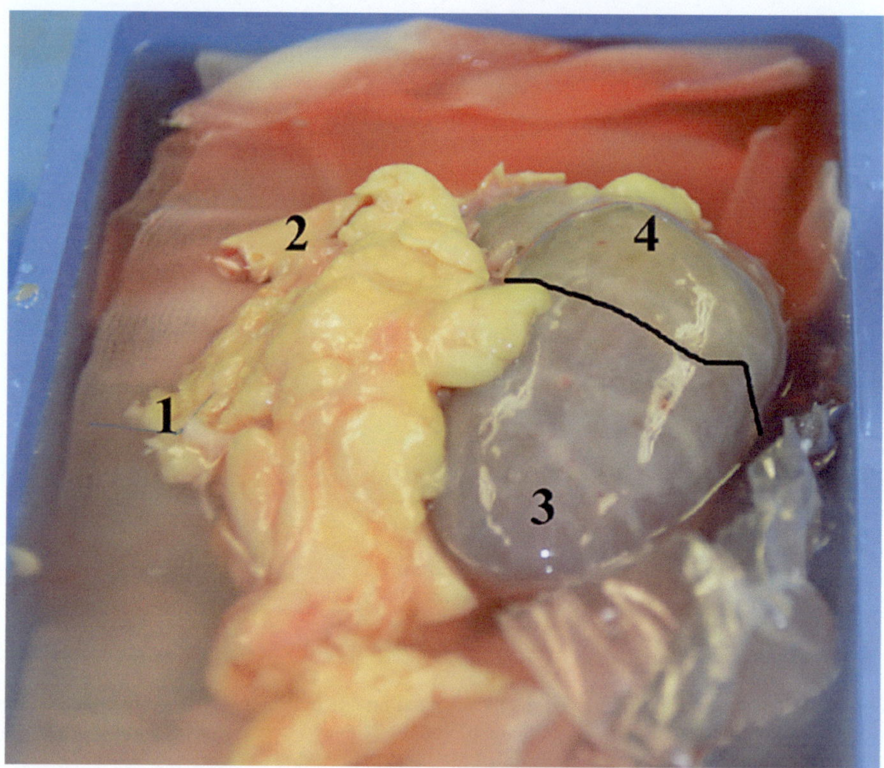

**Fig. 3.75** 1—Unnoticed, found and marked with suture aberrant renal artery to the lower pole of the kidney, 2—The main renal artery, 3—The lower pole of the kidney not washed out with blood, 4—The upper pole of the kidney is well flushed

The found aberrant renal artery to the lower pole was immediately perfused with cold preservation solution with added heparin (Fig. 3.76). The blood in the lower part of the kidney was washed out after a few minutes. The lower pole artery was reconstructed and implanted end to side in the wall of the main renal artery with nonabsorbable sutures 7/0 (Fig. 3.77). The presented kidney was successfully repaired and transplanted; after reperfusion the renal parenchyma had everywhere colored properly with a normal urine secretion during the whole postoperative period.

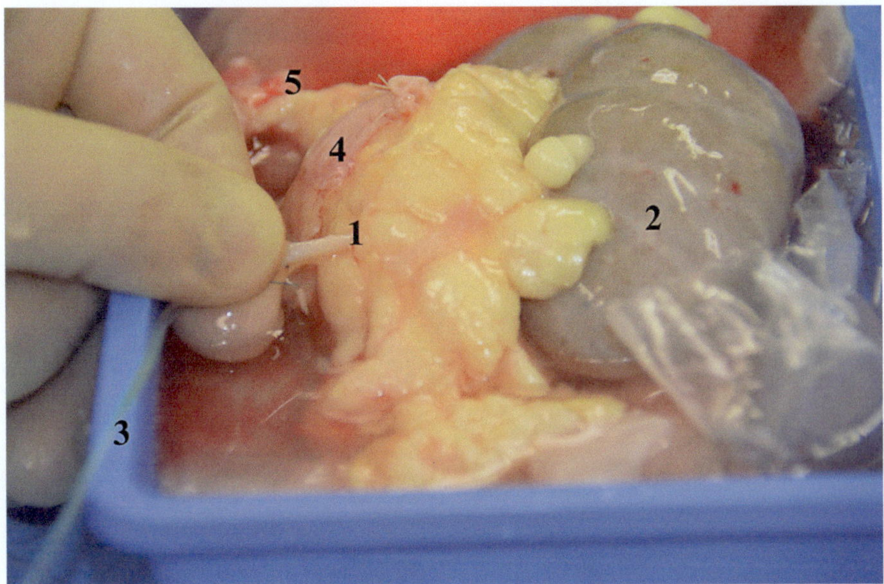

**Fig. 3.76**  The lower pole of the kidney is supplied with blood by a small accessory artery to the lower pole of the kidney. This artery was found incidentally during the inspection of the kidney. This artery was not listed as a damaged artery on the quality forms for the organs. 1—Flushing of the aberrant small renal artery leading to the lower half (pole) of the kidney and removal of residual blood from the lower pole of the kidney supplied by it, 2—After a few minutes of flushing the aberrant artery to the lower pole of the kidney together with the parenchyma of the lower pole of the kidney, when the blood is flushed out, the colour of the lower pole is normal and it no longer contains residual blood, 3—Thin silicone catheter inserted into the lumen of aberrant renal artery to the lower pole, 4—Renal vein, 5—Aortic patch

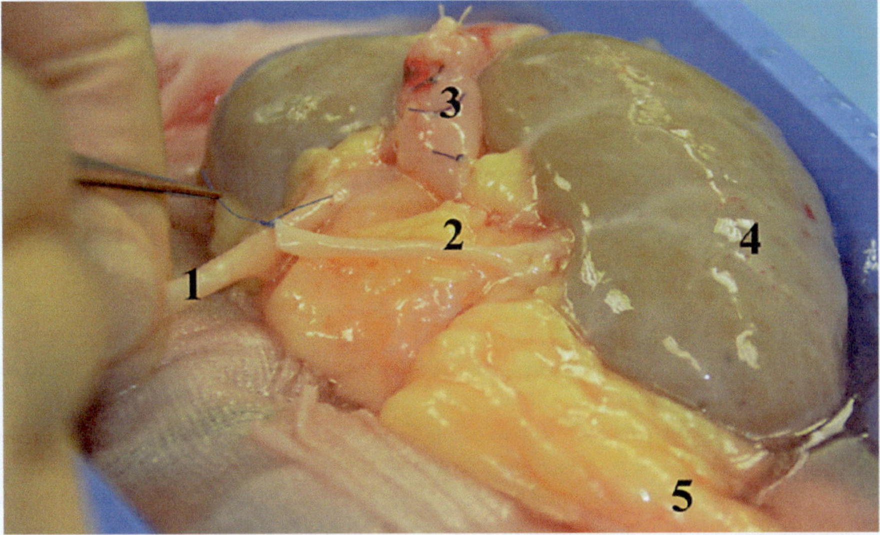

**Fig. 3.77**  The same kidney is already well rinsed. 1—Main renal artery, 2—An additional renal artery runs to the lower pole of the kidney and after careful dissection it was decided to anastomose its end to the side of the main renal artery trunk, 3—Renal vein, 4—Kidney, 5—Ureter

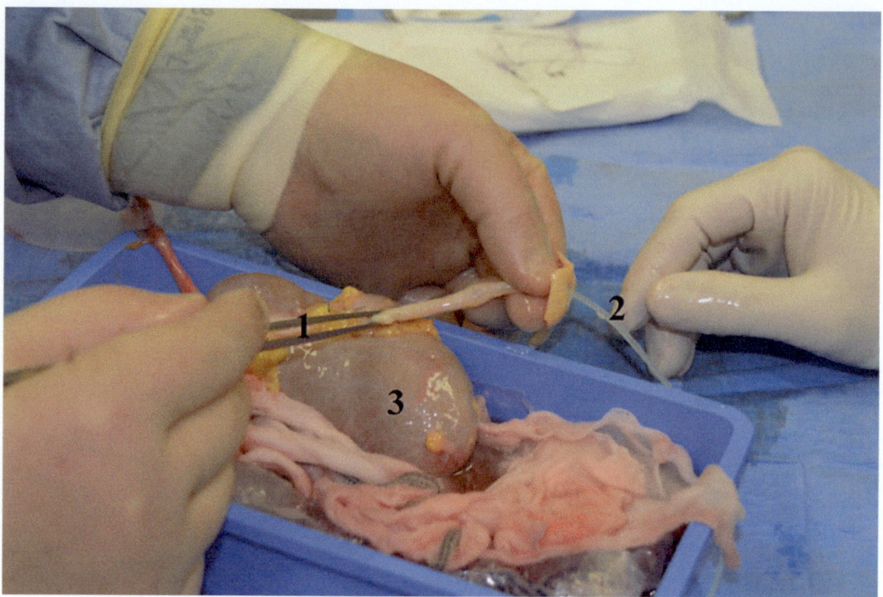

**Fig. 3.78** Sometimes pressure of the solution administered into the lumen of renal artery is insufficient to detect leakage; in order to find the leak in the renal artery, its branches or in the renal hilum, the renal artery can be gently closed using a small soft vascular clamp or soft vascular forceps or fingers. 1—Soft vascular forceps, 2—Small silicon tube inserted into the lumen of the renal artery, 3—Kidney

## Avoid Renal Artery Injury

If you think that the pressure of the applied cold sterile solution in the artery lumen is insufficient to detect a leak, in order to find the leak in the renal artery, its branches or in the renal hilum, the artery can be gently closed using soft vascular forceps (Fig. 3.78), your own fingers (best method) or a tiny vascular clamp (small bulldog). Please be very careful and avoid a lesion of the renal artery caused by a vascular clamp or forceps.

### 3.7.2.3  Simultaneous Testing of the Renal Artery and Vein

In principle, this kind of testing is 99% the same as previously described in Sect. 3.7.2.1. when the renal artery and renal vein are tested simultaneously, this means that before injecting the cold preservation solution into the lumen of the renal artery, the surgeon closes the end of the renal vein very gently with the fingers of one hand (Fig. 3.79), with fine and soft vascular forceps (Fig. 3.80) or with a fine bulldog which is a non-traumatizing vascular clamp (Fig. 3.81). Pay special attention to any type of leakage of the preservation solution from the vessel or its branches, and also in the hilum of the kidney. Any fluid leakage should be sutured or ligated preferably 6/0 or 7/0 with a non-absorbable suture. If the tightness of the vein does not seem to be sufficient to close it with a clamp, we can try very gently to close its lumen 2–3 cm in front of the renal hilum with our own fingers or very soft forceps (Fig. 3.82).

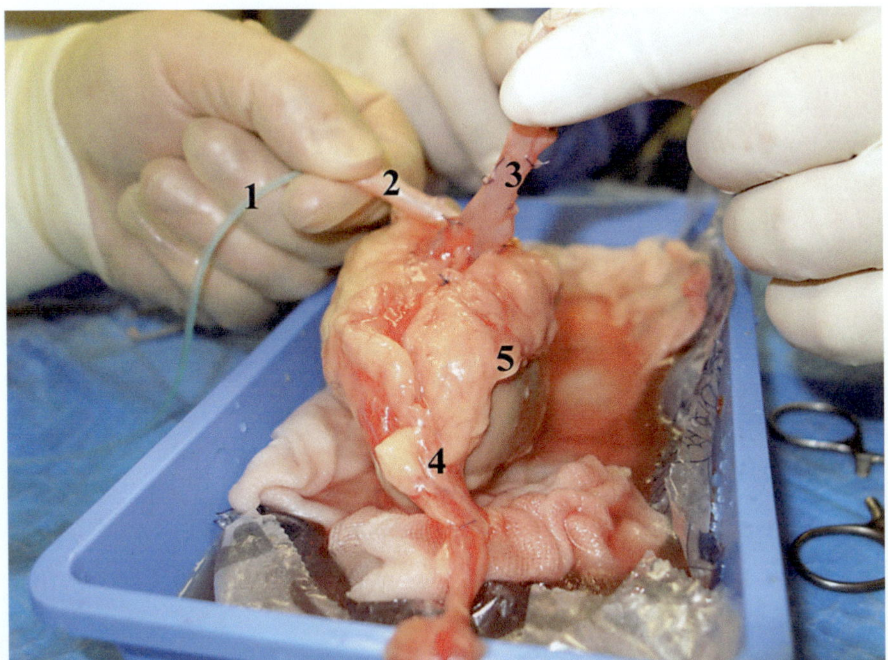

**Fig. 3.79** Another method for testing the tightness of the renal artery and vein. 1—Small silicone tube inserted into the renal artery closed with fingers, 2—Renal artery, 3—Renal vein closed with fingers of assistant, 4—Ureter, 5—Perirenal fat

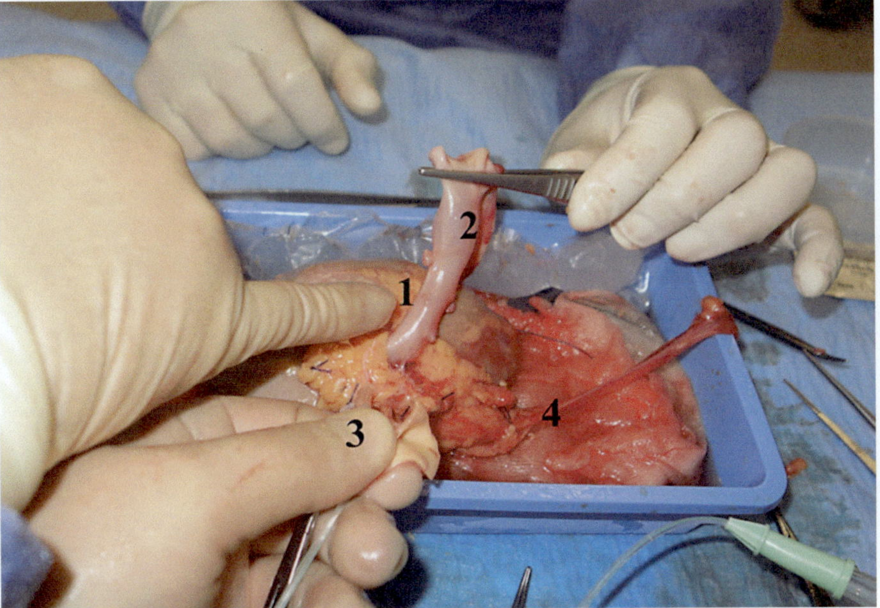

**Fig. 3.80** Testing the tightness of the renal artery and vein at the same time. Soft vascular forceps closes deep in the hilum renal vein. 1—Slight leakage of the preservation solution from the wall of the renal vein, 2—Renal vein, 3—Renal artery, 4—Ureter

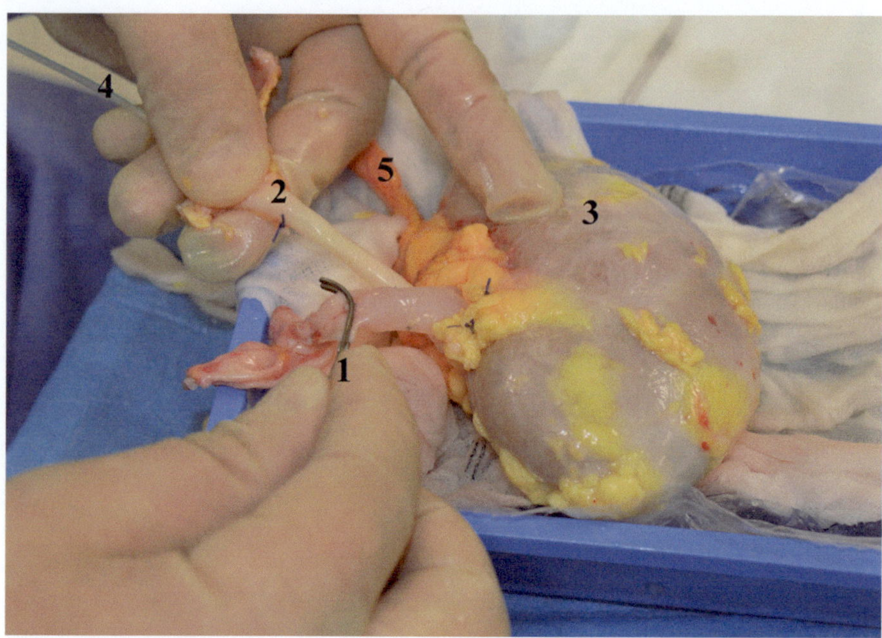

**Fig. 3.81** Right kidney. Simultaneously testing the tightness of the renal artery and vein. 1—Renal vein closed at the beginning with a small soft vascular clamp (small bulldog), 2—Renal artery with a thin silicon tube inserted into its lumen, 3—Kidney, 4—Thin silicon tube inserted into the renal artery, 5—Ureter

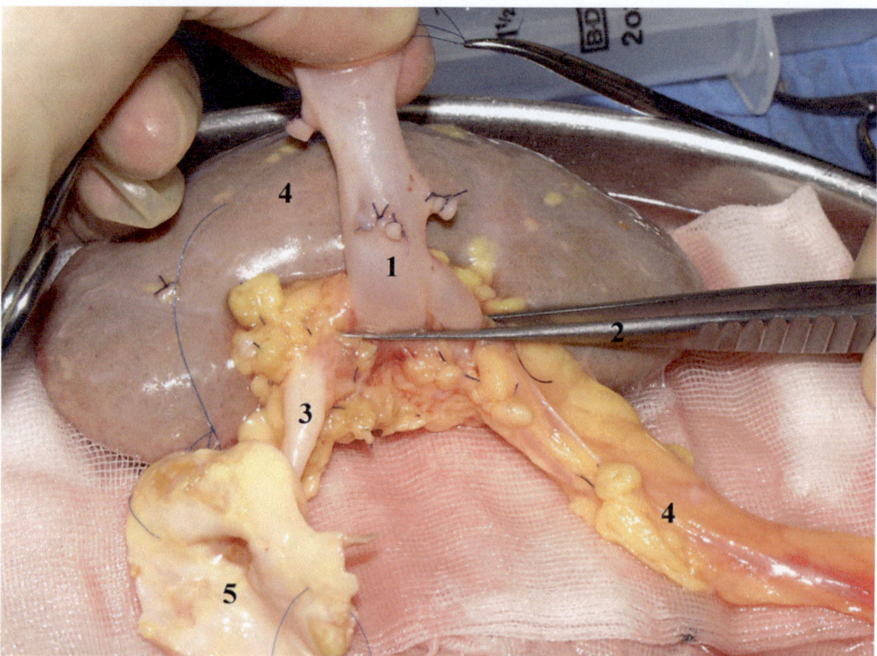

**Fig. 3.82** If the tightness of the vein does not seem sufficient, we can very gently close the vein before the kidney hilum with soft vascular forceps or a small soft vascular clamp (tiny bulldog). 1—Renal vein, 2—Soft vascular forceps, 3—Renal artery, 4—Ureter and kidney parenchyma, 5—Aortic patch

**Warning! (Short right renal vein—bleeding from the posterior surface)**
A very thorough preparation of the renal vessels is very important from the surgeon's point of view and the kidney recipient. When we are dealing with a short vein, when the kidney is reperfused and the blood flow through the kidney is restored, the kidney vein also starts to fills up with blood and at the same time the posterior surface of the kidney vein starts to bleed deep into the renal hilum. We have undertaken two repair attempts. If the bleeding is getting worse, remember that we have little chance or none to control the bleeding without removing the kidney, even if we are very experienced surgeons. A bad and careless preparation of the kidney may cost the recipient blood loss, kidney loss and finally loss of life. Such situations are not pleasant for the transplant surgeon, kidney recipient, kidney donor and also for their families, so be aware of them!

**Warning! (Be well prepared—avoid irreversible damage on the back table)**
Kidneys on the back table require a great deal of attention and experience in preparation, very good knowledge of surgical anatomy, and in some cases great surgical skills, which could be characterized in this way: surgical skills. Nobody wants to write about it, but it happens. How many well procured kidneys fail to be transplanted because they are so badly damaged on the back table that they cannot be repaired afterwards?—nobody knows. In my opinion, national or local transplant organizations should register such incidents and regardless of that train surgeons not only in procurement surgical techniques, but also in preparing (benching, the back table) organs for transplantation.

### 3.7.3  Control of the Ureter for the Presence of Diseases or Mechanical Injuries and Constrictions

After the preparation of the ureter and the kidney for transplantation, the ureter and renal pelvis should be carefully examined by palpation for tumors and urinary stones. In my opinion the ureter and the renal pelvis must be checked every time for:

– patency of the pelvic-ureteral junction (often the narrowing of the ureter)
– surgical lesions of the ureter and renal pelvis which are not noticed during the procurement (not mentioned in the quality form) and preparation for transplantation (cuts and burns).

This is a very unpleasant complication: if you did not check it and did transplant it, you have a urine leak in most cases on the second or third day after the transplantation but when you open the patient you see nothing, everything looks beautiful and normal. You wonder where the leak is, you examine, test, finally close the patient, leave the drain and on the same or second day urine appears again in the drain.

The ureter and renal pelvis are very sensitive to high temperatures. Coagulation at a distance of less than 1 cm from the ureter or renal pelvis may cause small burns and after a few days necrosis of its wall measuring a few millimeters. Please remember that sometimes the necrosis of the ureter or a small hole due to a cut is so small that it is difficult to localize it during first reoperation, even by a very experienced surgeon armed with magnifying surgical loupes. Very small renal pelvis and/or ureter diathermy burns during surgery (procurement and/or attempted haemostasis after transplantation) are undetectable because the wall of the ureter or renal pelvis is intact and does not yet pass urine into the area of the transplanted kidney (Fig. 3.83).

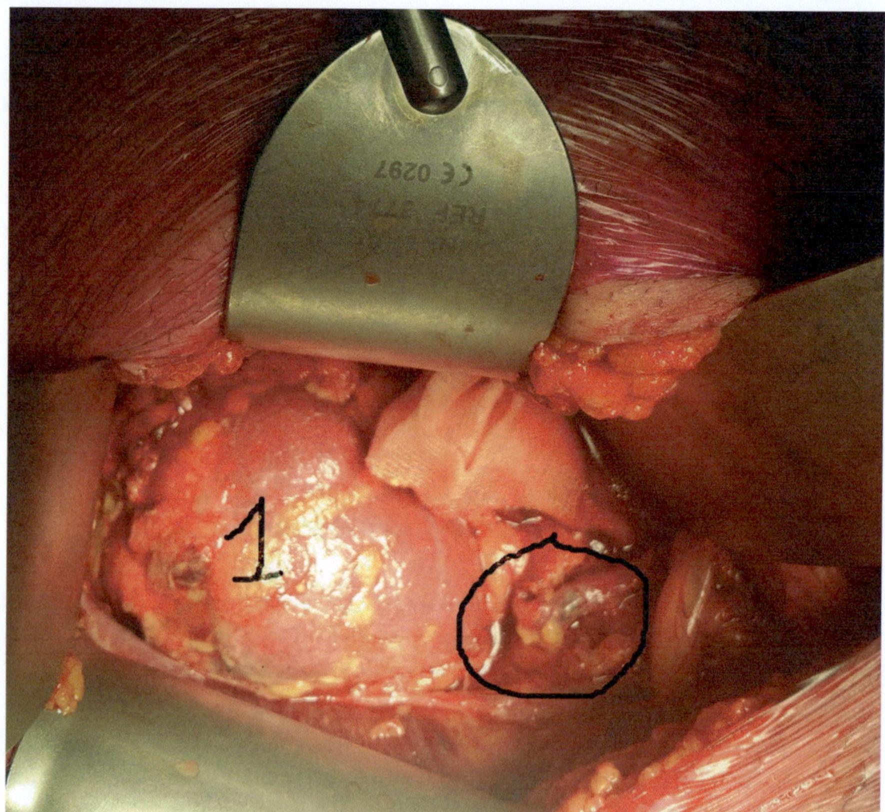

**Fig. 3.83** Slight thermal damage to the ureter during kidney retrieval. Leakage of urine on day 3 after kidney transplantation. The diagnosis was made on the basis of the high creatinine value based on the examination of the fluid drained, by the drain on the left, around the transplanted kidney. 1—Transplanted kidney. The initial part of the ureter is about 2–3 cm below the renal pelvis with slight necrosis of 2 × 3 mm is marked with a black circle

To properly prepare the ureter and renal pelvis for transplantation, follow these steps:

1. Find the cross-section of the ureter and insert very slowly the thinnest catheter into the ureter lumen (its cross-section must be much smaller than the cross-section of the ureter), stretch the ureter slightly and move the catheter very slowly up to the renal pelvis (Fig. 3.84).
2. Very gently, a few centimeters from its end, close the ureter around the catheter with your fingers and then slowly inject 10–20 ml of cold organ preservation solution or cold 0.9% NaCl solution or lactate Ringer's solution into the renal pelvis. When administering the fluid in a renal pelvis and ureter, observe carefully the increase in volume and consequently the distention of the renal pelvis and ureter, inject cold preservation solution very carefully, and try to locate the leak. Remember that filling the pelvis and ureter with force may cause severe damage to the epithelium located inside the renal pelvis and the ureter and/or severe damage of the renal pelvis and/or ureter wall.

If we still have doubts about the ureteral or renal pelvis damage, a small amount of sterile methylene blue can be added to the cold organ preservation solution which probably can help to locate the damage.

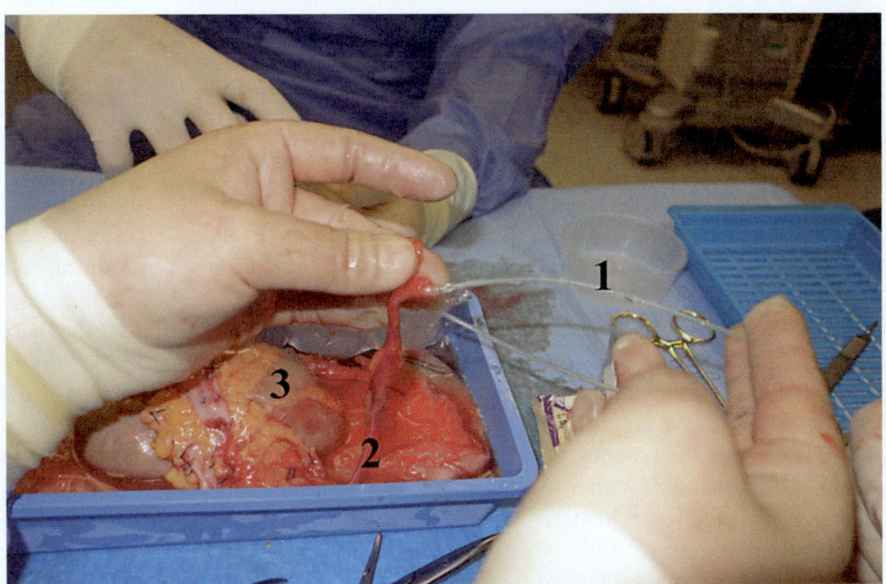



**Fig. 3.84** Ureter and renal pelvis leakage and stenosis testing. Gently insert a thin catheter into the ureter and renal pelvis. 1—Thin silicone catheter, 2—Ureter, 3—Kidney

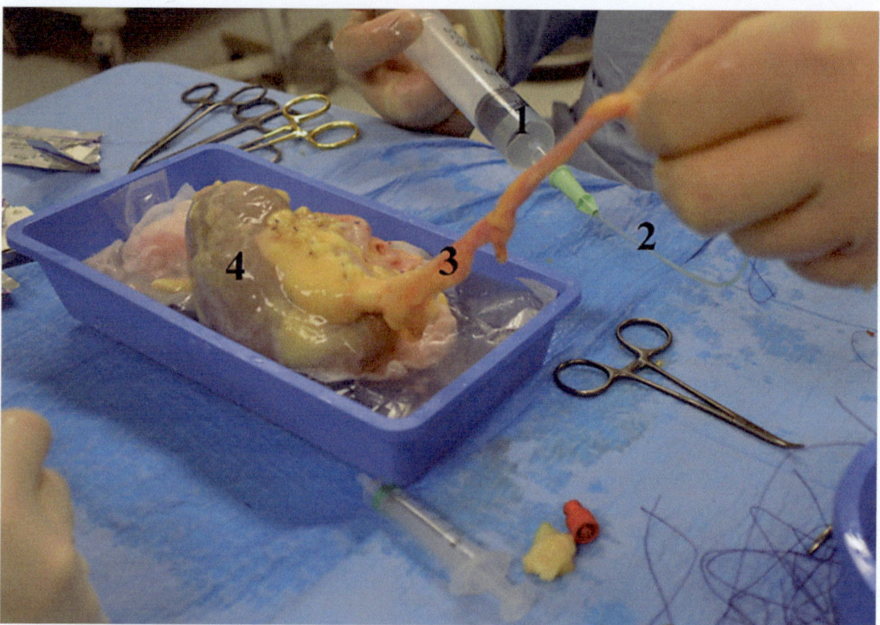

**Fig. 3.85** A thin silicone catheter inserted into the renal pelvis. Very slowly the pelvis and the ureter are filled with the cooled preservation solution. 1—Syringe with cold preservation solution, 2—Thin silicone catheter, 3—Preservation solution filled in ureter, 4—Kidney parenchyma

The renal pelvis and ureter should be once more subjected to a very gentle palpation. If we do not observe an obvious fluid leakage, we can conclude that the renal pelvis and ureter are not damaged (Fig. 3.85).

My proposal to control the ureter and renal pelvis may appear controversial, but I actually introduced ureter and renal pelvic controls after I failed twice to notice a surgical renal pelvic injury and once a ureteropelvic junction stenosis during the preparation of the kidney for transplantation. The problem is that in the cases mentioned above, this could have been prevented. In this book I will describe these cases, so you can (hopefully) remember them for the rest of your life in order to prevent similar complications. At that time we did not use the JJ catheter for the decomposition of the ureter urinary bladder anastomosis. I remember a case when we did not check the patency of the ureter during kidney preparation due to which an anuria occurred a day after the transplantation. An ultrasound scan revealed the renal pelvic distention which we had to drain with a radiological drain due to a significant enlargement. After administration of the contrast to the renal pelvis, it turned out that we missed during the preparation of the kidney an almost complete narrowing of the ureteropelvic junction. Finally the patient was treated surgically with the plastic of the ureteropelvic junction. An anatomopathological examination, in the form of a frozen section of the narrowing place, did not reveal any malignant tumor changes. Another case of an inadequate preparation of a kidney for transplantation is the one of a surgeon who forgot to check the patency of the ureter while inspecting the kidney. After the transplantation, when 50% of ureter urinary bladder anastomosis had already occurred, the surgeon could not insert the JJ catheter into the renal pelvis—despite many attempts.

The stenosis ureteropelvic junction (UPJ) was immediately operated on.

According to the principle of "prevention is better than cure", the cases I cited above introduced a habit in our transplant team to control the renal pelvic and ureter during kidney preparation for transplantation.

### 3.7.4   Assessment of the Severity of Atherosclerosis of the Abdominal Aorta Wall and Ostium of the Renal Artery

The renal arteries that arise from the lateral wall of the aorta below or above the level of origin of the superior mesenteric artery (SMA) of the superior mesenteric artery, are the only ones that supply vascular blood to the kidneys located in the retroperitoneum. They are approximately 4–6 cm long and have a diameter of 5–6 mm. They run posterior to the renal vein and enter the renal hilum anterior to the renal pelvis. The renal artery also supplies the adrenal gland and ureter on the ipsilateral side. Renal artery stenosis is a narrowing of one or both renal arteries. In most of the common cases, it occurs bilaterally due to atherosclerosis or fibromuscular dysplasia. Renal artery stenosis is a common cause of renovascular hypertension. In elderly individuals, the usual etiology of renal artery stenosis is an atherosclerotic disease. As the lumen of the artery narrows, the renal blood flow drops and this compromises the perfusion of the kidney.

Atherosclerotic lesions in the renal artery usually originate at the renal ostium, often as a result of the progression of lesions at the aortic entrance to the ostium. Studies of humans have established that these lesions initiate on the caudal side of the aortic entrance to the renal artery (Fig. 3.86). Little is currently known about the determinants of increased atherosclerosis observed at this site. The narrowing of the diameter of the ostium of the renal artery is usually caused by atherosclerotic plaque (Figs. 3.87 and 3.88) located at the beginning of the renal artery. Sometimes the renal artery ostium into the lumen of the abdominal aorta wall is not narrowed but the quality of the aortic wall is very poor (Figs. 3.89 and 3.90). In both presented cases of atherosclerosis, the kidney cannot be transplanted with the aortic patch. In this case, the renal artery should be reconstructed, for example cut in a healthy location outside the atherosclerotic plaque and anastomosed "end to side" or "end to end" with one of the renal or iliac vessels (Fig. 3.91).

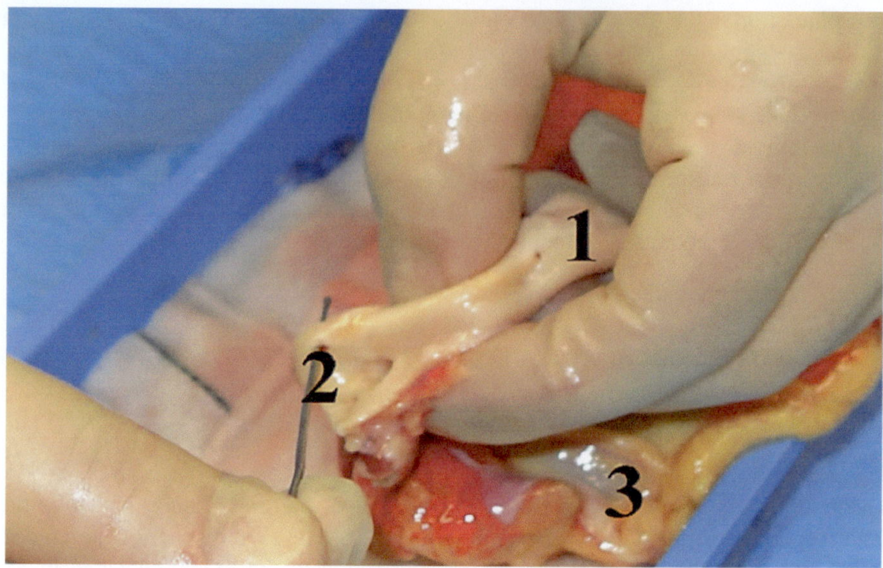

**Fig. 3.86** Normal aortic patch and renal artery ostium: both unchanged atherosclerotic. 1—Unchanged atherosclerotic aorta patch, 2—Unchanged atherosclerotic renal artery ostium, 3—Kidney

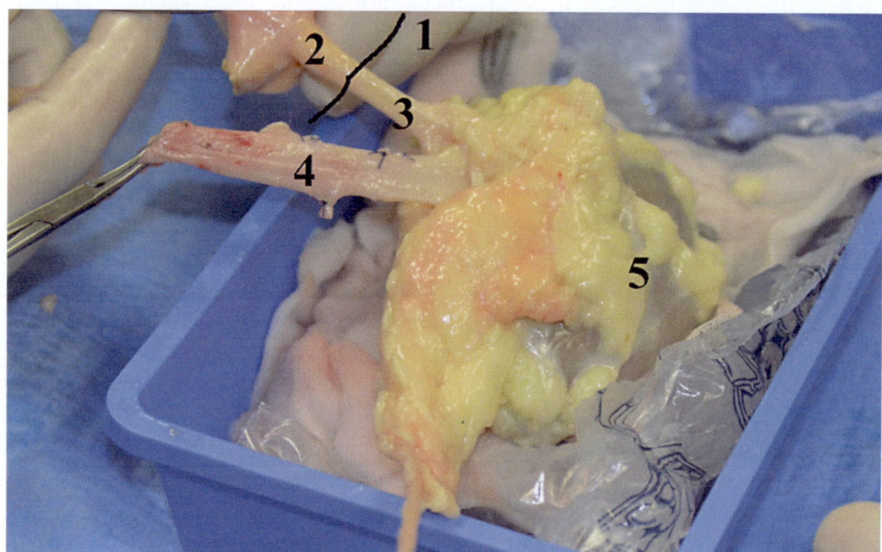

**Fig. 3.87** 1—The black mark draws the line between the atherosclerotic plaque situated from the ostium side in the first 1 cm of the renal artery. The plaque closes more than 50% of the lumen of the artery, so this kidney is not suitable for transplant with an aortic patch. In transplantation, the renal artery must be cut and implanted with "end to side" anastomosis of one of the iliac arteries, 2—Yellow color of atherosclerotic plaque, 3—Distal part of the renal artery not affected by atherosclerosis, 4—Renal vein, 5—Kidney

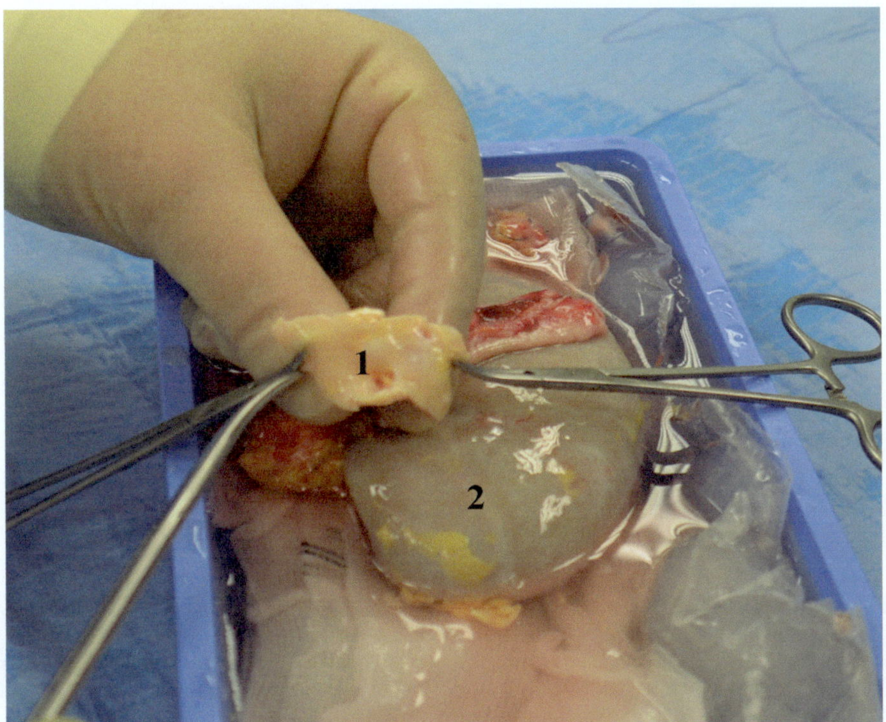

**Fig. 3.88** 1—Almost complete closure of the renal artery ostium due to atherosclerotic plaque, 2—Kidney

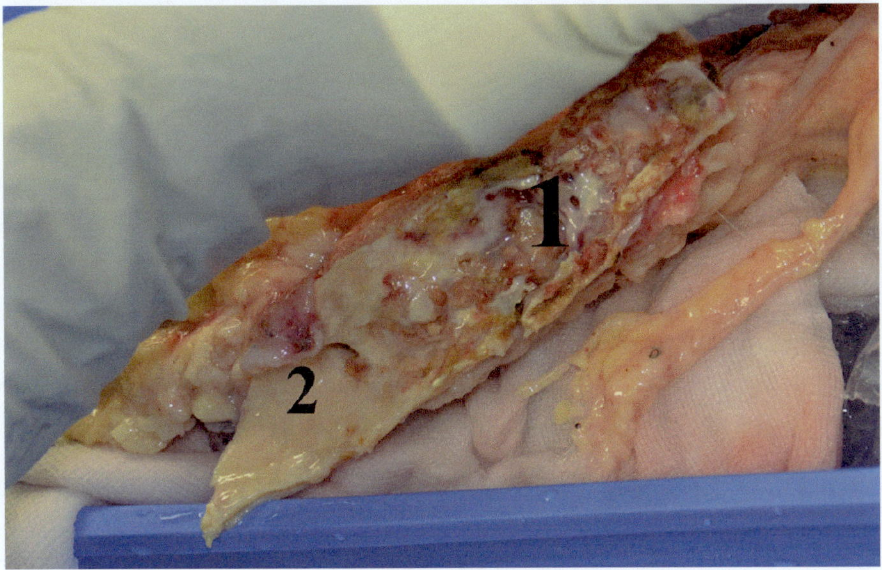

**Fig. 3.89** 1—Extremely advanced atherosclerotic lesions in the abdominal aorta wall, 2—Atherosclerotic lesions in the renal artery ostium area to the aorta with a visible onset of ulceration. No narrowing around the renal artery ostium is observed, but due to changes in the lumen and the wall of the abdominal aorta, an aorta patch was not used to transplant this kidney. This kidney was successful transplanted without an aorta patch

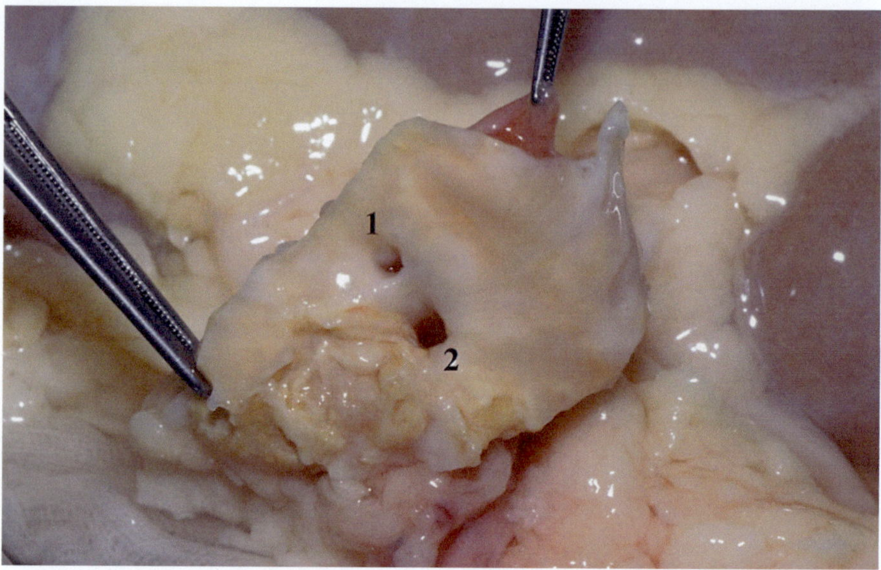

**Fig. 3.90** Advanced atherosclerosis of the aortic wall. Kidney with two arteries. 1—Kidney artery ostium almost completely closed with atherosclerotic lesions 2—Second renal artery: this is where atherosclerotic lesions and ulcerations enter the arterial lumen. This aorta patch is not suitable for transplantation together with the renal arteries; before transplantation of this kidney, arterial reconstruction seems to be essential

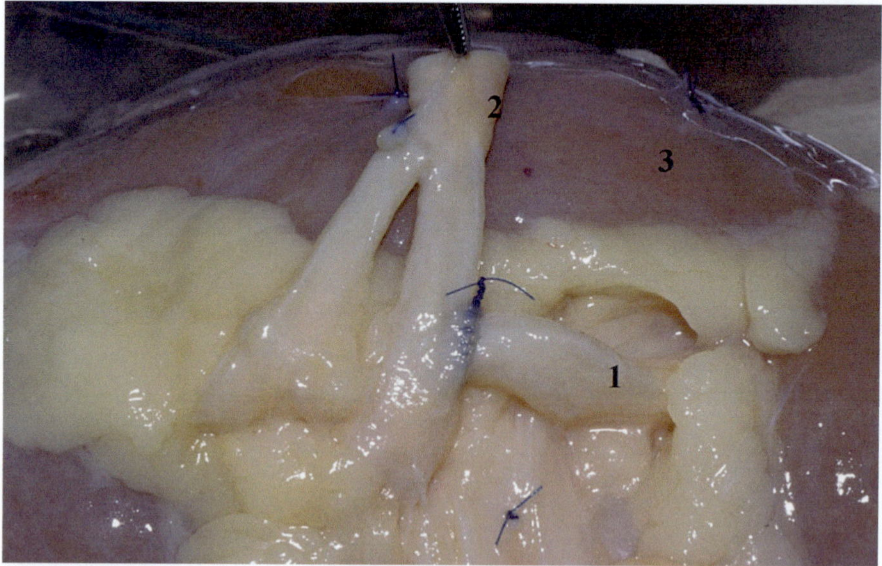

**Fig. 3.91** The renal arteries were reconstructed during the preparation of the kidney for transplantation. 1—"End to side" anastomosis between a second on the aorta patch accessory renal artery with the main stem of renal artery. Aortic ostium of implanted artery was almost completely closed. 2—Main trunk of the renal artery: at the beginning of the renal artery you can see a cream-colored plaque shining through the wall. 3—Kidney parenchyma

### 3.7.5   Sterile Repacking of the Kidney

1. The inspected kidney is packed in the first bag, which is completely submerged with a cold organ preservation solution (the kidney must be on all surfaces completely covered). The bag should be tightly tied and should not contain air (Fig. 3.92).
2. The first bag is placed in the second bag which is larger than the first. The second bag is filled up with 500 ml of cold 0.9% NaCl saline or Ringer's solution. The air is released from the second bag and the bag is tied (Fig. 3.93).
3. The two previous bags are inserted into the biggest bag, the air is released and the bag is tightly tied. The third bag is the largest. In Eurotransplant jargon it is called a "dry" bag, as it is not filled up with any liquid or solution (Fig. 3.94).
4. In some teams procuring abdominal organs in some countries it is still customary that the last "dry bag" or third bag is wrapped in a special sterile disposable surgical napkin normally used to wrap the operating field. Many procurement teams in a lot of countries have stopped doing this, so, in my opinion, wrapping in a napkin before transportation is not necessary. The prepared and packed kidney is placed in a donor transport organ box and covered with ice (Fig. 3.95—wrapped in a special disposable surgical napkin and Fig. 3.96—not wrapped).

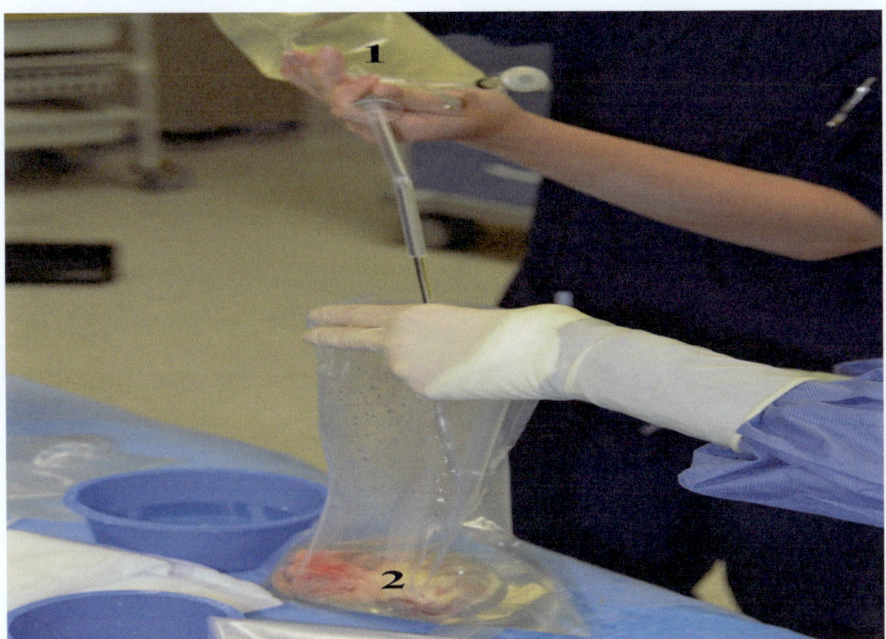


**Fig. 3.92** Prepared kidney packed in first bag. Pour fresh, cooled preservation solution onto the kidney, placed in a sterile bag. 1—Kidney container with fresh cooled preservation solution. 2—Kidney in sterile bag poured over with fresh cooled preservation solution (300–500 ml)

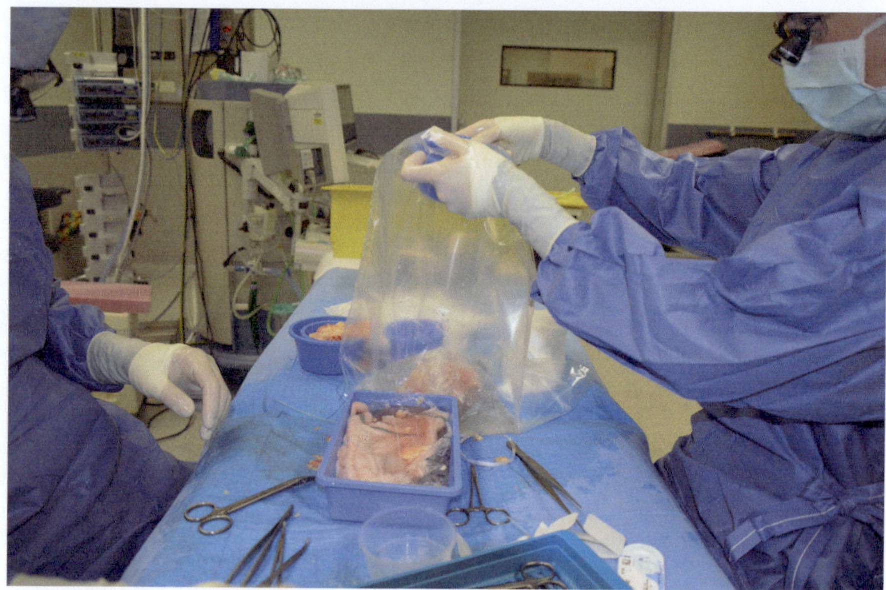

**Fig. 3.93** Pack the first bag into a second bag which is filled with 500 ml of 0.9% NaCl physiological natrium chloride solution

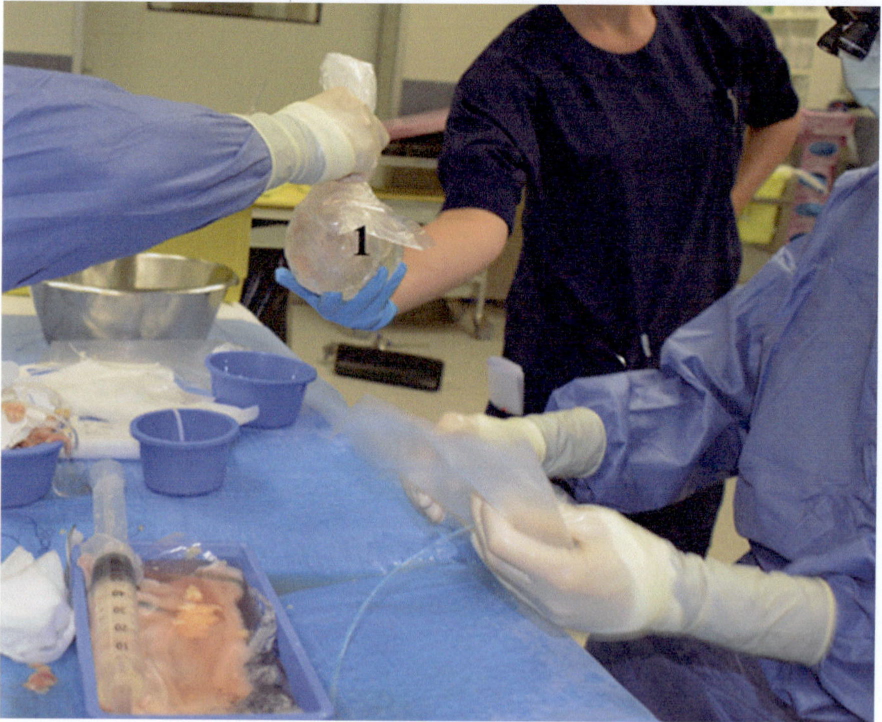

**Fig. 3.94** 1—The kidney, packed in a third "dry" bag, is handed over to one of the scrub nurses to be placed in the transport box

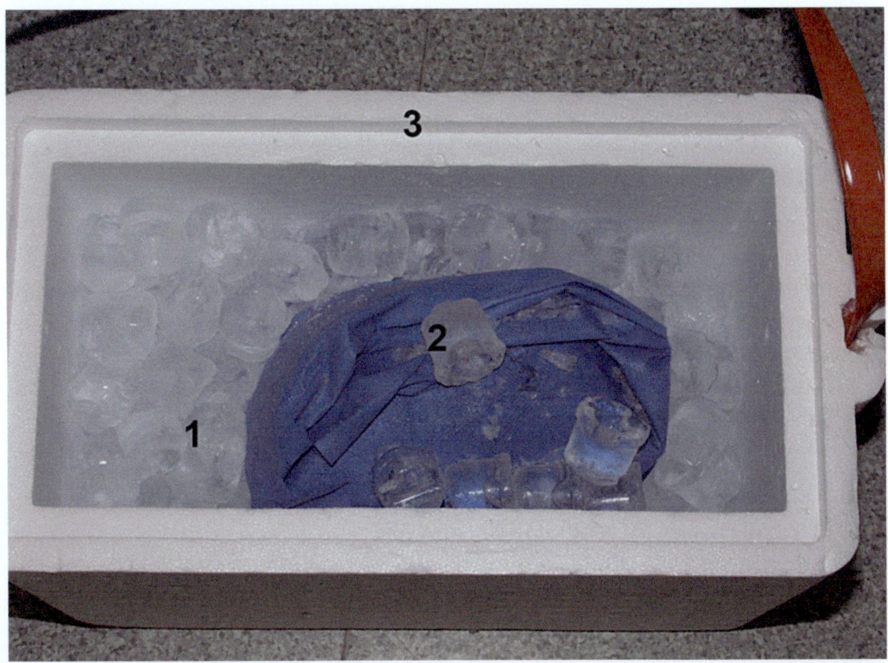

Fig. 3.95 Kidney placed in a transport box on ice. 1—Ice, 2—Pack according to the kidney protocol; kidney wrapped in a surgical drape, 3—Transport box

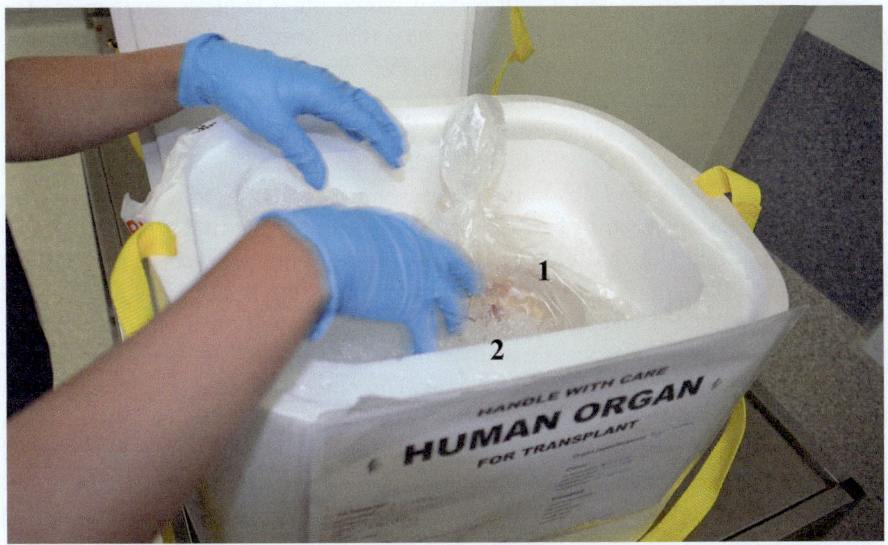



Fig. 3.96 The kidney, after preparation for transplantation, is placed without wrapping in a transport box. 1—Kidney, 2—Transport box

**Warning! (To wrap or not to wrap the kidney?)**

I would like to give you an argument in favour of wrapping, because if the fluid bag is damaged, e.g. during transport, the leakage is immediately visible on the napkin because it is wet. Without the napkin, you will not be able to see it so quickly because in the transport box the entire kidney is surrounded by ice and the fluid slowly leaks out and collects at the bottom of the container.

The kidney is transported to the recipient's hospital in a transport device which allows for continuous hypothermic kidney perfusion. Shortly before the transplantation in the recipient's hospital, the kidney is removed from the transport device and prepared. After preparation, the kidney is not put back in the machine, but in three (sterile) bags and an organ transport box which is filled with ice.

The three bags are sometimes wrapped in a special, disposable surgical napkin which is useful for recognizing a leakage of (one of) the bags.

## 3.8  Preparation of the Right Kidney

### 3.8.1  Introduction

In general, inspection and preparation the right kidney for transplantation does not differ from preparation of the left kidney. Once again, I would like to remind you that from the same donor two kidneys are different in the length of the renal vessels. A normal left kidney has a longer vein and a shorter artery, while the right kidney has a longer renal artery and a shorter vein which often requires elongation. The posterior wall of the right renal vein is very thin, brittle and prone tearing and injuries when short; it is procured without an IVC patch or without an IVC segment. After kidney revascularization, the right renal vein can become very vulnerable and easily tear when the right kidney is lifted or the renal vein is twisted to a place after transplantation kidney's vessels in an optimal position. The right renal vein is usually lengthened by the IVC. In many cases, however, the right renal vein is long enough and does not need to be extended (Fig. 3.97). If the right kidney is transplanted to the right side and the anastomosis of the right renal vein is made to the right common iliac vein or to the IVC, in most cases the right renal vein will not need to be lengthened and the recipient's iliac vessels will not need to be totally prepared. The right renal vein is usually lengthened, if necessary, using an IVC or another suitable donor's or recipient's vein. The elongation of the right renal vein with veins taken from the recipient (for example the inferior mesenteric vein (IMV)), one of the gonadal veins or the greater saphenous vein can be difficult and requires surgical experience and the consent of the recipient. In this section I will not deal with the transport of the kidney or the technique of its removal from the transport container, unpacking and repacking into individual bags, because all these

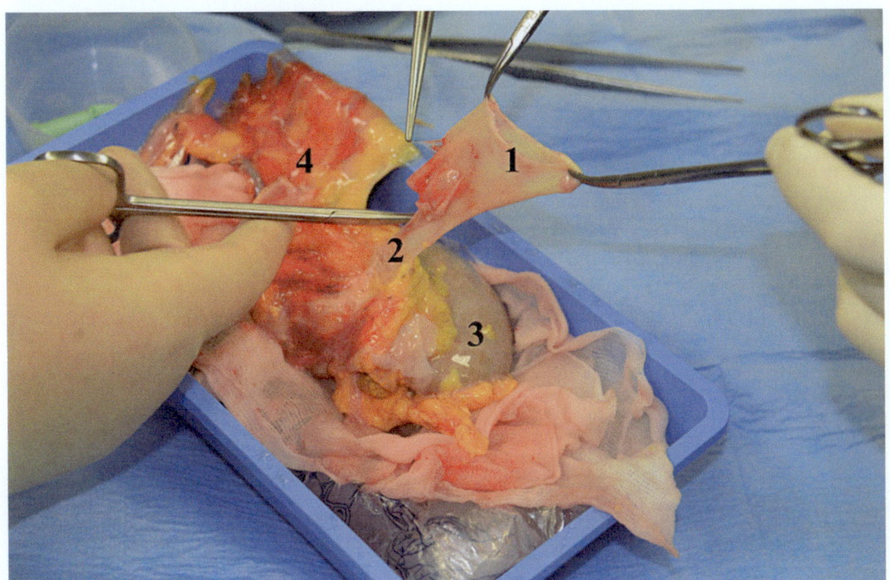

Fig. 3.97 Right kidney. The renal vein is long enough and can be transplanted to the right side without elongation of the renal vein by the IVC. 1—IVC, 2—Right renal vein, 3—Kidney, 4—Ureter

above mentioned steps are the same for both left and right kidney. The discussion of the common elements of preparation of the right and left kidney for transplantation was described in the previous section, therefore I will now limit myself to a minimal description of its preparation. In the right kidney, accessory renal veins are much more common than in the left kidney therefore, in order to discuss the topic of accessory veins, I will describe step by step the preparation of the right kidney with two veins retrieved from the IVC with a patch and the related decision making (Fig. 3.98).

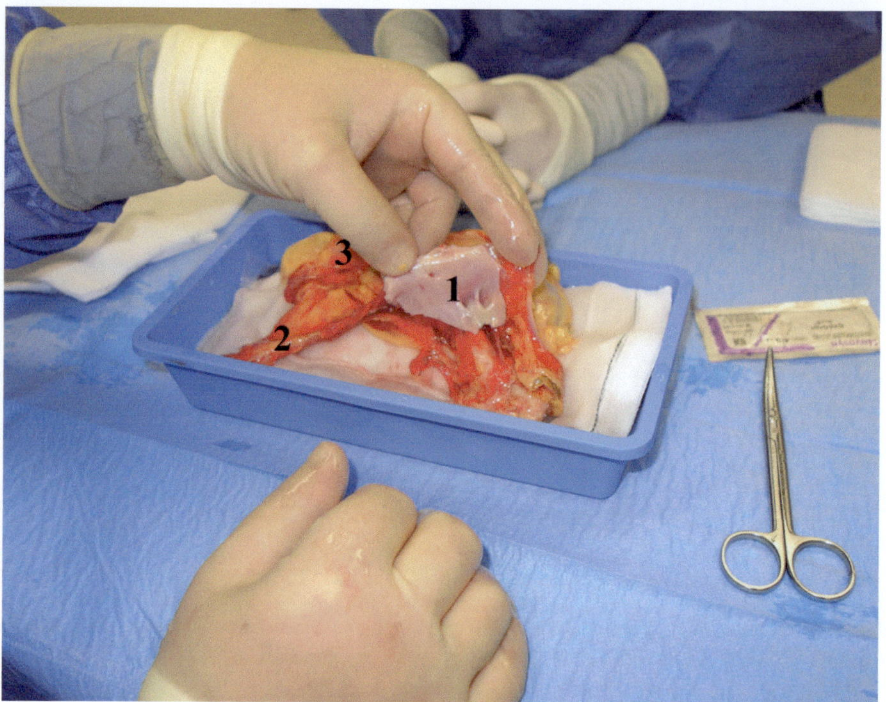

**Fig. 3.98** Right kidney with two renal veins on the IVC patch. 1—Ostia of the renal veins procured with IVC patch, 2—Ureter, 3—Kidney

## *3.8.2  Right Kidney Inspection: The Most Important Steps*

1. The sterile container is filled with preservation solution, sterile ice and covered by gauze. The right kidney is placed in the container in such a way that the first vessel from above is the right renal vein and IVC (if procured with the IVC); an aorta patch with renal artery(-ries) faces the surgeon; the right ureter is turned to the left side facing the surgeon's left hand (Fig. 3.99).

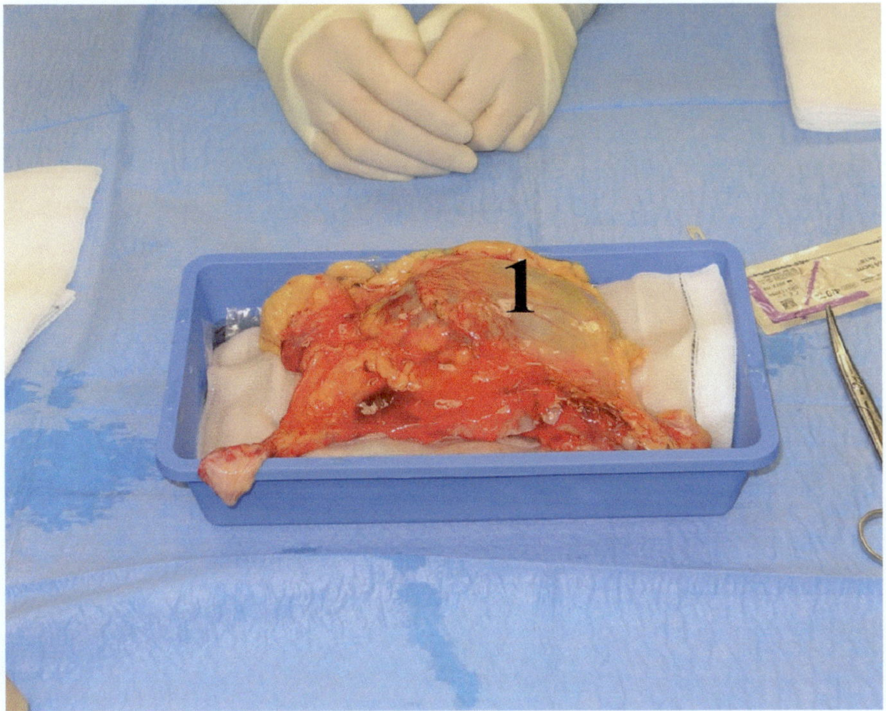

**Fig. 3.99**  1—Right kidney prepared for inspection. The ureter faces thesurgeon's left hand, the first vessel from the top is the right renal vein with or without the IVC

2. We examine the right renal vein which has been cut off from the IVC with an IVC patch; we also examine the aorta patch. If retrieved there is a possibility of additional renal veins reaching the IVC or additional renal arteries coming from the aortic patch; before preparation we control their course with a probe or a small catheter (Fig. 3.100).

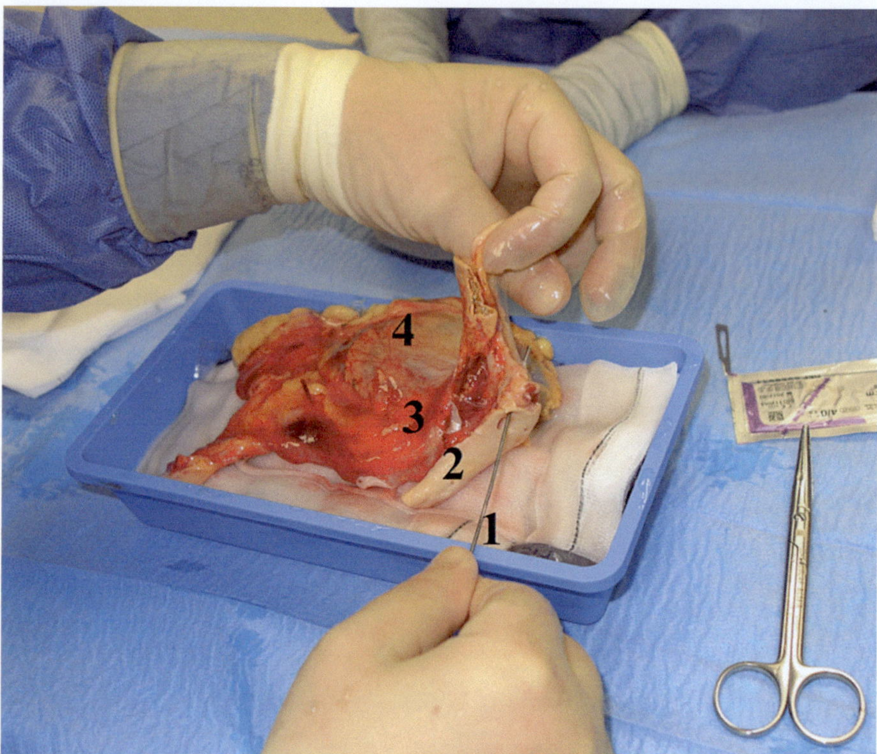


**Fig. 3.100** 1—Special vascular probe to control the number of veins and arteries and their branches arising from the abdominal aorta and coming into the IVC during kidney inspection, 2—Aortic patch, 3—The cut branch from the renal artery, which is the upper pole artery, 4—Kidney

3. The preparation of the right kidney begins with the placement of two "stay sutures" inside the patch retrieved from the IVC. We finish the preparation of the vein 2.5–3.0 cm in front of the renal hilum. During the inspection of the right kidney, the dissected IVC patch with the right renal vein(s) are placed vertically on the anterior surface and hilum of the kidney to make them more visible (Fig. 3.101).

4. The next step in preparing the kidney for transplantation will be to prepare the renal artery. Begin the preparation of the renal artery from the aortic patch with a placement of two stay sutures or two small Mosquito clamps on the aortas patch on the left and the right side of the renal artery. Use small preparation scissors, and start separating the fat from the wall of the renal artery by very gentle horizontal movements of the scissor blades. Cut the mobilized tissues along the long axis of the artery while holding the preparation scissors and their bladers vertically. We finish the preparation of the right renal artery 2.5–3.0 cm in front of the renal hilum. The freed renal artery(-ies) with or without the aortas patch are then placed next to the vein on the upper anterior surface of the renal parenchyma (Fig. 3.102).

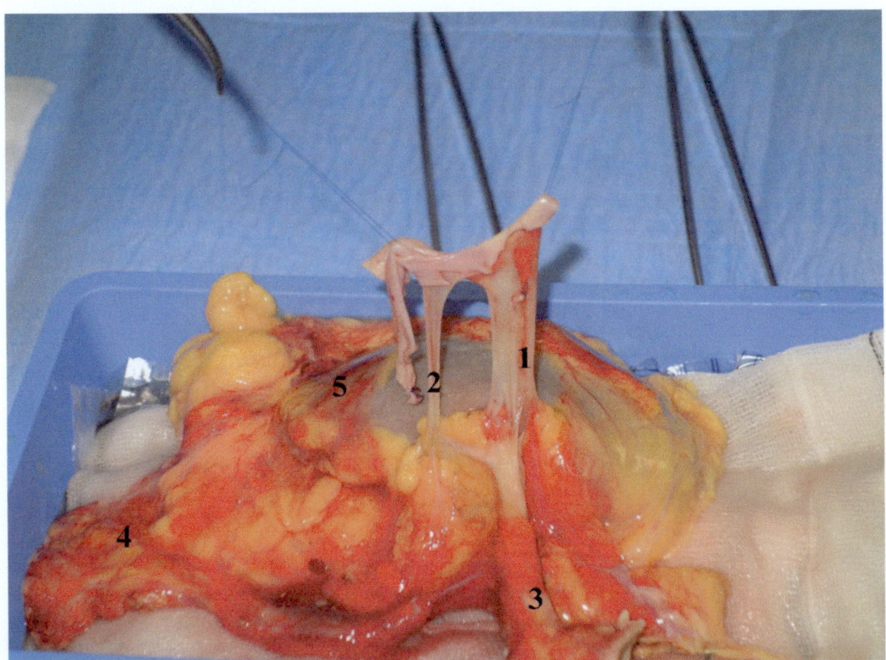

**Fig. 3.101** Right kidney with two renal veins entering a patch of IVC. IVC patch with two "stay sutures". 1—Major renal vein, 2—Aberrant renal vein, 3—Renal artery, 4—Ureter, 5—Kidney

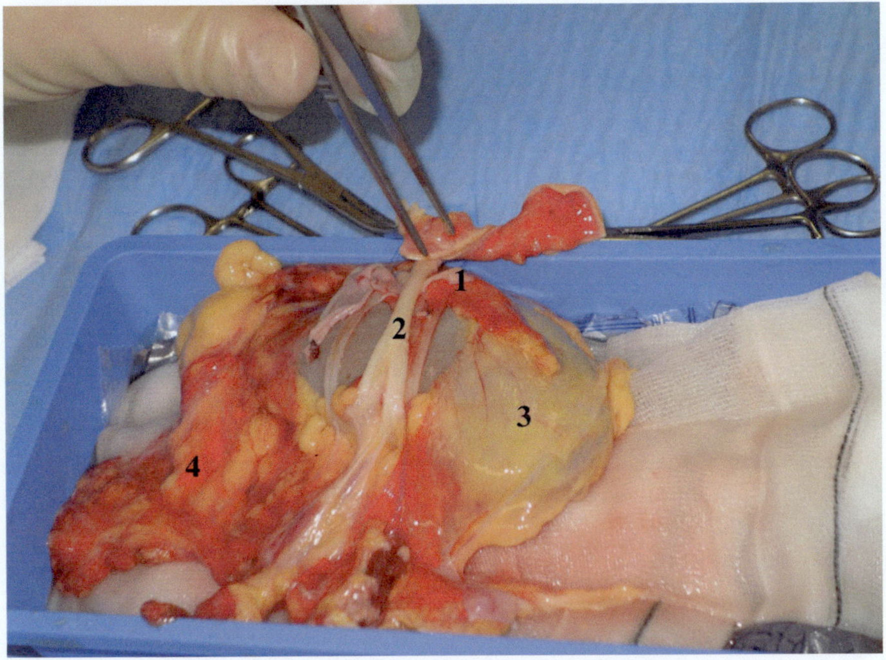

**Fig. 3.102** Prepared right renal artery and vein placed on the kidney's parenchyma. 1—Main right renal vein, 2—Main stem of the renal artery, 3—Upper right kidney pole, 4—Ureter

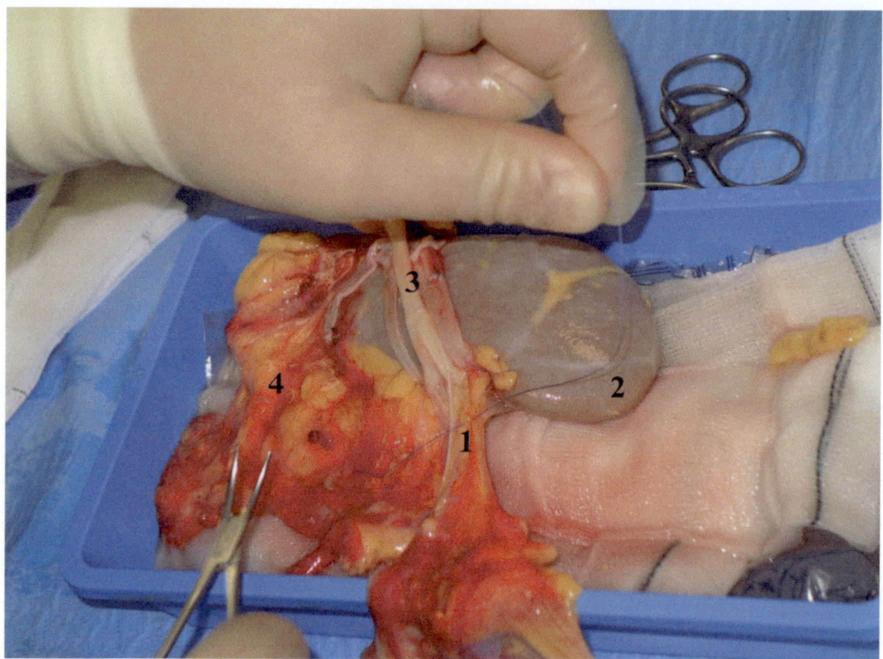

**Fig. 3.103**  1—Tissue and lymphatic vessel ligation at a distance of 2.5–3.0 cm from the hilum, 2—Upper pole of the kidney, 3—Renal artery, 4—Golden triangle ureter area

5. Ligate the fat tissue and all the lymphatic vessels which are hidden in them and run for a distance of 2.5–3.0 cm from the kidney hilum. Ligate them from the right side (upper pole) to the left, towards the ureter (Fig. 3.103).

6. Localize and stretch the ureter slightly. Look for its end and locate its star shaped lumen. At this point try to distinguish the ureter from the gonadal vessels. Excess fat in the ureter area is removed in such a way that the largest amounts of fat and tissues are left close to the lower pole, around the renal pelvis, kidney hilum and ureter. Moving from the renal pelvis to the end of the ureter, we systematically reduce the amount of fat and tissues around the ureter so that at the end, after checking the amount of tissue around the ureter, there is no more than 0.4–0.7 mm. We take care to preserve the so-called: there is golden triangle of the kidney blood supply. The whole philosophy is to maintain moderation in the reduction of fat in the area of the kidney hilum, renal pelvis, lower pole and at the beginning of the ureter. Because of the preparation of the kidney in this way, we maintain proper blood supply to the ureter and prevent its massive fibrosis or even necrosis after transplantation (Fig. 3.104).

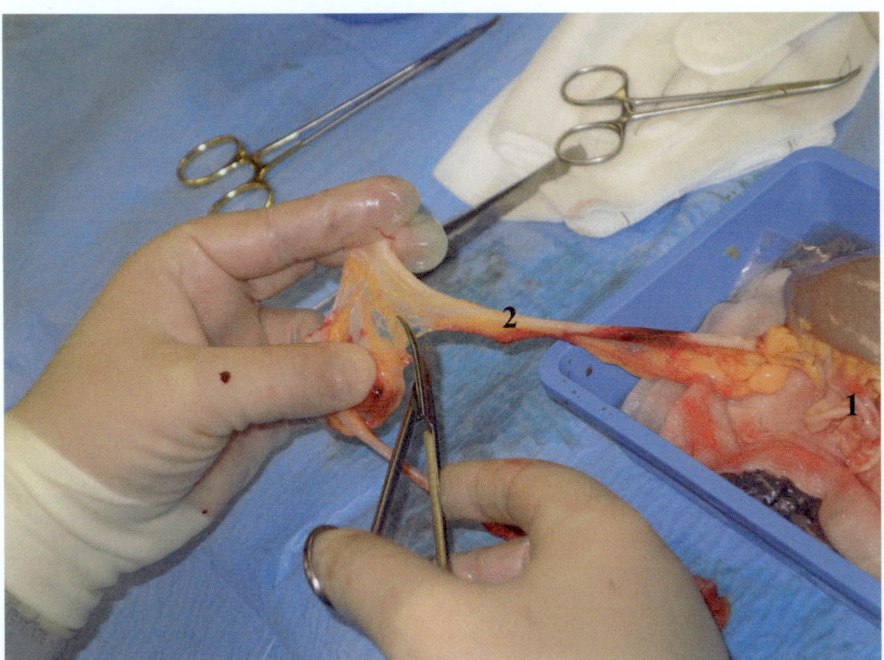

**Fig. 3.104** Preparation of the right ureter for transplantation. Going from the renal pelvis towards the end of the ureter, more and more tissues surrounding the ureter are reduced. 1—Right renal vessels, 2—Ureter

7. Test the renal vessels, renal pelvis and ureter to locate the leak or damage of their walls or strictures resulting from the patient's medical history or the procurement process. The artery and renal vein have been placed in a physiological position. At this point, ask the scrub nurse to pour fresh, cold organ preservation solution into a sterile container situated on the preparing table. Take the liquid into the syringe, connect the syringe to the thin silicone drain (0.6 or 0.8 F), remove air from the entire system. Gently insert the thin silicone tube into the lumen of right renal vein to a depth of 2–3 cm, then with your fingers close the lumen of the right renal vein gently around the thin drain and begin to fill it very slowly with cold organ preservation solution, check the tightness or weakness of the vein wall, look for leaks and connections between the two veins, if any.

8. In our case (see Fig. 3.105), two right renal veins were procured together with the IVC and had different diameters. As a next step, we had to check if the two renal veins were connected together at the level of the kidney parenchyma. If you face a similar situation, inject cold preservation solution into the lumen of both renal veins and observe if the solution comes out from the lumen of another vein.

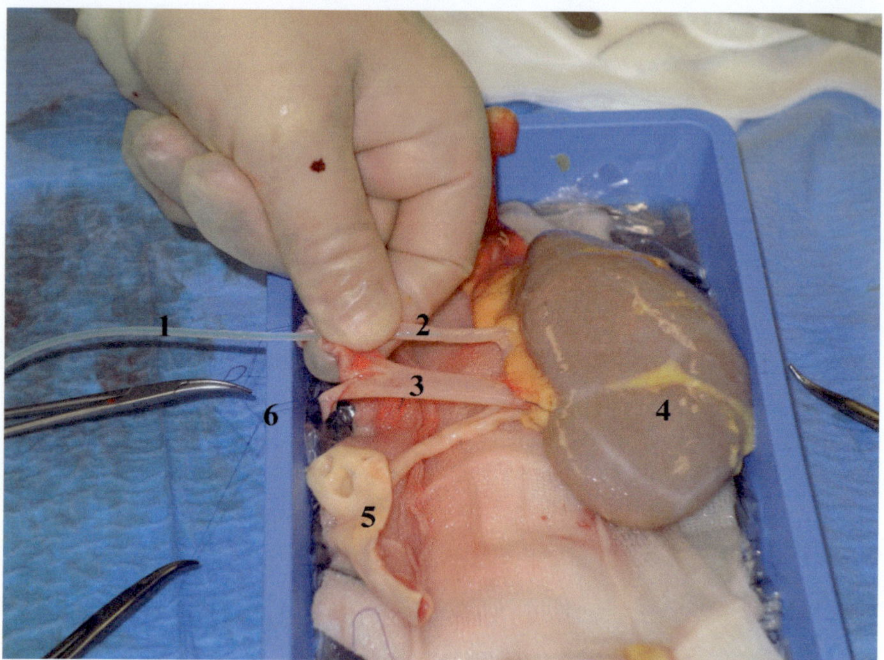

**Fig. 3.105** Tightness and connection testing of the lesser renal vein and its connection to the other large renal vein at the level of the renal parenchyma. 1—Thin silicon tube used for tightness and venous connection testing is placed into the lumen of a smaller renal vein, 2—Smaller diameter renal vein, 3—Main renal vein filled with cooled preservation solution, there is no resistance during preservation solution injection (good connections between two renal veins), 4—Kidney, 5—Aorta patch with the right renal artery ostium, 6—Stay sutures placed on the wall of the IVC

9. Now, change the position of the catheter and place it in the lumen of the other vein, just like before. Close gently the lumen of the renal vein on the thin drain and slowly, without using force, apply a fresh cold preservation solution to its lumen. Just like before, look for leaks or for a weakening of the wall of the renal vein. If there is no resistance during the injection of the preservation solution into the lumen of one of the renal veins, it means that there are very good connections between the two veins at the level of the renal parenchyma (Fig. 3.106).

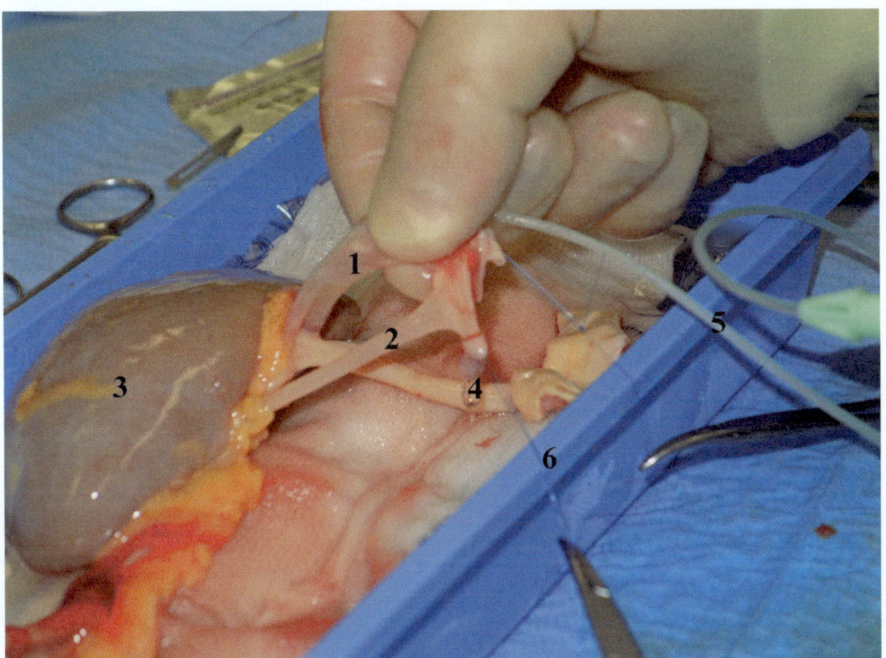

**Fig. 3.106**  1—Cannulated right main renal vein filled with chilled preservation solution injected into its lumen, 2—Leakage of preservation solution from the lumen of the lesser renal vein: there is no resistance whatsoever during administration of the cold preservation solution, 3—Kidney, 4— Renal artery and flowing cold preservation solution from the lower vein indicating good connections between the veins at the level of the renal parenchyma, 5—Silicone tube for kidney perfusion and probing vessels, 6—stay-suture

10. As you can see, on the basis of a very simple method of preservation solution administration, we can conclude that there are connections between the veins, in this case, the smaller diameter vein has excellent contact with the venous outflow of the larger diameter vein, so we do not have to implant it anywhere. It can be "tied with impunity", as it does not cause any disorders in blood flow or swelling of the kidney (Fig. 3.107).

11. The next step is testing the renal artery for the presence of pathological changes, mechanical damage as the result of procurement and/or during preparation. At the beginning of the renal artery, put into its lumen a thin catheter connected to a syringe filled with fresh, cold preservation solution. After placing the catheter into the lumen of the renal artery, use your fingers to close the lumen of the renal artery around a thin catheter to slowly fill the renal artery with the cold preservation solution. In this case, we can observe a leakage of the solution from, probably, a torn-off small branch of the renal artery wall (Fig. 3.108).

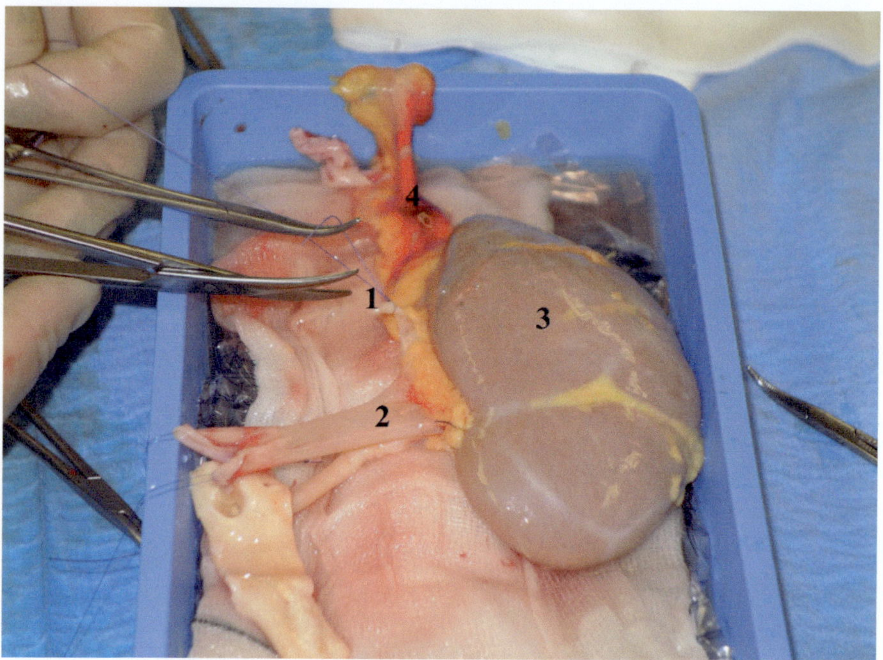

**Fig. 3.107**  1—An additional right renal vein of a smaller diameter was ligated near the hilum, 2—Main renal vein, 3—Kidney, 4—Ureter

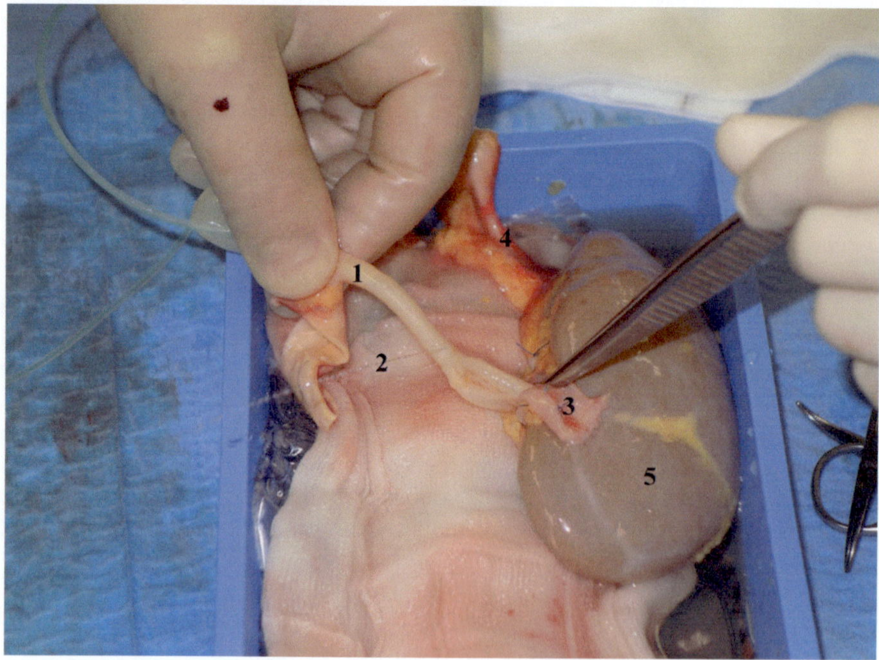

**Fig. 3.108**  Preservation solution leakage during right renal artery testing. 1—Right renal artery, 2—Small siding perfusion preservation solution leakage, 3—Renal vein, 4—Ureter, 5—Kidney parenchyma

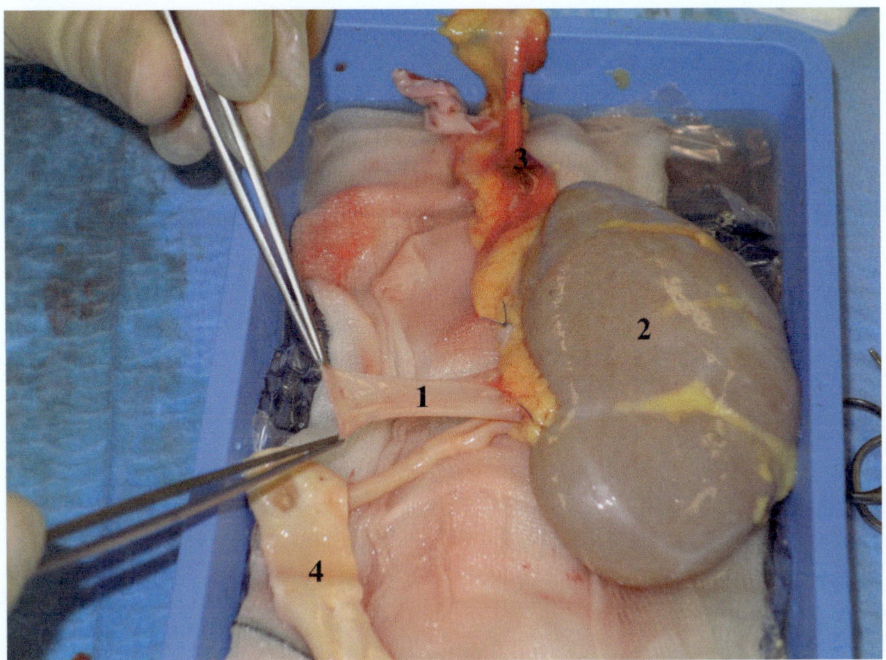

**Fig. 3.109**  1—Evaluation of right renal vein length after IVC removal, 2—Kidney, 3—Ureter, 4—Aorta patch

12. Assess the length of the right renal vein when it and the IVC are connected to each other. In the present case, you can see that the renal vein is long enough, so it does not have to be elongated, and therefore the kidney could be transplanted to the right iliac vessels of the young recipient. The IVC patch was cut off from the main renal vein (Fig. 3.109). After cutting the right renal vein one more time, we test the tightness of its walls again. Suture the areas of possible cold preservation solution leakage or where the vein's wall is weaked using surgical non-absorbable monofilament sutures 6/0 (Fig. 3.110).

13. The prepared kidney is transplanted to the right iliac fossa and the vascular anastomoses are performed in the next sequence, with the use of non-absorbable monofilament vascular sutures: the renal vein "end to side" with the common iliac vein (5/0) and the renal artery "end to side" with the common iliac artery (6/0). The warm ischemia time was 15 min. After reperfusion the kidney looked normal, its color indicated that it was very well supplied with blood. In spite of ligation of one of the veins, there was no swelling of the kidney and no impediment to the blood flow from the kidney, renal pelvis or ureter (Fig. 3.111). The ureter was implanted into the bladder using the Lich-Gregoir method with the use of absorbable 5/0 monofilament sutures. Ureter-bladder anastomosis was decompressed using the JJ catheter

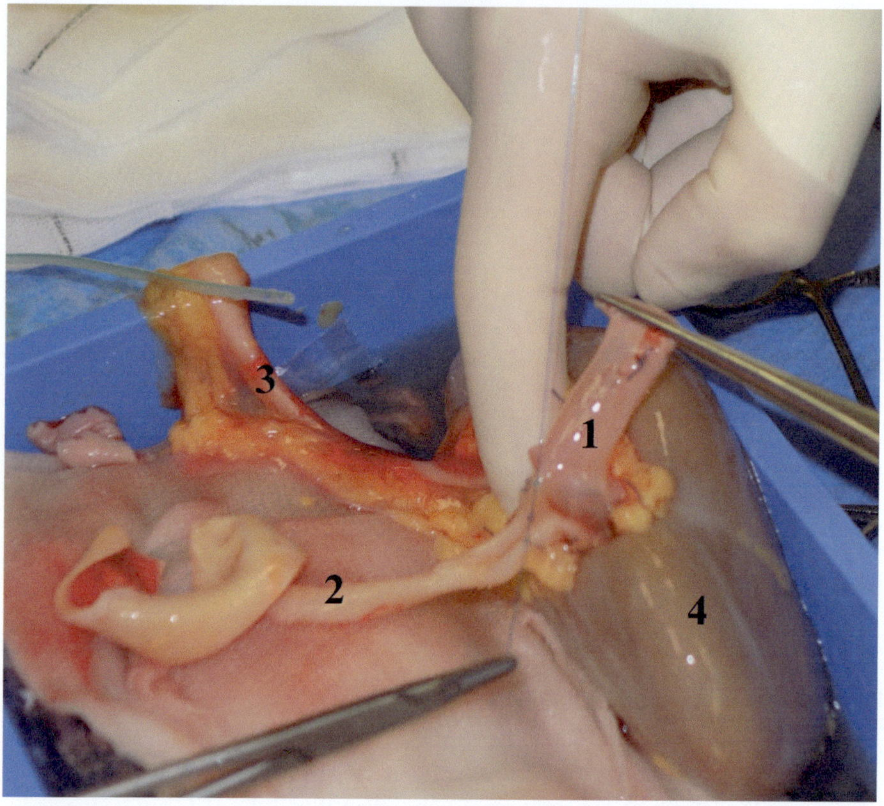

**Fig. 3.110** Testing the tightness of the right renal vein. A small leak in the vein wall was sutured with a 6/0 monofilament surgical suture. 1—Renal vein, 2—Renal artery, 3—Ureter, 4—Kidney

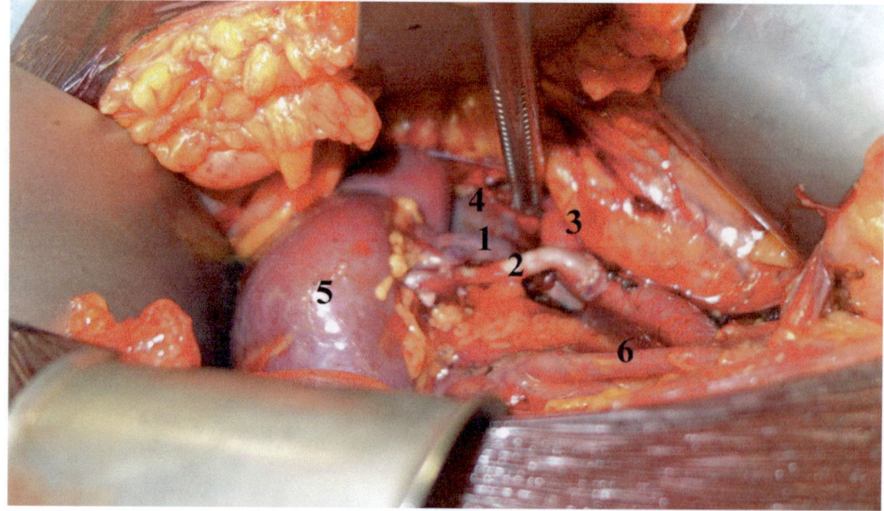

**Fig. 3.111** Transplanted kidney. 1—Right renal vein, 2—Right renal artery, 3—Common iliac artery, 4—Common iliac vein, 5—Kidney, 6—Transplanted kidney ureter

(each end of the catheter resembles the letter J, hence the name double J or pig tail). I will describe how to place the JJ catheter and how to handle it after renal transplantation in detail in the next chapter.

**Warning! (Try to recognize any kidney tumor in the donor's hospital before packing)**

During the preparation of the kidneys for transportation, pay great attention to a careful palpation of the perirenal fat and kidney parenchyma, because in this way the surgeon is able to detect a tumor localized within the parenchyma or within the fatty tissues (lipoma, liposarcoma) and protect the recipient from very serious consequences, that is transplantation kidneys with cancer and/or a transplantation lung(s) and/or a heart from a donor with renal cancer or fatty tissue cancer. We should remember that, as doctors, we are obliged to protect the recipient of an organ (s). If, during palpation, there is even the slightest suspicion that it may be cancer, then a problem arises—how do we advise the heart or lung recipients, the surgeons or transplant coordinator? How do they deal with this issue regarding the recipient of a heart or lungs when a few hours ago these have been transplanted? What do we have to do when during kidney preparation we find renal cancer confirmed by an anatomopathologist? And what happens if one of the patients was before the transplant in a very bad condition and he or she may not survive the second transplant or retransplantation? Then questions arise such as: What is the risk of developing renal cancer or fatty tissue cancer due to immunosuppression? How can we monitor the recipient after heart and/or lung(s) transplantation? What kind of immunosuppression should be used so that his/her survival is as long as possible? Unfortunately, these very difficult questions often have no clear answers. Therefore, it is also very important that a thorough inspection of the kidneys is carried out after they have been taken in order to detect any abnormalities early.

## 3.9  Surgical Methods of Elongation of the Right Renal Vein with the IVC

### 3.9.1  Introduction

As a rule, the right kidney with a short renal vein is considered to be a greater risk for vascular problems and graft thrombosis. An elongated right renal vein facilitates the surgical procedure and decreases the risk of complications, especially in obese patients whose veins are deeply situated in the pelvis. Vascular thrombosis occurred in 1–6% of all renal allografts and is one of the major causes of early graft loss [35]. I want to remind you once again that the right kidney has a shorter renal vein compared to the left kidney, and blood from the right kidney flows into the IVC through sometimes more than one renal vein and more often than in the left kidney.

The left renal vein, if it runs normally along the anterior surface of the aorta towards the IVC, is almost always sufficiently long and rarely requires lengthening (e.g. early division of the IVC, various anomalies of the IVC, anomalies of the renal veins). The most common indication for repair, and very rarely for lengthening of the left renal vein, is accidental damage during procurement or preparation (incision, complete dissection) or the course of the left renal vein on the posterior wall of the aorta towards the IVC. This vein, as we know, has a very thin wall and is easily damaged during retrieval. The most common material used to repair the renal veins originates from deceased donors. The following materials can be used for this purpose: the IVC, iliac or gonadal veins, the brachiocephalic vein, jugular veins and the portal vein (when the liver is not procured and the portal vein is open). There are also materials which originate from the recipient and can also be used for the repair, such as the great saphenous vein, or the inferior mesenteric or gonadal veins. It is not customary to attach a tool-kit (donor vessel for the repair and reconstruction of a recipient, organ or recipient vessel) to the kidney. If the procurement surgeon does not notice his or her error, the kidney will be sent to the donor's hospital with a damaged or very short renal vein, without any possibility of its extension or reconstruction [36–41]. The recipient surgeon has two options: either he/she will use the potential recipient's vessels (e.g. the great saphenous vein or the gonadal vein), or he/she will use vascular prostheses to reconstruct the renal vein. I personally recommend the donor or recipient or cryopreserved [42] human vessels as the first and best material for reconstruction. According to the literature the best choice of prosthesis is polytetrafluoroethylene (PTFE). PTFE is commonly used in most cases as a prosthesis for this type of reconstruction. Personally I have used PTFE prostheses several times, with good results but I have no experience with other vascular prostheses. In other articles you can read about other materials that have been used for the reconstruction of renal vessels, such as the Dacron or bovine arteria heterograft [43]. If you are unsure while on-call or you have no experience, consult a vascular surgeon or ask him/her to help you to perform the renal vessel reconstruction.

I would like us to consider for a moment the need to lengthen the right renal vein with the IVC. After studying the literature [35, 43–55], the following conclusions can be drawn: lengthening the renal vein is technically possible and does not increase the incidence of complications after transplantation, e.g. renal vein thrombosis; it shortens the duration of warm renal ischemia; it allows its implantation in patients without or with only minimal mobilization of the iliac vessels; it reduces the difference in length between the vein and the renal artery in the right kidney, which allows us to maintain the full length of the renal artery with an aortic patch during transplantation [32–34, 36–41, 44–51, 56–61].

## 3.9.2  *Kidney with a Short Renal Vein, Which Cannot be Lengthened*

### 3.9.2.1  Introduction

Everything I have written so far about the elongation of the right renal vein in kidney transplantation is true, but it is not the whole truth. Why? Because every day kidneys from living related donors are transplanted all over the world without the IVC and aorta patch and not in all cases has the surgeon the possibility of performing an elongation or reconstruction of the right renal vein or other renal vessels. This is the technique for implantation of the right kidneys with short renal veins without the need of reconstruction [35].

Try to transplant every first kidney, if technically possible, to the right side. Access to the iliac vessels on the right side, is quick, simple and does not require extensive vessel preparation of the recipient. The best and most physiological position of the kidney on the right side does not require long vessels. As a rule, 1.5–2 cm of the renal vein is sufficient, without mobilizing the recipient's iliac vessels, to connect the end of the renal vein to the side with the initial lower part of the IVC or with the upper part of the right common iliac vein. The attempt to transplant the kidney to the left side with an "end to end" anastomosis with the external iliac vein requires a much longer renal vein and thus its elongation. The external iliac vein has therefore to be fully mobilized with or without ligating the internal iliac vein.

### 3.9.2.2  Renal Transplantation with Recipient Iliac Vein Transposition

Molmenti et al. described their own interesting method [35] which consists of the dissection of the common and external iliac veins and arteries of the recipient by transecting the overlying and underlying tissues. The first step is to place the external iliac vein in a lateral position with respect to the external iliac artery. In case the length of the external iliac vein does not allow for comfortable anastomosis, the internal iliac vein may be ligated and transected. Ligation of the internal iliac vein provides much more common and external iliac vein mobility [35].

### 3.9.2.3  Right Kidney Placed in the Right Iliac Fossa in the Inversion Position

Zomorrodi et al. [52] proposed to transplant the right kidney "upside down" with the ureter pointing upwards. According to the surgical technique which the authors proposed, the anastomosing of the short length of the right renal vein may be compared with the left long renal vein. Twenty kidneys were anastomosed with the external iliac vein "upside down" and, before clamping the iliac vessels, 30 units of heparin per kilogram of the recipient's body weight were intravenously injected.

The follow-up period of six months showed that 100% of the patients and organs were in a good condition and that no thrombosis or any urological complications occured. Finally, the authors emphasize how important the perfect back table and dissection of the recipient's iliac vessels is in this method [52].

### 3.9.2.4 General Remarks: Short Renal Vein—Elongation Impossible

Regardless as to which side the kidney is going to be transplanted, if the need arises, perform a careful dissection of the iliac veins, ligate the iliac internal vein and other branches reaching the common and external iliac vein. After all these steps have been taken, you will achieve a complete mobilization of the common and external iliac vein. In some centers the ligation of the internal iliac vein and mobilizations of two others is part of the standard transplantation technique for each kidney. Please keep in mind that mobilization of the iliac veins and ligating their branches will be in many cases a long and quite difficult operation, sometimes combined with high blood loss. On the right side the length of the renal artery does not play any role. If the recipient's iliac vessels are not severely altered by arteriosclerosis, the renal artery can be shortened, or without shortening anastomosed "end to the side" to one of the iliac arteries—with or without the aortic patch and without renal vein elongation [55, 62–70].

**Warning! (A high kidney position needs a longer ureter—do we have a problem again?)**

(a) **High renal allograft position—right renal vein elongation impossible (thrombosis and/or severe atherosclerosis of one of the iliac vessels)**

The renal vein is  highly anastomosed when for example the initial section of the IVC, portal vein or superior mesenteric vein (SMA) lies in the extraperitoneal space in an ideal, almost physiological position. But nothing is free, as the proverb says— such a quite high (physiologically almost orthotopically) or an even higher position under the liver of the kidney requires slightly more extensive surgical access, which requires a longer incision and long ureter. The end of the long ureter is not always optimally supplied with blood which means that it has a much higher risk of fibrosis (stenosis) or necrosis and/or urine leakage. A solution for this problem is to shorten the kidney transplant ureter and to perform "end to end" or "end to side" anastomosis with the ureter of the recipient by inserting the JJ catheter to decompress the ureter-ureter anastomosis.

(b) **Or maybe a low renal allograft position (severe atherosclerosis, short-cut kidney ureter for transplantation, lack of own ureter) or the recipient's ureter is so pathologically altered that it is unsuitable for anastomosis with the donor kidney's ureter**

If we want to perform a venous anastomosis with one of the external right or left iliac veins (which are located much deeper especially in obese patients with a BMI

>35 or in patients who are very tall) and the external iliac artery, there is in many cases no need to totally mobilize both iliac veins on the same side. Only when the right renal vein is too short, will an elongation of the renal vein be needed with or without the mobilization of the iliac veins. It also should be remembered that the course of the external iliac vein, when approaching the inguinal ligament, rises upwards. This causes its distance from the kidney to be shorter and thus the incision will be smaller. However, in some cases the kidney may require special positioning (an inversion position if there is no possibility for vein elongation), for example in order to obtain the best physiological position and a proper inflow and outflow of the blood from the kidney. Renal vessels of the transplanted kidney must not be twisted or kinked. Twisting or kinking is usually responsible for the impeded blood inflow and outflow from the transplanted kidney, which may in turn lead to thrombosis. If elongation of the short renal vein for one reason or another is impossible to perform, the kidney transplant method of Momenti or Zamorrodi be used; or ligate and cut the iliac internal vein and mobilize totally the common and external iliac vein towards the vessels of the kidney [35, 52].

**Warning! (Help yourself)**
If the renal vein is short, and there is no possibility of its extension, it must be more than perfectly prepared for transplantation, that is the vessels must be 100% tight and during vascular anastomoses and reperfusion the position of the kidney must be the same. Remember that if there is bleeding from the back wall of the short right renal vein during the perfusion—for example somewhere high in the hilum—and the kidney has already increased its volume, even the best surgeon has little chance to control this bleeding without removing the kidney. After reperfusion of such a kidney, don't manipulate the kidney too much, as this can lead to a renal vein tear and a massive hemorrhage [69, 70].

Use professional automatic abdominal retractors for transplantation, such as Omnitrac or Thompson or Bookwalter. Learn how to use them as this will give you a stable surgical field and the possibility of an accurate and safe kidney transplantation and peace of mind, with one assistant and scrub nurse, without unnecessary shouting or stress.

**Author's Remark**
While writing this book, I have tried to count how many times in my life I was forced to elongate the right renal vein (not to be confused with the reconstruction of a short-cut renal vein). If I remember well, I have done it no more than 20 times. In most cases, the main reason for the vein elongation was that the right kidney, which had to be transplanted on the left side, had more than one renal vein and one artery or more arteries on the aortic patch. In the cases of the right kidney transplanted to the right side, I had to extend the right renal vein with the donor's IVC usually in obese, "deep", difficult and surgically demanding recipients.

### *3.9.3  The Most Popular Surgical Techniques for Lengthening the Right Renal Vein*

#### 3.9.3.1  Manual Lengthening of the Right Renal Vein with the IVC Using a Non-absorbable Continuous Suture (Author's Experience)

1. After a thorough kidney inspection, we determine the length by which the IVC right renal vein is to be extended. As a rule, we extend the right renal vein to a distance greater than 50–70% of the length of the right renal artery, but not more than the whole length of the right renal artery. Please do not forget also that the length of the elongated right vein or renal veins also depends on the quality and length of the procured IVC during organ retrieval.

2. The next step in the lengthening of the right renal vein is to ligate and/or sew tightly all the small open veins that reach the wall of the IVC, so that the walls of the IVC are tight. Put both (posterior and anterior) walls of the IVC on each other (slightly under tension), and then, with the use of vascular scissors, trim the anterior and posterior walls of the IVC to the desired width, 4–6 mm slightly larger than the width of the right renal vein or veins. When two or more renal veins are lengthened, the wall of the IVC should be an extension (alignment) of the outer walls of the renal veins. When the IVC is used for renal vein lengthening and suturing, the IVC should expand slightly towards its end. This slight expansion will help to prevent constriction and will be responsible for the good drainage of blood from the renal veins into one of the iliac veins of the recipient. My technique is that the diameter of lengthening of the right renal vein with the IVC, which runs from the renal vein towards the end of its lengthening, increases slightly its diameter by about 4–6 mm (Figs. 3.113 and 3.114).

**Warning! (The elongation at the end should be wider than the diameter of the renal vein)**
Remember that the diameter of the lumen cut from the IVC, before suturing its walls, must be at least 4–6 mm wider than the diameter of the renal vein after suturing. If we suture one side of the IVC during the renal vein elongation, 3–4 mm of the IVC will be absorbed by the suture. If we suture both sides of the IVC during the renal vein elongation, 6–8 mm of the IVC will be absorbed by the suture.

3. After the IVC has been cut and a new renal vein has been formed, before the anterior and posterior walls of the IVC are sutured together, the edges of the IVC should be lightly pressed against each other to make suturing easier.

**Attention! (How to reposition a knot or knots)**
In my opinion it is important to finish the suture 1–2 cm above the lumen of the "new renal vein" outlet, which means that the last 1–2 cm of the vein extensions will be sutured twice. When lengthening the renal vein with the IVC, it is possible

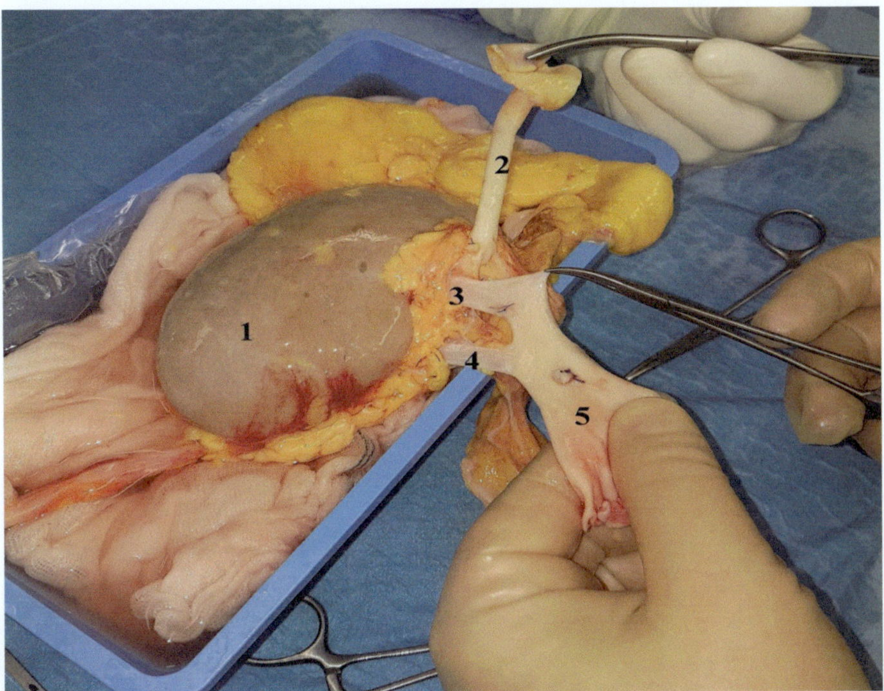

**Fig. 3.112** Right kidney with two renal veins of the same diameter taken with an IVC from the donor. 1—Right kidney, 2—Renal artery, 3 and 4—Renal veins, 5—IVC. With the Mosquito clamp, the wall of the IVC is grasped just above the cut opening in the IVC left after the left renal vein and the IVC patch have been removed. The anterior and posterior walls of the IVC are in contact, and the lower part of the IVC is stretched slightly downwards. After cutting to length and width, the Mosquito clamp is closed and the anterior and posterior walls of the IVC are sutured together

to suture its walls twice with the same suture from top to bottom, i.e. from the region of the renal tubule towards the lumen of the kidney, and then to suture the walls of the IVC again with the same suture, i.e. to return to the previous suture and to suture nothing with the suture close to the kidney, i.e. far from the lumen of the "new vein". Double suturing the walls of the IVC will result in better haemostasis and less blood loss when the kidney re-perfuses. In this case, my advice is that the surgical nerve should be placed away from the lumen of the new vein so that it and its cut ends do not interfere with the anastomosis, do not interfere with the anastomosis, and do not prolong the time required to anastomose the "new renal vein" to one of the recipient's iliac veins or IVC (Figs. 3.113 and 3.114).

4. The kidney has been transplanted to the left side. The two right renal veins were elongated with the donor's IVC (sewn on only one side), and anastomosed "end to the side" of the left external iliac vein, the end of the right renal artery was shortened and sewn "end to the side" of the left common iliac artery (Fig. 3.115).

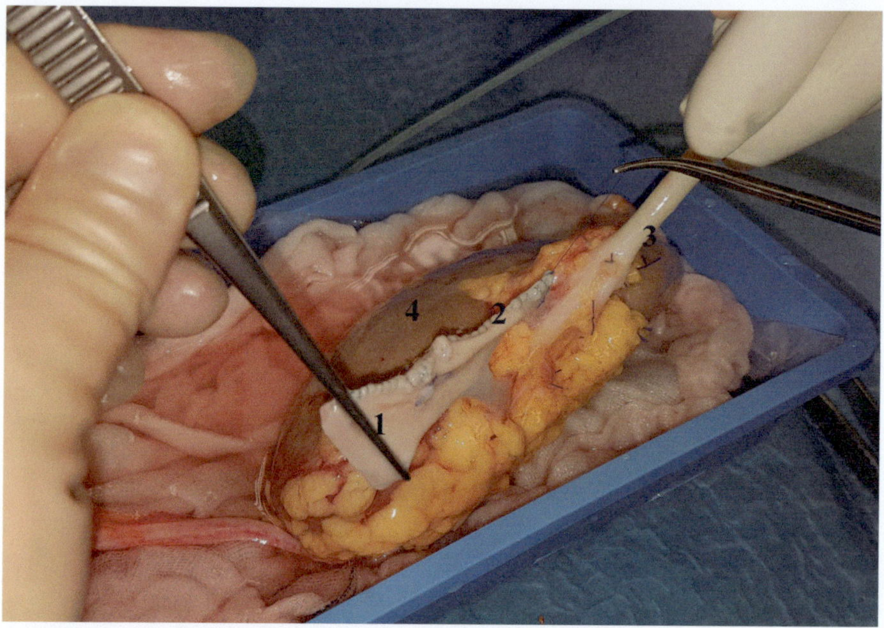

**Fig. 3.113** Stitched walls of the IVC to elongate two identical right renal veins. 1—Elongated right renal veins with IVC, 2—Suture site, 3—Renal artery, 4—Kidney

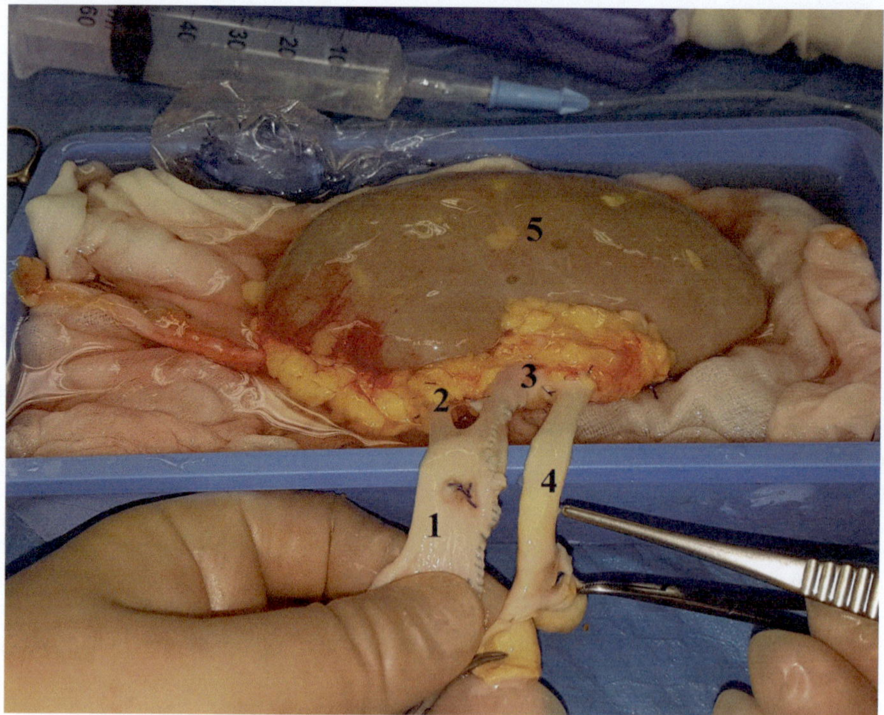

**Fig. 3.114** Elongated renal veins of the right IVC kidney: front view. 1—Sutured and elongated right renal veins with IVC slightly widening downwards, 2 and 3—Renal veins, 4—Renal artery, 5—Kidney

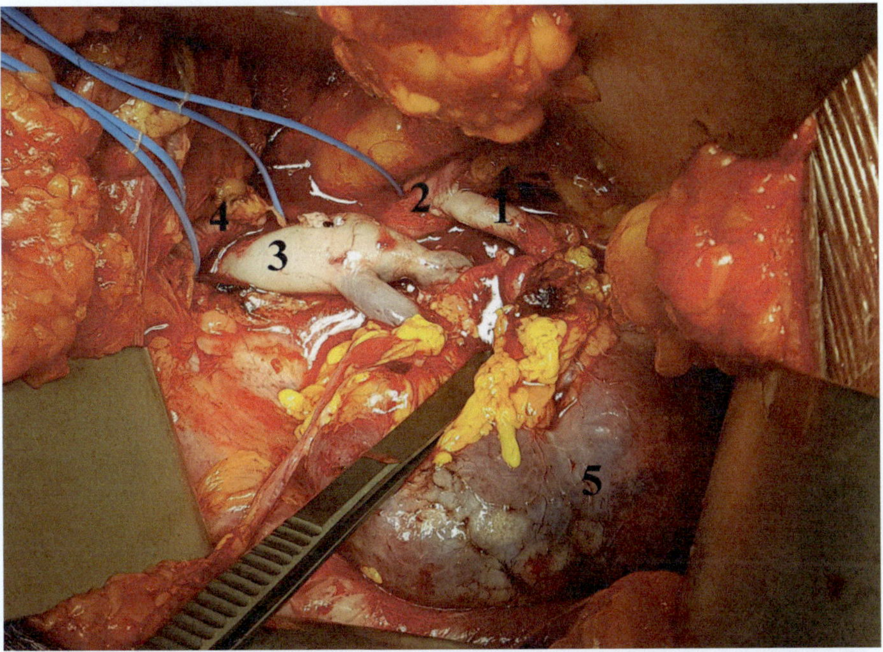

**Fig. 3.115** Right kidney with elongated veins, with the two IVC renal veins, anastomosed to the left iliac external vein of the recipient. 1—Renal artery, 2—Common iliac artery, 3—Donor IVC, which lengthened two renal veins, 4—Left external iliac artery, 5—Kidney

### 3.9.3.2   Elongation of the Right Renal Vein with IVC Using a Vascular Stapler

An elongation of the right renal vein with the IVC technique offers an expeditious and safe means of extending the cadaveric right renal vein for 3–5 cm while greatly minimizing the ischemic time of the kidney during back table [71]. We call this elongation of the right renal vein with IVC transverse lengthening, a transverse elongation by the diameter of the IVC.

The technique of elongation using a vascular stapler is step by step as follows:

1. The right kidney is to be transplanted for example to the left side. The renal artery, IVC, renal vein and ureter have been prepared. The renal vein is very short and quickly splits into two veins in the renal hilum.
2. The IVC and the right renal vein are pulled and stretched downwards using vascular forceps and the IVC is stretched sideways (Fig. 3.116).

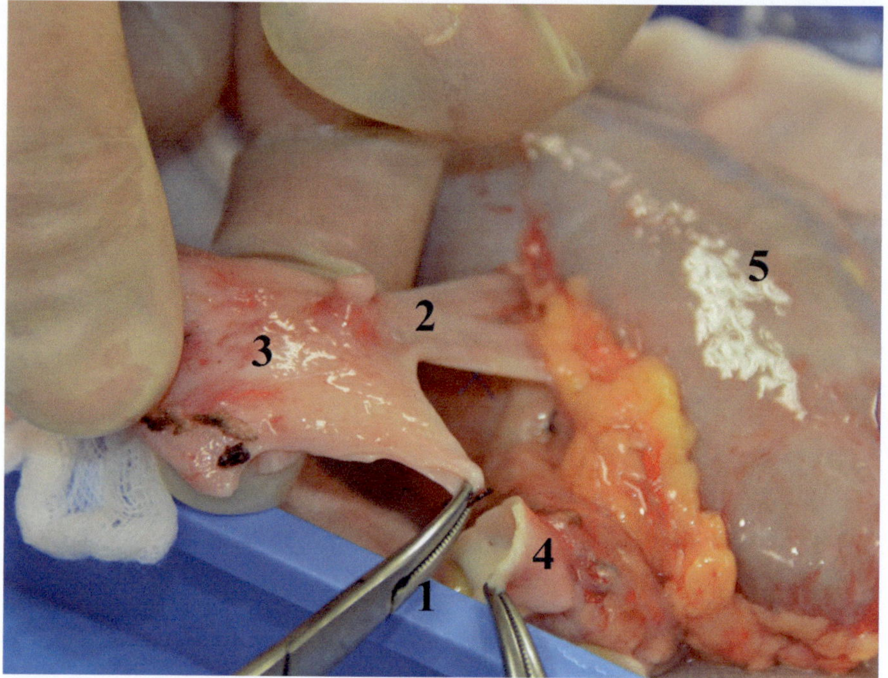

**Fig. 3.116** 1—Small vascular clamp slightly stretching the lower vena cava, 2—Short right kidney vein, 3—IVC, 4—Renal artery, 5—Kidney

3. Next, from the side of the renal hilum, a vascular stapler is inserted and closed across the IVC with on both sides a 2–4 mm extension of the renal vein. The lumen of the IVC is closed with the vascular stapler and its excess is cut off.
4. In the same way, the IVC is closed and cut off on the other side with an appropriate margin, according to the rule that the central renal vein extension should be on each side 2–4 mm larger in diameter than the main renal vein (Figs. 3.117 and 3.118).
5. Now, the elongated renal vein has no outflow. The renal vein opening should be cut from the lateral side of the IVC with sharp vascular scissors (Fig. 3.119).

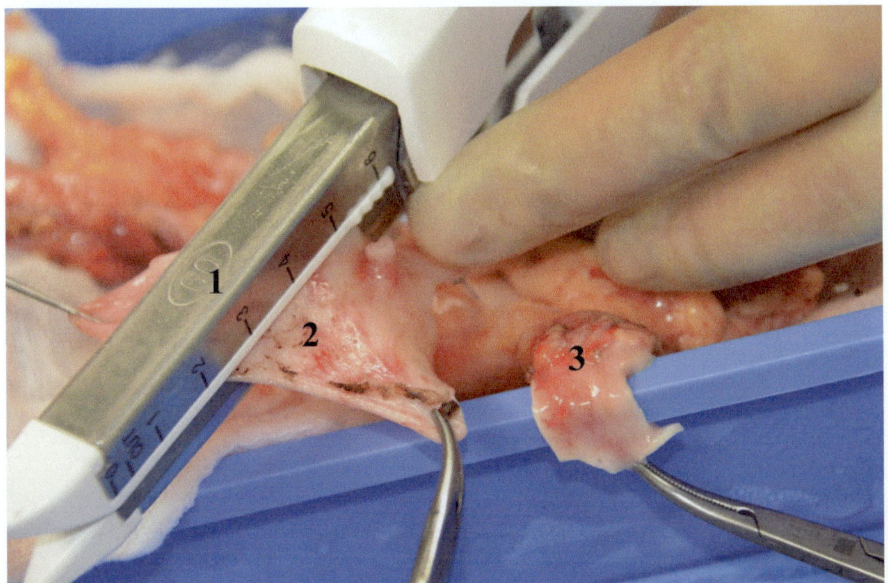

**Fig. 3.117**  1—Vascular stapler closed across the IVC, 2—Elongated with vascular stapler segment of IVC has to be 3–4 mm wider than the diameter of the renal vein, 3—Renal artery

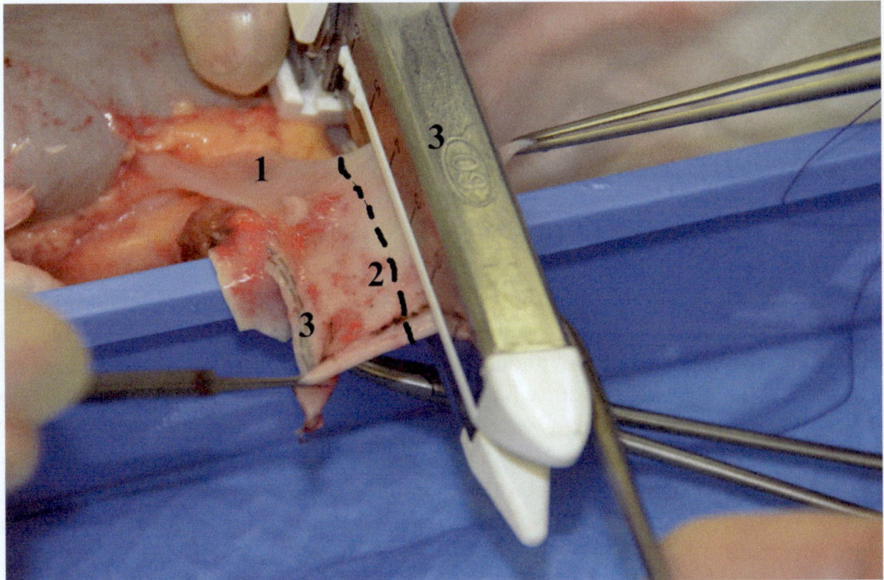

**Fig. 3.118**  1—Short right renal vein, 2—Elongated with vascular stapler segment of IVC has to be 3–4 mm wider than the diameter of the renal vein, 3—Vascular stapler (white cartridge) closed across the IVC

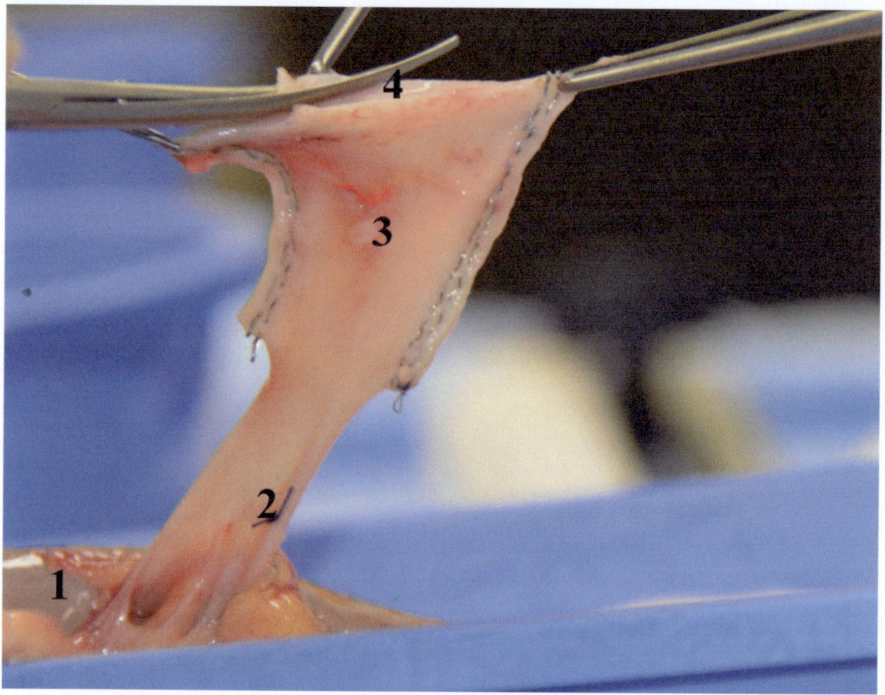

**Fig. 3.119** Right renal vein elongated with a vascular stapler technique. 1—Kidney, 2—Right renal vein, 3—IVC, 4—Cutting an opening in the lateral wall of the IVC with sharp vascular scissors. The lateral opening in the IVC was anastomosed end-to-side with the common iliac vein on the left side

**Warning! (Transverse elongation of the right renal vein is not always possible)**

Such transverse lengthening of the right renal vein with the IVC is possible when the IVC is completely preserved on both sides of the vein. Then in this technique the right renal vein can be extended by the width of the IVC. If on both sides of the right renal vein the IVC is not completely preserved and we want to elongate the renal vein with a stapler and without suturing, we have to apply the technique of lengthening the right renal vein which is similar to the "manual" method—where instead of a suture we use a vascular stapler to close one side of the IVC (Fig. 3.120) [42]. If you ask me which lengthening of the right renal vein is the most beautiful, I would answer you that it is the one done by hand. But if you ask me which extension of the right renal vein is the most useful, I would answer that it is the one made with a stapler. The handmade extension has to be made to measure,

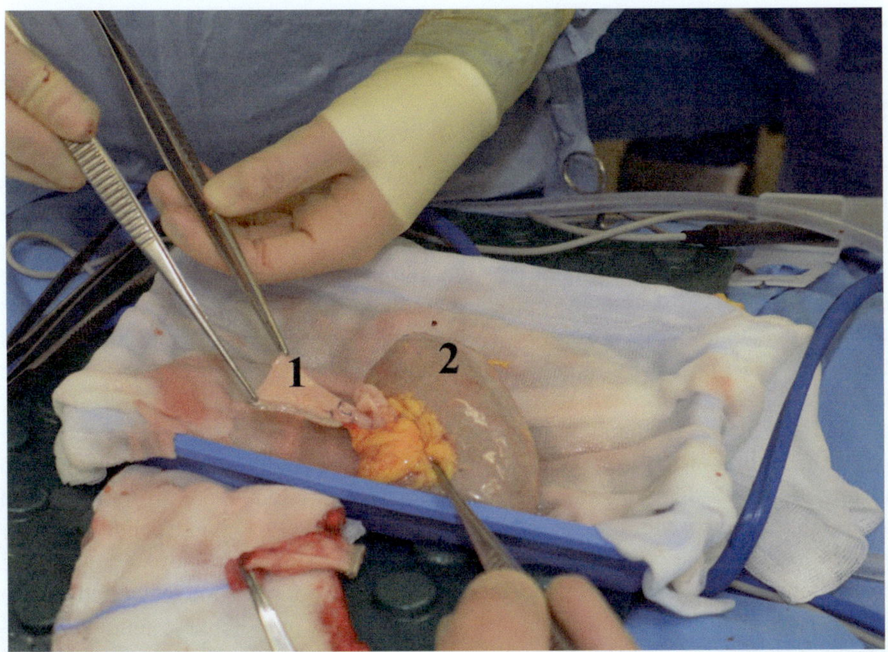

**Fig. 3.120** Another surgical technique for right renal vein elongation with the IVC. This technique consists of a manual elongation or cutting and stapling only one side of the IVC with a vascular stapler. 1—Elongated right renal vein with IVC shows closed anterior and posterior wall on one side only as you see on the picture from the ureter side, 2—Kidney

because the whole handmade construction cannot be shortened. Usually after lengthening of the renal vein, it is important to look for the best position for the elongated renal vein before performing the anastomosis. You have to be careful that the vein is not twisted and/or kinked in order to avoid a renal vein thrombosis. If the right renal vein is lengthened by the IVC with the help of a stapler, the whole structure can easily be shortened with very thick, coarse scissors and thus an optimal length and position can be performed without looking for the best place for anastomosis. This also means that the vein can be lengthened as long as possible. The big advantage of the stapler lengthening is that after opening the patient, it is possible at any time to shorten the vein to the desired length.

### 3.9.3.3   Short Cut Left Renal Vein: Reconstruction with Interposition Allograft

Introduction

The short renal vein is a technical inconvenience and a surgical challenge [36–38]. Such a situation limits the exposure of venues to anastomosis and compromises renal mobility and the final position of the kidney. Now we will analyze, step by step, how to solve the problem of a short renal vein—especially when we are dealing with the kidney which is procured without the IVC and/or with a very short renal vein. The first step is to mobilize the renal vein completely from the hilum of the kidney. If it is still not long enough, the iliac veins need to be totally mobilized by sacrificing the iliac internal vein and a renal vessels anastomosis with the IVC and/or one of the iliac veins and common and/or external iliac vein has to be performed without any tension. The second (difficult) step is to find an optimal position for the kidney and therefore, in some cases, to free all the iliac arteries and veins and to sacrify the iliac internal vessels. A too short or injured renal vein may benefit from elongation with a venous allograft—as described below—without the risk of thrombosis. Based on the literature, it can be concluded that renal vein reconstruction with an interposition allograft is a safe and effective modality [35–41, 44–54].

Brief Case Description

In this case, the left renal vein was accidentally cut off deeply in the renal hilum, its length did not exceed 1 cm. Fortunately, the surgeon retrieving the kidney discovered by accident that he had cut a renal vein and that the kidney would not be suitable for transplantation in this state. He was a very good and honest surgeon, as he informed the recipient kidney center about his accident, described the damage in detail and added a small section of the IVC to the retrieved kidney to reconstruct the left renal vein, adding a small piece of the vena cava superior (VCS) to the left kidney for reconstruction.

Ex Vivo Vein Reconstruction with Interposition Allograft Step by Step

1. The kidney was prepared for transplantation and a short-cut stump of the left vein was put on a non-absorbable 6/0 stay suture, then the left renal vein was mobilized from the surrounding tissues—deeply towards the hilum of the kidney.

2. After measuring the diameter of the renal vein stump, the donor's IVC was trimmed appropriately and sutured in the form of a cylinder. A new "renal vein" was thus produced, one end of which was anastomosed to the end of the left renal vein stump in the renal hilum with a continuous 6/0 non-absorbable monofilament suture (Fig. 3.121).
3. Then the tightness of the sutured IVC was checked, as well as the anastomosis. Only now do we see (Fig. 3.122) where the right renal vein was cut by the surgeon who procured the kidney. Fortunately, the kidney was reconstructed and transplanted without any complications, to the satisfaction of the recipient and recipient's family.

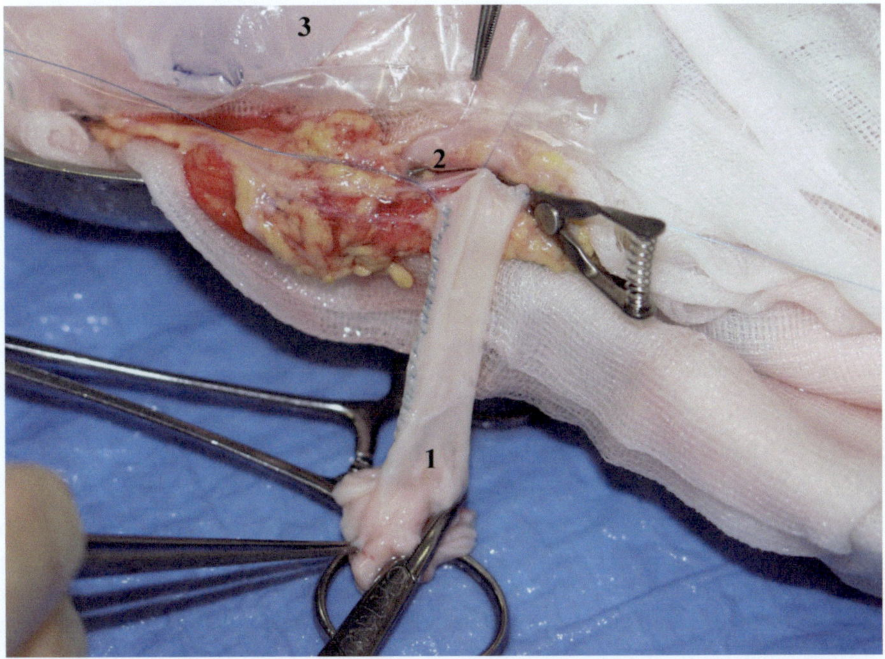

**Fig. 3.121** Procured left kidney with a very short renal vein as a technical mistake during organ procurement. Left renal vein formed from IVC with suturing end to end to the left renal vein. 1—A new left renal vein reconstructed from the IVC, 2—A very short cut left renal vein, deeply prepared in the renal hilum, 3—The kidney, in order not to warm it during reconstruction, was covered with sterile of ice

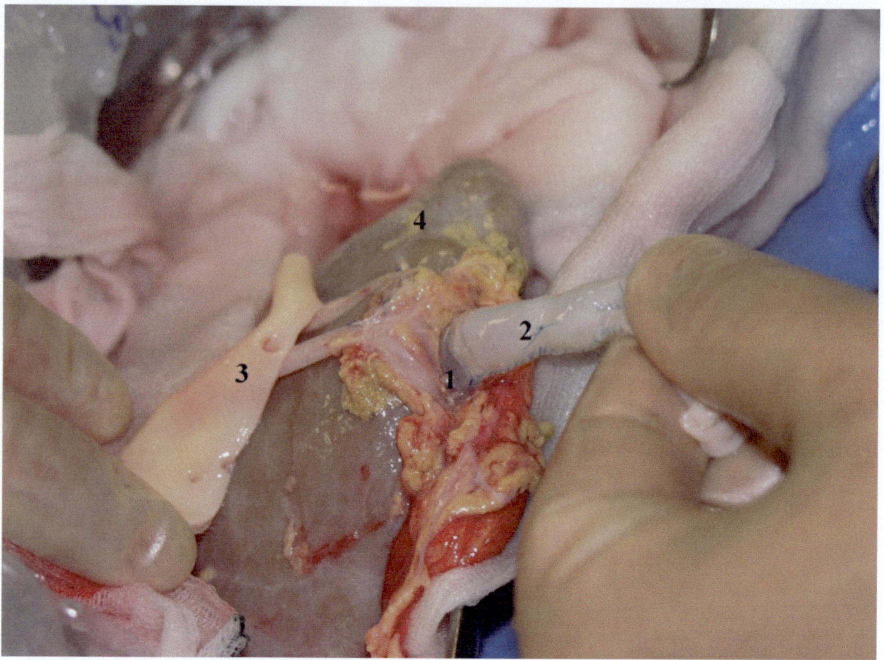

**Fig. 3.122** Leakage testing of left renal vein reconstruction with interposition allograft. 1—Own tiny margin of the left renal vein, 2—Donor inferior vena cava (IVC), 3—Aortic patch with two renal arteries, 4—Kidney upper pole

### 3.9.3.4   Other Techniques for Lengthening the Renal Vein

1. Barry et al. [47] described the "calm-shell technique" for the right renal vein extension using the IVC in a cadaver kidney transplantation in case the organ procurement team splits the IVC longitudinally. The split IVC is subsequently folded medially and sutured on its anterior and posterior surfaces to extend the right renal vein.
2. Other procured vessels from a deceased donor than the IVC can be used for extending the renal vein, such as: the iliac, subclavian and brachiocephalic vein(s) [54].
3. Feng et al. [48] described extending the renal vein using the ovarian or testicular vein. The use of the testicular vein can be controversial. Its removal has been associated with complications such as impaired blood and lymph drainage from the testis and temporary swelling. Disadvantages: small diameter; labor-intensive; as a rule, with a longitudinal incision, two or three sections of the vein are sewn

longitudinally; in order to reach the diameter of the renal vein, care must be taken not to narrow the lumen of the reconstructed vein and to ensure an optimal outflow of blood from the graft. Another approach is the spiral reconstruction, which is also laborious and requires extensive microsurgical experience—these reconstructions are complicated, non-routine and are associated with a greater risk of venous thrombosis.

4. A renal vein can be lengthened by using a specially prepared sterile and immunologically neutral bovine artery.
5. Extending the renal vein with an artificial prosthesis, for example made of PTFE or Dacron. This has been described in several cases as saving the kidney from being completely disqualified as an organ for transplantation [35–55, 71].
6. In situ patch in right renal vein elongation. Santangelo et al. [54] performed this right renal vein elongation during the procurement procedure abdominal organ perfusion phase with a substantial reduction of the back table time.

**Warning! (Some techniques can be dangerous)**
It should be remembered that some of the above mentioned methods are associated with a greater risk of thrombosis of the renal vein and infection, and thus septic hemorrhage from vascular anastomoses.

The currently most popular and safe method of lengthening the right renal vein (s), in general consists of:

- Always retrieving the right kidney with the IVC.
- Using the IVC or other vein(s) procured from the donor's body as needed to extend the right and, if necessary, also the left renal vein(s).

The methods of right renal vein elongation with the IVC as described above are characterized by the lowest number of complications. By extending the renal vein with the IVC or other donor veins, the graft of the patient's survival is the same as in the case of a classical kidney transplantation without vein lengthening.

The donor's IVC is the best and most easiest available material for a renal vein reconstruction. Other veins are also suitable for lengthening and reconstruction of damaged renal veins, but are more difficult to access. Remember that the reconstruction material in the form of different veins is normally not needed for the reconstruction of a renal vein. As a rule, the left kidney, if well procured, has a long vein which does not require elongation and the right kidney should always be procured with the IVC. The donor iliac veins—as a reconstructive material—should always be divided between the liver, pancreas and sometimes also the intestine, as these organs almost always require reconstruction. If during the procurement one of the renal veins is cut too short, other veins from the abdominal cavity or chest should be collected for its reconstruction.

**Warning! (Take care of the quality of the procured organs and fill in the quality form)**

Before packing the kidney, the procurement surgeon is obliged to examine the quality of the kidney perfusion, the number of renal arteries, veins and ureters and the advancement of abdominal aortic wall atherosclerosis and the degree of plaque in the renal arteries. The surgeon is also obliged to perform fat reduction around the kidney. After procuring and packing the kidney for transport, the procurement surgeon must describe the quality of the organs retrieved in the quality form, their possible damage before or during the procurement, as well as damage to vessels, parenchyma, renal pelvis and/or ureters thus all damages which the surgeon has seen during the removal or in kidney packaging.

## 3.10  Difficult Kidney Inspections and Preparation— Decision Making—Cases

### 3.10.1  *Right Kidney Procured with Three Renal Veins on a Patch from the IVC, but Without a Whole IVC from the Right Renal Vein up to Its Bifurcation*

The renal artery branches out into four, 1 cm after leaving the abdominal aorta's wall. In one case I dealt with, the lengthening of renal veins did not make sense because, firstly, we did not receive any material to lengthen the vein and, secondly, the distance between the first and third vein was about 8 cm. The kidney was of a good quality, each renal vein was intact and all veins were 3.0–4.0 cm long after mobilization and the recipient was a young, not obese man. After a thorough analysis of CT scans of the recipient's iliac vessels, I decided to transplant this kidney with a patch from the IVC on the right side. Please remember that the chance to transplant the kidney successfully was definitely only on the right side of the recipient (the venous anastomosis site: the IVC and right common iliac and external vein). The next challenge was to find a Satinsky vascular clamp which was long enough to allow for a more than 10 cm long venous anastomosis.

The preparation of three veins on a patch from the IVC and four renal arteries departing from the common trunk is not an easy task. The entire preparation of the kidney for transplant took over an hour and a half, with the use of microsurgical instruments, surgical loupes and cold lighting. The inspection of a kidney with many short vessels must be very thorough and requires not only a surgical but also microsurgical experience. Each, even the smallest, arterial and venous vessel must be very carefully dissected and the small venous branches must be carefully ligated and/or sewn with a non-absorbable monofilament. Do not forget that the wall of each prepared vessel (branch) must be leak tested. The kidney transplant operation was performed with a right pararectal incision. After the retroperitoneal space was exposed, the following vessels were dissected: the common iliac, external and the internal iliac artery—up to its first branch, close to its bifurcation and also the low segment of the IVC, the common iliac and half of the external iliac vein. The recipient's internal iliac vessels were not ligated. Prior to arterial anastomosis, the previously mobilized recipient's iliac arteries were very gently pulled to the left side with one of the specially designed Omnitrac renal blades in order to show the entire course of the previously prepared lower part of the IVC, common iliac and the external iliac vein. An open biopsy of the kidney was performed and then the kidney was placed in the right iliac fossa for several seconds in order to determine its best position and to select the most suitable places for vascular anastomoses. The beginning and the end of venous anastomosis were marked with an Argon Beamer coagulation. The kidney was placed in a container filled with cold organ preservation solution. With a Satinsky clamp, the lumen of the common iliac vein and the beginning of the IVC were partially closed. The clamped venous section was cut longitudinally along the long axis and rinsed from inside with a solution of physiological saline and heparin. To prevent cut left vein wall from closing the stay suture has been placed. As the next step, the kidney was placed in the previously chosen, best position in the retroperitoneal space on the greater psoas muscle. The "side to side" venous anastomosis (consisting of renal veins on the IVC patch to the side of the common iliac vein and the lower part of the IVC) was performed with a continuous, non-absorbable monofilament 5/0 suture. After the anastomosis, the iliac recipent arteries were released from the renal blade of the surgical retractor (Omnitrac). The renal artery was shortened and cut off about 20 mm after its exit from the aorta, because the ostium of the renal artery was narrowed by about 50% in the atherosclerotic plaque. The second reason to shorten the artery was that it was too long. Through shortening the artery, we have prevented the arteries from kinking. The renal artery with its branches was crossed over to the left side between the first and second renal vein, medially and to the left, towards the common iliac artery, counting from the top. Renal artery anastomosis was made end to side of the common iliac artery with a 6/0 continuous suture. After releasing the clamps, the kidney was supplied with blood properly and began to produce urine after a few minutes. The warm ischemia time was 30 min and the blood loss was about 100 ml. The patient was very stable all the time, no pressure drops were noted during reperfusion. If—theoretically—this kidney had to be transplanted to the left side for some reason, the operation would be much more difficult, if not impossible. This would involve a much greater loss of blood and would require the ligation of the internal iliac vein and possibly the artery as well, and numerous small veins extending from the lumbar region to the iliac vessels. The effects of the above-described operation are shown in (Figs. 3.123 and 3.124).

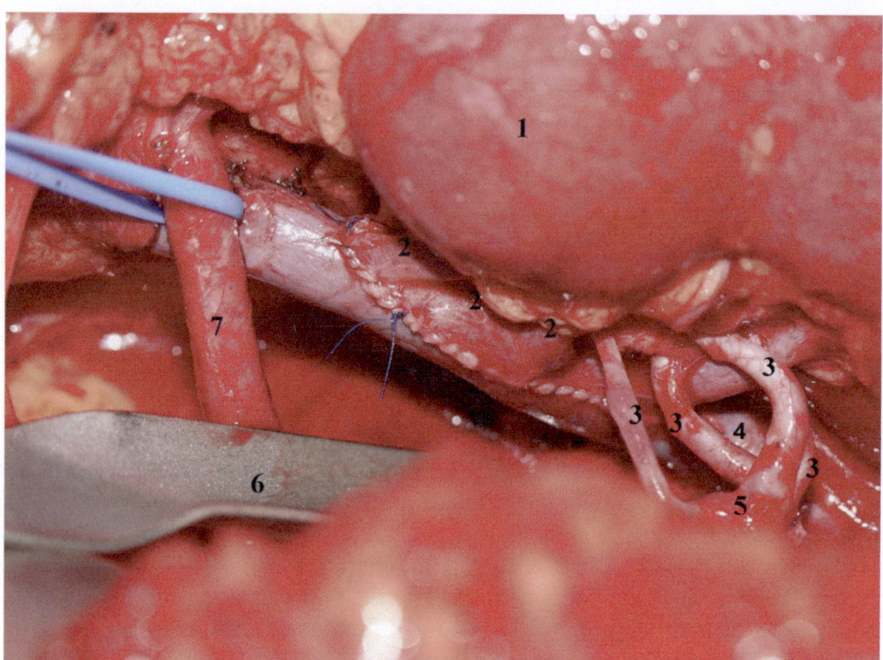

**Fig. 3.123** 1—Right kidney transplanted to the right side, 2—Three renal veins on theIVC patch, 3—Renal artery branches (four independent arteries), 4—IVC, 5—Renal artery main trunk, 6—Renal vein blade gently pulling the external iliac artery during venous anastomosis, 7—Right external iliac artery

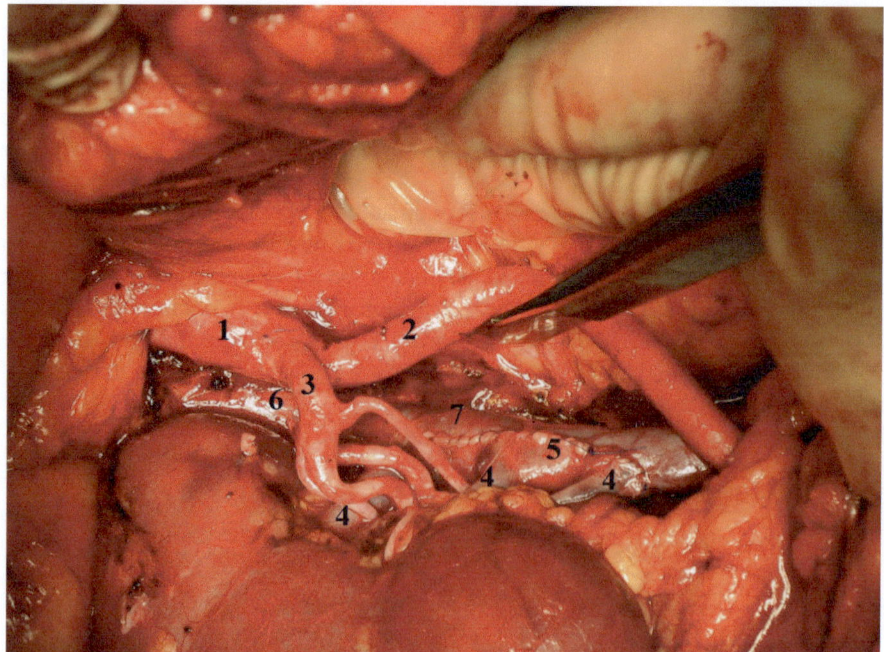

**Fig. 3.124** 1—Common iliac artery, 2—External iliac artery, 3—Main trunk of the renal artery, 4—Three renal veins on the IVC patch, 5—Patch of IVC, 6—Recipient IVC, 7—Common iliac vein

**Warning! (Learn to take the preparation of a kidney for transplant very seriously)**

Please remember what I mentioned earlier—a kidney qualified for transplantation, after proper preparation, must be safe not only for the recipient of the organ, but also for the surgeon. In my career as a transplant surgeon, I have seen various difficult situations resulting from poor preparation (poor back table) of a kidney for transplantation.

Usually they were the result of:

- an inaccurate, too fast or too superficial inspection of the kidney;
- overstepping the limits of all risks due to inexperience.

In all cases of poor kidney inspection and preparation, usually after vascular anastomosis and releasing of the vascular clamps, there was massive hemorrhage, severe blood loss, decompensation of the patient, significant prolongation of the warm ischemia time, delayed graft function and in some cases primary non-function, consequently a loss of the graft and return to dialysis.

## 3.10.2   Reconstruction of Two Renal Arteries of the Same or Different Diameter

### 3.10.2.1   Introduction

Most often such reconstructions are performed on renal arteries of the kidney taken from the living donor. Both arteries are taken without a patch from the abdominal aorta (Fig. 3.125). Sometimes such vascular reconstructions are also performed on the renal arteries procured from deceased donors. The best example of this type of reconstruction is the kidney with two renal arteries on a highly atherosclerotic patch from the abdominal aorta, where the ostias of both renal arteries are clearly constricted (Figs. 3.126 and 3.127). In this case, the renal arteries must be dissected from the patch towards the renal hilum and their quality assessed. As a rule, the walls of the renal arteries, which are located at a distance of 0.5–1.0 cm from the abdominal aorta, are in many cases—especially concerning elderly people—affected by severe atherosclerotic changes that are responsible for narrowing of the lumen of the renal artery. Beyond this distance, in most cases, the renal arteries are of a good quality (smooth and with an elastic wall) without any atherosclerotic changes and thus suitable for performing an arterial anastomosis.

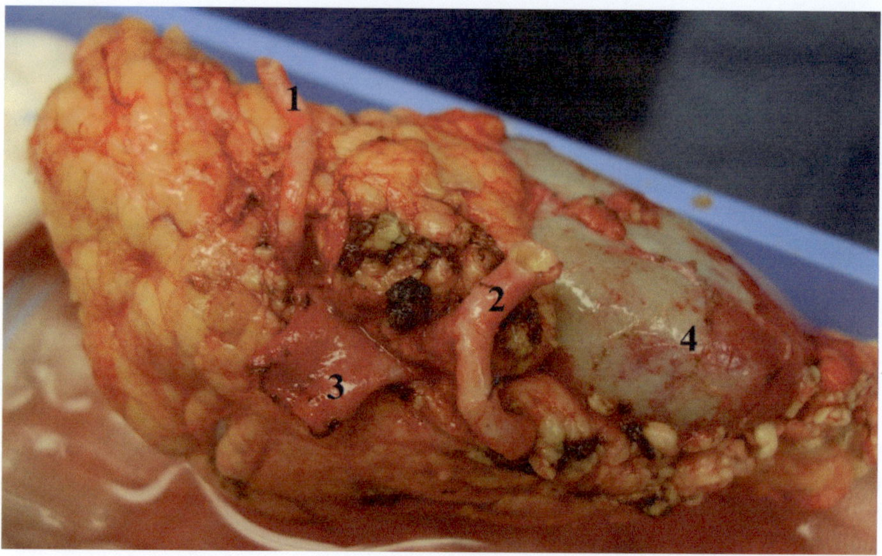

**Fig. 3.125** Left kidney with two renal arteries taken from a living donor. 1—Renal accessory artery to the lower pole, 2—Upper artery vascularizing the upper pole and middle kidney, 3—Renal vein, 4—Upper kidney pole

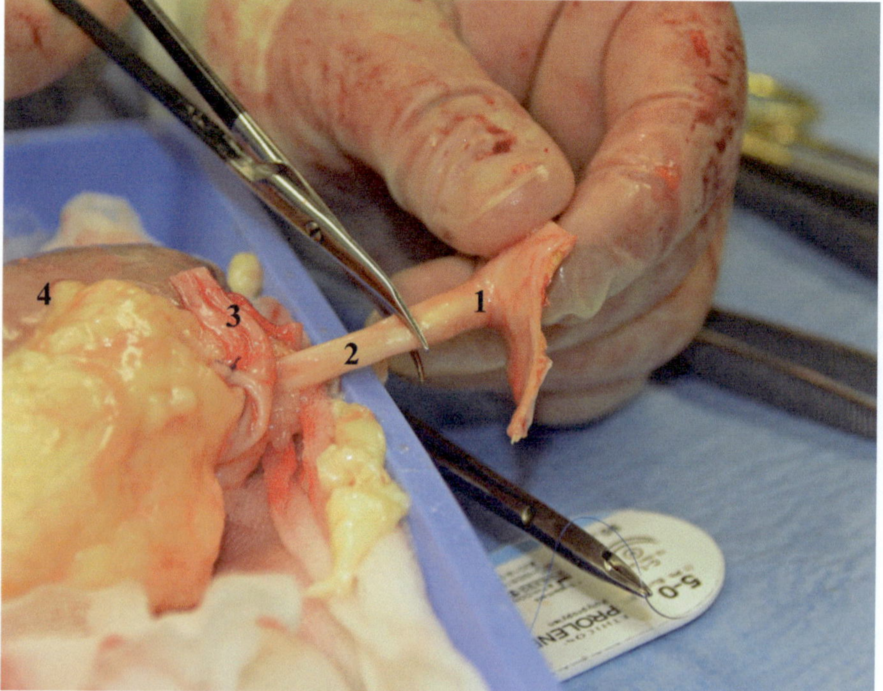

**Fig. 3.126** Renal artery immediately after leaving the abdominal aorta with a large artherosclerotic plaque causing a narrowing of the artery, starting at its origin. 1—Atherosclerotic plaque, 2—Segment of healthy renal artery, 3—Renal vein, 4—Kidney

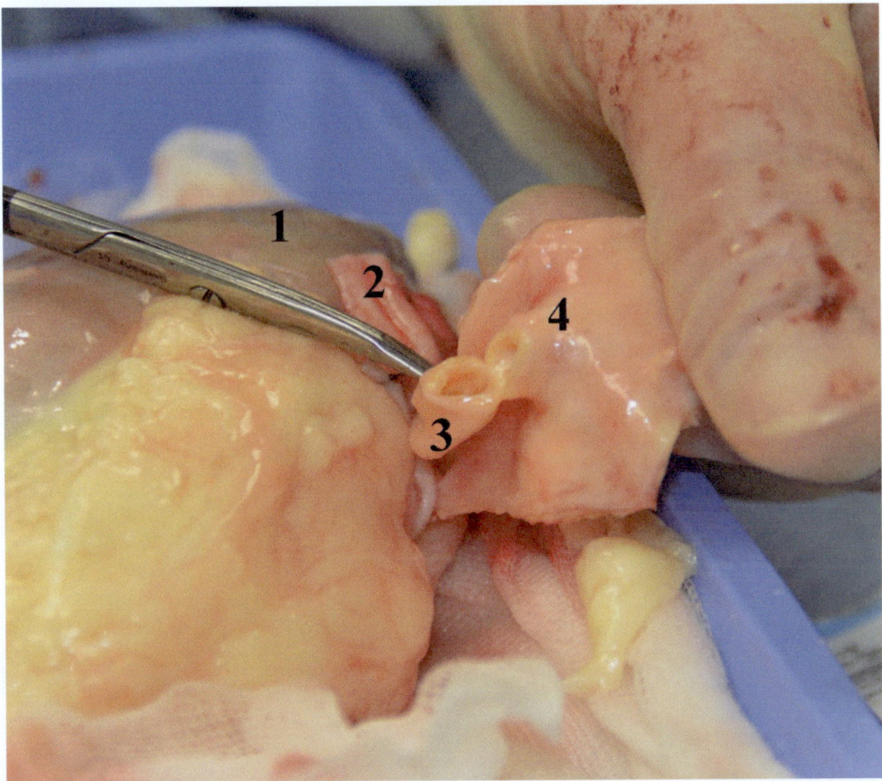

**Fig. 3.127** Renal artery cut with aortic patch at a distance of 0.8 mm from the abdominal aorta wall, with a large atherosclerotic plaque almost completely closed renal ostium in the aorta. 1—Kidney, 2—Renal vein, 3—Atherosclerotic unchanged proximal part of the renal artery, 4—Initial part of the renal artery lumen of its almost closed atherosclerotic plaque as seen

### 3.10.2.2   The Problem of Two Renal Arteries of the Same or Different Diameter Can Be Solved in Several Ways

These are the most common ones:

1. Both arteries can be implanted separately end to side in one of the iliac arteries. To minimize the risk of thrombosis, the recipient's iliac vessels must show no long term atherosclerotic lesions (Fig. 3.128). The argument in favor is that in the case of a thrombosis of one artery in difficult anastomoses, the recipient has another unobstructed artery and a half-active kidney.

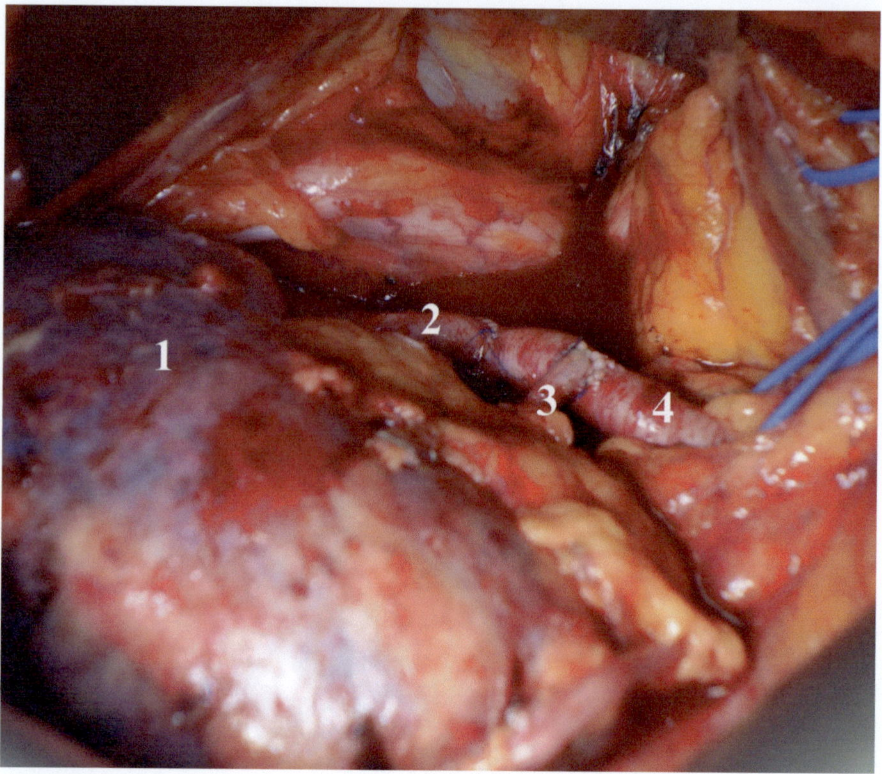

**Fig. 3.128** Living donation kidney transplant with two renal arteries. Two renal arteries implanted in without aortic patch. 1—Kidney, 2—Anastomosis of the spatulated upper renal artery to the side of the common iliac artery, 3—Second vascular anastomosis "end to side" between accessory spatulated renal artery and iliac external artery, 4—External iliac artery

2. During an arterial reconstruction, such as the "end to side" anastomosis between large and small renal arteries, you need to have microsurgical skills, surgical loupes and the possibility of using 7/0 and 8/0 surgical sutures. You can perform this anastomosis on a thin silicone catheter (I will describe the technique later). The disadvantages of the "end to side" anastomosis are that you have to deal with a long preparation time before the transplantation, an increased risk of thrombosis and in the case of arterial thrombosis (when both arteries are thrombosed) it is practically impossible to save the kidney. Advantages; cutting off atherosclerotic narrowed part of renal artery leaving healthy and unchanged renal arteries at the kidney, performing one arterial anastomosis. This is particularly important when the recipient's vessels show advanced atherosclerosis, where performing a long anastomosis with the aortic patch or performing two or more separate anastomoses would be impossible (Fig. 3.129) [25–33].

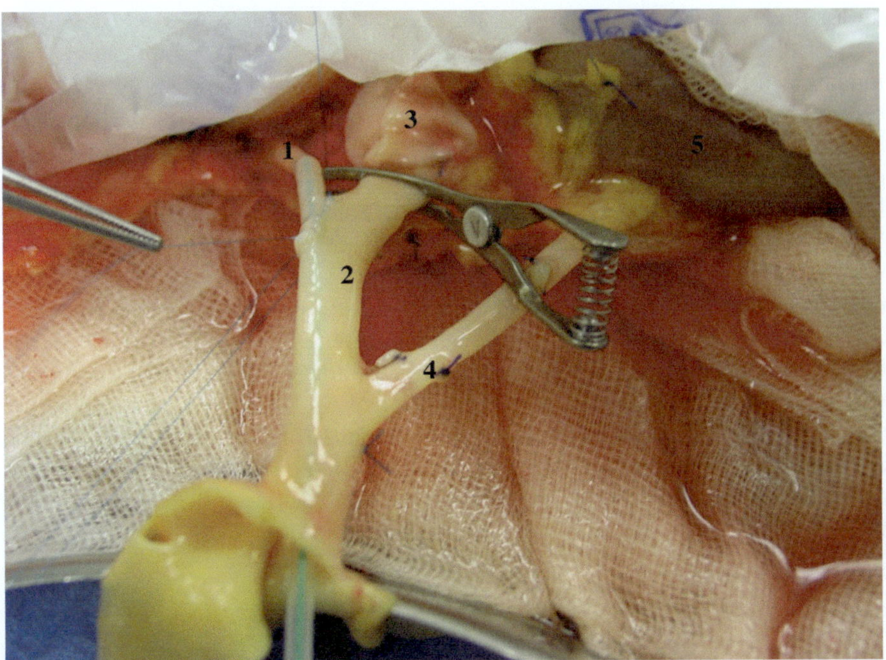

**Fig. 3.129** Kidney recipient with advanced atherosclerosis. It is impossible to perform long anastomosis of the two renal arteries on the long aortic patch. The smaller secondary renal artery was spatulated and sewn "end to side" to the main trunk of the renal artery (7/0). During anastomosis, a silicone tube was used, which was passed through anastomosis during suturing to prevent narrowing of the anastomotic site. During the entire renal vascular reconstruction the kidney was protected from heat by covering the entire surface of the kidney with wet gauzes and crushed ice. 1—One of the accessory renal arteries reaching the lower pole, 2—The main trunk of the renal artery, 3—Renal vein, 4—Accessory renal artery to the upper pole, 5—Kidney parenchyma

## Renal Artery Reconstruction Using the Recipient's Internal Iliac Artery

*Introduction*

As we know, kidneys with multiple renal arteries represent a surgical challenge. For these cases, the surgical strategy is to directly anastomose multiple renal arteries to the internal iliac artery or the common and/or external iliac artery. However, this approach is complicated by the difficulty in performing the anastomoses, bleeding, stenosis and a high incidence of false aneurysms.

*Reconstruction "Ex Vivo"*

By applying the method of ex vivo reconstruction of the donor renal arteries with the recipient's internal iliac artery, Pan et al. [62] repaired five cases of donor kidneys with more than three renal arteries and excessively short renal arteries during transplantation and treated three cases of renal aneurysms with renal auto-transplantation. In all the cases, the surgery was without complications. At a minimum follow-up of four years, all patients showed normal renal function, and also no thrombus or aneurysm formation or obstruction in the renal artery or its branches. The above mentioned method involves the complete ligation and excision of the internal iliac artery; first, the branches of the second or third degree of the internal iliac artery are ligated in the small pelvis and then the internal iliac artery is ligated just as it departs from the common iliac artery, or it is closed with a gentle vascular clamp, after which it is severed and the stump is closed with a non-absorbable vascular suture. The internal iliac artery, which has been completely cut out of the vascular space, is immediately transferred to a sterile bowl in which a kidney inspection is performed. The internal iliac artery and its branches are rinsed with a cold solution of preservative fluid with heparin. All vascular reconstructions are carried out in comfortable conditions by connecting the renal artery or renal arteries end to end or end to side with branches previously taken from the recipient's own internal iliac artery. The transplanted kidney arteries reconstructed in this way allow us to reduce the warm ischemia time [62, 69].

### Reconstruction "In Vivo"

Another method is that the internal iliac artery is dissected from the surrounding tissues with its distal branches. After ligation of the branches, the iliac internal artery is closed close to the common iliac artery (CIA) with a vascular clamp (a small bulldog), its lumen is rinsed with a heparin solution and two or more renal arteries are sewn end to end or end to side to the branches [45]. It is a good technique for the reconstruction of one or two renal arteries. When more than two renal arteries need to be constructed, the warm ischemia time will probably be prolonged and may cause irreversible and unnecessary injury to the kidney [63–65, 67].

## Common Ostium, Common Outlet, "Side to Side" Anastomosis: The Conjoined Technique is Possible Only When the Vessels Are of Sufficient Length and Similar Size

### Introduction and Surgical Technique

Side to side anastomosis of both arteries is performed over a space of 0.5–1.0 cm—creating a common outlet, i.e. a "common ostium".

To perform this type of anastomosis, the arteries must have approximately the same diameter and must not be too distant from each other. After a thorough inspection of the kidneys, in an ice bowl, we cut in the middle of the walls of both arteries at a length of 0.5–1.0 cm towards the renal hilum or cut out a small triangle in each artery from the medial side (I do not recommend this—this reduces the diameter of the anastomosis of the two arteries). Then, we proceed to the anastomosis of the walls of both arteries with continuous non-absorbable 7/0 surgical sutures. The anastomosis of the walls of both arteries should be performed from top to bottom using microsurgical instruments and magnification loupes or a microscope. Divide the suture in half, so that the front and back sutures of the walls of both arteries are of equal length. At this point, one of the sutures is chosen to create the anterior anastomosis and the other, once completed, to suture the posterior walls of the renal arteries. After completing the anastomosis of the walls of both vessels, place the knots as high as possible so that they do not enter into an anastomosis with one of the iliac arteries during kidney transplantation (Figs. 3.130 and 3.131) [68–70, 72–74].

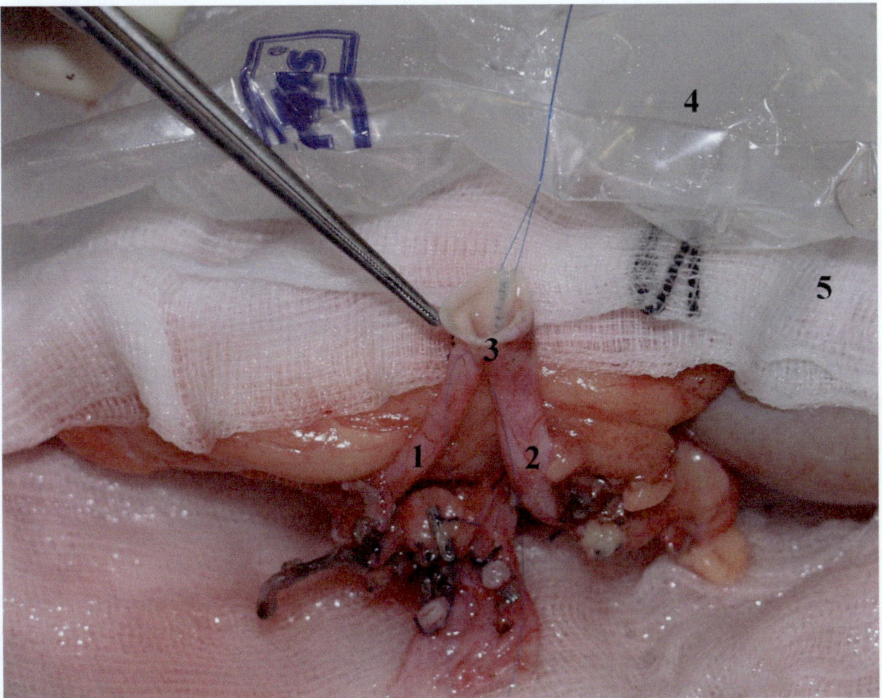

**Fig. 3.130** "Common ostium". 1—First renal artery, 2—Second renal artery, 3—Incised medially and stitched 7/0 walls of both renal arteries, 4—Ice, 5—Wet gauze protecting kidney from dry out and frostbite

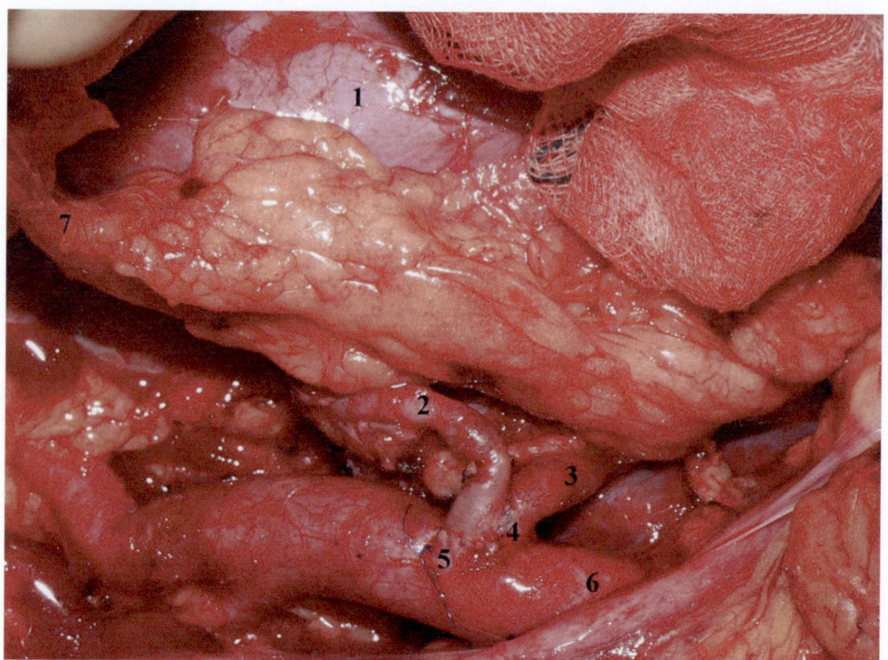

**Fig. 3.131** Transplanted kidney after suturing the beginnings of two renal arteries into one common ostium opening. 1—Kidney, 2—Lower renal artery, 3—Upper renal artery, 4—Anastomosis between medially incised renal arteries: creation common ostium, 5—Anastomosis "end to side" of the common ostium with a right common iliac artery, 6—Right common iliac artery, 7—Ureter

### *Advantages and Disadvantages of Common Ostium Between Two Arteries (Pantaloon—Side to Side Anastomosis)*

Advantages: short time of warm ischemia, possibility of kidney transplantation in a patient with advanced arteriosclerosis and only one vascular anastomosis—a small section of closure of one of the iliac arteries (in cases of advanced artherosclerosis where there is no room to perform two vascular anastomoses).

Disadvantages: when the anastomosis "thrombosed" the "whole kidney", the arterial anastomosis must be possible in the midline of the kidney (an attempt to move the anastomosis up or down may cause one of the anastomosed renal arteries to kink, and thus it may increase the risk of thrombosis) [68–70, 72–74].

### 3.10.3 Reconstruction of the Renal Upper Pole Accessory Artery Cut Close to the Capsule During Organ Procurement

Concurrently, different approaches have been applied according to the type of polar artery. Numerous studies have recommended the reconstruction of the lower pole artery (LPA) who branches are responsible for the arterial blood supply of the ureter and the lower pole of the kidney. The small branches of the lower pole renal artery are necessary to avoid uretal complications, such as leakage, stricture and necrosis. However, very few reports have discussed the importance of the safety of preserving versus ligating the upper pole renal artery in living-donor kidney transplantation. Only one recent study recommends routinely ligating the upper pole artery or arteries (UPAs) [74]. The study shows that if the area of the upper pole is infarcted by less than 10% of the entire area of the kidney, it has no influence on the immediate, postoperative kidney function. In the long term, there were no significant differences observed in the estimated glomerular filtration rate or serum creatinine concentration between the two groups analyzed: the arterial ligation group and the arterial reconstruction group. However, arterial complications and a prolonged total ischemic time were reported in the second group. Although the safety

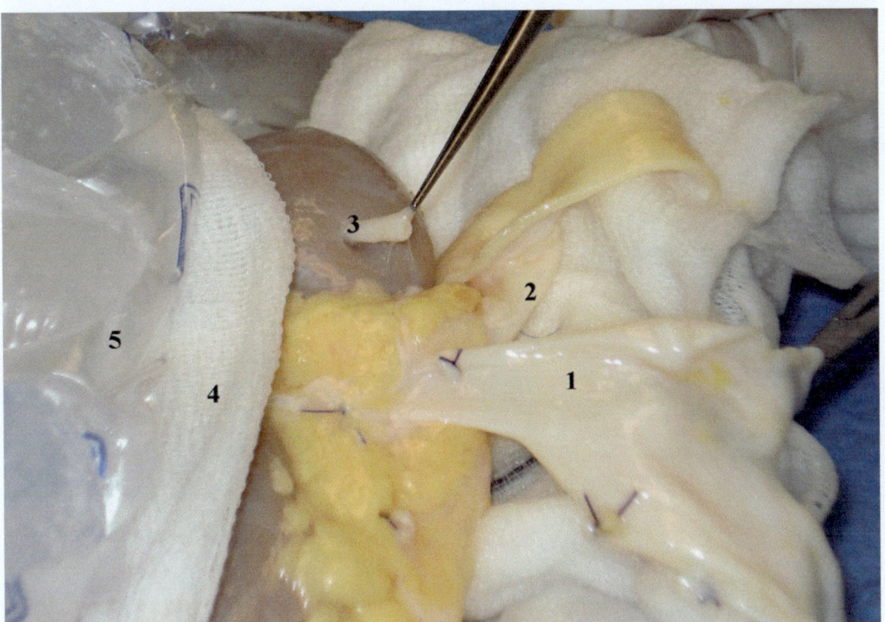

**Fig. 3.132** 1—VCI and right renal vein, 2—Renal artery, 3—Damaged accessory renal artery supplying the upper pole, 4—Gauze soaked in cold solution to prevent frostbite and dry out of the kidney, 5—Ice

of the arterial reconstruction was established, the authors do not provide criteria and indications for arterial reconstruction and optimum techniques for this procedure, stating only that the mean diameter of the 27 UPAs ligated in their study was 1.82 mm. Trying to draw conclusions from the articles I have read and from my experience, I can say that any renal artery over 2.0—2.5 mm in diameter should be reconstructed if possible. Ischemia (infarction) of less than or greater than 10% of the kidney is very difficult to predict, but it can be suggested that it increases with the diameter of the artery [74–76].

Surgical technique:

1. After unpacking, the kidney was placed in a container filled with ice and cold preservation solution. Due to the use of an operating lamp (no cold light source), in order to prevent unnecessary warming of the kidney, its front surface was covered with gauze and ice soaked in cold organ preservation solution.
2. The injured artery was dissected as far as possible in the kidney parenchyma. The major renal artery was directed towards the damaged upper pole renal artery to define the site of anastomosis. The main renal artery trunk was closed nearby the renal hilum with a small vascular clamp (bulldog) and then the renal artery

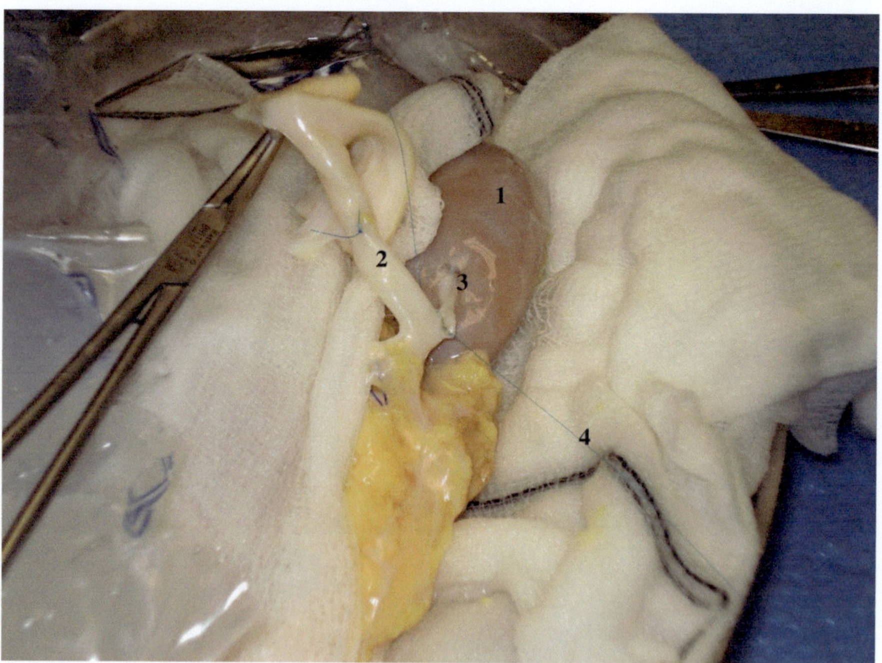

**Fig. 3.133** Sewing of the end of the injured upper pole artery "end to side" to the main trunk of the renal artery. 1—Upper pole, 2—Main trunk renal artery, 3—Injured upper pole artery, 4—Suture—anastomosis between arteries

was gently filled with the cold organ preservation solution. The place of anastomosis was marked.

3. The renal artery was incised longitudinally at a length of 3–4 mm in a previously selected place with a special surgical knife used in ocular surgery. In the wall of the main trunk of renal artery, after its longitudinal incision with rounded micro-scissors, a small semi-oval hole was cut on each side. The wall of the accessory (upper pole) renal artery was also incised on the side of the main renal artery over a length of 3–4 mm. Two 7/0 non-absorbable sutures (Fig. 3.133) were used to perform the anastomosis. In some situations, if we are not completely sure of the anastomosis, a thin catheter may be inserted from the side of the main renal artery lumen, passing through the anastomosis and entering the lumen of the cut accessory renal artery.

4. After the arterial anastomosis was performed and the arterial blood supply for the kidney upper pole was reconstructed, the anastomosis patency and tightness was checked with an injection of cold heparinized 0.9% NaCl (Fig. 3.134).

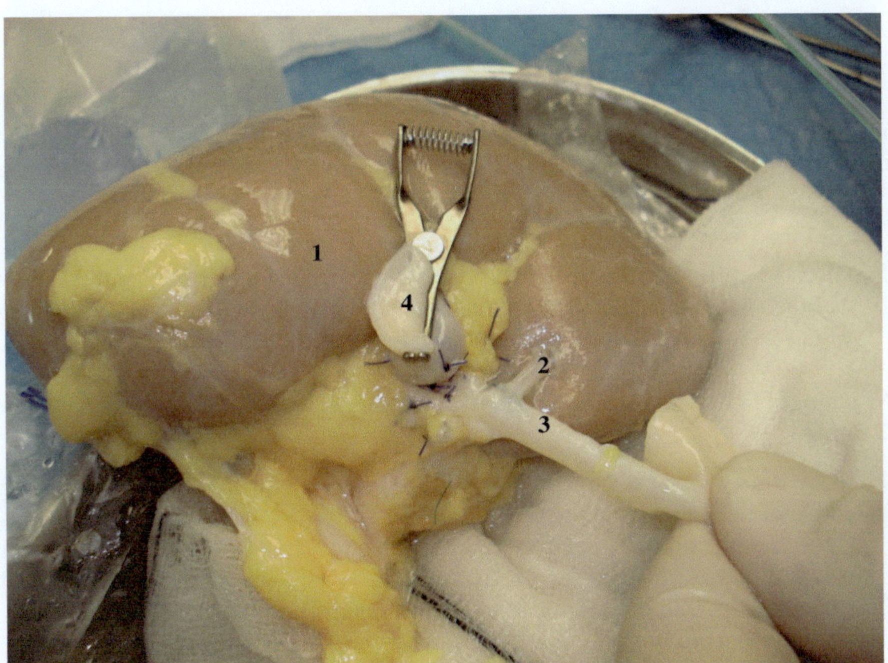

**Fig. 3.134** Testing the tightness of the renal artery and anastomosis. 1—Right kidney, 2—Reconstructed artery to the upper pole of the kidney, 3—Main stem of the renal artery, 4—Right renal vein closed with a vascular clamp: a small bulldog

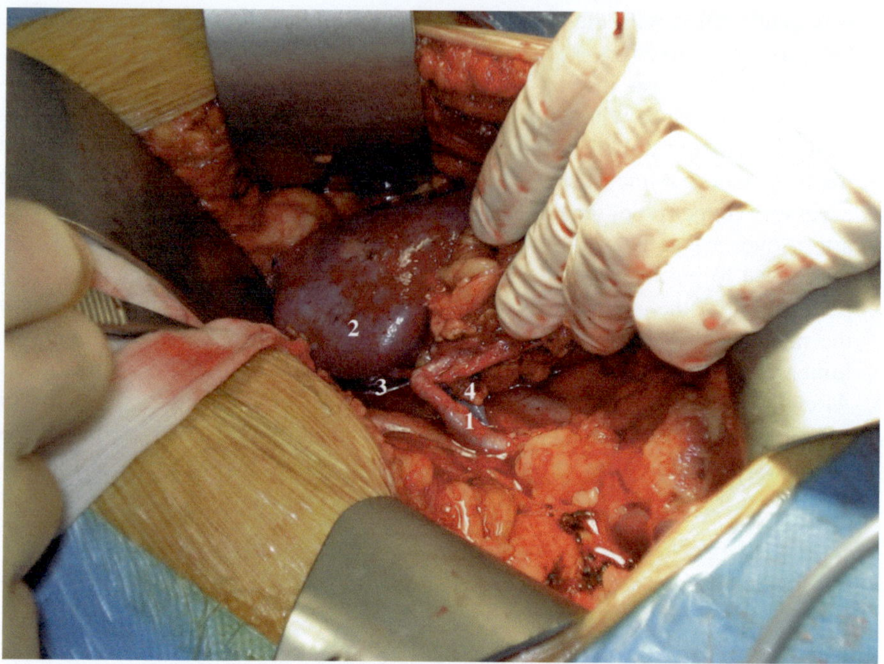

**Fig. 3.135** Kidney transplanted after reconstruction of the accessory renal artery carrying blood to the upper pole of the kidney; normal blood supply to the upper pole of the kidney. 1—Main stem renal artery, 2—Kidney, 3—Reconstructed renal artery, 4—Renal vein

5. After the transplantation the kidney looked normal, the upper pole of the kidney had the same color as the rest of the kidney parenchyma, the kidney took up work several minutes after the transplantation and started urinating (Fig. 3.135).

**Warning! (Try to save and reconstruct every UPA with a diameter bigger than 2 mm)**

1. In this situation, most surgeons would place a ligature on the stump of the artery and proceed with its transplantation. The following arguments support this procedure: the upper pole artery is not involved in the blood supply to the renal pelvis or ureter, a diameter of 2.0–2.5 mm is difficult for the microsurgical reconstruction and does not lead to a certain effect as there is a high probability of thrombosis in not only the UPA, but also in the main renal artery.

2. My arguments for the reconstruction are: the experience, availability of appropriate instruments, surgical loupes and cold light. I did several hundred reconstructions of renal arteries, liver and pancreas, without any thrombosis. Why should we sacrifice the entire upper pole of the kidney and cause ischemia? After all, the upper pole is one-third of the kidney surface. Different questions arise about what we will have if we do not reconstruct the upper pole artery: How long will the kidney work? How long will it survive? How much will the ischemia of the upper pole influence the survival of the kidney? Will the kidney function normally without the upper pole? How long will it last? Will the patient be dialyzed after the operation or will nothing happen so the patient can go home eight days after the operation? I think that I have listed enough arguments to encourage an attempt to save the blood supply to the upper pole and to take the action of reconstruction to the renal artery with a diameter greater than 2.5–3.0 mm [63–65, 74–76].

### 3.10.4   Preparation for Transplantation: Right Kidney with Four Arteries, One Renal Vein Procured with the IVC and One Ureter—Steps (From Author's Own Collection)

1. Four arteries on the aortic patch with very advanced atherosclerosis: after the general preparation of the kidney due to atherosclerosis, the aortic patch was cut off, leaving four healthy, non-atherosclerotic arteries at the kidney.
2. The two medial arteries were approximately 4 mm in diameter, and the two outside of them running to the upper and lower poles were approximately 2.5 mm in diameter. In order to avoid the necessity to perform four vascular anastomoses in the recipient, it was decided to implant two external arteries of smaller diameter into the side of the inner renal arteries of larger diameter. Vascular anastomosis was performed with a continuous non-absorbable 7/0 suture. The right renal vein was elongated with the IVC of the donor. Prior to transplantation, the tightness of the performed vascular anastomoses was tested (Fig. 3.136).
3. The right kidney was transplanted to the left side. First, an anastomosis of the elongated right renal vein was performed, end-to-side with the left common iliac vein of the recipient kidney. Then, after occlusion of the left, internal and external common iliac artery with two vascular clamps and after determining the optimal sites for arterial anastomoses, both vascular anastomoses of the renal arteries were performed with a 6/0 non-absorbable suture. Arterial anastomosis was performed by implanting the medial major renal arteries end to side of the common and external iliac arteries. Figure 3.137 shows the transplanted kidney prior to the release of the vascular clamps.

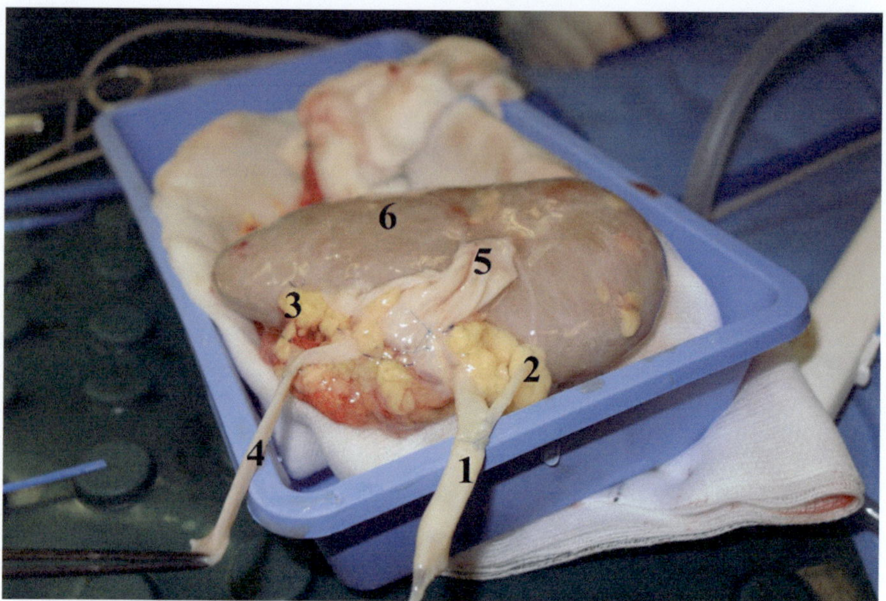

**Fig. 3.136**  Four renal arteries. 1—Upper major renal artery, 2—Secondary upper accessory renal artery implanted end to side to the upper major renal artery, 3—Secondary inferior renal artery to lower pole of kidney implanted end to side to the inferior major renal artery, 4—Inferior major renal artery, 5—Right renal vein, 6—Kidney

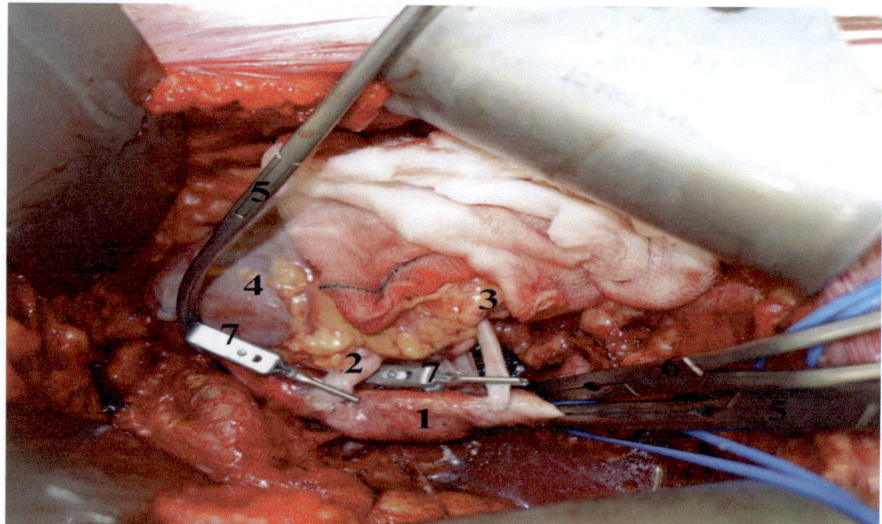

**Fig. 3.137**  A transplanted right kidney with four arteries just before reperfusion. 1—Common iliac artery, 2—Main upper renal artery, 3—Main lower renal artery with additional renal artery grafted to the side, 4—Kidney, 5—Upper and lower vascular clamps closing iliac arteries, 6—Satinsky vascular clamp closing iliac veins, 7—Very delicate bulldog vascular clamp

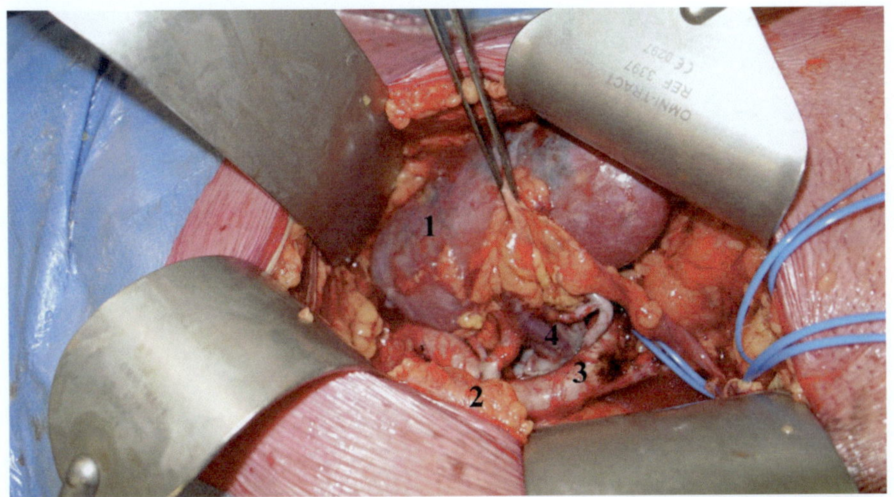

**Fig. 3.138**  Kidney transplanted with four renal arteries: two small implanted "end to side" in the main renal arteries and two main arteries implanted "end to side" in the iliac arteries. 1—Kidney, 2—Common iliac artery, 3—Lower pole renal artery, 4—Renal vein

4. After the reperfusion, the kidney started to excrete a small amount of urine. The color, consistency, position of the kidney and the reconstructed vessels were normal. Pulsation was clearly perceptible in all four renal arteries. The warm ischemia time was shortened by performing only two, not four, anastomoses with the common iliac artery of the recipient. The total duration of the warm ischemia was 35 min (Fig. 3.138).

**Warning! (I will repeat this ad nauseam: kidney back table is very important)**

Advantages of a good kidney inspection and preparation for transplantation:

- Ability to detect early and repair the damage done to the vessels (Fig. 3.139), kidney parenchyma, renal pelvis or ureter.
- If it is not possible to repair all the injuries that were made at the time of organ procurement during inspection, the kidney is disqualified and found not suitable for transplantation.
- Saves blood loss of the recipient after transplantation during reperfusion.
- Reduces the duration of warm ischemia, which in turn may contribute to a reduction in the frequency of the delayed graft function and the amount of dialysis after the kidney transplantation prior to complete kidney function.
- Reduction of the risk of kidney transplantation with the tumor due to a thorough organ check.

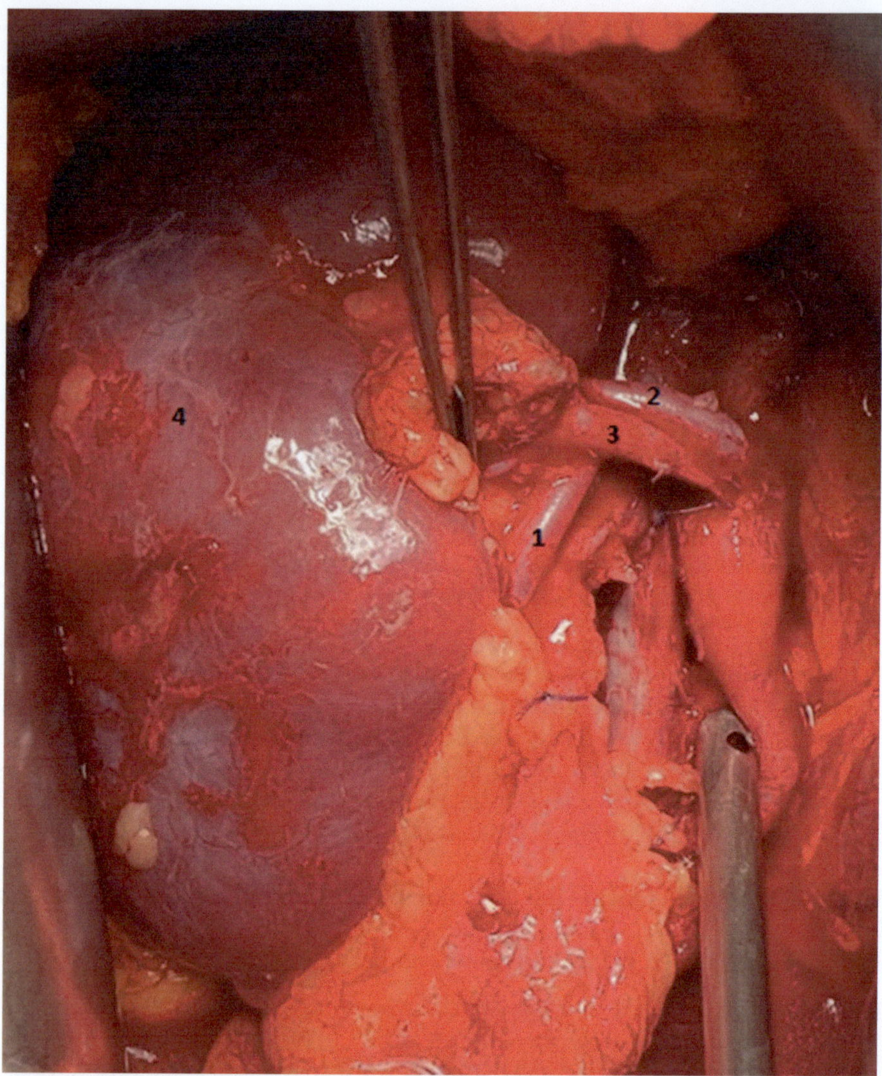

**Fig. 3.139** Kidney from DBD donor with three arteries (two damaged—cut without contact with the aorta, one renal artery on the aorta's patch). Reconstruction. 1—Lower pole renal artery anastomosed end to side to the artery number 2 in the picture, 2 and 3—Two renal arteries reconstructed as a common ostium and implanted end to side of the iliaca communis artery, 4—Kidney parenchyma

**Warning! (How a vascular surgeon can help in kidney transplantation)**
Lejay et al. [77] describe how a vascular surgeon can help at the different stages of a difficult kidney transplantation process in modern healthcare: (1) before kidney transplantation for recipient preparation in order to allow subsequent graft implantation, or stenting, either by performing percutaneous embolization of renal arteries in the setting of polycystic kidney disease or treatment of aneurysmal or occlusive lesions that would contra-indicate graft implantation; (2) Pre-transplant renal evaluation, when difficult vessel repairs (anastomoses) must be performed to prepare the kidney for transplantation so that a kidney transplant can be performed; (3) after surgery for long-term follow-up, including transplant renal artery or one of the iliac artery stenosis treatment or help with difficult transplant nephrectomy.

## 3.11  Conclusion

Not only the retrieval of the kidney, but also its mode of transport to the donor's hospital and the proper preparation of it for transplant, may significantly affect not only the quality of the transplant, but also the survival of the transplanted kidney and the patient. This is the case if only one of these circumstances is insufficient.

## References


1. https://dictionary.cambridge.org/.
2. https://www.thefreedictionary.com/.
3. Institute of Medicine (US) Committee on Organ Procurement and Transplantation Policy. Organ Procurement and Transplantation: Assessing Current Policies and the Potential Impact of the DHHS Final Rule. Washington (DC): National Academies Press (US); 1999. 4, Organ Donation. https://www.ncbi.nlm.nih.gov/books/NBK224655/.
4. https://www.eurotransplant.org/patients/eurotransplant-manual/.
5. Storage and transportation to processing facility. In: Guide to safety and quality assurance for organs, tissues and cell, 2nd ed. Council of Europe Publishing; 2014. p. 45–9. ISBN: 9287155186. https://www.coe.int/t/dg3/health/Source/GuideSecurity2_en.pdf.
6. Vila G-V, María J, Caralps A, Revert L, Andreu J, Carretero P, Figuls J. Extracorporeal renal surgery. Work bench surgery. Urology. 1975;5:444–51. https://doi.org/10.1016/0090-4295(75)90064-3.
7. https://4fetz713plu53drexe2d10ht-wpengine.netdna-ssl.com/wp-content/uploads/2019/12/755-00029-Rev-J-LKT100-Operators-Manual.pdf. Life Port Kidney Transporter. Operator's Manual 10.
8. Rossi M, Alfani D, Berloco P, Bruzzone P, Caricato M, Casciaro G, Poli L, Iappelli M, Pecorella I, Pretagostini R, et al. Bench surgery for multiple renal arteries in kidney transplantation from living donor. Transplant Proc. 1991;23(5):2328–9. PMID: 1926377.
9. Shih Y, Becker JA, Suster B, et al. Renal bench surgery. Urol Radiol. 1981;3:101. https://doi.org/10.1007/BF02927818.
10. Silverman SG, Pedrosa I, Ellis JH, Hindman NM, Schieda N, Smith AD, Remer EM, Shinagare AB, Curci NE, Raman SS, Wells SA, Kaffenberger SD, Wang ZJ, Chandarana H,

Davenport MS. Bosniak classification of cystic renal masses, version 2019: an update proposal and needs assessment. Radiology. 2019;292(2):475–88.

11. Muglia1 VF, Westphalen AC. Bosniak classification for complex renal cysts. Classificação de Bosniak para cistos renais complexos: histórico e análise critic. Radiol Bras. 2014;47(6): 368–73.

12. Israel GM, Bosniak MA. How I do it: evaluating renal masses. Radiology. 2005;236(2):441–50. https://doi.org/10.1148/radiol.2362040218.

13. Curry NS, Cochran ST, Bissada NK. Cystic renal masses: accurate Bosniak classification requires adequate renal CT. AJR Am J Roentgenol. 2000;175(2):339–42. AJR Am J Roentgenol (full text).

14. Warren KS, Mcfarlane J. The Bosniak classification of renal cystic masses. BJU Int. 2005;95 (7):939–42. https://doi.org/10.1111/j.1464-410X.2005.05442.x.

15. Park BK, Kim B, Kim SH, et-al. Assessment of cystic renal masses based on Bosniak classification: comparison of CT and contrast-enhanced US. Eur J Radiol. 2007;61(2):310–4. https://doi.org/10.1016/j.ejrad.2006.10.004.

16. Jessica L, Darcy M, Zuckerman DA. Renal cysts and urinomas. Semin Intervent Radiol. 2011;28(4):380–1.

17. Gawish AE, Donia F, Samhan M, et al. Outcome of renal allografts with multiple arteries. Transplant Proc. 2007;39(4):1116–7.

18. Lamers R, Zaccai K, Schoots I, et al. De Bosniak-classificatie voor niercysten: tijd voor een volgende verandering? Tijdschr Urol. 2016;6:2–14. https://doi.org/10.1007/s13629-015-0108-x.

19. Skandalakis JE. Scandalakis's surgical anatomy. The embryologic and anatomic basis of modern surgery. Chapter 23: Kidneys and ureters, p. 1291–344. Chapter 24: Urinary bladder, p. 1345–77, vol. 2. Paschalidis Medical Publication Ltd.;2004.

20. Panwar P, Bansal D, Maheshwari R, Chaturvedi S, Desai P, Kumar A. Management of donor kidneys with double renal arteries with significant luminal discrepancy: a retrospective cohort study. Indian J Urol. 2020;36:200–4.

21. Li Y, Song Y, Hu W, Wang X, Xiao Y, Huang C. Methylene blue usage for determining accessory artery ligation in donor kidneys. Surg Innov. 2020. https://doi.org/10.1177/1553350620971474. Epub ahead of print. PMID: 33124503.

22. Benedetti E, Troppmann C, Gillingham K, et al. Short-and long-term outcomes of kidney transplants with multiple renal arteries. Ann Surg. 1995;221(4):406–14.

23. Barry JM. Technical aspects of renal transplantation. In: Henrich WL, Bennet WM, editors. Atlas of kidney disease. Tom V; 2001.

24. Başaran O, Moray G, Emiroğlu R, Alevli F, Haberal M. Graft and patient outcomes among recipients of renal grafts with multiple arteries. Transplant Proc. 2004;36(1):102–4. https://doi.org/10.1016/j.transproceed.2003.11.012. PMID: 15013313.

25. Davari HR, Malek-Hossini SA, Salahi H, et al. Sequential anastomosis of accessory renal artery to external iliac artery in the management of renal transplantation with multiple arteries. Transplant Proc. 2003;35(1):329–31.

26. Merkel FK, Matalon TA. An en bloc method for use of small pediatric cadaver kidneys in adult recipients. Transplant Proc. 1990;22(2):405–6.

27. Boggi U, Vistoli F, Del Chiaro M, et al. A simplified technique for the en bloc procurement of abdominal organs that is suitable for pancreas and small-bowel transplantation. Surgery. 2004;1(35):629–41.

28. Nahas WC, Lucon AM, Mazzucchi E, et al. Kidney transplantation: the use of living donors with renal artery lesions. J Urol. 1998;160(4):1244–7.

29. Makiyama K, Tanabe K, Ishida H, Tokumoto T, Shimmura H, Omoto K, Toma H. Successful renovascular reconstruction for renal allografts with multiple renal arteries. Transplantation. 2003;75(6):828–32. https://doi.org/10.1097/01.TP.0000054461.57565.18. PMID: 12660510.

30. Chautems RC, Mourad M, Malaise J, Squifflet J. Inferior epigastric artery for revascularization of lower polar arteries in renal transplantation. Transplant Proc. 2000;32(2):441–2.

31. Mosley JG, Castro JE. Arterial anastomoses in renal transplantation. Br J Surg. 1978;65:60–3.

32. Yamanaga S, Rosario A, Fernandez D, Kobayashi T, Tavakol M, Stock PG, et al. Inferior long-term graft survival after end-to-side reconstruction for two renal arteries in living donor renal transplantation. PLoS One. 2018;13.

33. Wijayaratne DR, Sudusinghe DH, Gunawansa N. Multiple renal arteries in live donor renal transplantation; impact on graft function and outcome: a prospective cohort study. Open J Organ Transpl Surg. 2018;8:1–11.

34. Hernández-Rivera JCH, Espinoza-Pérez R, Cancino-López JD, Silva-Rueda RI, Salazar-Mendoza M, Paniagua-Sierra R. Anatomical variants in renal transplantation, surgical management, and impact on graft functionality. Transplant Proc. 2018;50:3216–21.

35. Molmenti EP, Varkarakis IM, Pinto P, Tiburi MF, Bluebond-Langner R, Komotar R, Montgomery RA, Jarrett T, Kavoussi LR, Ratner LE. Renal transplantation with iliac vein transposition. Transplant Proc. 2004;36(9):2643–5. https://doi.org/10.1016/j.transproceed.2004.10.012. PMID: 15621112.

36. Stratta RJ, D'Alessandro AM, Belzer FO. Renal vein reconstruction with interposition allografts in cadaveric renal transplantation. Transpl Int. 1988;1(2):86–90. https://doi.org/10.1007/BF00353825. PMID: 3076386.

37. Puche-Sanz I, Pascual-Geler M, Vazquez-Alonso F, et al. Right renal vein extension with cryopreserved external iliac artery allografts in living-donor kidney transplantations. Urology. 2013;82(6):1440–3.

38. Rahman AU, Tan LC, Walters AM, Sadek SA. Use of the inferior vena cava as a conduit in transplantation of the right cadaveric kidney. Transplant Proc. 1999;31(8):3131–2.

39. Launois B, Jamieson GG, Maddern G, et al. Venous allografts: a useful alternative to venous autografts in digestive surgery. Aust NZ J Surg. 1995;65:579–81.

40. Hammoudi Y, Benoit G, Bensadoun H, et al. Benefits of vena cava removal with the renal vein in cadaver kidney procurement: incidence of arterial complications. Transplant Proc. 1988;20:762.

41. Nakatani T, Takemoto Y, Kim T, Uchida J, Han Y, Tsuchida K, Yoshimura R, Kawashima H, Sugimura K. Results of cadaver kidney transplantation with right renal vein extension. Urol Int. 2003;70(4):282–5. https://doi.org/10.1159/000070136. PMID: 12740492.

42. Puche-Sanz I, Pascual-Geler M, Vázquez-Alonso F, Hernández-Vidaña AM, Flores-Martín JF, Espejo-Maldonado E, Cózar-Olmo JM. Right renal vein extension with cryopreserved external iliac artery allografts in living-donor kidney transplantations. Urology. 2013;82(6):1440–3. https://doi.org/10.1016/j.urology.2013.07.045. Epub 2013 Oct 2. PMID: 24094655.

43. Spees EK Jr, Oakes DD, Light JA, et al. Successful renal vein reconstruction with bovine arterial heterografts. Ann Surg. 1977;186:749–51.

44. Baptista-Silva JC, Medina-Pestana JO, et al. Right renal vein elongation with the inferior vena cava for cadaveric kidney transplants. An old neglected surgical approach. Int Braz J Urol. 2005;31(6):519–25.

45. Barry JM, Fuchs EF. Right renal vein extension in cadaver kidney transplantation. Arch Surg. 1978;113:300.

46. Barry JM, Lemmers MJ. Patch and flap techniques to repair right renal vein defects caused by cadaver liver retrieval for transplantation. J Urol. 1995;153:1803–4.

47. Barry JM, Hefty TR, Sasaki T. Clam-shell technique for right renal vein extension in cadaver kidney transplantation. J Urol. 1988;140(6):1479.

48. Feng JY, Huang CB, Fan MQ, et al. Renal vein lengthening using gonadal vein reduces surgical difficulty in living-donor kidney transplantation. World J Surg. 2012;36:468–72. https://doi.org/10.1007/s00268-011-1243-z.

49. Tan LC, Rahman AU, Walters AM, Sadek SA. The inferior vena caval conduit–a neglected technique in transplantation of the right cadaveric kidney? Transpl Int. 2000;13(Suppl 1):S60–3. https://doi.org/10.1007/s001470050276. PMID: 11111963.

50. Benedetti E, Fryer J, Matas AJ, et al. Kidney transplant outcome with and without right renal vein extension. Clin Transpl. 1994;8:416–7.

51. Janschek EC, Rothe AU, Holzenbein TJ, et al. Anatomic basis of right renal vein extension for cadaveric kidney transplantation. Urology. 2004;63(4):660–4.
52. Zomorrodi A, Kakaei F, Zomorrodi S. Novo techniques that facilitate the transplant of short right allograft kidney vein as left allograft kidney from live donor. https://doi.org/10.4236/ojots.2012.22002. Published Online May 2012. https://www.SciRP.org/journal/ojots.
53. Fabian MA, Herrin MK, Baxter J, Ackermann JR. Extension of the right renal vein in cadaveric renal transplants with use of the vena cava and the TA-30 V3 surgical stapler. Surg Gynecol Obstet. 1991;173(3):233–4. PMID: 1925888.
54. Santangelo M, Spinosa G, Grassia S, Clemente M, Caggiano M, Pelosio L, Scotti A, Tammaro V, Nappi R, Di Capua F, Renda A. In situ elongation patch in right kidney transplantation. Transplant Proc. 2008;40(6):1871–2. https://doi.org/10.1016/j.transproceed.2008.05.019. PMID.
55. Taylor RJ, Hakala TR, Rosenthal JT. Use of vena cava to extend the right renal vein in cadaveric transplants. Surg Gynecol Obstet. 1985;160(3):279–80. PMID: 3883553.
56. Kumar A, Gupta RS, Srivastava A, Bansal P. Sequential anastomosis of accessory renal artery to inferior epigastric artery in the management of multiple arteries in live related renal transplantation: a critical appraisal. Clin Transplant. 2001;15:131–5. PubMed.
57. Chin JL. Vena cava extension of right renal vein for cadaveric renal transplants. J Urol. 1988;139:552–3.
58. He B, Mitchell A. A novel technique for reconstruction of multiple renal arteries in live donor kidney transplantation: a case report and literature review. Transplant Proc. 2012;44(10):3055–8. The gonadal vein can be used as a Carrel patch for multiple renal artery reconstruction, in particular, for more than two renal arteries. This technique provides a new approach for the reconstruction of multiple renal arteries in living donor kidney transplantations.
59. Chopin DK, Popov Z, Abbou CC, Auvert JM. Use of vena cava to obtain additional length for the right renal vein during transplantation of cadaveric kidneys. J Urol. 1989;141:1143–4.
60. Yatawatta A. Vascular reconstruction in kidney transplantation. Clin Surg. 2017:1–3.
61. Panwar P, Bansal D, Maheshwari R, Chaturvedi S, Desai P, Kumar A. Management of donor kidneys with double renal arteries with significant luminal discrepancy: a retrospective cohort study. Indian J Urol. 2020;36(3):200–4.
62. Pan G, Chen Z, Liao D, Fang J, Li G. The application of the iliac artery in the ex vivo reconstruction of renal arteries in renal transplantation. Transplantation. 2010;89(9):1113–6. https://doi.org/10.1097/TP.0b013e3181d54b8e. Retraction in: Transplantation. 2019;103(8):1736. PMID: 20179665.
63. Pal DK, Sanki PK, Roy S. Analysis of outcome of end-to-end and end-to-side internal iliac artery anastomosis in renal transplantation: Our initial experience with a case series. Urol Ann. 2017;9(2):166–9. https://doi.org/10.4103/0974-7796.204176.
64. Daowd R, Al AA. Renal artery anastomosis to internal or external iliac artery in kidney transplant patients. Saudi J Kidney Dis Transpl. 2015;26:1009–12.
65. Fechner G, von Pezold C, Hauser S, Gerhardt T, Klehr HU, Müller SC. Impairment of long-term graft function after kidney transplantation by intraoperative vascular complications. Int Urol Nephrol. 2008;40:869–73.
66. Rayt HS, Bown MJ, Lambert KV, Fishwick NG, McCarthy MJ, London NJ, et al. Buttock claudication and erectile dysfunction after internal iliac artery embolization in patients prior to endovascular aortic aneurysm repair. Cardiovasc Intervent Radiol. 2008;31:728–34.
67. Mohamed IH, Bagul A, Doughman T, Nicholson ML. Use of internal iliac artery as a side-to-end anastomosis in renal transplantation. Ann R Coll Surg Engl. 2012;94:e36–7.
68. Tzakis AG, Mazzaferro V, Pan CE, Gordon RD, Todo S, Makowka L, Starzl TE. Renal artery reconstruction for harvesting injuries in kidney transplantation with particular reference to the use of vascular allografts. Transplant Int Official J Eur Soc Organ Transplant. 1988;1(2):80–5.
69. Dean RH, Meacham PW, Weaver FA. Ex vivo renal artery reconstructions: indications and techniques. J Vasc Surg. 1986;4:546–52.

70. Deterling RA, Claus RH. Long term fate of aortic and arterial homograft's. J Cardiovasc Surg. 1970;11:35–43.
71. Sterioff S Jr, Zachary JB, Williams GM. Dacron vascular grafts in renal transplant patients. Am J Surg. 1974;127:525–8.
72. Lacombe M. Surgical techniques in renal transplantation. In: Hamburger J, Crosuier J, Bach JF, Kreis H, editors. Renal transplantation: theory and practice, 2nd ed. Baltimore: Williams & Wilkins;1981. p. 325–7.
73. Novick AC, Magnusson M, Braun WE. Multiple-artery renal transplantation: emphasis on extracorporeal methods of donor arterial reconstruction. J Urol. 1979;122:731–5.
74. Vincenzi P, Gonzalez J, Guerra G, Gaynor JJ, Alvarez A, Ciancio G. Complex surgicalreconstruction of upper pole artery in living-donor kidney transplantation. Ann Transplant.2021;26:e926850. https://doi.org/10.12659/AOT.926850.
75. Zorgdrager M, Krikke C, Hofker SH, et al. Multiple renal arteries in kidney transplantation: A systematic review and meta-analysis. Ann Transplant. 2016;21:469–77.
76. Hiramitsu T, Okada M, Futamura K, et al. Impact of grafting using thin upper pole artery ligation on living-donor adult kidney transplantation. Medicine (Baltimore). 2016;95(42): e5188.
77. Lejay A, Thaveau F, Caillard S, Georg Y, Moulin B, Wolf P, et al. How can a vascular surgeon help in kidney transplantation. J Cardiovasc Surg. 2017;58:351–9. https://doi.org/10.23736/S0021-9509.16.09808-6.

## Further Reading

78. Manuals hypothermic machine perfusions:
79. A. LifePort Kidney Transporter 1.1 Operator's Manual: https://4fetz713plu53drexe2d10ht-wpengine.netdna-ssl.com/wp-content/uploads/2020/10/755-00002-Rev-P-LKT101-Operators-Manual.pdf.
80. B. Kidney Assist–Stark Medical Empower the Healer: https://www.starkmed.com.au/pages/kidney-assist-organ-perfusion-system.
81. C. Bridge to Life: https://bridgetolife.eu/wp-content/uploads/english-4088-eu-belzer-mps-ifu-070820.pdf.

# Chapter 4
# Kidney Transplant Surgery Techniques

## 4.1  Patient Position on the Operating Table

### 4.1.1  The Position of the Patient on the Operating Table and "Time Out"

The patient is placed on the operating table in a supine position with his or her arms placed at a 90-degree angle to the body (Fig. 4.1). The arms rest on specially designed supports. To prevent any kind of upper limb injuries during transplantation and to protect the hemodialysis access much padding is used. After safely positioning the patient all members of the operation team cease their activity and maintain a zone of silence during which the patient's safety is protected and confirmed [1–4].

**Warning! (Time out:maintaining high patient safety in the operating room) Participation in the patient's safety is one concrete expression of a foundational principle of medical ethics: first, do no harm—primum non nocere. Being an ethical professional requires taking action to prevent harm to patients in health care environments. Checklists and time outs have become common patient safety tools in the USA and other nations [5].**The "time out" is carried out after the kidney's recipient is placed on the operating table prior to general anesthesia. An optimal time out includes the following elements: (a) patient verification using two identifiers and in the presence of the patient himself; (b) together with the patient's verification of correct procedure, correct sites, correct position, (c) verification equipment is available including relevant images and scans displayed; (d) allergies, if any; (e) antibiotics: name, time and dose administrated and/or to be administered; (f) safety precautions based on fire, hazards, patient's history or medication use [1–5].

© The Author(s), under exclusive license to Springer Nature Switzerland AG 2023

A. Baranski, *Kidney Transplantation*,
https://doi.org/10.1007/978-3-030-75886-8_4

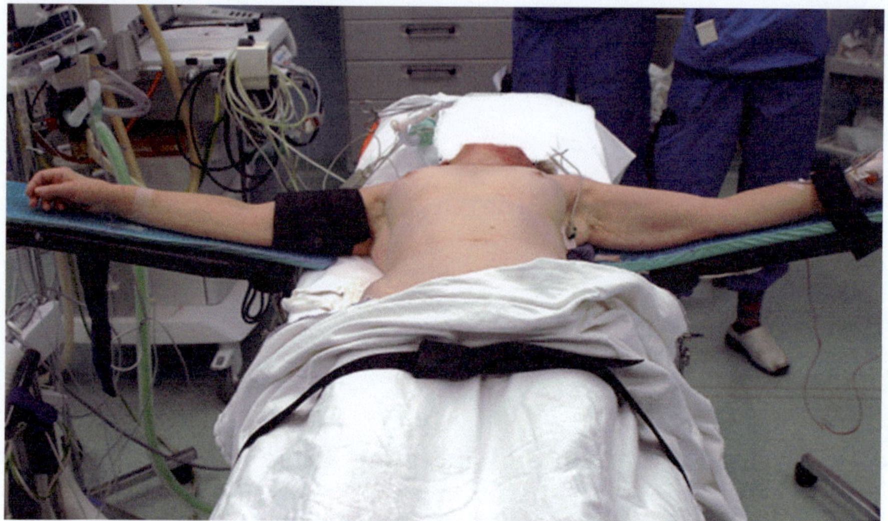

**Fig. 4.1** Placing a patient on an operating table before a kidney transplant

### 4.1.2 *General Anesthesia and the Last Time the Patient Is Repositioned on the Operating Table (Depending on the Surgeon)*

As a rule, general anesthesia is inducted. Depending on the general condition of the kidney's recipient one central venue catheter and one arterial line are inserted. The patient is being intubated, completely sedated and moved downwards on the operating table so that his/her feet are approximately 10 cm in front of the end of the table. Such a patient's positioning will provide the surgeon with excellent access to the retroperitoneal space, iliac vessels and provides maximum use of blades of the abdominal surgical retractor type: Bookwalter, Thomson or Omnitrac [6–8].

## 4.2  Urinary Bladder Catheter Placement and Its Availability During the Operation

The bladder catheter is inserted and then extended towards the patient's feet with a sterile silicon drain. This Foley catheter "elongation" drain must be long enough to run between the legs of the recipient, where it is attached to one of his/her legs in an atraumatic way. The idea is that everyone in the operating theatre, if necessary, has access to the urinary bladder at any time of the operation. During the operation, the entire system is connected at the end to the urine collecting bag. After the kidney reperfusion when the urinary bladder needs to be filled, the circulating nurse disconnects the urimeter linked to the drain and connects it directly to the end of a new drain attached to the scrub nurse's table. All bladder filling is carried out under the control and close supervision of the surgeon. During the filling of the urinary bladder, the surgeon has to control the degree of filling at all times with his/her hand in order to avoid causing a urinary bladder musosa injury and/or rupture. After the bladder is filled, the drain is closed with the clamp—but only at the sole request of the surgeon. After a ureter-bladder anastomosis, the urinary bladder is sometimes gently cleaned with warm Ringer's solution. The sterile drain under the operating table is disconnected from the scrub nurse's side and connected back to the urine collection bag (urimeter). The entire system of "silicone tube extensions" of the urinary-bladder catheter inserted into the bladder must be safe for the patient and tight enough to prevent leakage of urine or the fluid that fills the bladder during the transplant surgery (Figs. 4.2 and 4.3) [9–12].

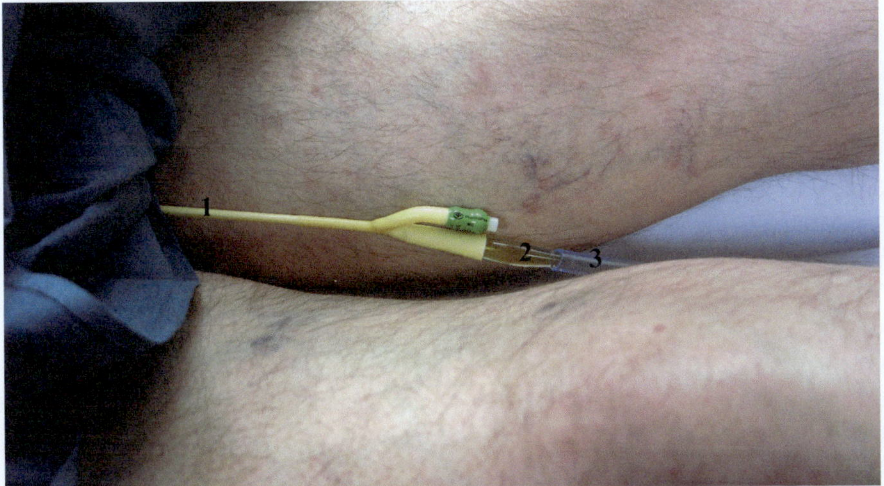


**Fig. 4.2** Extension of the urinary bladder catheter inserted into the bladder with a silicone drain. 1—Urinary catheter, 2—Connector between the silicone tube and the catheter placed in the urinary bladder, 3—Silicone tube as an extension of the urinary catheter ends in a urimeter

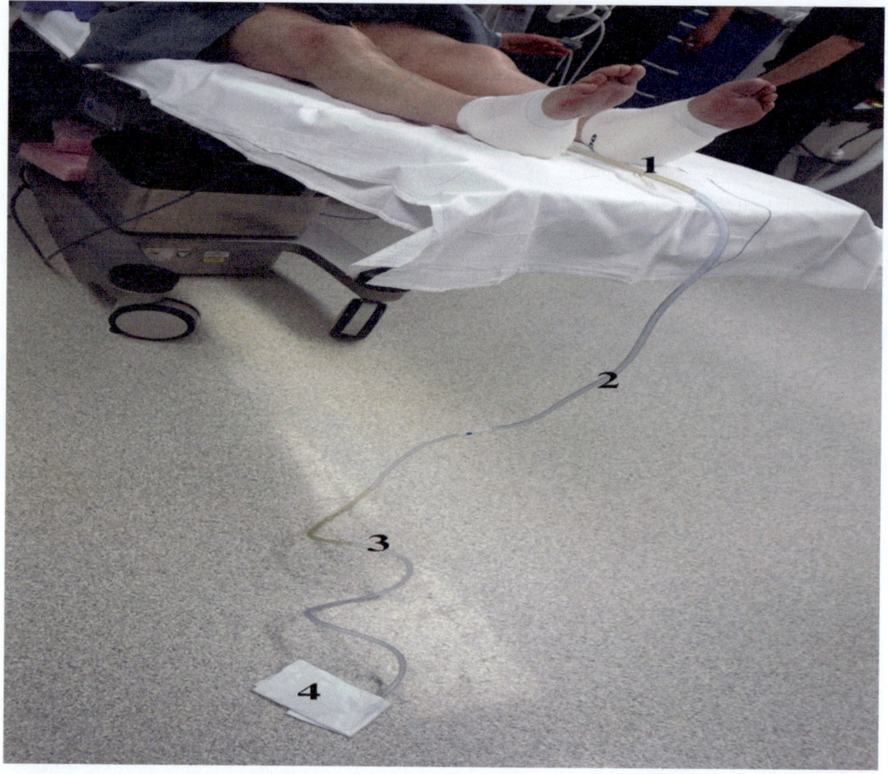


**Fig. 4.3** 1 and 2—Silicone drain connected with a catheter inserted into the urinary bladder, 2—Silicone drain connecting the urinary catheter with the urine bag, 3—One of the silicon tubes used for system lengthening, 4—Urine bag outside the operating table

**Warning! (Urinary bladder catheter—using it during surgery:options)**
In a few sentences, I will describe the most important ways of dealing with the urinary bladder after the insertion of a urinary catheter that I have encountered in the literature.

At the beginning of the operation, after bladder catheter insertion:

1. the bladder is flushed continuously from the beginning of the surgery, e.g. with sterile saline (a two-channel bladder catheter) until it is completed;
2. the bladder is continuously rinsed with a mixture of physiological salt and gentamycin (a two-channel bladder catheter) until surgery is completed;
3. do not rinse the bladder like a bladder—in this case the bladder is filled with sterile saline solution on the request of the surgeon, after the kidney reperfusion, but before the ureter implantation, to locate the urinary bladder [1–4].

**Warning!**

A. After opening the contents of the bladder, a bacteriological culture (examination) should be taken.
B. It is believed that the perioperative intravenous administration of antibiotics protects the patient much more against the development of urinary tract infections after surgery. According to other authors, a local continuous bladder flushing with a physiologic sterile salt solution or a mixture of sterile physiologic saline solution and antibiotic is not a goal because it does not fully prevent urinary tract infections (dual-channel urinary catheter).
C. If there are bloody contents from the bladder or blood-stained urine after transplantation, bladder irrigation may be continued for several days after surgery until all blood clots and blood are flushed out of the urinary bladder and the urine is clear (dual-channel urinary catheter).
D. Another option before transplantation is to inject 400–600 ml sterile solution into the urinary bladder, and to close its outflow with a clamp. In my opinion, this is—mainly for kidney recipients with a small bladder—not a recommended method. The reason for this is that the surgeon is confronted during the entire operation with a distended urinary bladder which reduces the area of the operating field which makes the transplant difficult [1–4, 9–12].

## 4.3   Cleaning and Sterile Draping of the Operating Field

### 4.3.1   Patient Preparation Before Operation

The patient should take a bath and wash the operation site and the area surrounding it with soap and water.

### 4.3.2   Skin: Operating Room

Prepare the skin with an antiseptic solution, starting in the center and moving out to the periphery. After disinfecting the surgical field, it is necessary to wait at least two minutes to keep the surgical site dry (before applying a check one more time to ensure that the patient is not allergic to any of the agents).

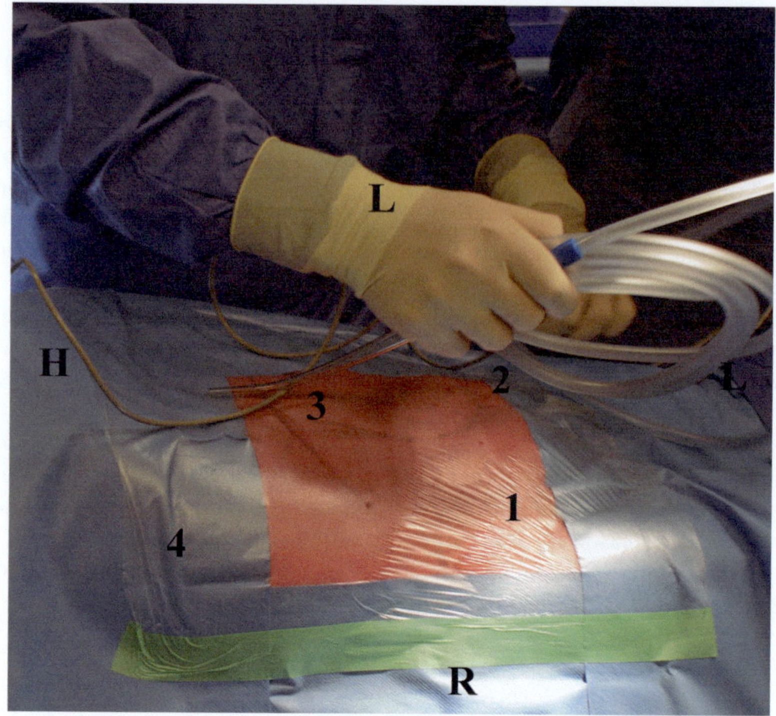


**Fig. 4.4** Disposable operating field draping materials, 1—Upper right anterior superior iliac spine, 2—Pubic bone, 3—Umbilicus level, 4—Adhesive foil, H—Head, L—Legs, R—Right side, L—Left side

### *4.3.3   Draping: Operating Room*

Do not place drapes on the patient until you are scrubbed, gowned and gloved. Leave only the operative field and those areas necessary for the maintenance of anesthesia uncovered. The surgical field is covered in a standard manner and as a rule with the use of disposable sheets. Self-adhesive sterile foil is applied over the previously disinfected and shaved skin to prevent wound infections (Fig. 4.4), [13, 14].

## 4.4   Choice of Surgical Access for Kidney Transplantation (Most Common Incisions)

### *4.4.1   Hockey Stick Incision*

The hockey stick approach (pararectal incision) has been advocated for renal transplantation in children because it yields excellent access to the iliac vessels and inferior vena cava, in the case of intraperitoneal transplantation and in other surgical options [15]. In recent years the incision, due to its simplicity and good access to the extraperitoneal space, is also gaining ground in kidney transplantation in adults.

The pararectal incision consists of cutting both sheaths of the abdominal rectus muscle just next to its the lateral border and the medial muscle offset. Nowadays the hockey stick incision is probably the most common one (Fig. 4.5). The line of incision is determined in the following way: from the navel, a continuous line is drawn to the anterior superior iliac spine, and then one-third of the distance between the anterior superior iliac spike and the navel is determined—this is the lateral edge of the abdominal rectus muscle. The incision is then made about 5–10 mm medially from the predetermined line to the bottom, two fingers above the pubic junction. The incision is finished at the level of the pubic junction, before or just outside it, depending on the patient's height and weight. The length of the incision depends on the size of recipient, how big the kidney is, the intensity and distribution of arteriosclerosis of the iliac vessels, and the length and quantity of the renal vessels. We can start the incision at different levels. The maximal length of this incision can be extended between the rib arch until or beyond the pubic bone. As a rule, the incision starts 1–2 cm below the level of the umbilicus, continues obliquely to the pubic

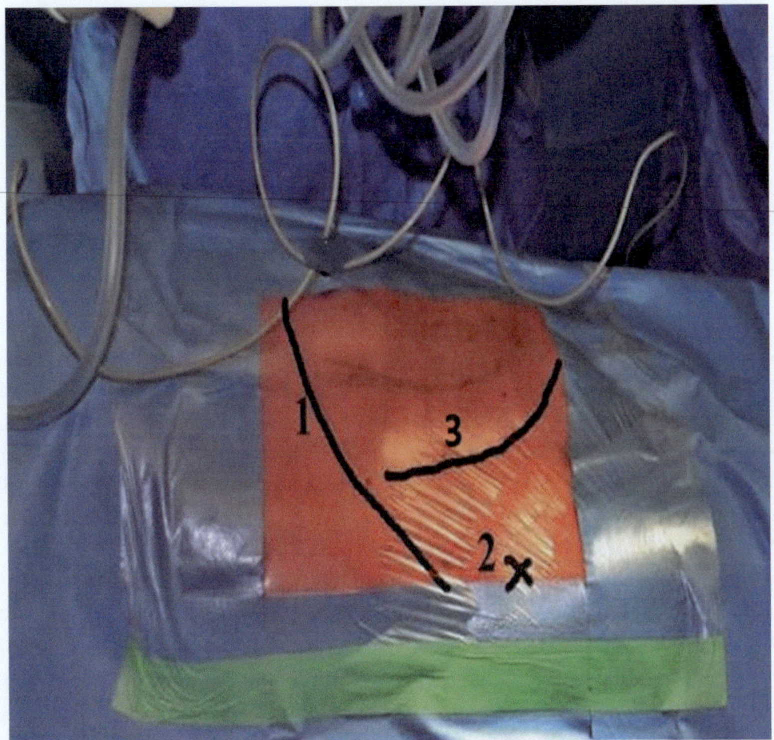


**Fig. 4.5** Operating field limited to the right lower abdomen. 1—Arcuate line, 2—Upper right anterior superior iliac spine, 3—Linea semilunaris: lateral border of the rectal muscle

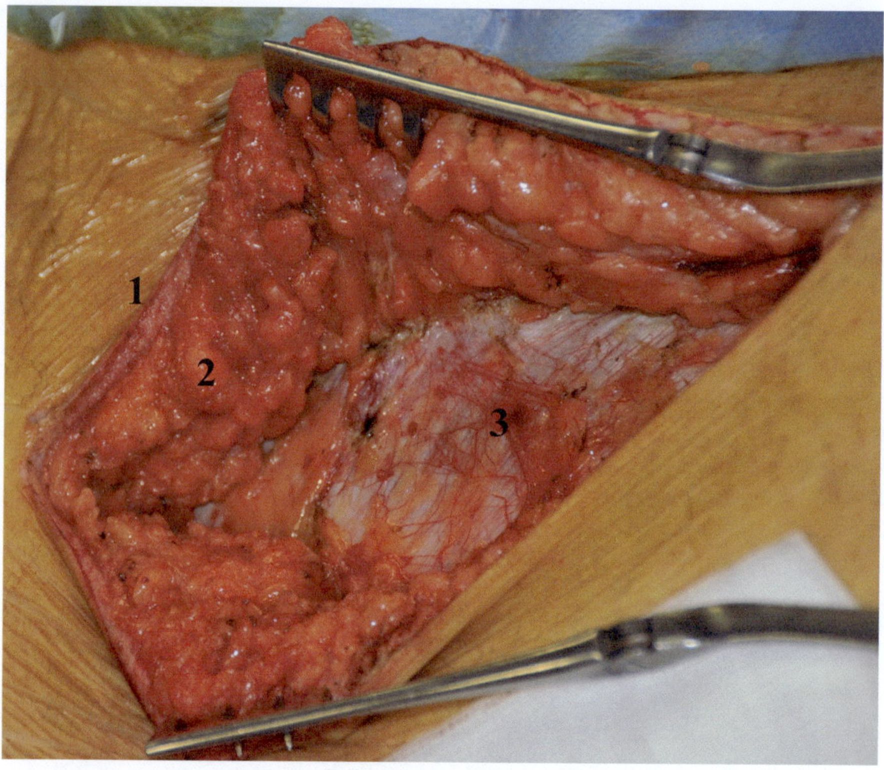

**Fig. 4.6** Incision in the shape of a hockey stick next to the abdominal rectus muscle. Cut the skin and subcutaneous tissue. 1—Skin, 2—Subcutaneous tissue, 3—Anterior abdominal rectus muscle sheath

symphysis and about two fingers above it. The incision is very safe and it can start below the arcuate line which occurs at about half the distance from the umbilicus to the pubic crest though this varies from person to person. It should be remembered that below the arcuate line the aponeuroses of all three muscles (including the transversus) pass in front of the rectus. The posterior wall of the rectus abdominal muscle below the arcuate line is separated from the abdominal cavity only by the parietal peritoneum. Above the arcuate line, the rectus muscle has an anterior and posterior sheath to which the parietal peritoneum is "glued".

To reach the peritoneum you have to incise the skin and the subcutaneous tissue (Fig. 4.6) 0.5–1.0 cm medially from the lateral edge of the rectal muscle at a distance of 5–6 cm from the anterior rectus abdominus sheath (Fig. 4.7). After 5–6 cm of opening the anterior rectus abdominus sheath, separate the anterior surface of the rectus muscle from the posterior side of the anterior sheath and pull it up and outside with two forceps in order to check whether you have properly opened the anterior rectus abdominal sheath or not. If you are inside, extend the incision downwards and upwards depending on the patient's weight and height, how high or

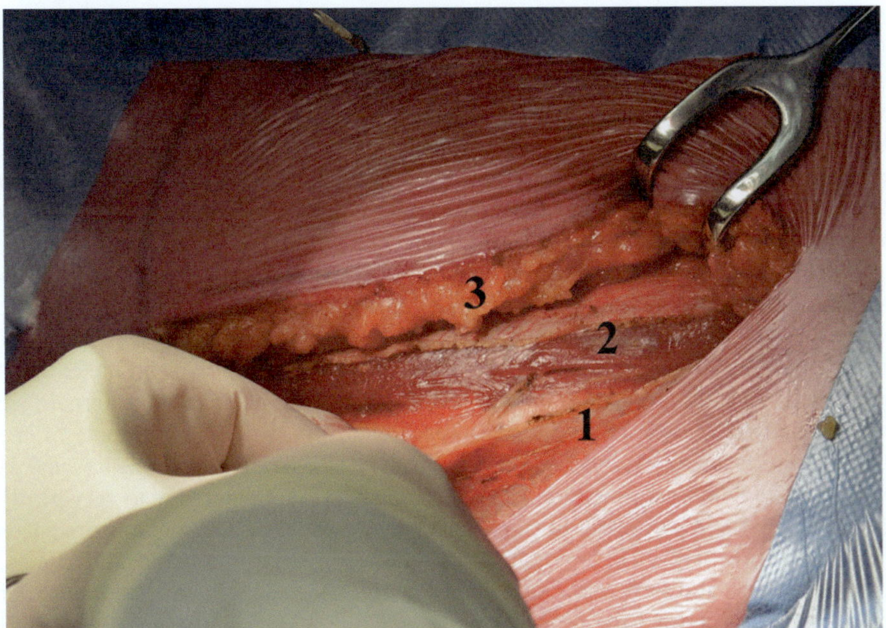

**Fig. 4.7**  1—The medially incised anterior sheath of the rectus abdominal, 2—Abdominal rectus muscle: lateral part, 3—Subcutaneous tissue

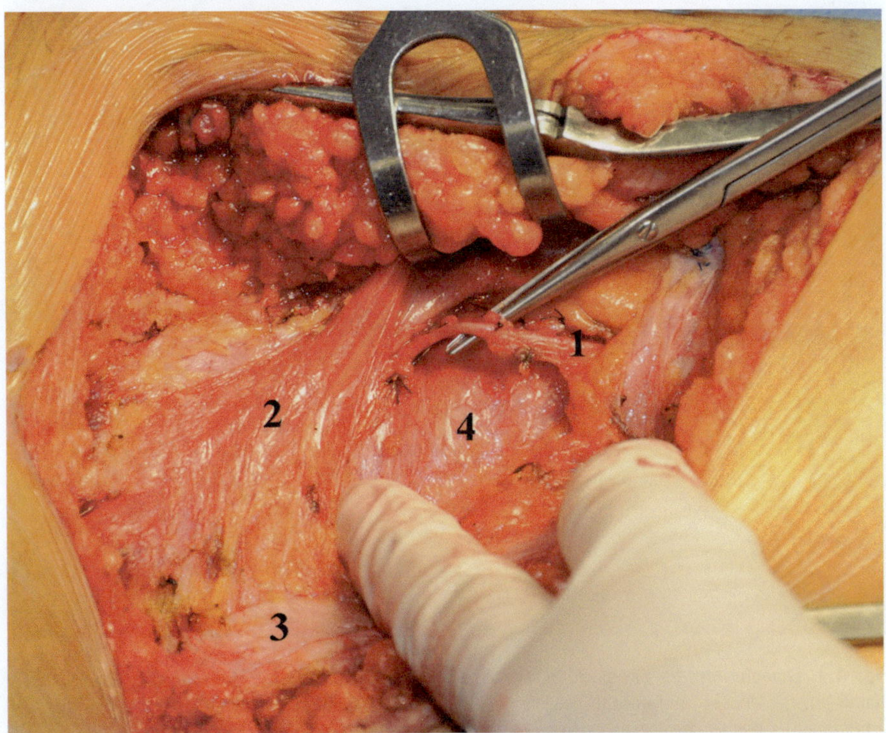

**Fig. 4.8**  1—Dissected inferior epigastric artery and vein 2—Rectus abdominal muscle, 3—Incised anterior sheath of rectus abdominal, 4—Peritoneum

low you want to go and as to whether you are forced to perform a vascular anastomosis. The location of the vascular anastomosis may be determined by: the stage of the iliac vessel's atherosclerosis; earlier vascular operations; by placing vascular devices, for example vascular stents; the length of the renal vessels; or the ureter (a short ureter forces us to transplant the kidney as low as possible and perform anastomosis with the external iliac vessels or to perform "end to end" or "end to side" anastomosis between the donor's kidney ureter and the ureter of the kidney recipient). The next step to reach the extraperitoneal space is to coagulate and cut the small vessels and nerves that run on the anterior side of the posterior sheath of the rectus abdominal above the arcuate line. Below the arcuate line, the posterior wall of the rectus abdominal directly contacts the parietal peritoneum. Ligate the inferior epigastric artery and the vein (the artery arises from the external iliac artery), which gives very good access to the urinary bladder, the external iliac vessels and the lower retroperitoneal space. Perform a blunt dissection of the peritoneum by using electrocoagulation and different surgical instruments such as your own fingers, forceps and/or a small gauze swab in a holder. Try to very gently detach the parietal peritoneum from the abdominal wall and retroperitoneum space and sweep it medially. The round ligament in women or the spermatic cord in men, the iliac vessels and 50% of the surface of the urinary bladder have to be free. After preparation, put around the round ligament or spermatic cord, the vessel loop and

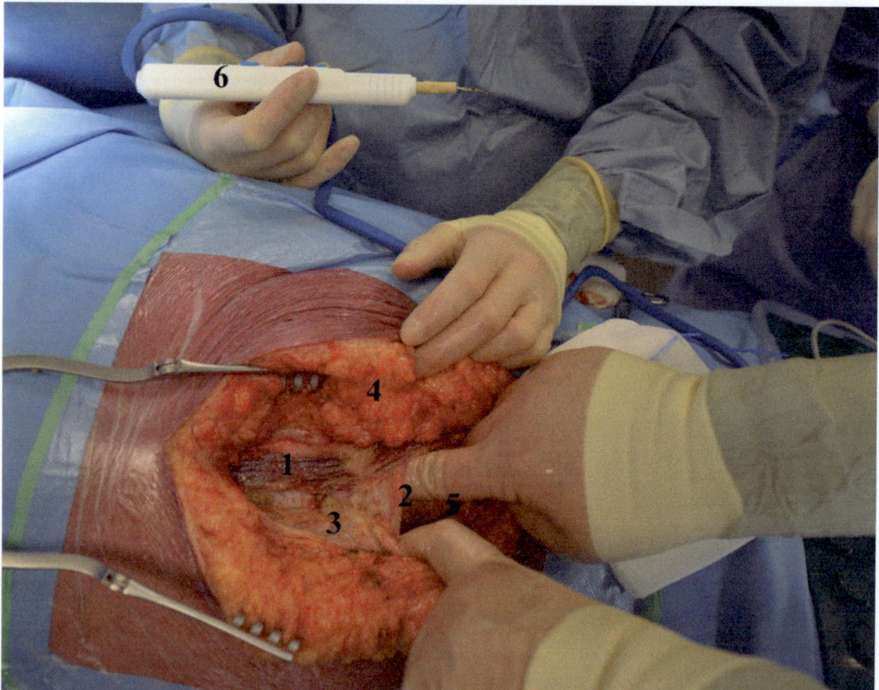

**Fig. 4.9** Detachment of the parietal peritoneum. 1—Rectus abdominal muscle, 2—Posterior sheath of the rectus abdominal muscle, 3—External oblique abdominal muscle tendon, 4—Subcutaneous tissue, 5—Retroperitoneal space, 6—Argon-beamer coagulation

fix it with a clamp. Then if necessary detach the parietal peritoneum from the posterior sheath of the rectus abdominal muscle upwards (Fig. 4.8). The posterior sheath of the rectus muscle is cut along the muscle with coagulation (Fig. 4.9). Detach the parietal peritoneum from the retroperitoneal space, revealing in turn the lumbar muscles, the inferior vena cava (IVC) (right side)and the common iliac and external vessels on the side of the graft [1–4, 14, 15].

**Warning! (Do not ligate—use if necessary the inferior epigastric artery for the reconstruction): inferior epigastric artery**

With each side incision for kidney transplantation, you always will be confronted with an inferior epigastric artery and the vein in the bladder area. Here everyone is asking themselves if it is needed, how and for what purpose it can be used, whether it can be cut and tied up or left uninjured.

In human anatomy, the inferior epigastric artery refers to the artery that arises from the external iliac artery and anastomoses with the superior epigastric artery. Along its course, it is accompanied by a similarly named vein, the inferior epigastric vein. The inferior epigastric artery gives off several side branches: the pubic branch, cremasteric artery (for males) and the artery of the round ligament of the uterus (for females). There is also an anastomosis formed between the inferior epigastric artery and the superior epigastric artery (from the internal thoracic artery). The inferior epigastric artery supplies blood to the muscles of the anterior abdominal wall, such as the rectus abdominal muscle and to the deep abdominal wall of the pubic and the lower umbilical regions.

If the diameter of the artery exceeds 2.5–3.0 mm, and the artery is not badly altered by atherosclerotic changes and has good blood flow and pulsation, we can use it—if necessary—to reconstruct, for example, a damaged accessory the renal artery running to the lower pole of the kidney. If we are going to use the inferior epigastric artery to reconstruct aberrant renal artery supplying inferior pole of the kidney. Let me tell you step by step what is important in its preparation for end-to-end anastomosis with the renal artery: The inferior epigastric artery can be identified midway between the anterior superior iliac spine and the pubic symphysis on its way to the umbilicus. The first step is to identify the inferior epigastric artery, separate it from the vein and ligate its small branches. It is important to dissect the artery as long as possible (on page 255, Fig. 4.8 shows a picture of the dissected inferior epigastric artery).Then ligate the artery close to the edge of the rectus abdominis muscle. Do not cut the ligature. Tighten the artery by pulling on the ends of the uncut garter, and make an incision 0.5–1.0 cm from the garter, halfway through the lumen of the vessel, using microsurgical scissors. The administration of papaverine in particular dilates the artery and widens its lumen. Once the vessel has been flushed and the blood drained, the artery is cut completely. Cutting the artery to half its lumen makes it much easier to cannulate and prevents damage to the artery during cannulation. May be perhaps this method of dealing with the inferior epigastric artery seems incomprehensible, but it must be remembered that the diameter of this artery is not always sufficient for anastomosis with the additional renal artery to reach the inferior pole of the kidney. The inferior epigastric artery may undergo atherosclerotic changes, when the flow from it to the lower pole of the kidney will not be sufficient. It should also be remembered that during qualification and examination of the recipient before transplantation, no examination of the recipient is ever assessed in terms of patency, diameter and atherosclerotic changes present in the inferior epigastric artery. The anastomosis with the epigastric artery is one of the technical solutions which, in order to perform it, two conditions must be met: the epigastric artery should be of the same diameter or larger than the diameter of the additional renal artery; and it should have a very good blood flow as we cannot perform anastomosis with the iliac artery. The usefulness of the inferior epigastric artery must be assessed at the time of surgery. What is the easiest way to do this if we want to use it for an anastomosis? Well, you have to dissect it very carefully, ligate it branches (if it has them), and ligate it at the rectus abdominal muscle to keep its as long as possible. The outflow or inflow of blood from the artery should be checked by cutting its lumen in half close to the rectus abdominal muscle before closing it with a tiny microsurgical bulldog vascular clamp. After releasing the bulldog, we observe the flow of blood from the artery: if it is good and the artery is usable, we rinse it with a 0.9% NaCl saline solution with heparin and close it with the bulldog, and then cut the artery completely. Due to its diameter, cannulating an artery and flushing it is much easier when its diameter is only incised; however it is not completely cut and the artery is still in contact with the remaining tissues from the side of the rectus abdominal muscle. I am an advocate of the following treatment of epigastric vessels: if I do not use the inferior epigastric artery to reconstruct the renal vessel I cut it and ligate it. If the epigastric inferior vessels are not suitable for

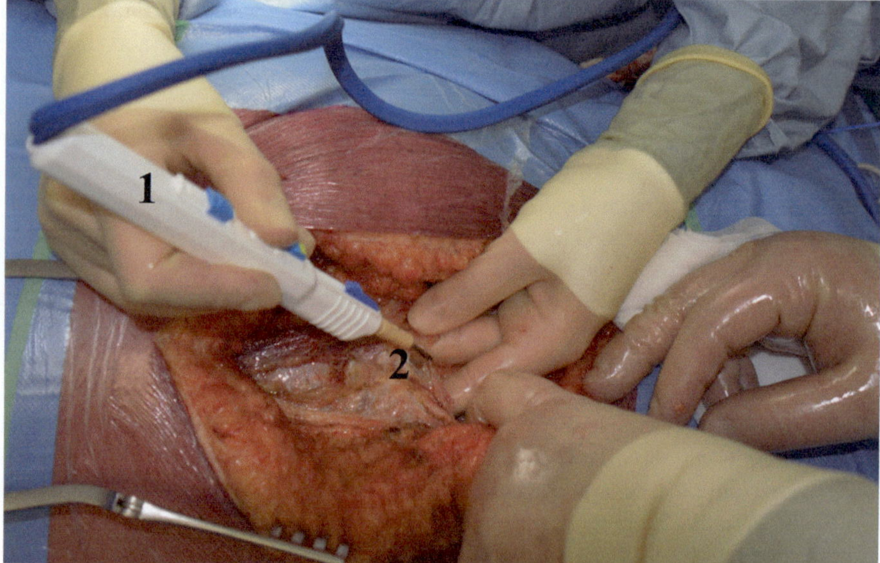

**Fig. 4.10** Above arcuate line. Cutting the posterior sheath of the rectus abdominal muscle. 1—Argon coagulation, 2—The posterior sheath of the rectus muscle, located above the arcuate line

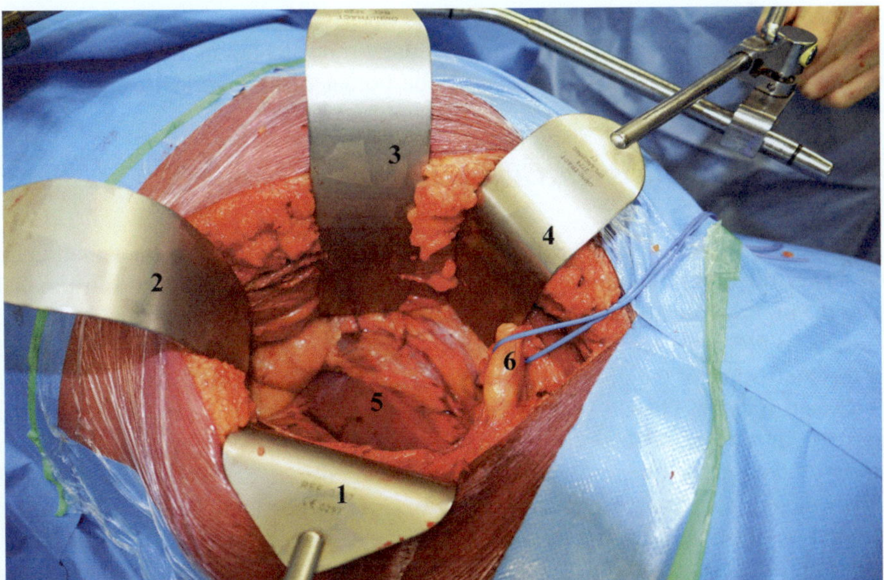

**Fig. 4.11** Installation of a professional abdominal retractor during kidney transplantation. 1, 2, 3, 4—Different blades of the professional abdominal retractor, 5—Right psoas major muscle: retroperitoneum, 6—Spermatic cord with a vessel loop around them

anastomosis, in my opinion it should also be cut and tied from both sides. This gives you much better access to the bladder and eliminates one more factor that may be responsible for any ureteral strictures that may develop in the post-operative period. In the recipient's kidney transplantation with multiple arteries, anastomosis of the lower pole artery to the inferior epigastric artery after declamping avoids prolongation of warm ischemia time that occurs with other surgical and microsurgical techniques of intracorporeal and ex vivo surgeries [16, 17]. Install a professional abdominal retractor (Fig. 4.11). The surgeon should avoid entering the peritoneal space and any defect in the peritoneum should be repaired before continuing the incision or after kidney transplantation.

**Warning! (Round ligament of the uterus—ligamentum rotundum—ligamentum teres uteri)**

When exposing the retroperitoneal space, try always in every case—if possible—to keep the round ligament whole and do not cut it through, especially in young women. A complete ligament transection may be responsible for future urine instability and could be manifested by discomfort or pain in the abdominal cavity. Try also, of course, if it is possible, to save the ligament in women who are planning to become pregnant in the future. Cut the round ligament of the uterus only if it is necessary, for example during a difficult reoperation or urological complications related to the urinary bladder and/or ureter and/or in women over 60 who have no intention of becoming pregnant.

There is no recommendation to cut the spermatic cord as this may lead to testicular necrosis or infertility. During a kidney transplantation the spermatic cord is simply retracted medially by releasing the border of the inguinal canal.

### 4.4.2   Oblique Incision (Gibson Incision—Gibson Cut)

An oblique or curvilinear Gibson incision is made on the side of the implantation, in the lower quadrant beginning almost in the midline extending upward in parallel with the inguinal ligament. The external oblique muscle and fascia are then divided. To expose the peritoneum, the internal oblique and transverse muscles are divided or the confluence of the oblique muscles and the rectal sheath is divided medially. It is a small incision (15–17 cm) ending at the lateral edge of the rectus abdominal muscle, running parallel to the inguinal ligament (Fig. 4.12). The Gibson incision starts at the pubic tubercule and continues laterally transverse to the inguinal ligament and then upwards in a curvilinear manner in the lateral border of the rectus abdominal muscle up to 1–2 cm above the level of the umbilicus. In larger adults extension up to the anterior superior iliac spine may be enough. This incision is performed in slim kidney recipients. The retroperitoneal space is reached in the same way as when making a pararectal incision under the arcuate line by cutting the two anterior rectus sheaths. This incision is used in kidney transplants in slim people, without any vascular anomalies, and also in kidney recipients with a very advanced atherosclerosis in the common iliac region. The peritoneum is swept

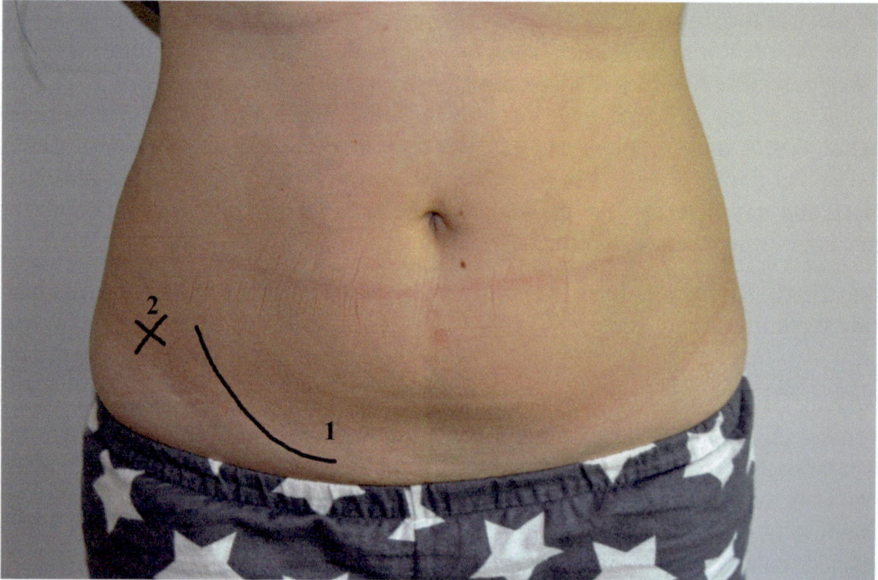

**Fig. 4.12**  Transversal cut (Gibson incision) running parallel to the inguinal ligament and 1—ending at the lateral edge of the rectus abdominal muscle, 2—Upper right anterior superior iliac spine

upwards to expose the iliac vascular system. Lymphatics over these vessels may be ligated to prevent the formation of a lymphocele [1–4]. Nani et al. compared the oblique incision with the hockey stick incision and the conclusion in their article was that the scar of 20% of the patients with the hockey stick incisions had widened —particularly in the upper vertical branch of the J incision. The article concludes that the final outcome of the oblique surgical incision was better than the hockey stick incision because of the lower incidence of hernia and abdominal wall relaxation and the more favorable cosmetic results [15].

### 4.4.3   Horizontal Incision Lengths of 10–12 cm for Use in Young Slim Recipients

With the advent of minimally invasive surgery, surgeons are driven to minimize or modify the incisions. A transverse suprapubic incision is a popular incision owing to its excellent cosmetic effect and decreased morbidity. Most of the open gynecological procedures are performed by this route. Urological procedures (such as radical prostatectomy) have also been performed through this incision [20–22].

This incision begins below the anterior superior iliac spine, then crosses the midline as far as the pubic symphysis (Fig. 4.13). The incision is modified in such a

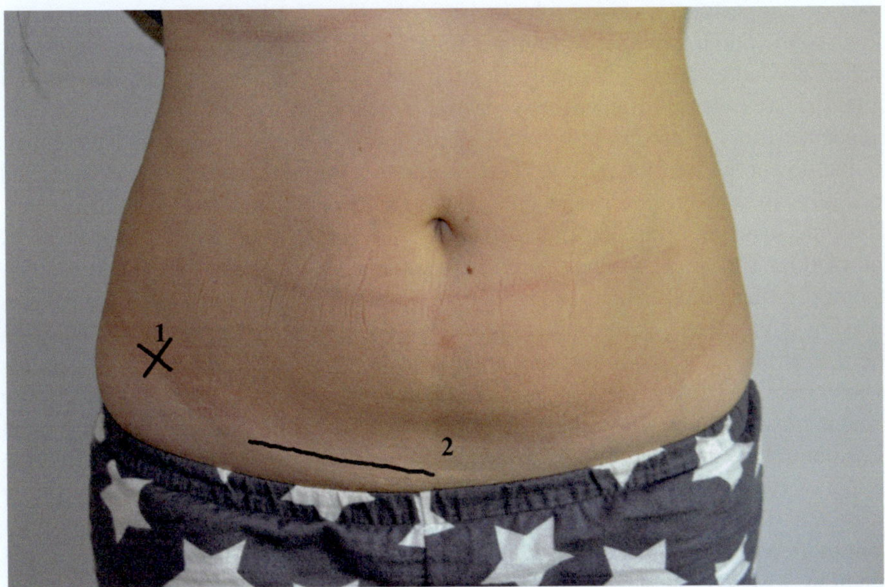

**Fig. 4.13** 10–12 cm long transverse incision used in young slim women and 1—Upper right anterior superior iliac spine, 2—Incision below upper right anterior superior iliac spine running right above the inguinal ligament, extending to the midline and ending at the level symphysis pubis

manner that two-thirds of the incision fall on the side of the graft placement. The incision in the skin is deepened through the subcutaneous fat, Scarpa's fascia and the anterior rectus sheath. The anterior rectus sheath is incised in the line of the incision. Rectus sheath flaps are raised superiorly and inferiorly up to the umbilicus and pubic symphysis, respectively. The rectus muscles are separated by the midline. For adequate exposure, the inferior flap of the rectus muscle can be divided by the midline, up to the superior border of the pubic symphysis. The underlying fascia transversalis is incised, and the inferior epigastric vessels are ligated and divided. The round ligament, if necessary, is ligated in females; the vas deferens is dissected and retracted medially. If required, further mobilization of the vas deferens is achieved by dividing the obliterated umbilical artery. The peritoneum and bladder are now swept super-laterally to expose the external iliac vessels. By sweeping the peritoneum cephalad, a space is created in the right or left iliac fossa to accommodate the kidney [23]. This incision is used in simple kidney transplants in very slim people, without any vascular anomalies, and in kidney recipients with very advanced atherosclerosis in the common iliac region [23].

### 4.4.4   Classic Incision: Rutherford Morison Incision

This incision begins 2 cm or two fingers above the anterior superior iliac spine—its length depends on the height and weight of the recipient kidney and how high we want or can perform renal vascular anastomosis (Fig. 4.14). The incision continues down to the pubic tubercle. A 20-cm extraperitoneal Rutherford Morison incision is made. The anterior rectus sheath, not the rectus muscle, is cut, and the inferior epigastric vessels are divided between silk ligatures. A long stump of the inferior epigastric artery is preserved if it will be necessary to make a separate anastomosis to the lower pole renal artery. The spermatic cord is preserved and retracted medially. In women, the round ligament is divided between heavy silk ligatures. The iliac fossa and retroperitoneal space are developed until the lateral surface of the bladder and the ipsilateral sacral promontory are exposed. The Bookwalter or another professional abdominal retractor is placed. The inconvenience of this incision is the need to cut the transverse muscles and their fascia, which increases the risk of bleeding into the wound and/or around the kidney, especially in patients whose kidneys are not working properly immediately after transplantation and the patient must undergo dialysis. It should be remembered that every patient treated with hemodialysis receives heparin which prevents the formation of clots inside the drains of the artificial kidney which may make the patient more prone to bleeding from the wound, retropertoneal space or transplanted kidney. Low molecular weight heparin (LMWH) is excreted by the kidneys—if the kidney does not function, LMWH can accumulate in the recipient's body, which increases the risk of bleeding from the abdominal wall muscles, the kidney itself or vascular anastomoses [1–4, 24].

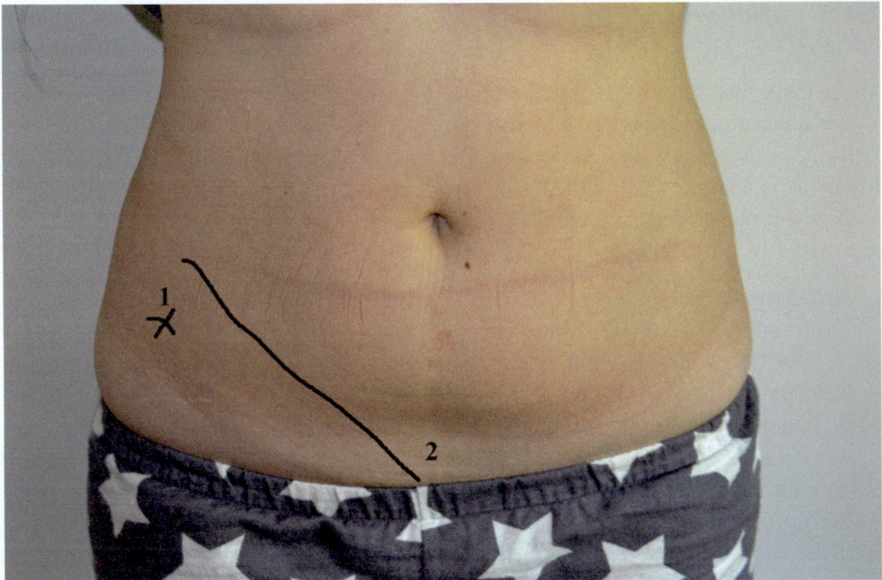

**Fig. 4.14** Classic oblique incision, one of the first incisions. 1—Starts above the anterior superior iliac spine and runs obliquely, ending above the tubercle of the pubic bone, 2—Tubercle of the pubic bone area as a point of attachment for the medial aspect of the inguinal ligament

**Warning! (I have pain after the kidney transplantation!)**
The patient's satisfaction and mortality as well as the graft function are not influenced by the incision length. With the patient and graft safety being paramount, especially in times of organ shortage, the incision length should reflect the requirement for a successful transplantation and not be a measure of feasibility [18].

The incidence and impact of chronic inguinal pain after kidney transplantation is not clearly established. Chronic inguinal neuropathic pain after kidney transplantation is common and seems to have a similar etiology as observed in inguinal hernia repair. Detection of the inguinal nerves is advised after hernia repair and leads to a decrease in chronic pain and an improvement of the quality of life. The same approach may be considered during kidney transplantation, although it is unclear whether the same positive effects are obtained. Zorgdrager et al.'s study aims to increase awareness among kidney transplantation surgeons to properly inform the kidney recipient, especially the obese patients, about the risk of chronic pain and to consider appropriate measures [19].

### *4.4.5  Midline Incision*

An incision that follows the linea alba (almost a avascular structure) to access most of the abdominal viscera is performed in a wide variety of abdominal surgeries, including emergency procedures, as this incision causes minimal blood loss; the downside is a susceptibility to significant scars. It is a very safe incision (Fig. 4.15), used in the massive calcification of the iliac vessels on the sides, as well as in the next, usually third, kidney transplant in the following situations:

– simultaneous pancreas and kidney transplantation (intraperitoneally).
– liver and kidney transplantation (intraperitoneally).
– if there are old renal transplants on both sides and one of the transplanted kidneys has to be replaced with a new one.
– in patients after pancreas and kidney transplantation, when the kidney is not working and must be replaced with a new organ; or the new kidney, if there is enough space, is to be grafted on the right or left side to an existing kidney.
– both procured kidneys must be transplanted on both sides of the abdomen.
– if the patient has advanced atherosclerosis on both sides, and based on the tests performed, we cannot decide on which side we want to transplant the kidney. After opening the abdominal cavity from the midline incision, by palpating, we can carefully assess the iliac arteries from the aorta to the inguinal ligament on both sides and choose the best place or places for aretrial anastomosis.
– reoperation in the case of ureteral necrosis, when we want to connect the ureter of the transplanted kidney with the recipient's own ureter lying on the opposite side.

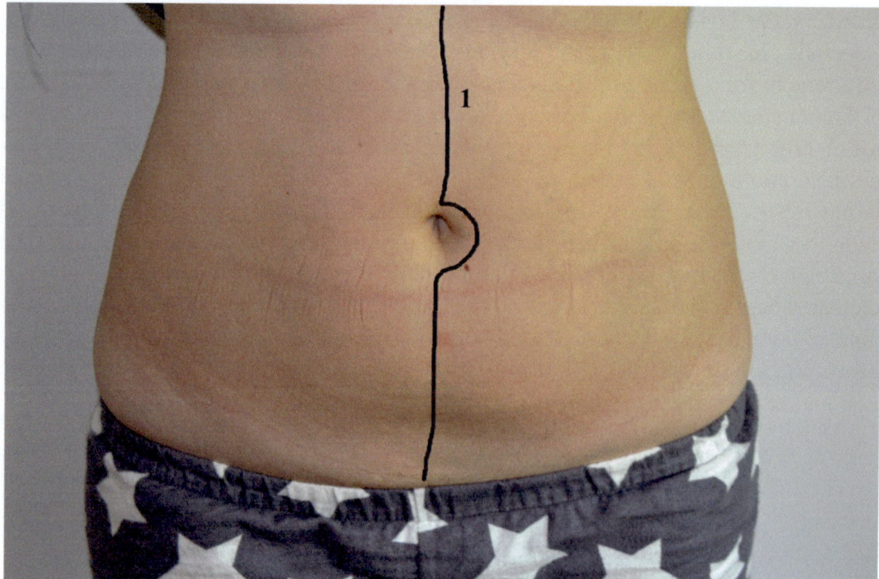


**Fig. 4.15**  1—Middle line incision

- if connecting the ureter with the intestine (ureteroenteric anastomosis but also revision of this anastomosis due to stricture, closure or necrosis of the ureter).
- surgical treatment of some laparoscopically untreatable lymphocele [1–4].

## 4.5   Installation of a Professional Abdominal Retractor

### 4.5.1   Introduction

Nowadays, there are thee professional abdominal retractors being used worldwide for kidney transplantation: OmniTrack from OmniTrack Surgical, Thompson from Thompson Surgical Inc., and Bookwalter from Symmetry Surgical Acquired O.R, Company. They have one common feature which is based on independently working arms and full mobility of individual parts which allow it to be adapted to any type of operation field. A professional abdominal retractor, although expensive, provides great comfort to the surgeon in the form of a stable, clear operating field, allowing large operations to be performed safely, significantly reducing the number of intra- and post-operative complications.

### 4.5.2   Installation Step by Step

1. In most kidney transplant procedures, I used OmniTrac which generally consists of a sterile field post, standard wishbone frame, extension arm, blade holders, clamps, retractors, many sizes and shapes of blades, all which adapt to the surgical field during the operation. We need to assembling them in such a way that the surgical field is as stable as possible, i.e. to give the surgeon the greatest possible comfort (Fig. 4.16).
2. After shaving, scrubbing and covering the recipient's abdomen with sterile operating sheets and incision drapes, one of the above mentioned kidney transplantation incisions is made when the extraperitoneal space is reached. After that, a professional abdominal retractor is installed.

   (a) determine the location of the Omni-Clamp Sterile Field Post (vertical post) Fig. 4.16 relative to the surgical field. Place the post on the O.R. table rail over the sterile drape. Rotate the knob (the first from the top on a vertical post) clockwise to secure it to the table, 10–15 cm above the upper pole of the incision or at the level of the xiphoid process.

   (b) adjust the wishbone (arms) of the Fast System Frame to the post and secure it. The arms of the wishbone have to be spread for the distance we want from the wound secured and turned towards the recipient's legs.

   (c) the wound is expanded in different directions to obtain a very good view of the structures prepared (iliac and lymphatic vessels, urinary bladder) in the extraperitoneal space.

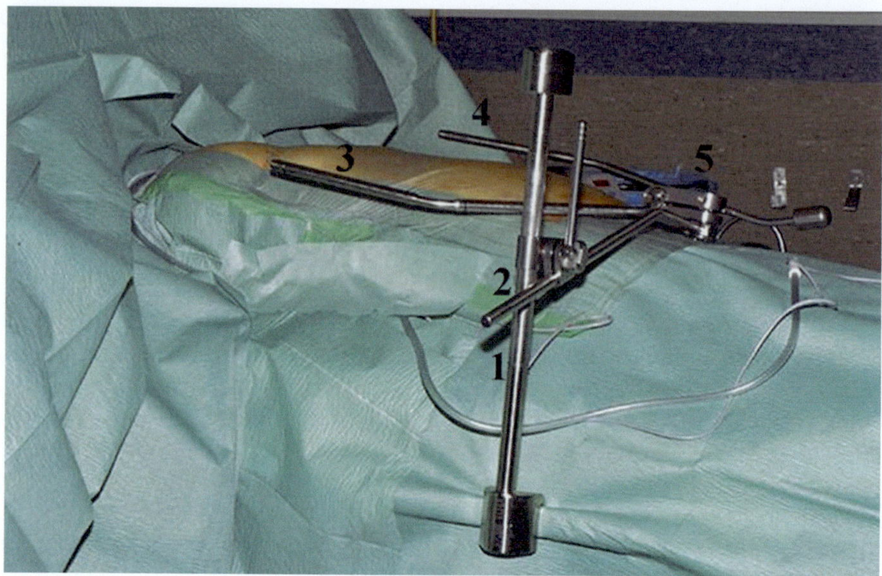

**Fig. 4.16** Abdominal retractor type Omni-Trac, 1—Vertical part (Sterile Field Post) attached to the operating table, 2—Horizontal part attached to the vertical part, 3 and 4—two movable arms that can be freely moved apart and to approach each other, 5—Lock securing retractor arms in any position

### 4.5.3   *My Personal Settings of Retractors and Blades on the Wishbone Frame*

During a kidney transplantation I use four to five abdominal wall tissue and vessel retractors with different blades:

- the first rounded retractor pulls the abdominal wall outside (Fig. 4.17—No. 1).
- the second retractor is placed along the long axis of the common iliac artery, 1–2 cm above it, and I move the peritoneal contents away until the abdominal aorta bifurcation is visible. (Attention! The retractor has to be placed in such a way that it does not compress or even touch any artery or vein during the entire operation). (Fig. 4.17—No. 2).
- the third retractor with the long blade is used to move the intestines upward towards the liver and further expose the upper iliac fossa, especially the lumbar muscle, on which in most cases the kidney transplant is placed (Fig. 4.17—No. 3).
- the fourth retractor has long or short blade which is wide or narrow, depending on the recipient's weight and height; its task is to move the contents of the peritoneal sac to the middle of the abdominal cavity in order to give a very good exposure to the artery and the internal and external iliac vein on the left, and to

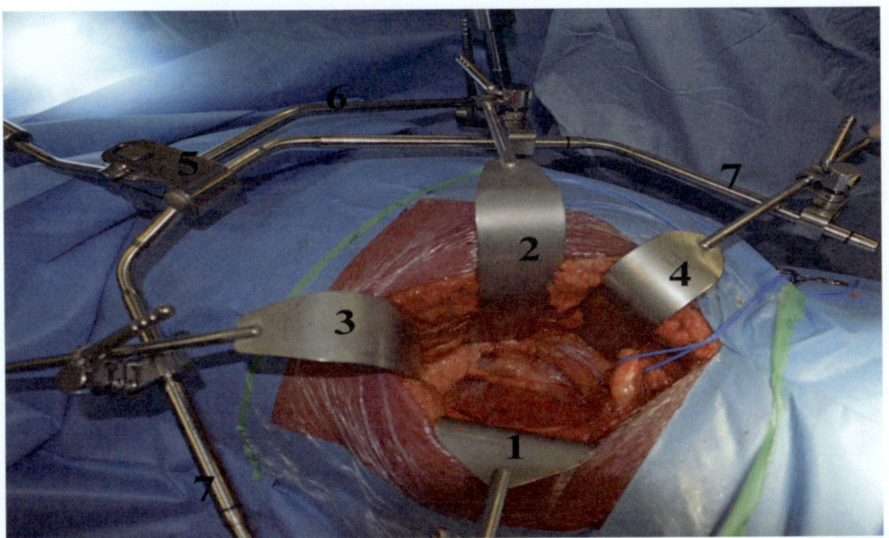

**Fig. 4.17** Omni-Trac in kidney transplant operation. 1—The first semicircular blade is responsible for pulling outside the abdominal wall, 2—The second blade is responsible for pulling the abdominal wall together with the peritoneal sac along the long axis of the common iliac artery, aorta and its bifurcation, 3—The third blade is used in order to move the abdominal muscles and the peritoneum bag with its contents upwards towards the collarbone, 4—The fourth blade is responsible for pulling the abdominal wall and the peritoneal bag towards the middle line, and is used during the operation to visualize the external and internal iliac vessels, 5—The lock which immobilizes the retractor arms, 6—The horizontal arm of the Omni-Trac is attached to the vertical post (section), which is attached to the side rails on one or both sides of the OR table, (7)—The horizontal arm is connecting using lock system vertical part (post) abdominal retractor. attached to the side rails on both sides of the operating table with a lock securing the retractor arms (7) in any position, 7—The arms of a professional abdominal retractor stabilized in any position by the lock (5)

the right iliac vessels and the inferior vena cava (IVA) of the lower and final abdominal aorta (Fig. 4.17—No. 4).

- when performing vascular anastomoses, I often use a long, thin retractor called the "Renal Vein Swivel Retractor" to gently move back the iliac arteries towards the midline of the abdominal cavity which have been dissected from the retroperitoneal space. The Renal Vein Swivel Retractor is a very delicate retractor which is usually used to gently move the iliac arteries towards the body's midline for good exposure of the iliac veins during venous anastomosis (Fig. 4.18).
- after the anastomosis, in order to visualize the urinary bladder, I use a retractor with a semicircular blade which pulls the abdominal wall outside the urinary bladder (Fig. 4.19).

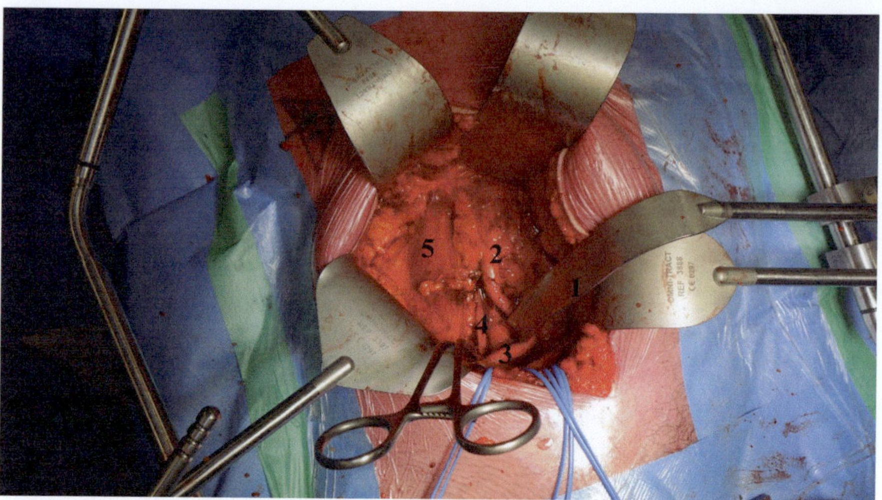

**Fig. 4.18** 1—Thin blade or renal vein blade of a professional abdominal retractor; the blade is used to gently pull towards the midline the iliac arteries during venous anastomosis, 2—Common, internal and external arteries gently pulled to the median line, 3—External iliac artery, 4—Common iliac vein—right side, 5—Psoas muscle major

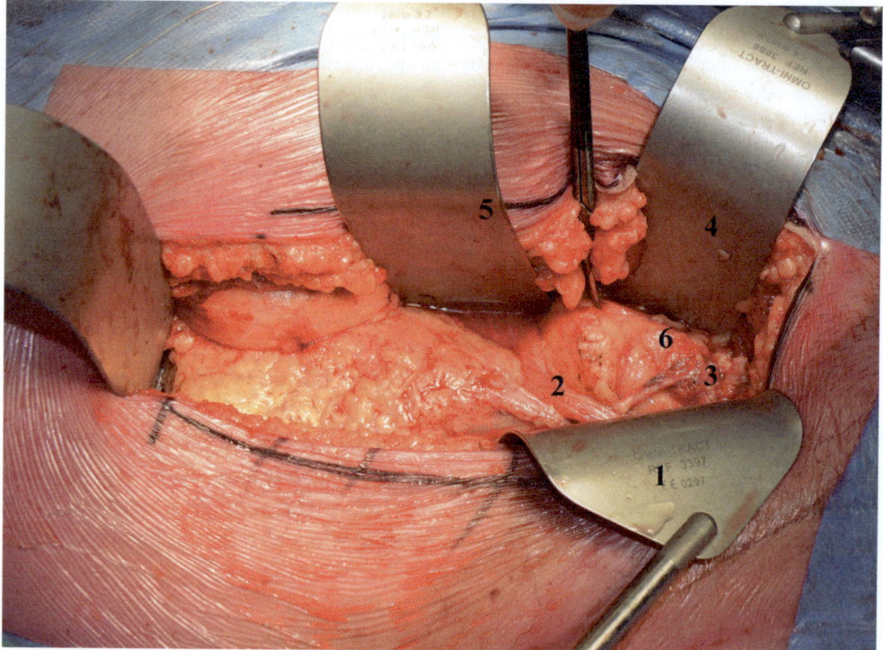

**Fig. 4.19** During uretero-bladder anastomosis, the blades of the abdominal retractor are moved towards the urinary bladder. 1—Semicircular blade, 2—Spermatic cord or ligamentum rotundum, 3—Ureter-urinary bladder anastomosis, 4 and 5—Blades have been placed at the beginning of the operation in the upper part of the wound and at this stage of the operation have been replaced below to increase the visibility area of ureter-urinary bladder anastomosis, 6—Urinary bladder

### 4.5.4   *Iliac Vessel Preparation*

- the gentle prepartion of the right common, internal and external iliac artery and vein mainly comes down to a gentle separation of them from each other, the surrounding muscles and overlying lymphatic vessels.
- the lymphatic vessels, which were cut during preparation, have to be ligated or coagulated to avoid postoperative lymph leakage (Fig. 4.20).
- the differences between the anatomical position and the course of the right and left iliac vessels I will explain in Sects. 4.9 and 4.10.

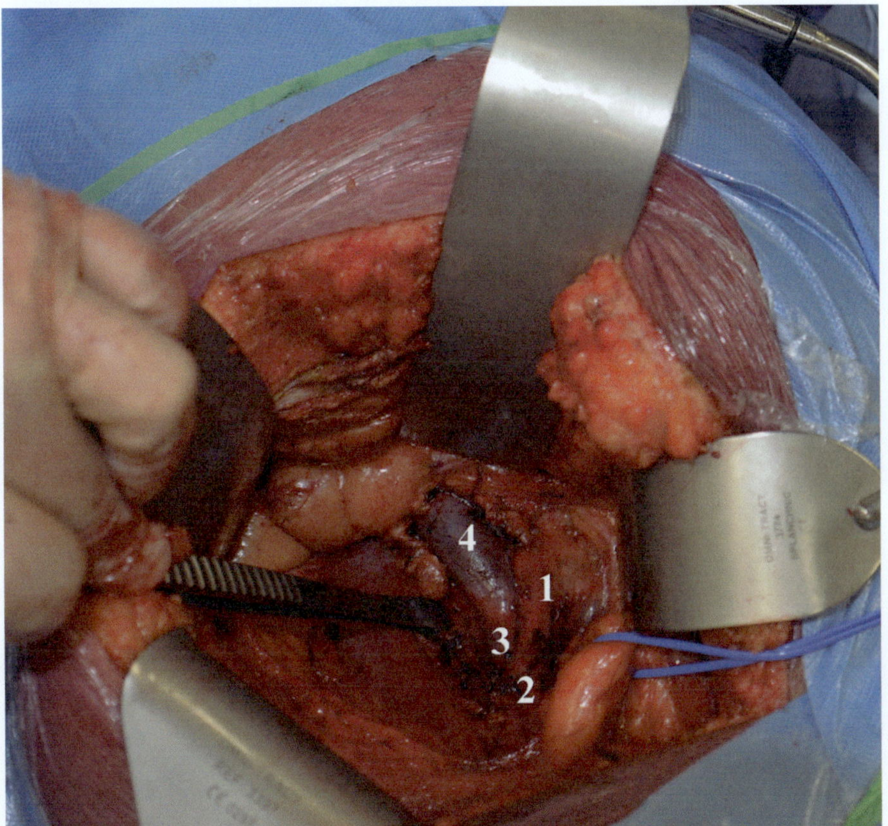

**Fig. 4.20** Dissected right iliac vessels before kidney transplantation. 1—Common iliac artery, 2—External iliac artery, 3—Common iliac vein, 4—Inferior vena cava

## 4.6  Kidney Inspected, Packed and Taken to Operating Theatre

The circulating nurse removes the inspected and on the newly packed kidney from the transport box (static cold storage). The nurse who removed the kidney from the box is responsible for the sterile opening of the first bag (Fig. 4.21) and its sterile administration (Fig. 4.22) by the scrub nurse. The scrub nurse's task is to sterilely remove the kidney from the first 'dry' bag and place it on the operating table in a sterile ice-filled bowl for further sterile unpacking (Fig. 4.23). The final step in unpacking the kidney is to completely remove the first (last) bag and place the kidney in a bowl of ice and immerse it in cold preservation solution (Fig. 4.24).

The sterile instrumentation nurse, standing in a sterile position, cuts the sterile ribbon that ties the last bag containing the kidney and preservation fluid and then the kidney, after removal, is transferred to a special container with ice and than poured over with fresh and cold preservation solution (Fig. 4.24).

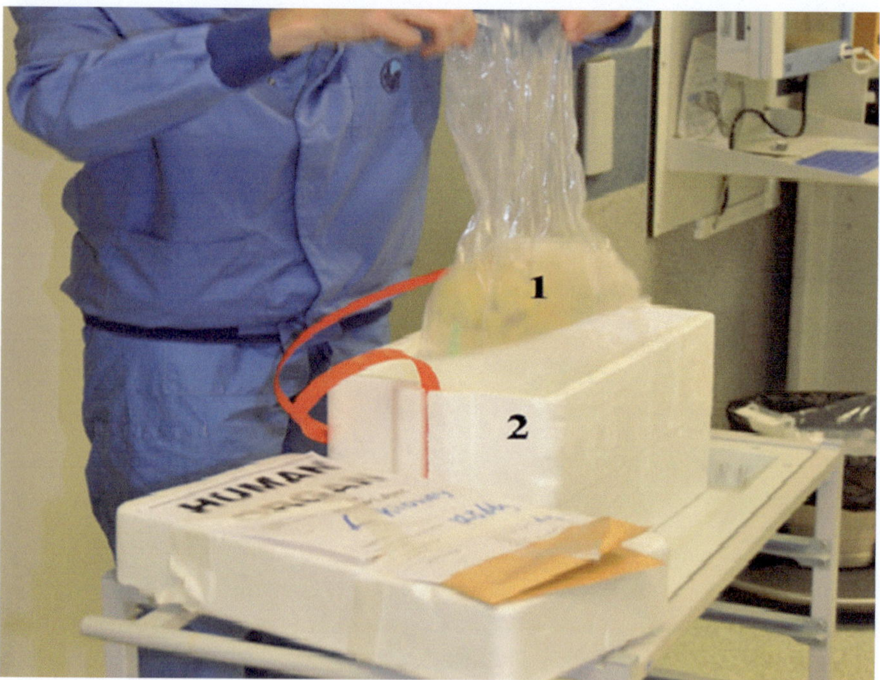


**Fig. 4.21** The circulating scrub nurse or scrub nurse removes the kidney from the transport box. Remember that the first bag from outside is only sterile on the inside. 1—Open the first "dry" bag from outside, 2—Transport box

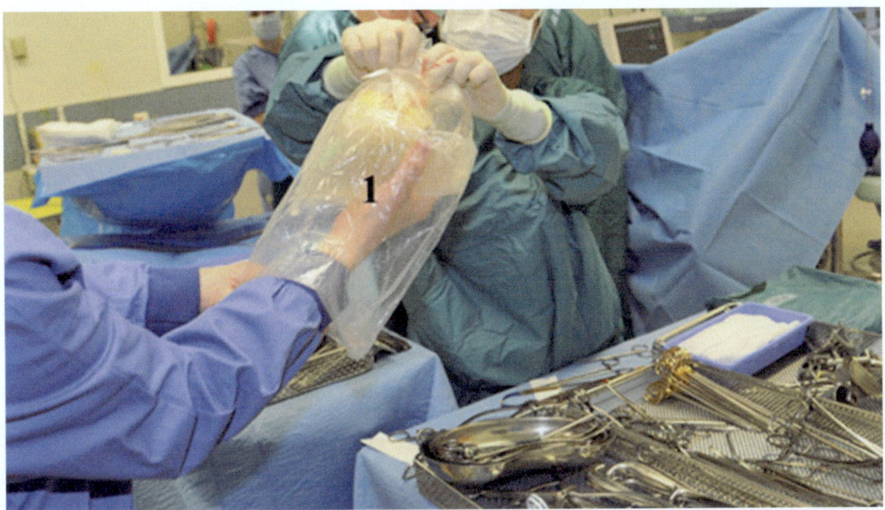


**Fig. 4.22** The circulating nurse administers the packed kidney in a special way while preserving sterility to the sterile dressed scrub nurse for further sterile unpacking and placement in a special container of ice and cold preservation solution. 1—One of the methods of preserving sterility when donating a kidney for transplantation is to fold up the walls of the bag on the hinge containing the kidney packed in the last bag. In a bag the kidney is immersed in a cooled preservation fluid

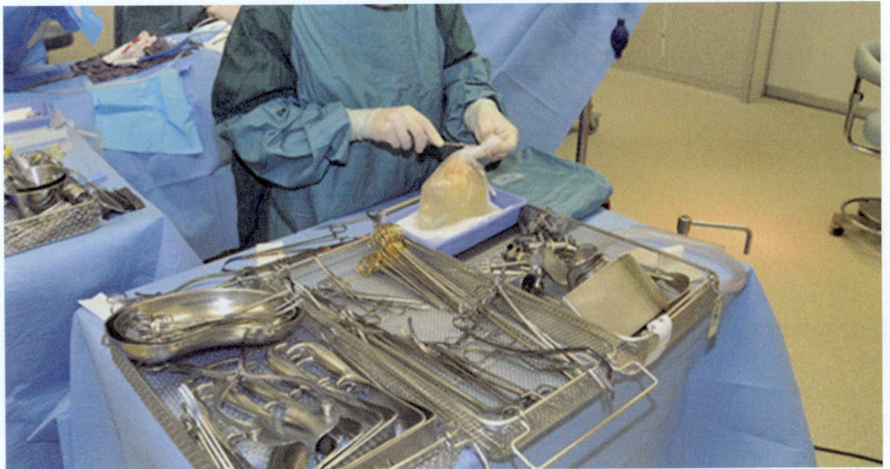

**Fig. 4.23** Sterile unpacking of the kidney in the operating room. At this point the kidney is only packed in one bag and immersed in cold preservation fluid

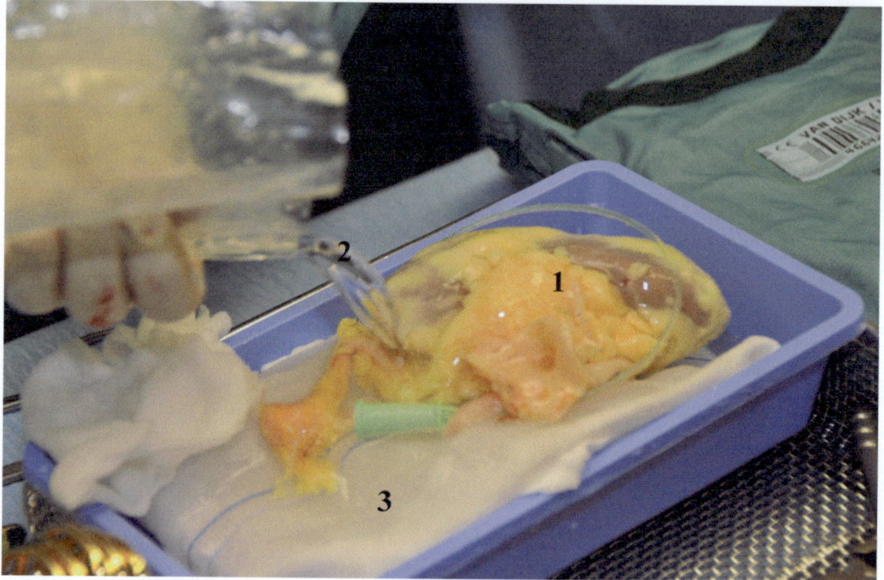

**Fig. 4.24** Sterile unpacked kidney placed in a container with ice, and then poured over with cold preservation solution. 1—Kidney, 2—Chilled conduction fluid, which is poured over the kidney in a special box just before transplantation, 3—Ice covered with wet gauze to protect the kidney against frostbite

## 4.7   Biopsy of the Renal Allograft and of the Transplanted Kidney

### 4.7.1   Introduction

Renal biopsy remains the gold standard by which essential diagnostic and prognostic information is obtained after kidney transplantation. A renal allograft biopsy is the gold standard to accurately establish the cause of renal allograft dysfunction. Biopsy methodologies have been devised to assess the acceptability of an organ before transplantation and to assess and predict renal allograft performance after implantation. Renal transplant biopsy samples are analyzed by the same traditional and modern techniques as are used to assess samples from native kidney.[25–27].

### 4.7.2   Open Biopsy

A pretransplant kidney biopsy is used to judge the quality of a deceased donor organ at excision and, before transplantation on occasion, to rule out the possibility of disease in live donors.

The biopsy is performed under sterile conditions during back table or after removal of the kidney from the bag, before vascular anastomosis. Usually the biopsy is taken from the upper pole of the kidney by use of a sterile surgical scalpel (No. 15). An example of the dimensions of the kidney biopsy taken from the tissues of the renal parenchyma, by a cone-shaped cut, are 8–10 mm long, 4–6 mm wide, and 7–10 mm deep (Fig. 4.25). The excised defect of the kidney parenchyma is sewn with a 4/0 or 5/0 absorbable monofilament suture. I personally use half of the 4/0 absorbable monofilament suture with no needle at the end. The kidney parenchyma defect is closed with two rows of the same suture using the back and forth technique (Fig. 4.26). My method is to make the first insertion of a needle about 2–3 mm before the defect, as I mentioned above I always use half of the suture, and at the end of it. I fix it with a very delicate vessel clamp with jaw covers. During suturing the cone-shaped cut that occurred as a result of performing a biopsy, the surgical suture passes 1–2 mm under the bottom of the defect and is gently pulled so that the edges begin to touch each other. The surgical suture used to close the renal tissues should not be pulled too strongly and after the completion of suturing the suture should not be tied under high tension. If the suture is to be tied under high tension during reperfusion, the volume of the kidney will significantly increase and instead of closing the biopsy place, surgical suture may cut through the kidney's

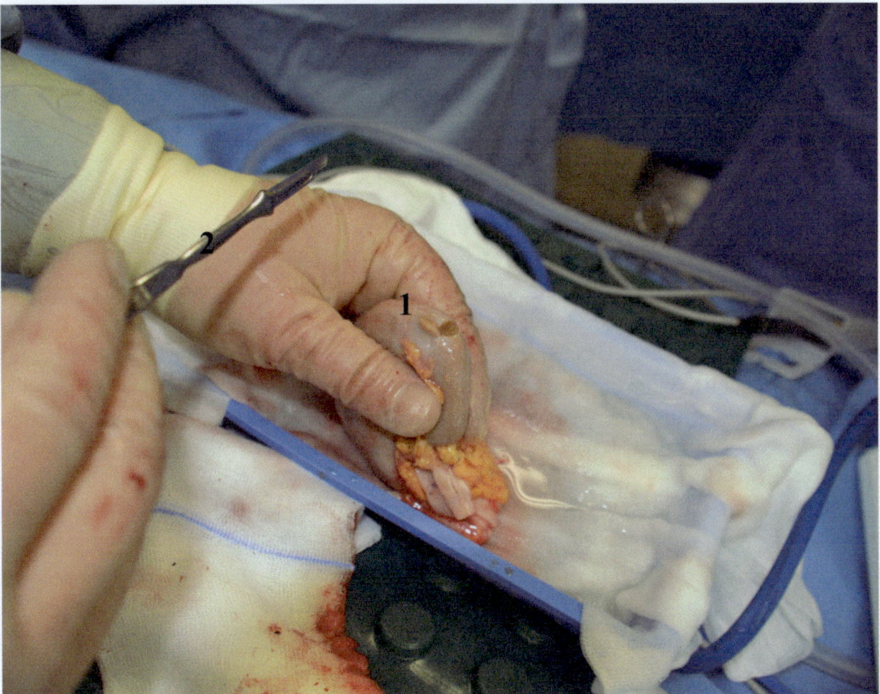

**Fig. 4.25** Upper pole open kidney biopsy before transplantation. 1—A cone-shaped scalpel cut a small piece of kidney parenchyma from the upper pole of the kidney, 2—Surgical scalpel No. 15

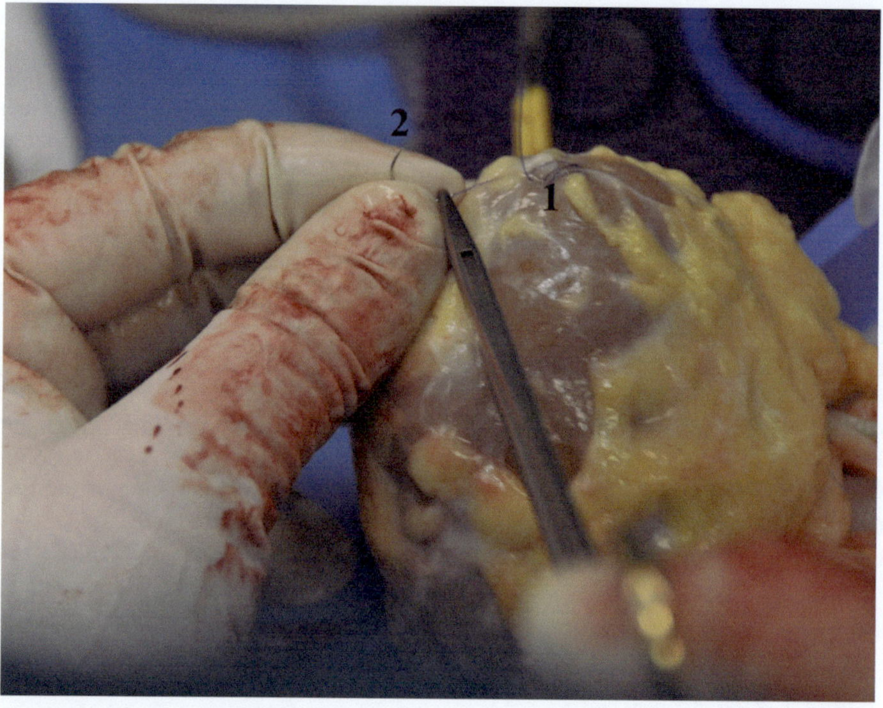

**Fig. 4.26** The defect in the upper pole of the kidney parenchyma is sutured with a continuous absorbed suture back and forth, 1—Suturing the kidney biopsy site, 2—Suture 4/0 absorbed monofilament

parenchyma and cause significant bleeding. This biopsy is called a zero biopsy or an initial biopsy. This biopsy is very important because it compares every subsequent biopsy taken after transplantation. Performing an open biopsy after a renal reperfusion can be dangerous and usually involves considerable bleeding from the site where it was taken. If the parenchyma of the kidney is brittle or even normal, we have sometimes additional problems with hemostasis, because tying and tightening the sutures on already very tense renal tissues often causes the parenchyma to cut through, which only increases the bleeding from the biopsy side. If you have trouble stopping the bleeding, I recommend tying a suture on one of the topic hemostatic materials, filling the biopsy site (see Sect. 5.2 "Renal Allograft Rupture and Surgical Treatment"). The open biopsy is mostly a superficial one. The ideal site for it is the upper pole of the kidney (Fig. 4.27). The biopsy can also be taken from the posterior surface of the lower pole, but you must remember that the arterial blood supply of the ureter and renal pelvis—the "golden triangle"—must remain intact and that there is less access in the case of bleeding due to the tissues which surround the ureter and renal pelvis [1–4, 25–27].

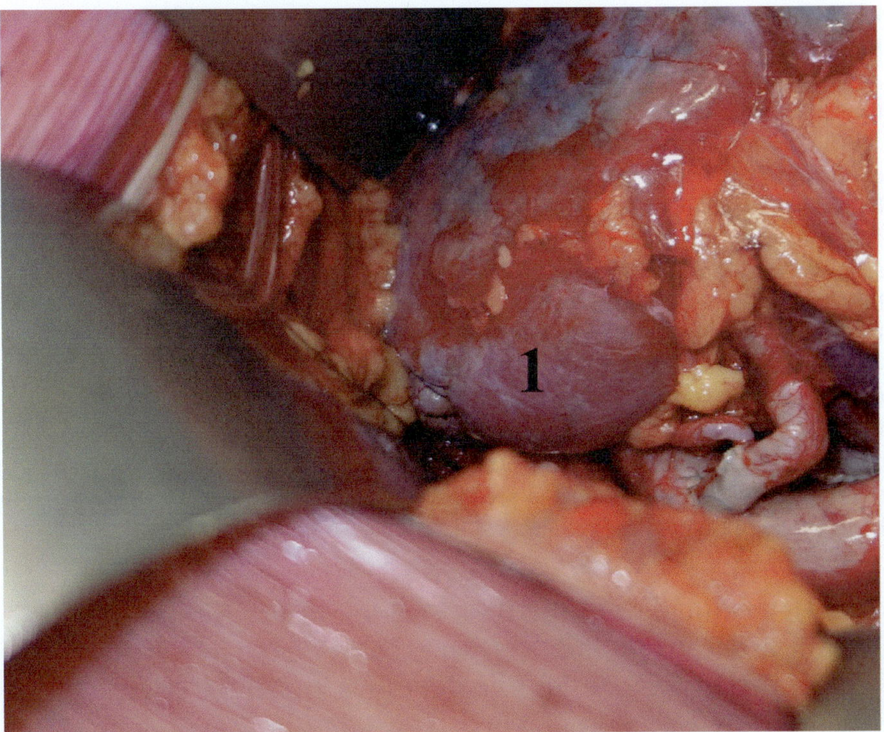


**Fig. 4.27** Picture taken after kidney transplantation. 1—Place where an open kidney biopsy was performed and sutured

### 4.7.3   Deep Needle Biopsy

Percutaneous renal biopsy (PRB) is a safe and effective modality for sampling kidney tissue. In limited circumstances, alternative methods for kidney biopsy may be indicated. Historical contraindications for PRB such as bleeding diathesis, morbid obesity and solitary kidney have been called into question in the literature.

The biopsy can be performed both before and after renal reperfusion, from the lower or upper pole of the kidney. The depth of the biopsy can be adjusted. The surgeon must take care of his own fingers and hands when performing the biopsy. Biopsy after kidney reperfusion is usually accompanied by more bleeding. In the case of bleeding and stopping, we can use coagulation, sew the biopsy hole, seal the biopsy hole with tissue glue or use superficial hemostatic contact agents.

You can also use an Argon Beamer or Aquamantys. Indications for kidney biopsy are as follows: (1) continuous anuria and oliguria; (2) serum creatinine keeps increasing or stabilizes above normal level during regular reexamination; (3) recurrent and unexplained abnormal renal function; (4) increasing blood pressure or persistence of albuminuria and hematuria. A quick description of the kidney biopsy will now follow. The patient is lying down in a supine position, so the transplanted kidney can be easily reached. The skin over the biopsy site is disinfected. After that, local anesthetics are injected into the skin, through the subcutaneous tissue and down to and around the kidney. Under the guidance of a Doppler ultrasound biopsy the needle is inserted into a kidney [28–34].

The most common complication of the renal biopsy is in most of cases: damage to an intrarenal artery (bleeding). The consequence of damage to the artery is a fistula between the renal pelvis and the renal vessel leading to transient and sometimes mass and/or chronic hematuria; hemorrhage into the abdominal cavity or extraperitoneal space and an arterio-venous fistula in the kidney parenchyma leading to a decrease in blood filtration capacity and thus an increase in serum creatinine concentration. Bleeding may occur in three distinct locations within the kidney: into the collecting system, under the renal capsule or into the perinephric space. If the bleeding enters the collecting system, blood is seen in the urine and can cause pain and obstruction. If the bleeding is subcapsular, it can create enough of a mechanical compressive effect onto the kidney to cause hypertension owing to an increase in the release of renin, which is a hormone that is secreted by the juxtaglomerular apparatus of the kidney in the proximal convoluted tubule to increase systemic blood pressure [1–4].

## 4.8 Determination of the Best Position of the Kidney in the Retroperitoneal Space, Determination of the Length of the Renal Vessels and the Ureter, and the Location of Their Anastomosis

Wrap the kidney in fine and thin sterile gauze soaked in cold preservation or 0.9% NaCl solution previously immersed in crushed ice or slush. Place the kidney in the right or left iliac fossa in a best (my preference is always to be as high as possible, if that is possible) retroperitoneal position.

The purpose of temporarily placing the kidney in the iliac fossa is:

- to determine its best permanent position in the extraperitoneal space.
- to determine the best position for the anastomosis of the renal vessels with the recipienyt's aorta, IVC, iliac or/and inferior epigastric vessels (can be marked with a sterile marker or argon coagulation) and the correct length of the renal vessels.
- to determine the length of the ureter (urethral shortening) only after vascular anastomoses have been performed and blood flow to the kidney has been fully restored should the ureter be shortened especially at the time when at a given moment we are forced to with the ureter upwards (kidney inversion position) with implantation of the ureter into the isolated loop of the intestine (the Bricker operation—an operation utilizing an isolated segment of the ileum to collect urine from two of its own ureters or one ureter from a transplanted kidney and conduct it to the skin surface).

After determining the final position of the kidney in the retroperitoneal space and establishing the places of vascular anastomoses and the length of the renal vessels, remove the kidney from the retroperitoneal space and place it back in the container box with ice and cold preservation solution.

### 4.8.1  Confrontation with a Short Ureter; A Kidney You May Receive for Transplantation; Some Tips and Tricks

- if necessary due to the severity of intravascular calcifications, try to perform vascular anastomoses with the external iliac vessels towards the inguinal ligament, with or without urinary bladder mobilization; the anastomosis between the ureter and the urinary bladder must be without any tension; (with or without the bladder psoas hitch). If the anastomosis between the urinary bladder and the ureter was performed under tension then keep the catheter in the urinary bladder for about seven to ten days after the operation.
- perform vascular anastomoses high above the internal iliac artery and vein with the use of the Boari-flap or psoas-bladder hitch technique—which requires a normal bladder wall and bladder capacity exceeding 400 ml. After psoas-bladder hitch surgery, patients require a Foley catheter in the urinary bladder for 10–14 days.
- perform a vascular anastomosis high above the internal iliac artery and vein. As the next step, perform an end-to-side or end-to-end anastomosis between the donor's and the recipient's ureter, depending on the immunosuppression and the amount of urine excreted by the own recipient's kidneys. The ureter can be repaired by sewing the two cut ends together as long as the gap between them is less than 3 cm. At the time the ureter is sewn together, a stent (plastic tube) is also placed in the ureter. The stent helps the ureter to heal and is typically removed three to four weeks after repair.
- perform vascular anastomosis very low below the iliac internal artery and vein after properly mobilizing the iliac external vessels as close as possible to the inguinal ligament so that, the anastomosis of the ureter with the urinary bladder will not be under tension. Check also that the kidney vessels do not bend and the inflow and outflow of blood from the kidney are guaranteed without any obstruction.

**Warning! (Mark the places of every anastomosis)**
If it is difficult to remember the places of vascular anastomoses, but you can mark them with a sterile marker or an Argon Beamer coagulation.


## 4.9  Kidney Transplantation on the Right Side of the Retroperitoneal Space

### 4.9.1  Introduction

As I emphasized before, if there were no previous grafts on the right side and the iliac vessels are in good condition, without advanced atherosclerosis, and this is the first transplant, I always transplant each kidney "high", trying to perform an anastomosis with the common iliac vessels. Transplantation on the right side is technically easier due to the location of the iliac vessels. The IVC and the common

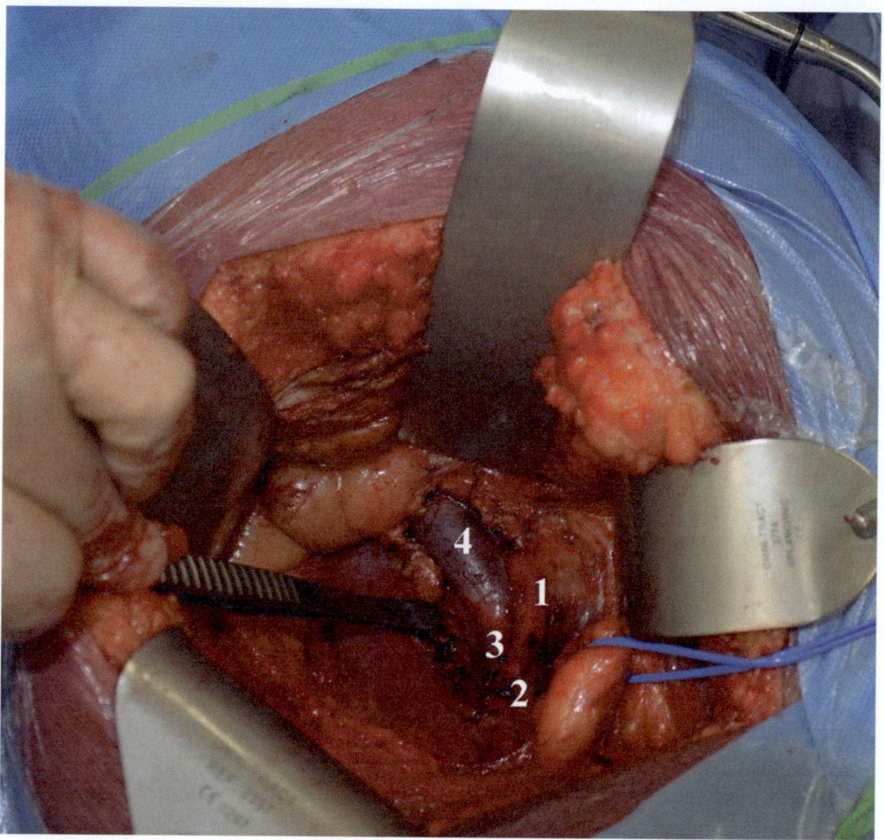

**Fig. 4.28** Location of the iliac vessels on the right side. Behind the forceps is the psoas major muscle. 1—Common iliac artery, 2—External iliac artery, 3—Common iliac vein, 4—IVC

iliac vein are partially located outside and parallel just behind the common iliac artery and, viewed from the right, in front of the common iliac artery (Fig. 4.28). The second advantage of a high anastomosis of the renal vessels with the IVC or common iliac vessels is the position of the kidney in the retroperitoneal space. It can be said that the position of the kidney on the psoas major muscle is almost ideal because of the distance to the iliac vessels. Another argument for the renal vessel anastomosis with the iliac vessels being as high as possible, apart from the perfect position (if they are normal and unchanged), is the fact that the formation of lymphocele, as a complication after kidney transplantation, is relatively rare. This is due to the fact that, when preparing the common iliac vessels, the lymphatic vessels overlying the common iliac vessels are mostly split rather than cut over a very small distance. The preparation of the common iliac vessels is shorter and less traumatic, especially for lymphatic vessels. Someone will say: but you will need a longer ureter. I will answer—yes, but you can mobilize the bladder, you can also perform uretero-ureteral anastomosis "end to end" or "end to side" with the ureter of the recipient kidney. Regarding the number of complications, it can be concluded from the literature that uretero-ureteral anastomoses do not differ from uretero-bladder anastomoses in terms of postoperative complications. If the iliac vessels are healthy without or with slight calcifications, then there is no problem to transplant the right kidney with a short right renal vein on the right side. A problem may arise when the iliac vessels are sick and have a lot of calcification, where all over the iliac vessels there is only one healthy place to close it with one or two vascular clamps. This is a difficult anastomosis, because the renal artery is short and situated behind the renal vein. If you do not have experience with transplanting the kidney on the right side, perform the transplant on the left side.

### 4.9.2  How Long Does the Renal Vein Have to Be in a Renal Allograft just Before the Anastomosis?

After placing the kidney in the best position in the retroperitoneal space; look first of all for the best place to perform a venous anastomosis; mark it and try to measure the best length of the renal vein. The best length of the renal vessels should end 2–3 mm before the place of the planned vascular anastomosis. If you have measured it and if the renal vein is still too short and a venous anastomosis cannot be made between the renal vein and the IVC and/or one of the iliac veins, the right or left common iliac vein should be dissected, The right or left common iliac vein should be dissected, with the internal iliac vein ligated on both sides if necessary, to maximise mobilisation of the iliac veins towards the kidney. Kinking and/or twisting of the renal vessels increases the risk of their thrombosis, which can even lead to kidney loss. Sometimes operators, especially those who love implanting kidneys with long vessels, without any kind of measuring or trying them on during transplantation, following vascular anastomosis push the kidney into the retroperitoneal space. I am not a supporter of this technique and I have never taught anyone to transplant a kidney in such an irresponsible manner. Several times I had the opportunity to observe surgeons transplanting kidneys in such a way that when the vascular anastomosis was due to be performed, an unprotected kidney was hanging outside the recipient's body. These surgeons were usually technically very skilled, and quickly performed vascular anastomosis and released the vascular clamp(s); most of them held the kidney into their hands during reperfusion, and then by pushing the kidney in different places of the extraperitoneal space they tried to find the best position for it, that is the one in which there was no folding of the vessels of the transplanted kidney or there was the least folding of the renal vessels. I must admit that in most cases they succeeded in finding the best position, but the number of thromboses of the transplanted kidneys in such centers was on the borderline of the upper limit accepted by international organizations.

**And now a little anecdote:**

When I was abroad, I was watching a kidney transplant. After it was completed, I asked the surgeon if he had seen that the transplanted kidney's vessels were slightly tortuous before he closed the abdominal wall. The surgeon stated that it was just such a "momentary fold" and that the kidney will able to move and will "find" an optimal position in the retroperitoneal space where it will have an ideal inflow and outflow of blood to prevent graft thrombosis. Slightly irritated I asked him when this would happen. He replied that would happen within the next four hours after closing the abdominal wall. However, I kept annoying him with my questions and asked him why (already) his third kidney transplant had become thrombosed this month. He politely replied: "Because the kidney could not find a good position for itself".

**I have quoted Surgeon this here to warn potential transplant surgeons against this type of thinking: of making a positive interpretation of negative facts.**

### 4.9.3   Surgical Technique for Kidney Transplantation on the Right Side of the Pelvic Girdle

#### 4.9.3.1   Prepare the Right Iliac Vessels

The iliac vessels are completely freed around from the overlying tissues and lymphatic vessels. Enough length and depth of each vessel is needed for a proper clamp(s) placement and to perform vascular anastomosis.

#### 4.9.3.2   Preparing for Renal Vein Anastomosis

The dissected iliac artery or arteries are slightly moved with a thin renal vein retractor of the OmniTrac towards the midline. After one of the iliac arteries has been moved, check the pulse on the external iliac artery near the inguinal ligament and iliac internal artery. The pulse on the iliac arteries should be checked regularly and also during venous anastomosis. A too movement of the artery behind the retractor towards the midline and its pressing force may lead to a decrease or even stopping of the blood flow to the lower limb.

#### 4.9.3.3   Iliac Vein Clamping

If possible the right common iliac vein clamping is for me always a first choice (Fig. 4.29).

Some adult and a lot of pediatric kidney transplant surgeons prefer to give heparin intravenously at 50 IU/kg before placing a vascular clamp, though there are many who do not [36].

#### Administration of Heparin Before Vessel Clamping: Is It Really Necessary?

Renal graft thrombosis (RGT) is a serious complication after kidney transplantation and a major risk factor for impaired graft function and graft loss. Although RGT is rare, varying from 0.5 to 8.0%, it has high morbidity and mortality and accounts for up to 45% of graft loss in the first post-transplantation phase. Known risk factors for RGT are: donor age of less than 6 or more than 60 years; recipient age of less than 5 or more than 50 years; cold ischemic time (CIT) of more than 24 h; atherosclerosis in

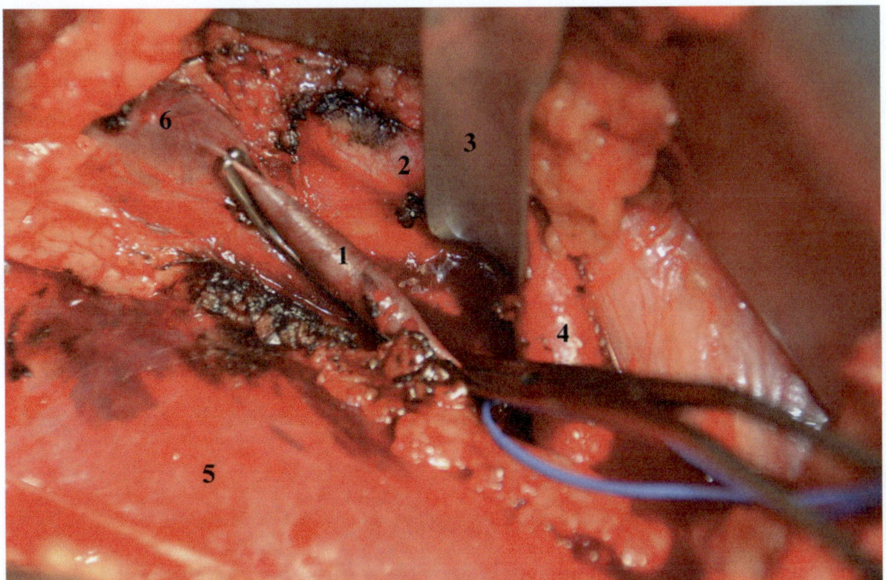

**Fig. 4.29**  1—Common iliac vein closed in the Satinsky vascular clamp, 2—Common iliac artery gently moved away with thin renal vein blade, 3—Thin renal vein blade is designed to gently pull the vessels, 4—External iliac artery, 5—Psoas major muscle, 6—IVC

the external iliac, common iliac or renal artery or the right donor kidneys; prior peritoneal dialysis; diabetes mellitus; previous thrombosis in the recipient; technical difficulties and hemodynamic instability during transplantation. RGT, deep venous thrombosis (DVT) and pulmonary embolisms (PE) are collectively known as thromboembolic complications (TEC) [34]. The incidence of TEC after kidney transplantation is reported to vary between 0.6 and 9.1% [34]. The wide ranges reported are because of the differences in study populations, with the highest incidences found in pediatric kidney transplantation and the lowest in studies involving living donor kidney transplantations. In the kidney transplantation population, the risk factors for DVT are age more than 40 years, diabetes mellitus, previous DVT and simultaneous pancreas–kidney transplantation. Since more elderly patients with higher comorbidity are being transplanted, the incidence of TEC is likely to increase. Primary RGT was related to presentation with delayed graft function (DGF) and was significantly associated with extrarenal TEC. There was no association between primary RGT and recipient's age; sex; number of previous transplants; type of dialysis; pretransplant treatment with erythropoietin, antiplatelet agents or oral anticoagulants; or donor's age, sex and number of graft vessels. In vascular surgery, intraoperative administration of heparin is common with the aim of avoiding thrombus formation at the anastomosis and clamp sites [35]. In kidney transplantation no consensus or protocol for antithrombotic prophylaxis exists. Therapeutic use of heparin increased the risk of bleeding among renal transplant recipients, but there were no cases of thrombosis. Prophylactic use of heparin did not increase the risk of bleeding and prevented proportionately more cases of thrombosis relative to no anticoagulation; this result supports the continued use of prophylaxis. Intraoperative heparin and antiplatelet therapy were not associated with increased bleeding risk. These regimens appear to be safe for the possible prevention of TEC without increasing the risk for bleeding after kidney transplantation [34, 35].

RGT is one of the main causes of early graft loss in pediatric kidney transplantation. Despite the lack of evidence-based recommendations, antithrombotic prophylaxis is used to prevent RGT, which occurs mostly within the first week following transplantation. The reported incidence of RGT varies between 2.3 and 5.1%, mainly due to differences in study populations and associated risk factors [36]. The risk of developing a thrombotic episode seems to be higher in pediatric than in adult renal transplantation. Hence, antithrombotic prophylaxis with anticoagulants and anti-platelets is widely used to prevent RGT in pediatric kidney transplantation [36].

**Arguments Against the Administration of Heparin Before Vessel Clamping**

*Introduction*

(a)  Heparin-induced thrombocytopenia (HIT).

HIT is an adverse drug reaction characterized by thrombocytopenia and a high risk of venous or arterial thrombosis. The frequency of HIT ranges from 1 to 5% of patients receiving heparin with exact frequencies ranging between specific agents. Interestingly, this immune-mediated syndrome is ironically associated with thrombosis, not bleeding, with thrombin formation playing a major role. It is caused by heparin-dependent, platelet-activating antibodies that identify a self-protein, PF4, bound to heparin that results in antibody formation. The resulting platelet activation is associated with increased thrombin generation. Typically, the platelet count fall begins 5–10 days after starting heparin, although a rapid platelet count fall can occur in a patient who has antibodies from recent heparin use [37].

HIT type II is an immunologically mediated reduction in platelets that increases the risk of arterial or venous thrombosis. Unlike other thrombocytopenic coagulopathies, HIT is associated with a high risk of thromboembolic events if not treated with an appropriate anticoagulant alternative. The diagnosis depends on the assessment of platelet reduction, identification of previous heparin exposure, detection of thrombotic complications and evaluation of laboratory assays. HIT has been well described in surgical patient populations; however, the abdominal organ transplant population is an exception. HIT should be included in the differential diagnosis of patients presenting with thrombocytopenia after transplantation in order to prevent or treat thrombotic complications that can pose a risk to patient or graft survival. Laboratory assays, such as platelet factor 4 (PF4) which is a small cytokine belonging to the CXC chemokine family that is also known as chemokine (C-X-C motif) ligand 4 (CXCL4 PF4 and SRA, aid in the diagnosis, but cannot provide absolute certainty about the presence of HIT antibodies or their association with clinical HIT. Appropriate treatment includes avoidance of heparin, administration of a DTI and proper transition to long-term oral anticoagulation [38]. HIT II—especially in combination with TEC—represents a medical-economic burden for the hospital. Although this is only an orientation guide, it shows that HIT II syndrome is not adequately cost-covered by the G DRG (diagnosis-related groups) system. An early thrombosis prophylaxis with argatroban/danaparoid for HIT II risk patients should therefore be taken into account for medical-related as well as patient safety-relevant aspects. From experience, the pharmaceutical supply for these medically needed products (anticoagulants) should be ensured for reasons of patient safety [38].

(b)  Coagulation disorders in uremia—the most common—impaired platelet function

The association between kidney dysfunction and bleeding was made more than 200 years ago. However, there remains an incomplete understanding of the underlying pathophysiology. Impaired platelet function is one of the main determinants of uremic bleeding. This impairment is due to largely and incompletely defined inhibitors of the platelet function in the plasma of patients with markedly reduced kidney function. An increased bleeding risk has been described for patients with an end-stage renal disease. Bleeding occurs in about 50% of patients with an end-stage renal disease reaching from minor events, such as bruises and bleeding at venipuncture sites, to menorrhagia, gastrointestinal blood loss, severe perioperative bleeding and retroperitoneal as well as intracranial hemorrhage. Bleeding can significantly contribute to mortality and morbidity and blood transfusions can lead to alloimmunization and thereby limit options for transplantation [39].

Although predisposition to bleeding seems obvious, recommendations for risk determination are missing as no single factor or test has been established to detect individual bleeding risk in patients with an end-stage renal disease [39].

### Conclusion

Chronic kidney disease (CKD), acute kidney injury (AKI) and nephrotic syndrome (NS) are called renal diseases in which hypercoagulation prevails (and which lead to an increased risk of deep vein, renal vein and/or arterial thrombosis). Antiphospholipid syndrome (APS), due to which the autoantibodies are directed against phospholipid-binding proteins, is associated with a high risk of vascular thrombosis. Based on the literature it is not clear, though it seems one can find some strong suggestions, that in kidney recipients at medium and high risk of thrombosis, perioperative anticoagulation therapy has its scientific justification and in many cases is advisable/indicated [34–39].

### Vessel Clamping With or Without Heparin: Vein is Clamped First

If necessary, heparinization of the patient should be performed five minutes before closing one of the iliac veins to prevent thrombosis. Heparin has a half-life of 1.0 to 1.5 hours and lasts approximately 3 to 4 hours. Adequate anticoagulation can be followed with activated clotting time (ACT). For peripheral vascular operations, an ACT in the 250 to 350 second range is adequate [40].

If you have given intravenous heparin before inserting a clamp, wait five minutes before closing the vessel. Remember that heparin needs five minutes to fully work in the human body.

Depending on the predetermined best place for the renal vein anastomosis, grasp the already gently prepared iliac vein with forceps and carry it slightly upwards and then with the help of a Satinsky vascular clamp close the vein partially along its long axis. Assure that during the vein clamping with the Statinsky clamp only IVC or one of the iliac vein is being clamped (selectively partial closure) and not the vein together with all surrounding tissues. Closing the lumen of the vein with the surrounding tissue will result in inadequate closure of the vein and when the vein is cut for anastomosis, the area will bleed, making the anastomosis difficult to perform or forcing the operator to correct the position of the vascular clamp closing the vein. Clamping the IVC and/or one of the iliac veins which is not well dissected from the surrounding tissues will be responsible for bleeding after venotomy, because the vein with too much tissue around it will not be properly closed. The place on the right side for the renal vein anastomosis may include a segment from the IVC up to the end of the section of the external iliac vein which ends at the level of the inguinal ligament. In our case the right common iliac vein appears to be the fastest accessible and the most exposed place for the renal vein anastomosis. After clamping, use the sterile scalpel with surgical blade No. 15 or 11 on the top of the bulge of the closed common iliac vein wall, and make a 3–4 mm incision along its long axis. After opening the vein and suction of blood, rinse the vein lumen from inside out with a 0.9% NaCl (Natrium Chloride) with heparin. Then the wall of the common iliac vein is further cut lengthwise with vascular scissors (angled scissors) —the vein is cut to the width of the renal vein diameter (Fig. 4.30). I recommend

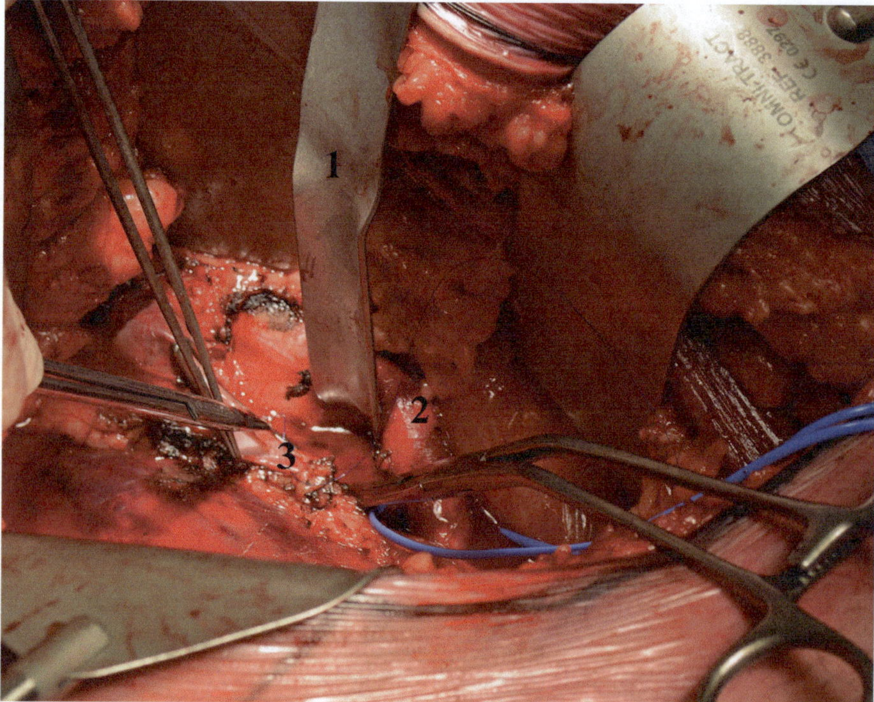

**Fig. 4.30** Before applying the stay suture which will be pulling the medial vein wall towards the middle line. 1—Thin renal vein blade has been designed for gently pulling the vessels, 2—Pulled by the renal vein blade inwards to the common iliac artery, 3—The wall of the common iliac vein is cut lengthwise with vascular scissors. The length of the incision of the common iliac vein is slightly 2.0–3.0 mm longer than the circumference of the renal vein

that the incision in a partially clamped iliac vein should be 2–3 mm larger than the diameter of the renal vein. Some authors suggest making the venotomy in the IVC or one or the iliac veins 10–15% larger than the diameter of the renal vein [1–4].

**Warning!**

A.  Do not close the arteries before completing the venous anastomosis.
B.  The diameter of a renal vein can be measured by very gently placing the jaws of closed vascular forceps inside the renal vein (3–4 mm above the renal vein outlet), which is then opened very slowly until the resistance of the vein wall is reached. The distance between the ends of the jaws' of the vascular forceps will determine the diameter of the renal vein.

In the middle of the medial wall of the right common iliac vein place a non-absorbable auxiliary or stay suture 5/0 (Fig. 4.31). This suture is pulled towards the left side of the recipient's midline and fixed at the end with a delicate, "jaws armed" (Suture-Boots), small vascular clamp.

**Warning!**
Suture-Boots™ small surgical clamp jaws are special plastic covers which are designed to hold the finest suture without damage or slippage. Covers during operation are placed on the instrument's jaws in order to prevent cutting, crushing and thus weakening of the surgical sutures (Fig. 3.44).

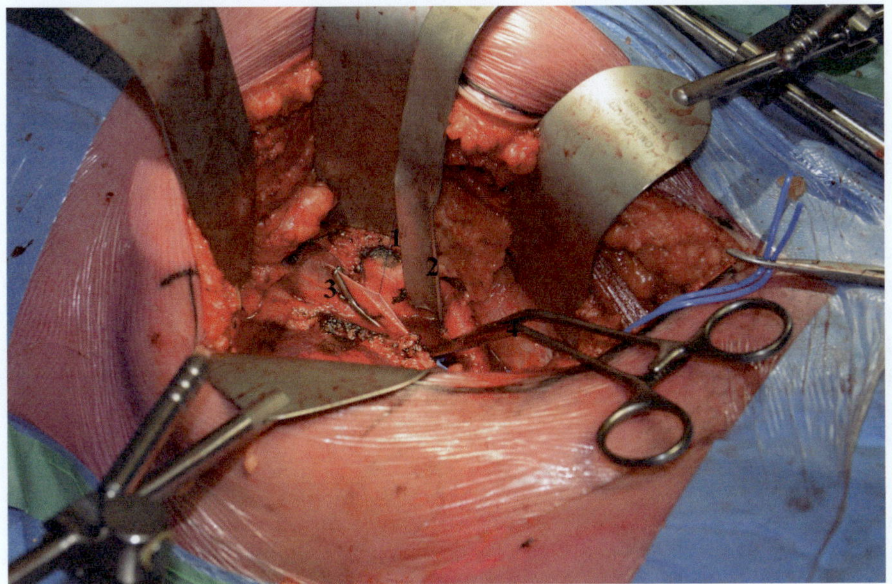

**Fig. 4.31** 1—Stay suture pulling medial wall of the right common iliac vein to the left side, 2—Renal vein thin blade pulling the common iliac artery to the left side, 3—Closed with vascular clamp common iliac vein with placed on the medial wall stay suture, 4—Satinsky vascular clamp closed along the long axis

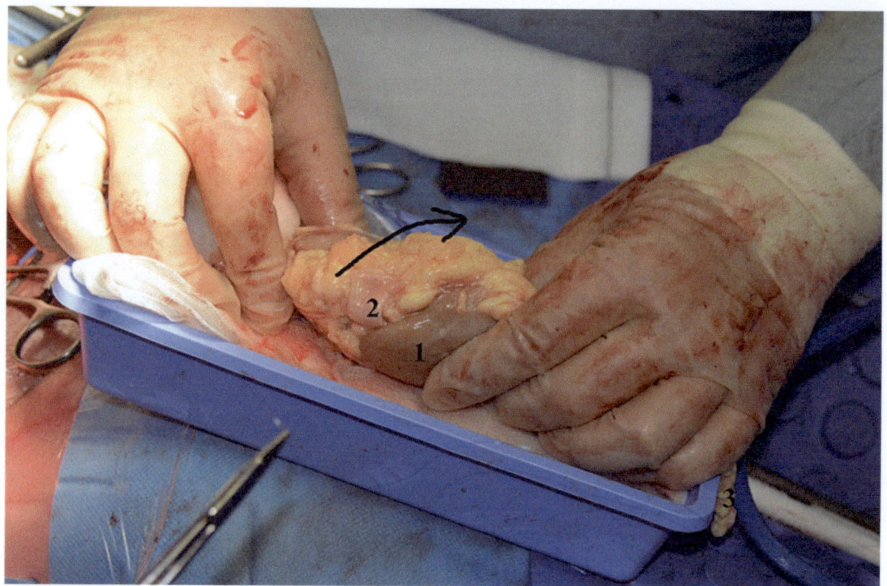

**Fig. 4.32** Positioning the kidney in its container before transplantation. The arrow indicates that the kidney will be rotated to the left in the recipient's body. 1—Kidney, 2—Renal vein, 3—Ureter is turned down

## Detailed Description of the Surgical Techniques for Venous Anastomosis

*Putting the kidney in a container in the right position*

In a container with ice and cold organ preservation solution, the kidney is positioned as it will be transplanated into the retroperitoneal space, that is with the ureter downwards (sometimes the ureter is being transplanted upwards in the absence of a bladder or if a Bricker's method is used, i.e. the ureter is implanted into an isolated loop of the small intestine) (Fig. 4.32). There are a number of surgical techniques describing renal vein anastomosis to the IVC or one of the iliac veins. Here I describe a surgical technique to anastomose a renal vein to IVC or one of the iliac veins, which I perform myself.

## Renal Vein Corner Sutures

Venous anastomosis of the renal vein end to side of the IVC or one of the iliac veins is usually performed with the use of two monofilament, unabsorbable 5/0 or 6/0 sutures. Each suture is armed with two needles. The assistant is asked to provide a good visualization of the renal vein and its corners. If the assistant is not experienced, the operator slowly injects heparin-saline solution into the lumen of the renal vein to establish the physiological position of the renal vein. After filling the renal vein lumen, the end of the renal vein is closed with a small vascular clamp approximately 10 mm from the end of the renal vein lumen. The assistant now

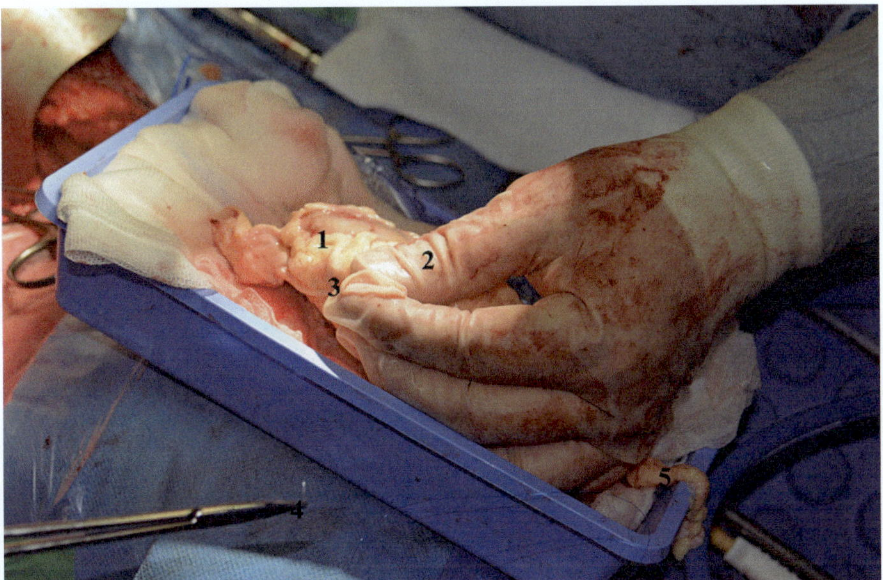

**Fig. 4.33** Renal vein without corner sutures; inexperienced assistance. The operator had to trace the correct position of the renal vein himself and stabilized it between the fingers of his left hand. This is the moment where two non-absorbable monofilament sutures will connect the superior and inferior corner of the renal vein with the superior and inferior corner of the opening in the common iliac vein. 1—Kidney, 2—Surgeon's fingers holding the renal vein in the correct position (not twisted), 3—Superior corner of the renal vein, 4—Needle holder ready to pierce the needle in the superior corner of the renal vein, 5—Ureter turned down

grasps the right and left parts of the renal vein wall with two forceps so that the wall length is the same on both sides. The vein is now taken over by the surgeon and held between the thumb and forefinger of the left hand (Fig. 4.33). This position of the end of the renal vein makes it possible to distinguish the position of its wall in the lower corner (ureter side), the upper corner (upper pole side) of the kidney and the two walls of the renal vein anterior and posterior.

*Vena iliaca corner sutures*

Move the container with the kidney, ice and preservation solution as close as possible to the retroperitoneal space and right iliac vessels. The assistant's task is to keep the container with the kidney placed in the physiological position as close as possible to the right iliac vessels. A surgical needle with an non absorb-able suture 5/0 is used to pierce the suture of the upper corner of the renal vein from the outside to the inside or vice versa. It is important to remember that after piercing the wall of the upper corner of the ICV or one of the iliac veins, the suture should be tied to the outside. The second suture is placed in the same way—the inferior corner of the renal vein is pierced. Both ends of this suture are fixed outside the operating field, 5 cm before the needles, with small vascular clamps. In the same way, the inferior

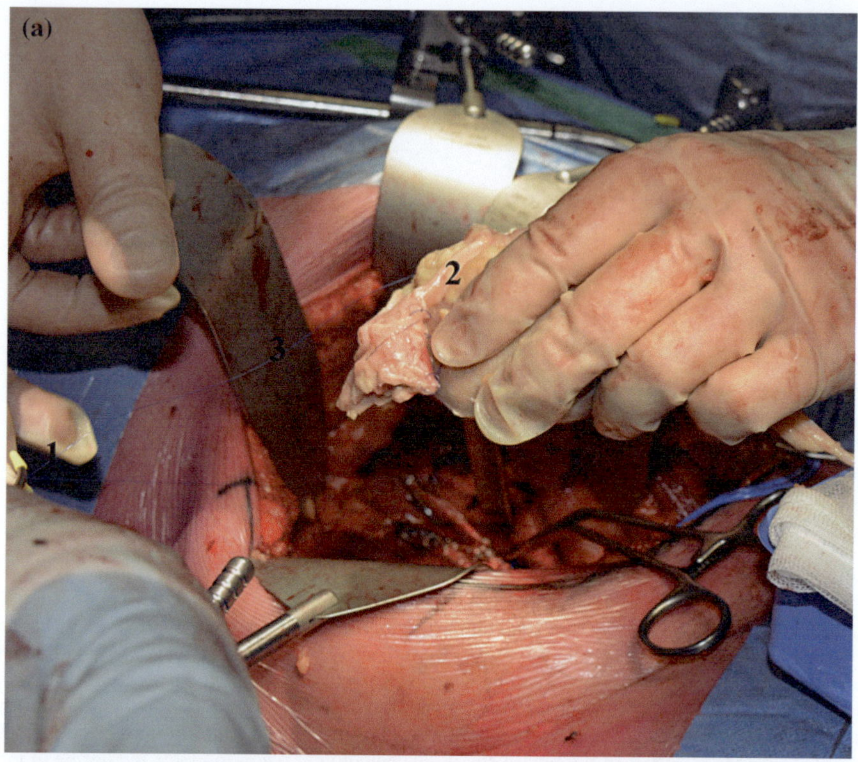

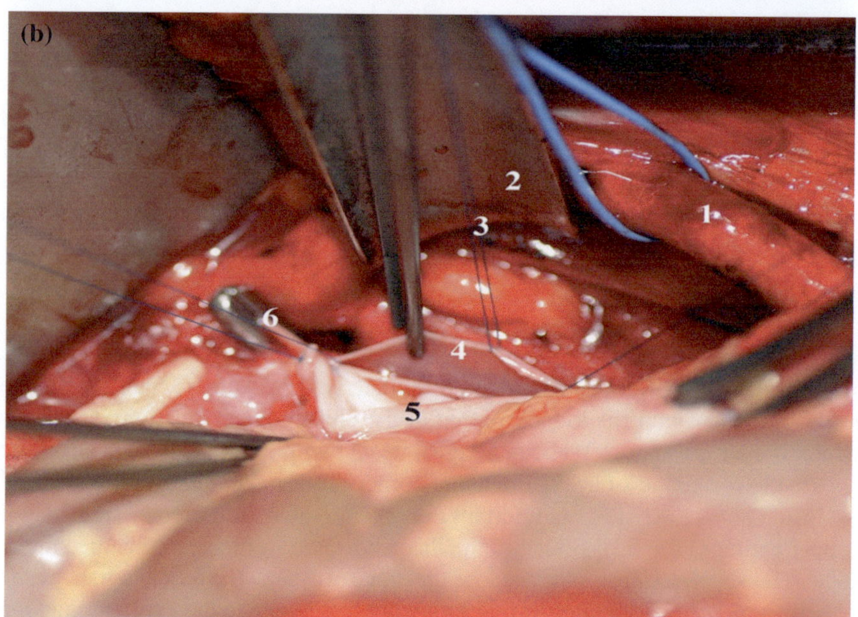

◄**Fig. 4.34** (a) By the assistant gently pulling both corner sutures, and by the surgeon gently moving the kidney towards the retroperitoneal space, the kidney will be correctly positioned in the extraperitoneal space. 1—Surgical suture connecting both superior corners of the venous anastomosis: picture shows the ends of the suture is fastened with a special small jaw covered vascular clamp, 2—Kidney, 3—Blade of the abdominal retractor. (**b**) 1—Common iliac artery gently pulled inwards by the thin blade of the renal vein retractor, 2—Blade of the "renal vein" retractor, 3— Stay suture pulling the medial common iliac vein wall inwards to the left side, 4— The anterior wall of the common iliac vein, which is closed with a vascular clamp, is opened with a visible stay suture, so that the walls of the common iliac vein, which is cut along its axis, are not glued together. Anterior wall is cut off to the left with and suture, the lumen of the dissected vein is perfectly visible, which greatly facilitates correct anastomosis, 5—Renal vein, 6—Satinsky vascular clamp and superior corner suture

corners of the renal and iliac vein are connected with the second suture whose ends are also fixed outside the operation field.

*Final kidney position*

Keep the same kidney graft position during the veneus, arterial and ureteral anastomosis. Try to not change the position of the kidney over time. Venous anastomosis is made by using two non-absorbable vascular sutures that connect the two upper and lower corners of the renal and iliac vein with each other. Because the posterior wall is sewn from the intraluminal space of the anastomosis site, this technique avoids any possibility of the posterior or anterior wall being caught up in the suture line. [41].

Then the assistant very gently grasps the clamps that are fixed on the sutures connected to the superior and the inferior corners and pulls them slightly up and towards himself/herself. At the same time, the surgeon takes the kidney out of the container and goes very slowly with it towards the iliac fossa and anastomosis side. The assistant begins to lightly pull both stitches fastened with small clamps, and at this point the renal vein is very slightly strained. The operator slowly positions the kidney towards the retroperitoneal space in the previously determined best place for end to side anastomosis. The operator puts the kidney then in the correct position on the psoas muscles (Fig. 4.34a, b). Now the assistant stretches the superior and inferior sutures slightly and the edges of the renal vein wall contact (kiss) the edges of the iliac vein wall; the renal vein is slightly stretched, the kidney is already placed and positioned in the lumbar region. When the kidney is properly positioned, the corner sutures are stretched so that the posterior wall of the renal vein is against the posterior wall of the iliac vein at the anastomosis site (Fig. 4.35).

End-to-side anastomosis of the renal vein to the inferior vena cava (IVC) or one of the iliac veins, anastomosis of the posterior wall of the IVC or one of the iliac veins from the inside of both veins. Two non-absorbable sutures are used to create the anastomosis. The sutures are passed through the upper and lower corners of both veins. The upper suture is tied off and the lower suture is used to pull the renal vein so that its posterior wall is closely attached to the posterior wall of the IVC or one of the iliac veins. The anastomosis is performed with one of the half sutures tied at the upper corner (Fig. 4.36).

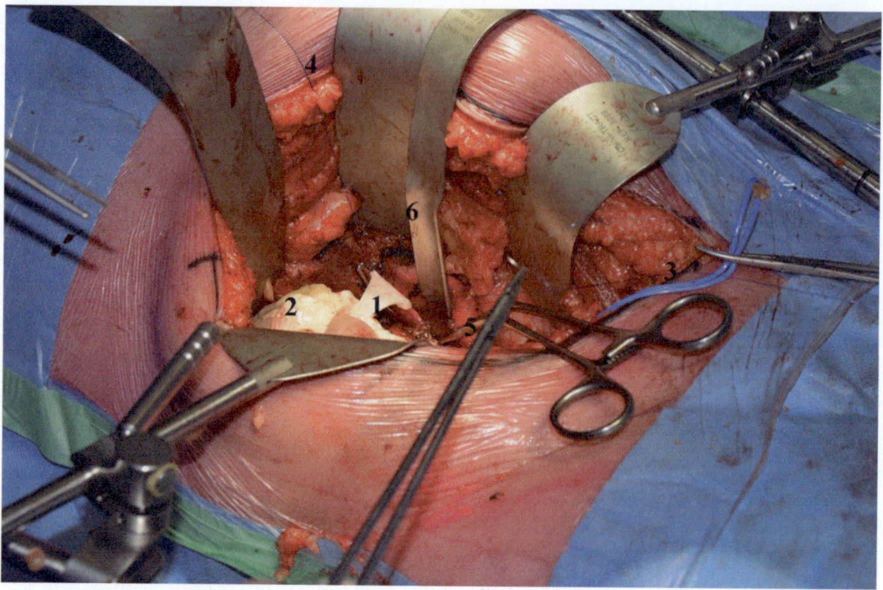

**Fig. 4.35** The vascular sutures placed on the superior and inferior anastomotic corners are now slightly stretched by the assistant at this point. The diameter of the renal vein opening must be the same or slightly smaller than that made in the common iliac vein. 1—Renal vein, 2—Kidney, 3—Untied suture connection of the lower corners of this anastomosis fixed with small vascular clamp on its ends and kept under slight tension, 4—Two tightly connected superior corner sutures (if you have enough surgical skills you can try to perform venous anastomosis without tying the superior corners suture), 5—Satinsky vascular clamp, 6—Renal vein thin blade pulling the common iliac artery inward

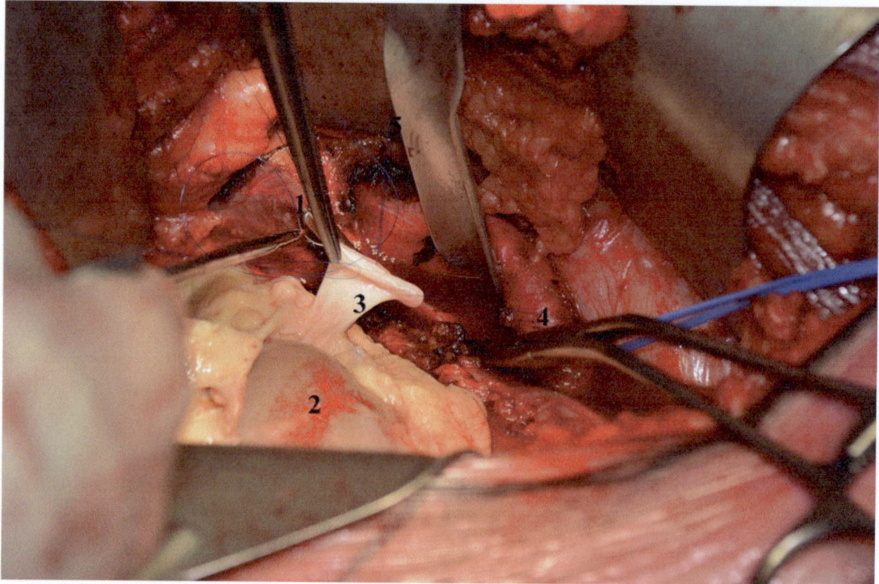

**Fig. 4.36** The anastomosis begins with tying (or not) the surgical suture placed on the superior corner of the renal and common iliac vein, 1—Half of the suture is pierced with a needle from the outside to the inside through the wall of the renal vein, 2—Kidney, 3—Renal vein under slight tension, 4—Right common iliac artery, 5—Thin, narrow renal vein blade gently pulling to the right common iliac artery

The second half of the upper suture is then fixed with a clamp with jaw cover. Next, take the needle of the unattached superior suture in the needle holder and insert the needle from the outside to the inside of the renal vein. Pierce the wall of the renal vein from the outside to the inside with the needle so that it and the suture are inside the lumen of the renal vein, very close to the upper corner. If a seam has a knot or if it is not knotted and if both parts of the suture should be of the same length when sewing. Then the second half of the superior suture is fixed with a clamp and the other half-suture from the superior corner. Take it in the needle holder and place the needle from the outside to the inside of the renal vein. Pierce the renal vein wall from the outside to the inside with the needle so that it and the suture are inside the lumen of the renal vein and very close to the superior corner. The anastomosis of the posterior venous walls is made from the inside; the needle is inserted every 1.5–2.0 mm, touching the back walls of both veins in the vascular suture (Figs. 4.37 and 4.38). An assistant guides the suture by holding it between the index finger and thumb. While sewing from the inside, the assistant tightens the suture and at the same time pulls it up gently so that the sewing line converts to the lumens of both stitched veins. The inferior suture corner is not tied but only stretched towards and along the external iliac vein during the anastomosis by the scrub nurse. The lower corner suture should be stretched, so that the back walls of the anastomosis are in full contact with each other ("they are kissing together"). If you are at the level of the inferior corner sewing

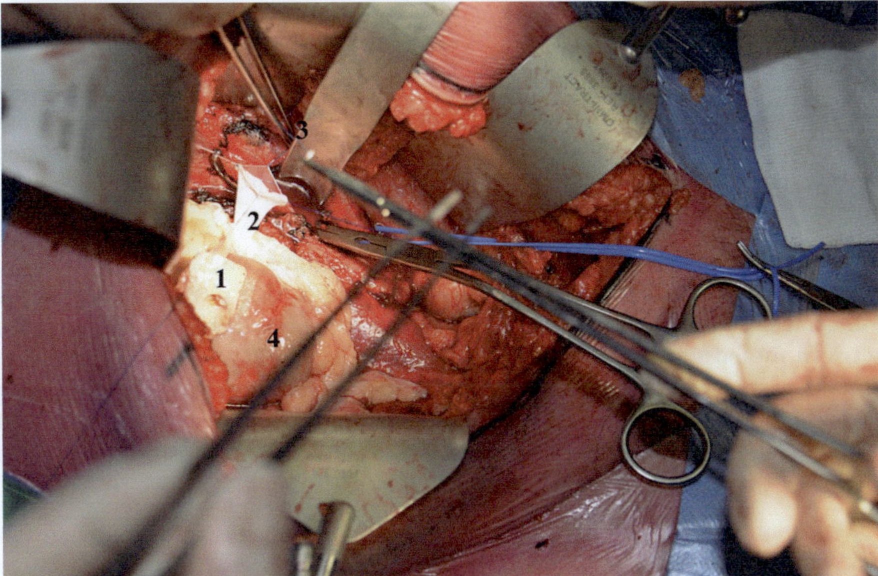

**Fig. 4.37** Needle and suture have pierced inside the lumen of the renal vein close to the superior corner of the renal and iliac vein: from now the anastomosis between the renal vein and the common iliac vein is performed from the inside. The kidney is placed in a fixed position. After venous anastomosis the kidney can be moved anywhere and the operator will not seek the best position for it. 1—Renal artery, 2—Renal vein, 3—Stay suture pulling the middle wall of the common iliac vein to the left side, 4—Kidney

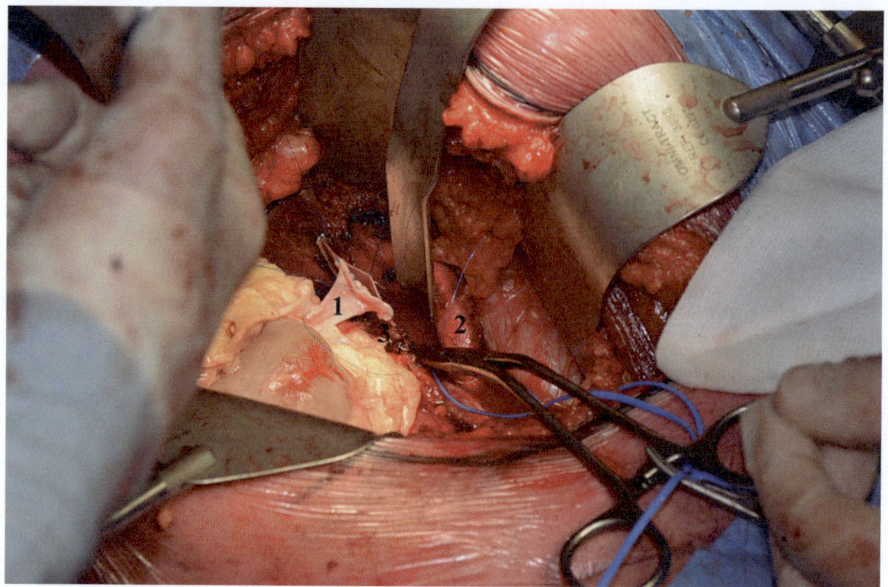

**Fig. 4.38** Posterior side of vascular anastomosis between the posterior walls of the renal and common iliac vein has been performed. 1—Renal vein, 2—Common iliac artery, 3—Inferior corner of anastomosis

with a continuous suture, you can do two things: you can remove the inferior corner suture or tie it and fix it outside the operation field. The sutures are continued until they meet on the anterior wall of the renal and iliac vein. The same end to side veno-venous anastomosis can be performed without tying any suture, but during suturing by pulling and holding the renal vein under tension.

**End to side renal vein anastomosis with one suture, one knot - parachute technique; detailed description. Veno-venous end to side parachute technique with anastomosis from the inside: during the anastomosis, the distance between the posterior walls of the renal vein and the IVC, or one of the iliac veins is preserved. This means that when they are sewn together, their backs walls do not stick to each other as tightly as they should as with the classical technique described above. In parachute technique no suture is used that fixes the lower corners of the renal and IVC, of one of the iliac veins.**

The superior corner suture is placed from the outside to the inside of the renal vein and with another needle from the inside to the outside of the iliac vein. The suture that comes out of the superior corner of the iliac vein is pulled and fixed with a small clamp outside the operating field. This means that in the middle of the renal vein lumen there is a suture near the superior corner. In this case, the suture was not placed on the inferior corners of the renal and iliac veins. This parachute anastomosis is performed as follows. First the stitch from the superior corner is already inside the renal vein; the sutured suture was not tied and very loosely sutured in the posterior wall of the veins by the continuous intra-luminal anastomosis. After suturing the posterior wall, each suture was pulled towards the other side along the orifice and then the anastomosis of the posterior wall was accomplished. Another superior needle suture was used for suturing the anterior wall. Before both sutures were finally loosely tied, the renal and iliac veins were rinsed with heparinized 10–30 ml 0.9% saline chloride solution. For the last time the physiologic position and anastomosis of the renal vein were checked.

The technique of end-to-side anastomosis of the renal vein to the external iliac vein consists of the one suture and one knot. The same method can be used for end-to-end or end-to-side anastomosis of the renal artery, with or without spatulation. The anastomosis begins with an in–out and out-in suture at one corner of the venotomy incision. Then, the posterior wall is sutured in a running fashion from the intraluminal space of the external iliac vein. After finishing the anastomosis of the posterior wall, the anterior wall is sewn with the same suture material while pulling the edge of the graft side and the recipient's side. This is done without putting any knot at the other corner of the venotomy incision. Finally, the anastomosis is finished at the start point. After the last suture, both ends of the suture material are pulled gently, though making the knot is delayed until the unclamping of the external iliac vein (or the artery, in the case of an arterial anastomosis). This permits the anastomosis site to become expanded to its widest size, and prevents a purse-string effect at the anastomosis site [41].

**Warning! (I consider my vein anastomosis technique the best)**
The correct execution of a renal vein anastomosis with the parachute and one-suture, one-knot surgical technique requires experience and very good surgical skills and a quite an experienced assistant. In the one-knot surgical technique, the lower corners of the vascular anastomosis are not joined by a surgical suture so that the edges of the veins cannot be arranged in such a way that they adhere to each other when the suture is pulled. While sewing, pull the renal vein with forceps down for each stab, especially when sewing the back wall; if you do not do this you can easily narrow the anastomosis. With the second inferior corner suture, the posterior walls of the renal vein and the illiac vein kiss each other which gives the surgeon the possibility to focus on the sewing and not pulling the renal vein downwards. I personally like and prefer this technique of anastomosis.

**Warning! (The last inspection of the position of the renal vein)**
If we are not yet sure of the physiological position of the renal vein, to avoid a technical error, you can inject 0.9% natrium chloride solution with heparin into the lumen of the vein and observe how it fills and whether it is twisted or bent, which would mean that it is too long. You have to follow the renal vein from the anastomosis up to the renal hilum. If the venous anastomosis is ready and tied, then you have no access to inject the heparinized solution into the renal vein. Another solution is to slowly inject the heparinized solution into the renal artery, and then to observe the behavior and positioning of the renal vein under the influence of the injected solution (it is very important not to twist the vein and implant it too long, because then it will bend). When performing the anastomosis, I check the position of the renal vein two to three times so as to be 100% sure that the vein is not twisted

and does not bend after releasing the vascular clamp. If it is too long, cut and shorten it. Remember that, theoretically, with complete closure of the anastomosis, the kidney and also the renal vein may simply rupture when the vascular clamps are released.

**Warning!**

The best hemodynamically end-to-side vascular anastomosis between two vessels is when an angle of 90 degrees is maintained between the anastomosed vessels [86].

**Warning!**

I know that there are a few surgical techniques for veno-venous end-to-side anastomosis, and that I have demonstrated only two. I believe that the demonstrated techniques are the quickest, the easiest to learn and, in my opinion, a very small number of mistakes are made when performing them.

## *4.9.4  Arterial Anastomosis: The Renal Artery with the Iliac Artery End to Side*

### 4.9.4.1  Introduction

Kidney transplant is the treatment of choice for most cases of end-stage renal disease. Transplant surgeons use different techniques for arterial and venous anastomoses in the recipients. In 1902, Carrel described a three-point anastomosis technique for allograft arterial anastomosis. Since then, others have described a two-point anastomosis, a four-quadrant technique, a corner-saving technique, a non-suture technique and other methods for vascular anastomoses. Most of these techniques were invented to reduce the warm ischemic time of the allograft to the minimum, while providing good patency, especially in the case of arterial anastomoses [2, 41–50].

The renal arteries carry a large portion of the total blood flow to the kidneys. Up to a third of the total cardiac output can pass through the renal arteries to be filtered by the kidneys. In the physiology of the kidney, RBF is the volume of blood delivered to the kidneys per unit time. In humans, RBF is about 1.0–1.3 L/min. This constitutes 20–25% of the resting cardiac output through tissue that constitutes less than 0.5% of the body mass. Considering that the volume of each kidney is less than 150 ml, this means that each kidney is perfused with over three times its total volume every minute. It passes about 94% to the cortex [49, 50].

Mital et al. in 1996 performed arterial and venous anastomoses in a kidney recipient using four-stay sutures and several vascular clips for each anastomosis. The time taken for each anastomosis was 8 min, and the authors concluded that it was a safe, easy and rapid method for a renal vascular anastomosis [50].

Haberal et al. used a corner-saving technique for the arterial anastomosis of allograft kidneys in 183 recipients. In only one patient was renal arterial stenosis

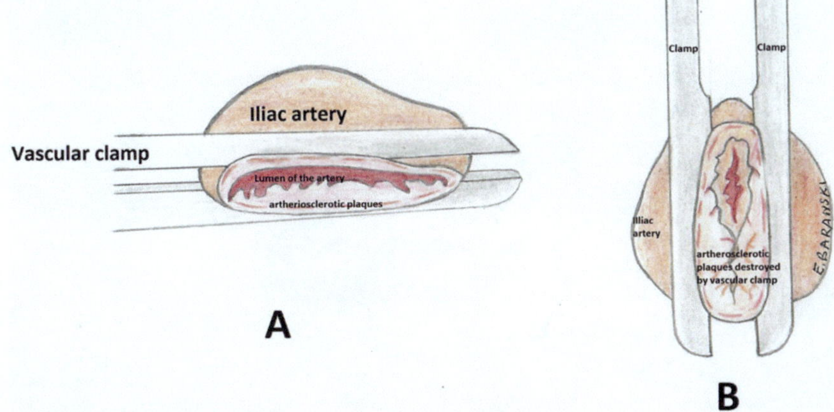


**Fig. 4.39** (**A**) The atherosclerotic plaques are usually located dorsally in the artery. The clamp should be placed horizontally to avoid plaque injury (fracture and/or fragmentation). (**B**) Atherosclerotic plaques located dorsally with a vascular clamp placed vertically and closed without any artery examination. Artery injured—fractured and fragmented atherosclerotic plaque located dorsally. To avoid such an injury first locate the position of the atherosclerotic plaque (dorsally, aslant—inclined or twisted to one side or vertically—in a vertical direction). Vertically and aslant are semantically related across topics. In some cases you can use "vertically" instead of the adjective "aslant"

seen, and no case of arterial thrombosis was encountered. They concluded that this technique was a safe and which, when applied, has reduced the number of vascular complications [46, 48].

Atherosclerotic plaques are usually located dorsally in the artery. The clamp should be placed horizontally to avoid plaque fracture and/or fragmentation (Fig. 4.39).

The preferred arterial anastomosis is end to end or end to side between the renal artery and the other artery, which is made at the end of the renal artery to the end of the iliac internal artery. This kind of arterial anastomosis carries a lower incidence of stenosis.

### 4.9.4.2  Renal Artery Anastomosis with the One-suture, one-knot, Parachute Technique Is Also Preferred by the Author: Detailed Description of the Best Technique for the Artery

During venous anastomosis, the iliac arteries are totally dissected from the retroperitonal space and gently pulled medially with the aid of the renal vein thin blade (one of the retractor's blades). During arterial anastomosis, the iliac arteries are released from the renal vein thin blade and returned to their physiological

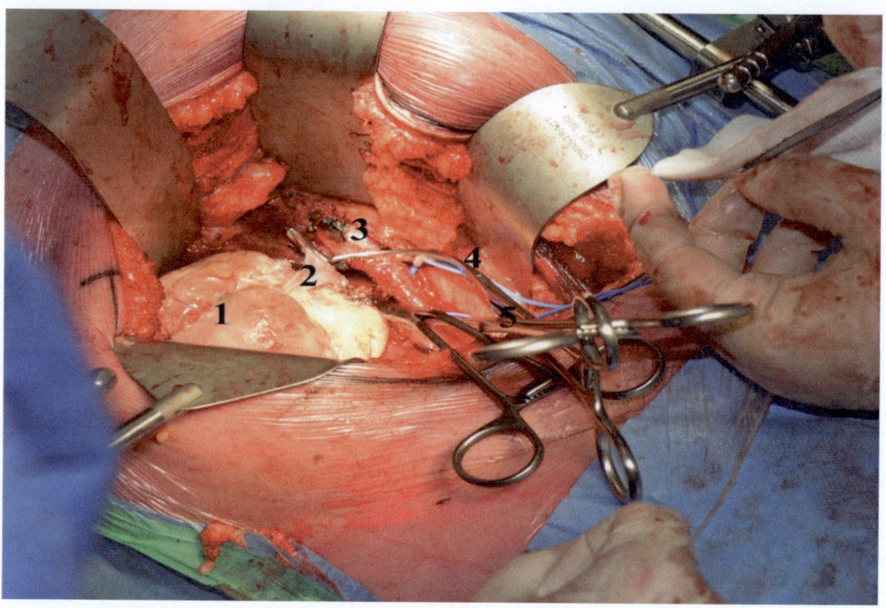

**Fig. 4.40** The iliac artery is closed with two soft vascular clamps. 1—Kidney, 2—Completed and checked venous anastomosis, 3—Common iliac artery, 4—Placed in horizontal position at the beginning of the common iliac artery and not affected by the arteriosclerosis vascular clamp, 5—Closed in the vertical position and placed in the distal part on the common iliac artery vascular clamp

position. Before the anastomosis the iliac arteries are completely freed from the retroperitoneum, examined by delicate palpation for having calcifications and are marked with "vessel loop(s)". The best place for arterial anastomosis between the renal artery and one of the iliac arteries or the abdominal aorta has already been selected and are marked. The soft vascular clamps have been placed horizontally above and below the previously designated place for the renal artery anastomosis (Fig. 4.40). After closing the clamps, check by palpation the artery pulsation below the proximal clamp. If the artery is well closed with the clamp(s), you cannot feel the pulsations or blood flow below the vascular clamp which is closed the lowest on one of the iliac arteries. The renal artery is very gently rinsed with heparinized saline to check its position and how it will arrange itself after releasing the vascular clamps. The next step is to measure the length of the renal artery to the site of the anastomosis (Fig. 4.41); if the artery is too long and there is a necessary need, we shorten it with very sharp scissors (Fig. 4.42). The renal artery should be anastomosed with a little tension, should be as short as possible, ideally positioned, and

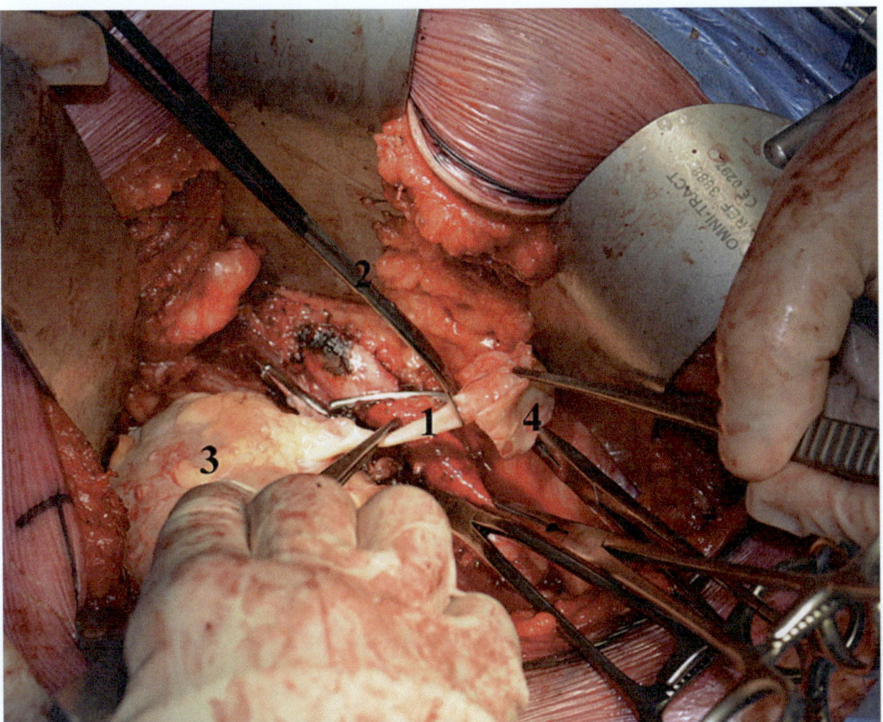

**Fig. 4.41** Shortening the length of the renal artery to the desired length. 1—Renal artery, 2—Sharp scissors, 3—Kidney, 4—In this case, the end of the renal artery is narrowed. The narrowing consists of an atherosclerotic plaque and occurs 1.5 cm from where the renal artery enters the aorta. The rest of the renal artery is of very good quality. Before the renal artery is anastomosed to one of the iliac arteries, the aortic patch and the first 2 cm of the renal artery are cut off. The remaining part of the renal artery is healthy and will be anastomosed end-to-end to the common iliac artery in the next step patch

not twisted. The best hemodynamically end-to-side anastomosis is one made at a 90 degree angle. Personally I cut the renal artery 2–3 mm from the anastomotic site (Fig. 4.42). The iliac artery is now punctured with a No. 15 or 11 scalpel over a length of 4–5 mm and flushed with cold heparinized saline. Then the aortic punch is introduced into the lumen of the artery (Fig. 4.43). This is a disposable tool that cuts straight, oval holes. You can choose to use it, depending on the renal artery's diameter from 2 to 8 mm [46]. Personally, I use a 4 mm. Using a cutter, cut an oval opening in the wall of the iliac artery, and rinse the lumen with a physiological saline solution with heparin. Depending on the diameter of the artery, I always use the cutter once or twice if I want to enlarge the first cut by 2–3 mm. Sometimes the

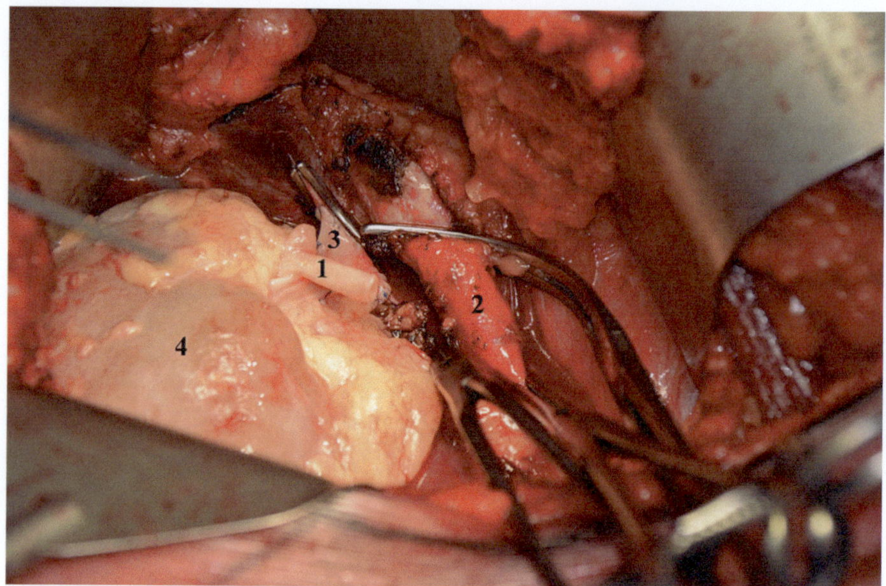

**Fig. 4.42** 1—Shortened renal artery, 2—Common iliac artery, 3—Venous anastomosis, 4—Kidney

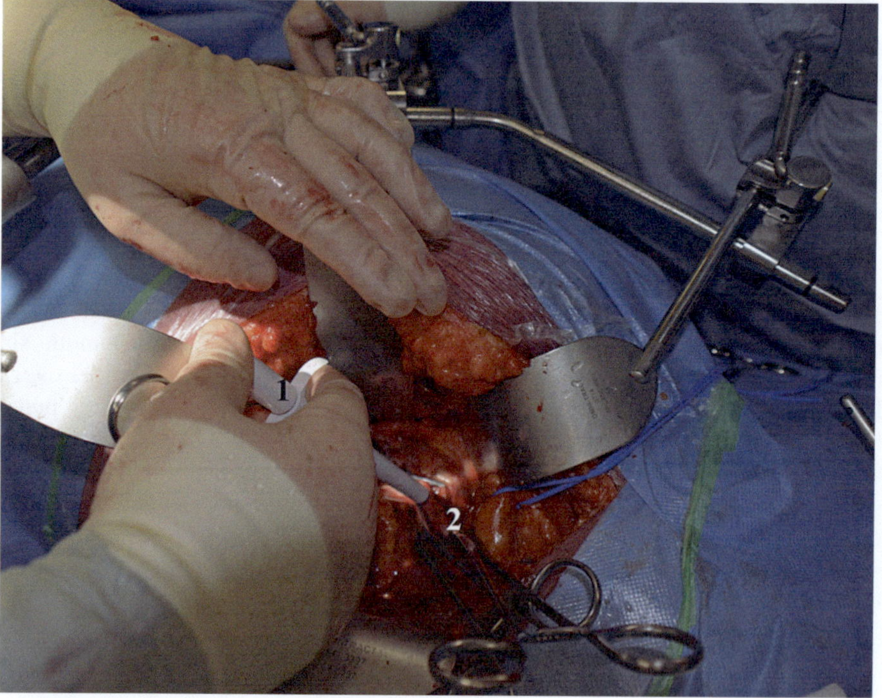

**Fig. 4.43** 1—Punch inside the lumen of the common iliac artery: a circular cutter to cut a perfect hole in the artery with a diameter of 4 mm, 2—Iliac artery

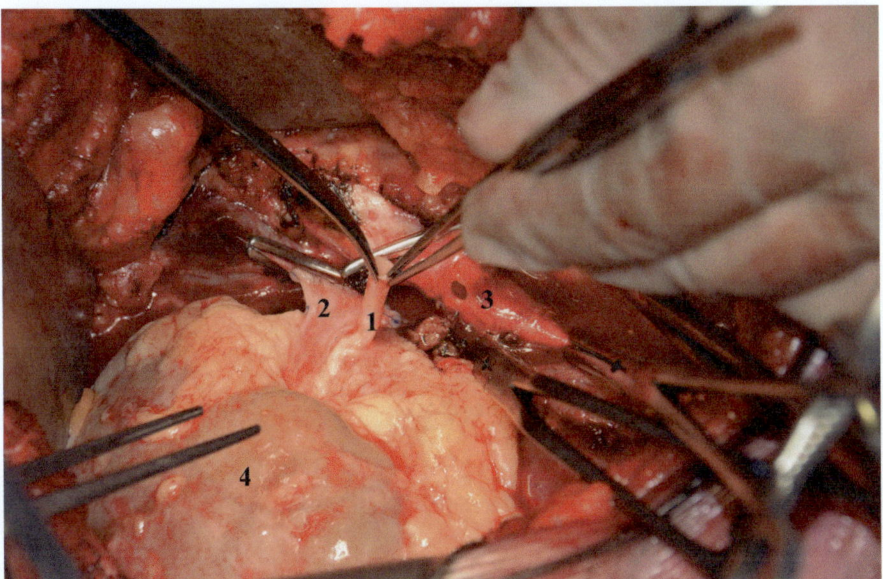

**Fig. 4.44**  1—The renal artery wall slightly incised (spatulated) to enlarge the diameter of its anastomosis, 2—Completed venous anastomosis: renal vein, 3—Oval opening in the common iliac artery made with a cutter, 4—Kidney

diameter of the cut hole in the iliac artery is larger than the diameter of the renal artery. To solve this problem, I cut the renal artery wall 2–3 mm towards the renal hilum (Fig. 4.44). I do this in almost every transplant to avoid the renal artery and its anastomosis stenosis at the anastomosis place. Now we ask the scrub nurse for a needle holder with a vascular suture (Fig. 4.45). For renal artery anastomosis, I always use one thin unabsorbed monofilament suture at least 6/0 or 7/0 depending on the diameter and quality of the renal artery. I start the vascular anastomosis by inserting both needles one by one from the inside to the outside into the superior corner of the punched hole [46]. This is like two halves of the same suture extended outside the illiac artery: the distance between the two, separated surgical sutures is about 2 mm. The ends of a suture are not tied. On the medial or left suture a small vessel clamp arm is fastened. This half-suture is placed outside the retroperitoneal space towards the left side of the recipient under a little tension. The needle from the operator's side is inserted from the outside to the inside into the superior corner of the renal artery. This is a parachute anastomosis, so it is performed at a certain distance from the walls of the renal and iliac arteries. After almost half of the

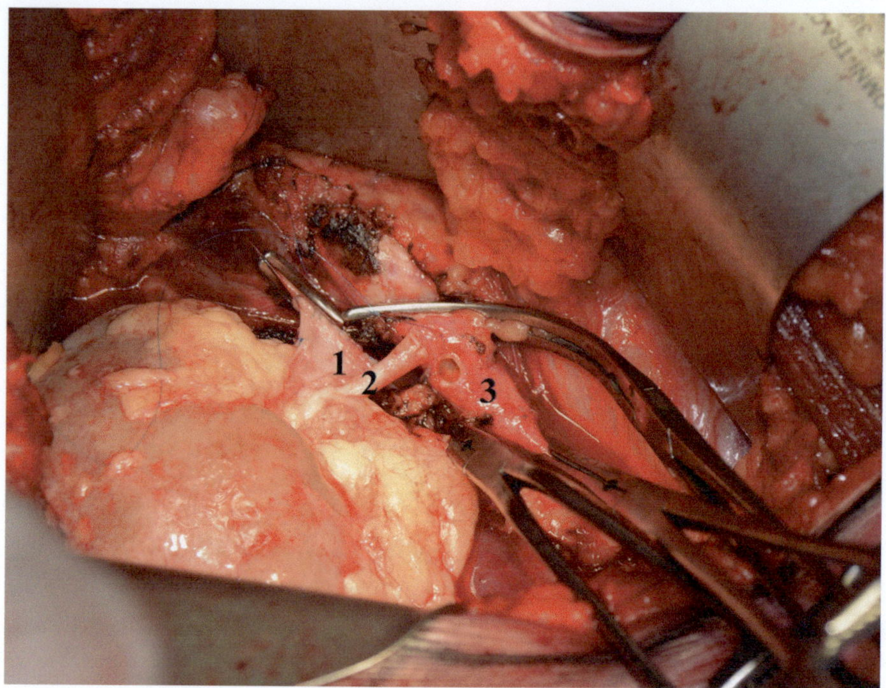

**Fig. 4.45** 1—Completed venous anastomosis, 2—The renal artery is shortened to the correct length and with a slight vertical incison of the wall of the artery to prevent the narrowing of the anastomosis, 3—Common iliac artery with opening. If the iliac artery is healthy, to obtain very good access to the lumen of the iliac artery, the artery should be clamped so that the upper clamp above the anastomosis closes the artery horizontally, while the clamp below the anastomosis closes the artery vertically. This position of the clamps above and below the anastomosis gives you a good view into the lumen of the artery and prevents the walls of the artery from sticking together during the anastomosis: this makes the arterial anastomosis easier and error-free

anastomosis (posterior walls sutured from the inside) is made, we pour a large amount of heparinized cold saline solution over the suture and both ends of the suture material are pulled gently so that the posterior walls of the two sutured vessels can come closer to each other (Fig. 4.46). Continue sewing the inferior corner and anterior walls until 3–4 mm above the inferior corner. When sewing, be very careful with the inferior corner so that blood does not leak from there when the clamps are released. The inferior corner area is almost always the source of anastomotic bleeding. Now we release the second vascular clamp from the upper corner suture, fasten it with the lower one and continue sewing from top to bottom towards the inferior corner. We finish the vascular anastomosis between the renal and iliac

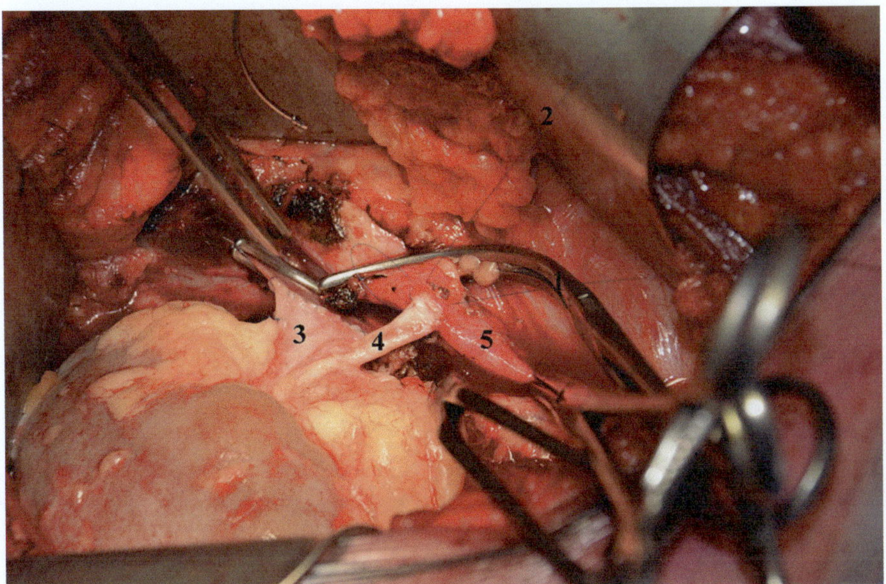

**Fig. 4.46**   The vascular anastomosis end of the renal artery to the side of the common iliac artery was performed using the parachute technique, with a single non-resolvable vascular suture. 1—The suture with which the posterior wall anastomosis of both arteries was performed; with this suture the anterior wall anastomosis was started from bottom to top, 2—Superior corner of the vascular suture, 3—Venous anastomosis, 4—Renal artery, 5—Common iliac artery

artery 1–2 mm before the end of the anastomosis; the lumen of the arteries is flushed with heparinized saline solution (Fig. 4.47); during the next step anastomosis is finished, needles are cut off and the sutures are tied six to eight times very gently so as not to tear them and the vessels. The first knot is tied not too tightly, about 1–2 mm from the walls of both arteries, to allow the anastomosis to grow and thus prevent it from narrowing (Fig. 4.48). Then we ask the scrub nurse for a small vascular clamp, e.g. a small delicate bulldog, with which we close the renal artery 3–5 mm above the anastomosis. To test the tightness of the anastomosis, the vascular clamps closing the segment of the iliac artery below it are opened first. The renal artery is then closed so that blood does not flow towards the kidney. If everything is all right (there is no blood leakage) we release the upper vascular clamp and close the common iliac artery in this case—now the blood flows freely to the lower limb. Before removing the bulldog from the renal artery we once again check the tightness of the arterial anastomosis (blood pressure and blood flow in the

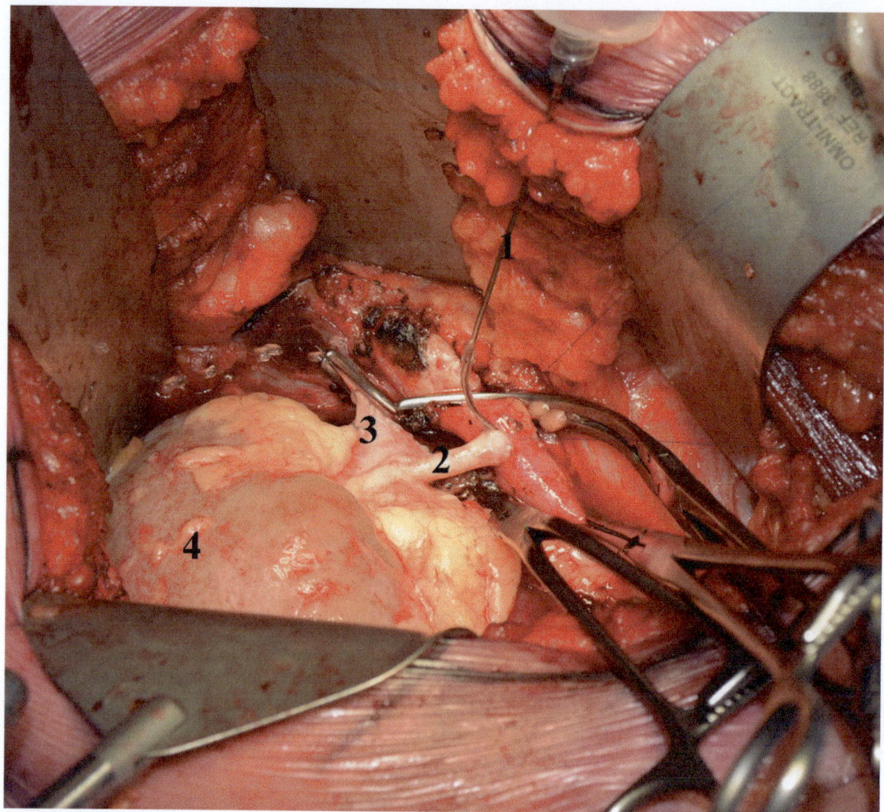

**Fig. 4.47** At the end of the anastomosis, both lumens of the arteries are flushed with heparinized saline solution. 1—A special curved needle connected to a syringe with heparin solution used to flush out the lumens of both arteries, 2—The filled up renal artery shows proper length and position: as you can see the renal artery is not twisted or kinked, 3—Venous anastomosis, 4—Kidney

area of the anastomosis are now much higher than the backflow of blood from the lower limb) (Fig. 4.49). If the arterial anastomosis is tight, slowly remove the bulldog clamp that is occluding the renal artery. Then we observe a slow filling of the renal artery and kidney with arterial blood. When the renal vein starts to fill in completely with venous blood, slow down, take away the Satinsky clamp, check the tightness of the anastomosis and the renal vein wall (Fig. 4.50).

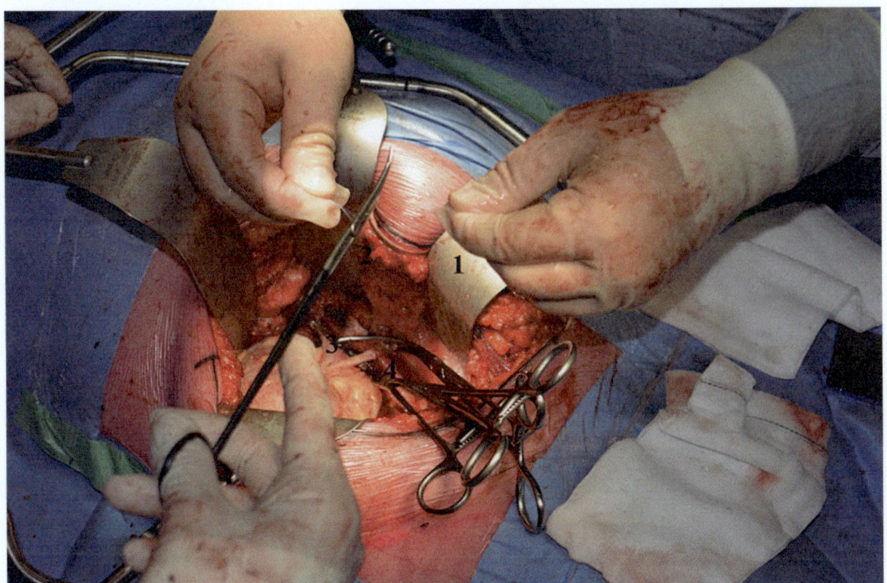

**Fig. 4.48** End of arterial anastomosis. 1 and 2—Two ends of a monofilament nonabsorbable suture; needles were cut to avoid injury, both ends of the sutures will be tied, 3—Venous anastomosis, 4—Common iliac artery

Then we ask for a warm sterile solution of Ringer's solution, which we pour into the extraperitoneal space. This solution or physiologic natrium chloride is intended to warm up the organ; secondly, it can be very helpful in obtaining proper hemostasis in the surgical field (under water it is easier to locate the bleeding). We warm up the kidney a few times until the hemostasis is complete and the kidney is colored correctly. Special attention is paid to the anastomoses, the position of the kidney, the course of the renal vessels, bleeding under the kidney capsule and blood supply to the ureter. Each bleeding vessel is coagulated, tied or sewn. Lift the kidney very gently up and turn it sideways so that the hemostasis can be performed optimally. After the complete hemostasis, place the kidney in the best position chosen beforehand and proceed to the ureter hemostasis. Any bleeding from the ureter wall or tissues surrounding the ureter must be treated at the same time due to the danger of a hematoma which may later cause ischemia (necrosis) or a narrowing (fibrrosis) of the urine leading to impaired urine drainage from the transplanted

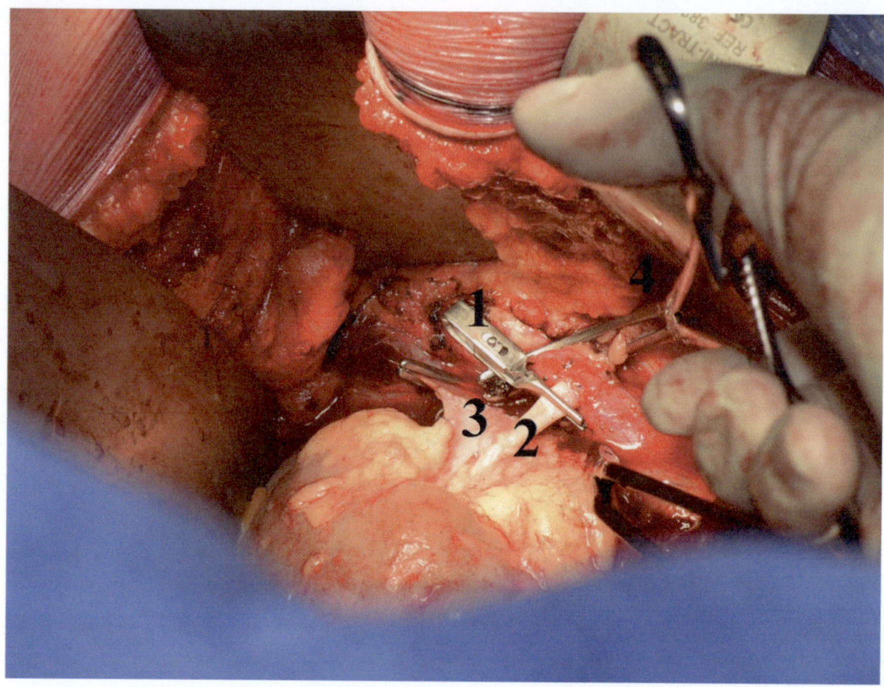

**Fig. 4.49** 1—Small bulldog vascular clamp placed on the renal artery, 2—Renal artery: end-to-side anastomosis with the common iliac artery, 3—Venous anastomosis. The moment of removing the superior vascular clamp closing the common iliac artery above arterial anastomosis. The first (inferior) clamp was removed, closing the distal part of the common iliac artery, 4—slow release of the superior vascular clamp, which is closed proximally to the right common iliac artery above the anastomosis site during anastomosis

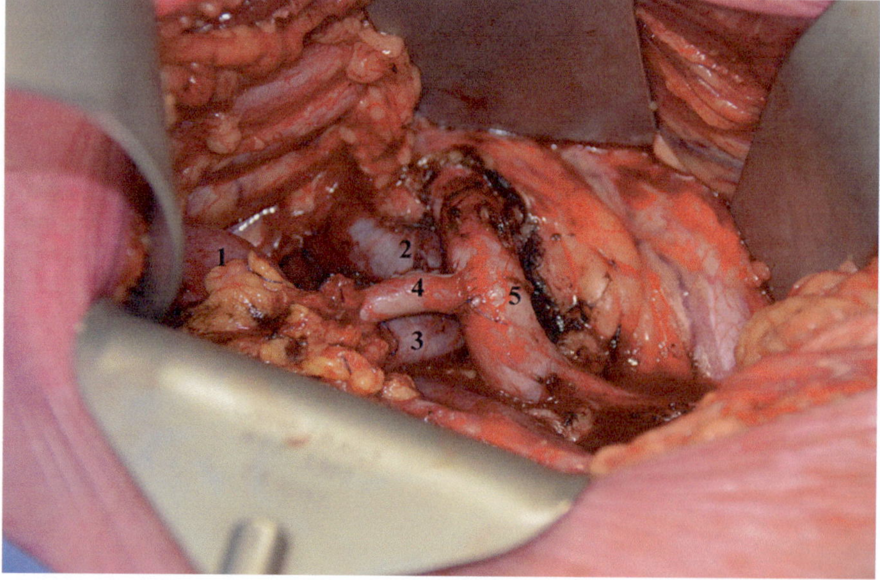

**Fig. 4.50** All vascular clamps removed: renal reperfusion, complete hemostasis. 1—Kidney, 2—IVC, 3—Renal vein, 4—Renal artery, 5— Common iliac artery

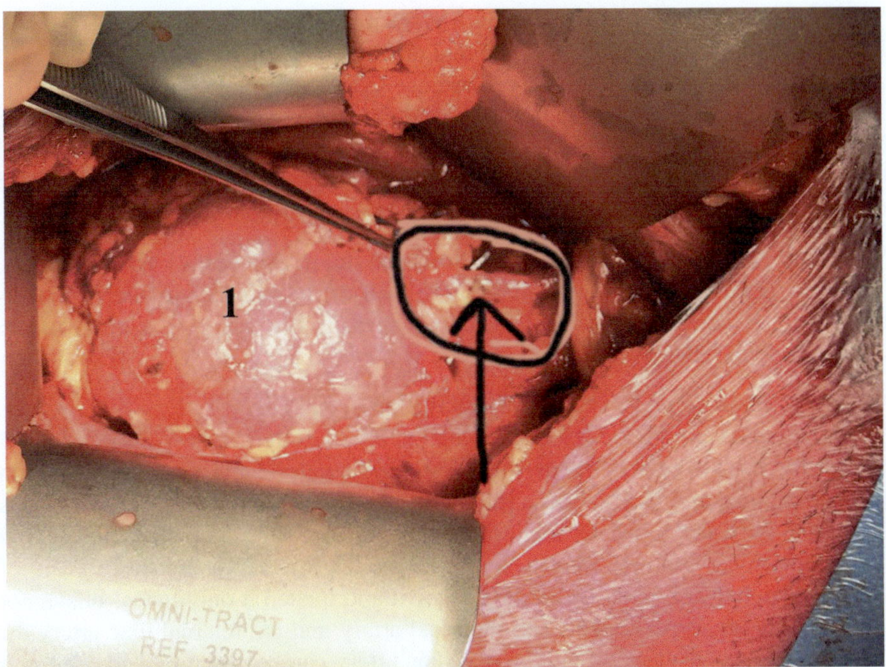

**Fig. 4.51** 1—Kidney: the arrow shows a leakage of urine on a very small area of 2 × 2 mm. Living donor kidney. Two days after transplantation, most likely due to unintentional and unnoticed burns, coagulation developed ureteral wall necrosis and urine leakage. Necrosis was treated with the excision of the ureter to a level above the urine leakage, mobilization of the transplanted kidney and bladder, and reimplantation of the unchanged part of the ureter into the bladder

kidney, renal pelvis volume enlargement and finally with radiologic drain from outside renal pelvis drainage. To control bleeding from tissues around the ureter, we can make use of Argon Beamer coagulation. I would certainly advise against classical coagulation because the wall of the ureter is sensitive to heat and coagulation on and/or around the vessels, even to a small extent, can lead to partial or total necrosis of the ureter wall and leakage of urine (Fig. 4.51) [41]. If you are not using an Argon Beamer to achieve hemostasis of the bleeding tissues surrounding the ureter, my advice is to tie or suture every bleeding vessel in the ureteral area, rather than trying to coagulate it.

**Warning! (Leaning on the abdominal retractor must be avoided)**
Remember that it happens quite often that during renal reperfusion and removal of all vascular clamps, despite good pressure, the kidney does not fill and a weak pulse is felt on the renal and iliac arteries. At this point the surgeon's first reaction should be to check whether the assistant is leaning on one of the hooks or leaning on one of the arms of the abdominal retractor causing complete or partial occlusion of the vessels and thus a weak or zero arterial blood supply to the transplanted kidney.

**Warning! (During hemostasis don't overheat the ureter and/or renal pelvis)**
The renal pelvis and ureter and mainly the wall of the ureter, hate high temperatures, so they are easily burned and damaged and it is therefore easy to obtain necrosis which leads to leakage.

**Warning! (End to end with the internal iliac artery)**
When I started learning kidney transplantation 35 years ago at the Warsaw Medical University, the leading technique was end-to-end renal the artery anastomosis with the internal iliac artery. This was a long time ago and the arguments in favor of this technique were the threat of septic hemorrhage from the place of assembly and saving the lower limb. Currently, septic hemorrhage is very rare. In 25 years of work experience at Leiden University, I saw it and treated it only twice. I have not performed an anastomosis between the renal artery and the internal iliac artery for 20 years and I consider that the internal iliac artery can be procured and used as a tool-kit for the reconstruction of the kidney's arteries from a living or deceased donor. We should remember that the internal iliac artery, as a rule, is the first of all iliac arteries to undergo atherosclerotic changes and rapid narrowing and then closure.

**Warning! (After reperfusion is there low blood pressure?)**
When the patient following kidney reperfusion has low blood pressure and the kidney does not fill with enough blood and is soft and in order to direct more blood to the kidney, we can close the iliac artery below the renal artery anastomosis for a few minutes and thus direct more blood to the newly transplanted kidney.

**Warning! (After anastomosis try to avoid the purse string effect)**
After finishing the venous and arterial anastomoses, the first knot is tied at a small distance from the joint made—in most cases this distance is one-third to one-sixth of the joint diameter (1–2 mm). It is important to prevent the formation of a narrowing at the site of anastomosis and/or prevent the effect of a purse string suture, which consists in damaging or even cutting through the walls of the veins or arteries sutured with it.

**Warning! (When you are tying do not cross the sutures)**
Be careful not to cross the sutures when tying, as the knots containing the crossed sutures are much weaker and significantly reduce the strength of the suture. Rupture of the suture may threaten the patient with massive hemorrhage, which may lead to kidney loss and even the loss of the patient's life.

## 4.9.5   Ureter Implantation into the Wall of the Urinary Bladder: Own Modified Lich-Gregoir (LG) Technique

### 4.9.5.1   Introduction

The most important surgical aspects of renal transplantation are the vascular and the ureterovesical anastomoses. The ureterovesical anastomosis is the most frequent source of morbidity following kidney transplantation. The mean prevalence of urological complications ranges between 3 and 5%. However, prevalences between 1 and 30% have also been described. Urological complications are urinary leakage, ureteral stricture, vesicoureteral reflux or significant hematuria [51]. The ureterovesical anastomotic technique is an important aspect of kidney transplantation, which can influence the urological complication rate. Since the start of renal transplantation, a number of different ureteroneocystostomy techniques have been developed. The most frequently used techniques are the intravesical Politano-Leadbetter (PL), the extravesical Campos Freire technique, better known as Lich-Gregoir (LG) and the Taguchi or U-stitch (U) technique. Several studies have compared these techniques. However, the effect of the ureterovesical anastomotic technique on the development of urological complications and the preferred technique continue to be a subject of discussion. Additionally, the stenting of the ureterovesical anastomosis has been recognized as an independent protective factor in preventing the development of urological complications after kidney transplantation. Unstented techniques are often compared with stented or partly stented techniques which could introduce the bias. Indirectly or directly, based on studies, people try to say which ureter urinary bladder anastomosis can be considered the best one [51, 52].

Performing the LG technique for ureteroneocystostomy in conjunction with stenting the ureter seems to be the most favorable procedure in the setting of renal transplantation. By choosing this technique, major postoperative complications can be minimized, resulting in a positive outcome for the patient and the graft function. However, there is no consensus about the optimal stent removal time. Further research needs to be done concerning the stent removal time and other methods for ureteroneocystostomy [55].

### 4.9.5.2   The Ureter Implantation LG Own Modified Technique: A Detailed Description (Fig. 4.52)

Implantation of the ureter begins with exposing the area of the urinary bladder by using the appropriate blades of a professional abdominal retractor. After exposing the area of the bladder under visual control, through a previously prepared system,

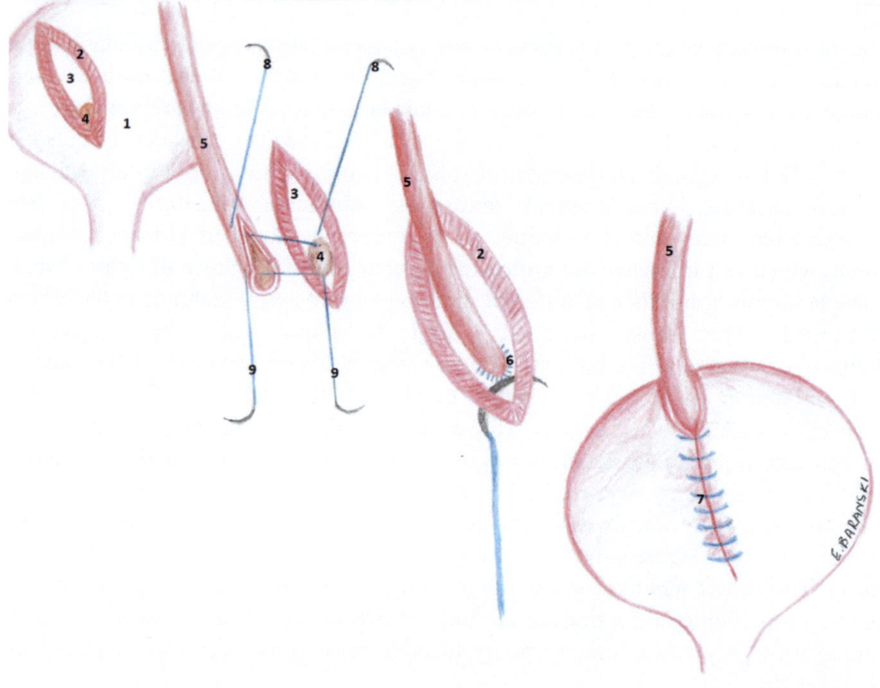

**Fig. 4.52** The ureter implantation LG technique. 1—Urinary bladder, 2—Urinary bladder wall detrusor muscle, 3—Mucosa, 4—Opening in mucosa, 5—Spatulated ureter, 6—Anastomosis between ureter and mucosa (if bad quality mucosa with a little detrusor muscle), 7—Ureter-bladder anastomosis: anti-reflux urinary bladder wall treatment which consists of bringing the previously cut bladder detrusor muscle tissue closer together above the anastomosis, 8—Posterior suture connecting posterior corners of urinary bladder and ureteranastomosis, 9—Anterior suture connecting anterior corners anastomosis between urinary bladder and the ureter

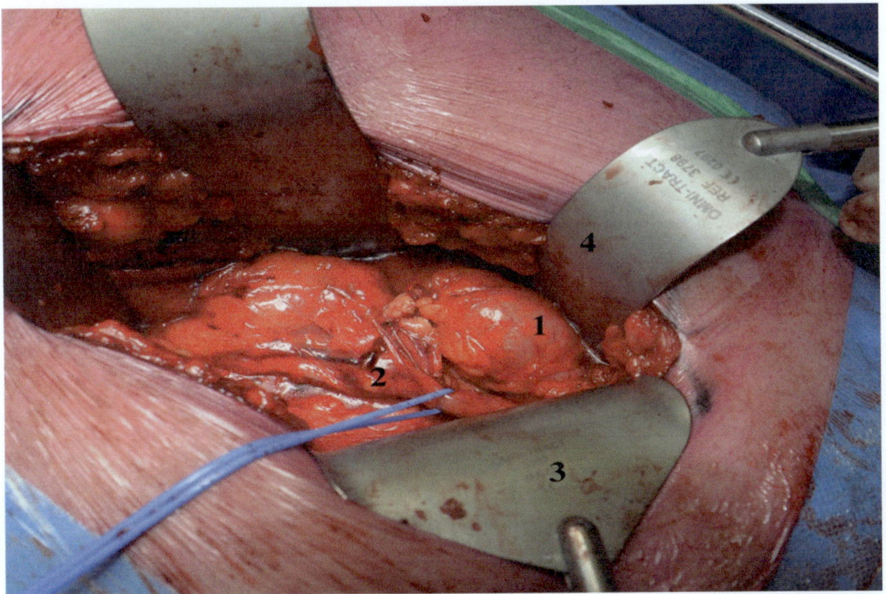

**Fig. 4.53** 1—Bladder filled with warm physiological saline solution, 2—Spermatic cord, 3—Semicircular blade of the retractor moved towards the urinary bladder, 4—Lower blade of retractor moved downwards for better exposure of the urinary bladder area

the surgeon or scrub nurse will inject warm Ringer's solution or physiologic natrium chloride solution into the urinary bladder of the recipient. Then, after filling the bladder and localizing it, we proceed to the preparation of its wall from the surrounding fat. I would like to introduce you to the technique of uretero-bladder anastomosis using the LG method (with my own small modification) with the use of a JJ catheter stent. The steps are as follows.

(a) As I mentioned above, bladder filling is usually done under the surgeon's visual and manual control and requires frequent checking with the finger(s) for the degree of its filling (Fig. 4.53).

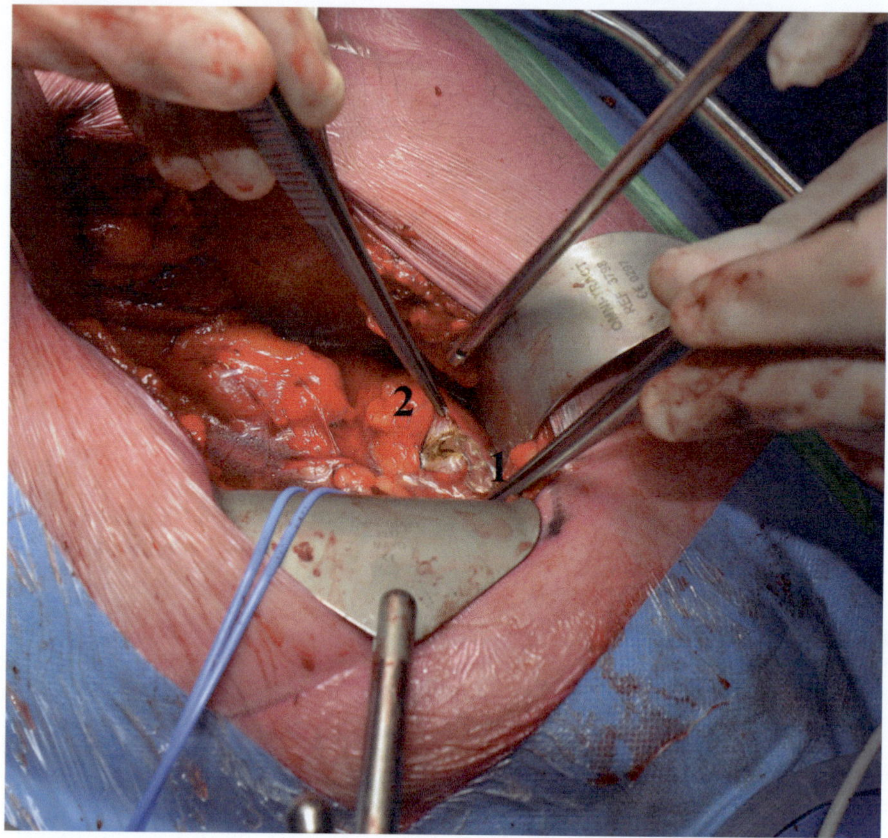

**Fig. 4.54** 1—Opening in the urinary bladder wall along the muscles with a small part of the mucosa. From inside of the urinary bladder there is a warm saline solution that was previously injected into the bladder, 2—Urinary bladder

(b) During urinary bladder filling, try to locate its wall with your finger, and then very carefully and gently dissect it with the parietal peritoneum, thus making its upper and lateral surface visible. After the fat has been removed from the external surface of the urinary bladder wall, use diathermy to cut the muscularis propria (the detrusor of the urinary bladder), muscle and submucosa over a distance of 2.5–3.0 cm, so that the mucosa remains intact. Then, open and cut the mucosa with scissors over a distance of 1.5–2.0 cm (Fig. 4.54).

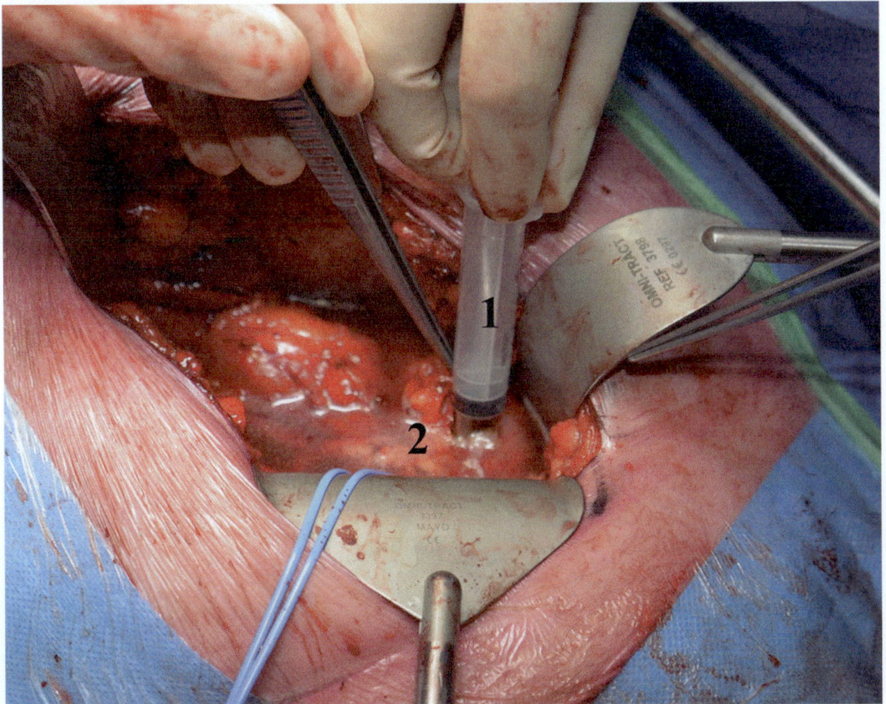

**Fig. 4.55**  When the wall of the bladder and its mucous membrane are cut, the fluid mixed with urine starts to flow out into the bladder area. The bladder fluid is taken into the syringe for bacteriological examination. 1—The syringe, 2—The fluid is coming out from the urinary bladder

(c) Now, the fluid is flowing outside from the opening made in the bladder wall into the retroperitoneal space and is collected inside the sterile syringe for bacterial examination in order to assess its sterility. In the case of confirmation of bacterial content, the fluid should be cultured. If necessary, antibiotic therapy is applied after surgery (prolonging or changing the antibiotics given during transplantation depends on the result of the bacterial culture) (Fig. 4.55).

(d) Start the vesicoureteral anastomosis by placing bladder sutures. For this purpose, use 5/0 or 4/0 absorbable monofilament sutures. Two sutures are placed on the bladder wall. The proximal suture is placed from the side of the spermatic cord or the round ligament (posterior) and the distal suture (anterior) is placed from the side of the pubic bone. Each suture is armed with two needles. The end of the anterior and posterior suture is fastened close to the needles with

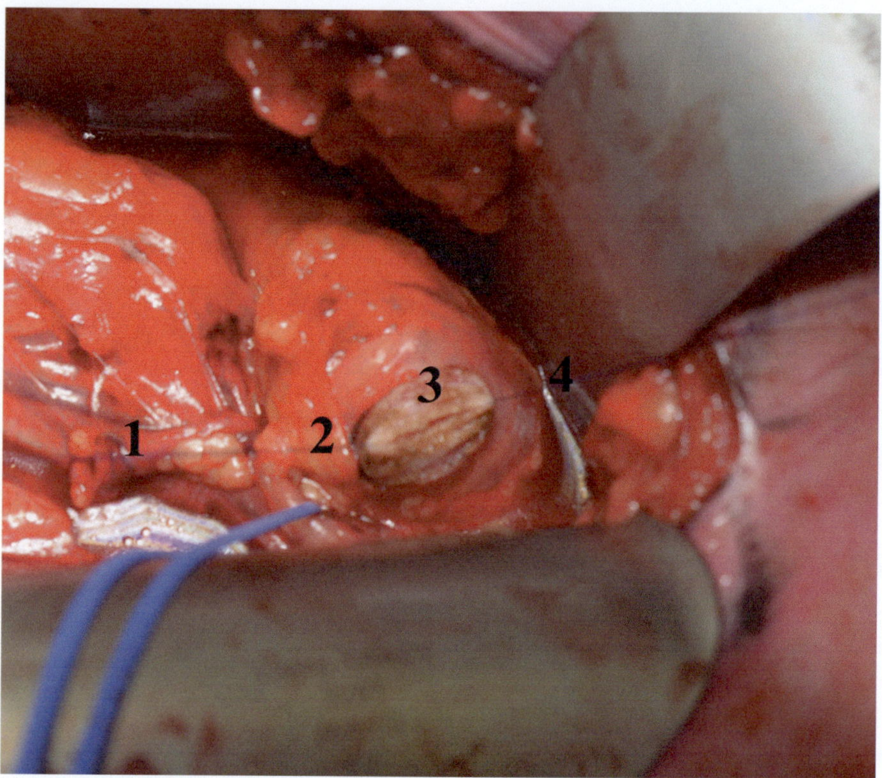

**Fig. 4.56** 1—Ureter, 2—Monofilament absorbable suture 5/0 placed on the posterior corner of the ureter-urinary bladder anastomosis, 3—Open bladder place of ureter-urinary bladder anastomosis, 4—Monofilament absorbable suture 5/0 placed on the anterior corner of the ureter-urinary bladder anastomosis

vascular clamps with armed jaws. The suture thickness covers the bladder mucosa and about a quarter to a third of the thickness of the muscularis propria of the urinary bladder. If the bladder mucosa is thin or sick and bleeds easily or is short or is of a poor quality, I would never recommend anastomosis of the ureter but only the mucosa itself. I believe that the mechanical value of such an anastomosis is almost none. The two stretched sutures in the cephalic direction and in the direction of the pubic symphysis form a straight line, and the bladder intersection line is an extension of the ureter (Fig. 4.56).

(e) Find the physiological position of the ureter. If it is twisted, unscrew it, then pull it under the spermatic cord or the round ligament of the uterus and adjust its length from the kidney to the anastomosis with the bladder. Before starting anastomosis, remember to properly prepare the end of the ureter, which includes removing excess tissue while maintaining its good blood supply. Use sharp scissors to shorten the ureter to the desired length or, if it is long enough, cut it a few millimeters, refreshing its end. After cutting the ureter if it is

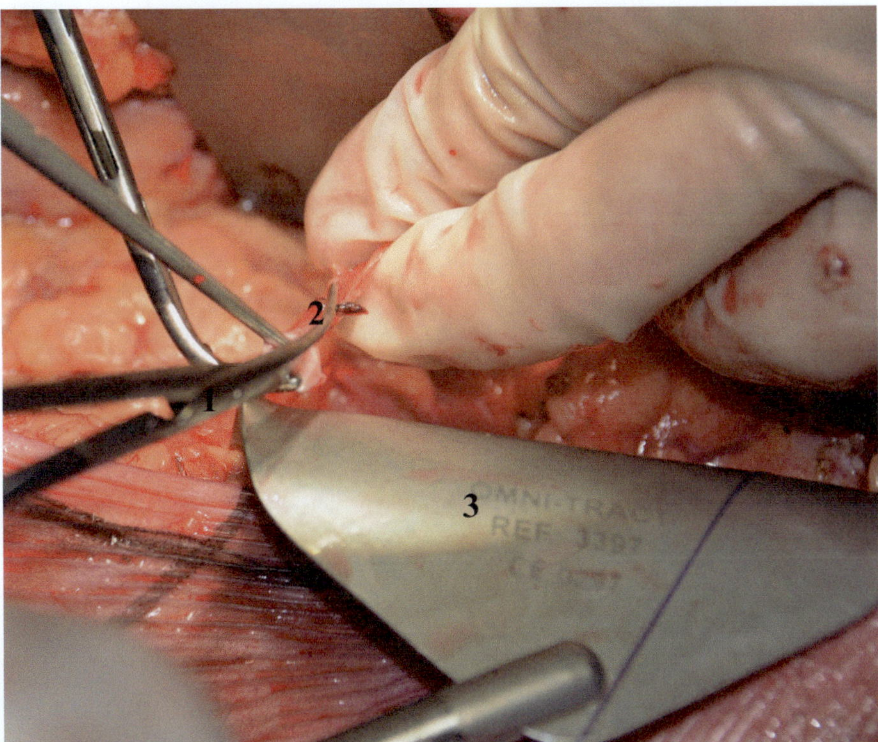

**Fig. 4.57** 1—Sharp vascular scissors, 2—The end of the ureter, after shortening or refreshing the end, is incised along its long axis (spatulated), 3—Semicircular blade of retractor is moved to the bladder region

needed, perform a perfect hemostasis of the bleeding tissues around the ureter. Please note that each anastomosis of the uretero-bladder must be performed without tension and bleeding from the ureter and/or surrounding tissues.

(f) The end of the ureter is cut 1.5–2.0 cm along its long axis and adjusted to the hole previously made in the bladder (Fig. 4.57).

(g) Start the uretero-bladder anastomosis with the posterior suture, which has initially punctured into the bladder wall. So, first open the vascular clamp that holds the two ends of the proximal suture. Choose the suture coming from the lumen of the urinary bladder, and then grab the needle of the same suture in a needle holder. At the same time, the assistant lifts the ureter upwards with forceps, and the operator—if necessary—inserts the forceps very gently into the lumen of the ureter and punctures it from the inside to the outside with the needle through the wall of the ureter at a distance of 2–3 mm from the posterior corner of the ureter. Both ends of the suture are fixed with a vascular clamp armed with plastic sheaths near the needles. Now we select the suture inside the bladder in the distal corner, release the suture from the vascular clamp, take it in a needle holder and puncture it from the inside to the outside in the distal corner

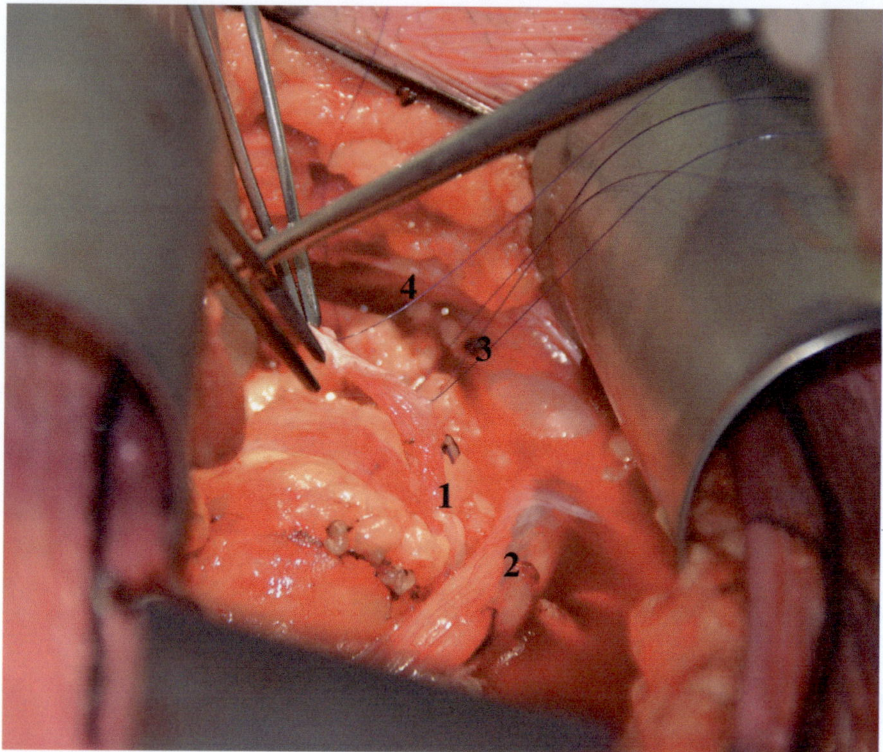

**Fig. 4.58** The ureter is tied on and cut to length. Incised anti-mesenteric ureteral wall. 1—Ureter, 2—Spermatic cord, 3—Posterior suture connecting the posterior corners of the urinary bladder and ureter anastomosis, 4—Anterior (distal) suture connecting the anterior corner anastomosis between the urinary bladder and ureter. 3 and 4—The anterior and posterior sutures shown in the photo are pierced through the ureteral wall

of the ureter. Fasten both ends of the suture with a small vascular clamp with a plastic or rubber band (Fig. 4.58).

(h)  At this point, the transplant surgeon introduces a delicate guidewire through the side opening into the catheter, the purpose of which is to facilitate insertion of the catheter into the pelvis of the transplanted kidney (Fig. 4.59).

(i)  The anterior and posterior sutures between the ureter and bladder are not tied, allowing the ureter to be moved at considerable distance from the bladder for the safe insertion of the JJ catheter through the lumen of the ureter into the renal pelvis (Fig. 4.60).

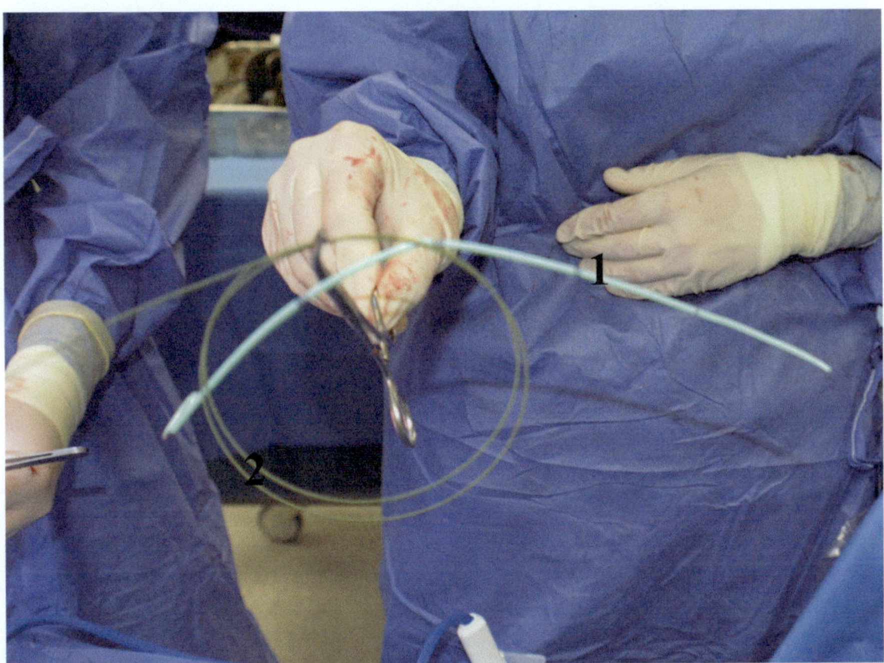

**Fig. 4.59** 1—JJ Catheter with the guide inserted into the lumen, 2—A very delicate catheter guide is constructed in such a way that one end of the catheter is quite stiff and the other end is soft

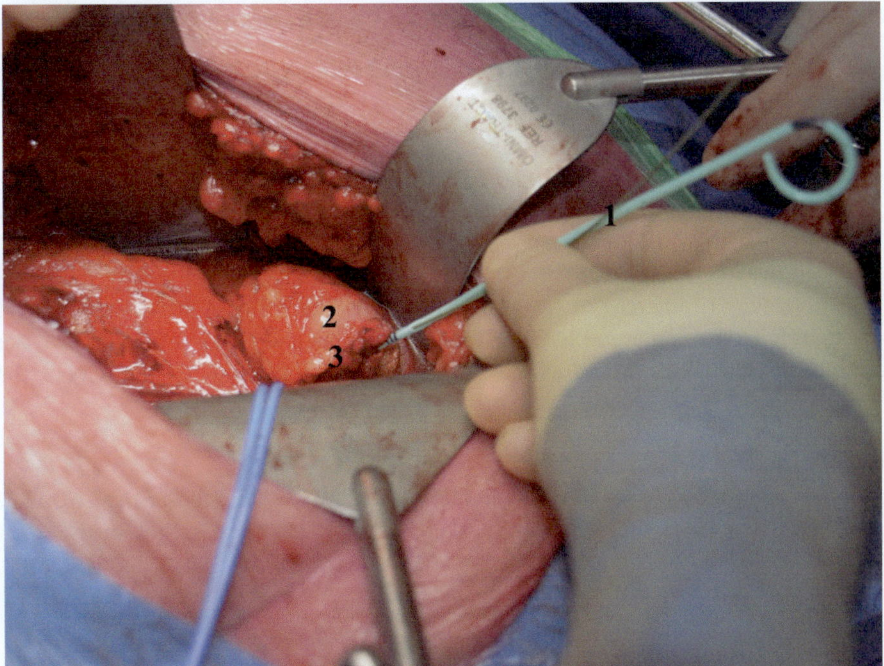

**Fig. 4.60** 1—Placement of the JJ catheter into the ureter and renal pelvis of the transplanted kidney, 2—Urinary bladder, 3—One of the sutures, between the bladder and ureter, of the posterior corner suture

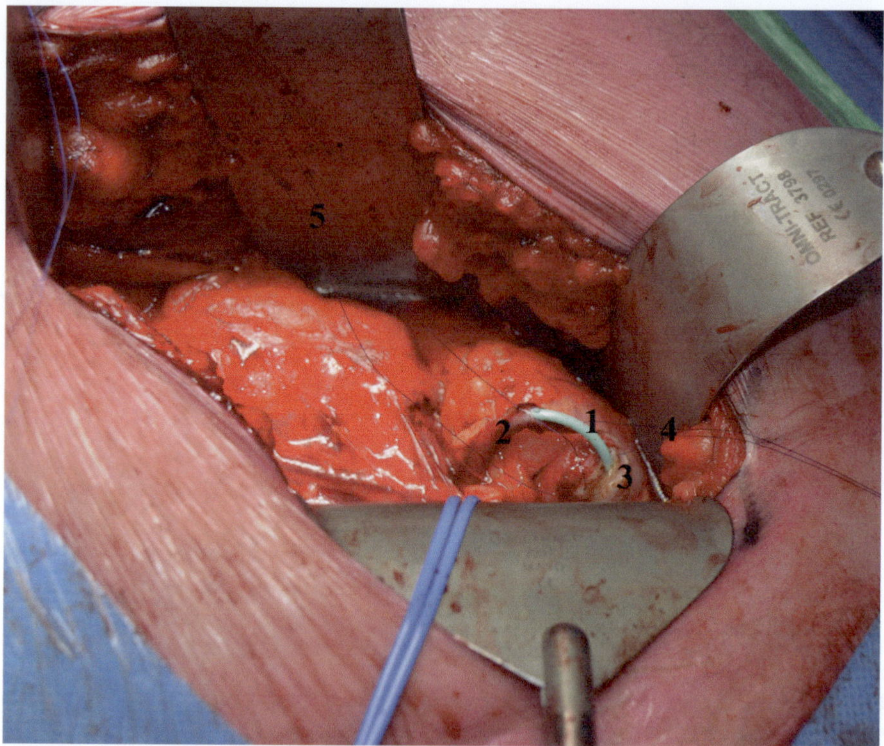

**Fig. 4.61** Placing the JJ catheter into the lumen of the urinary bladder. 1—JJ catheter, 2—Ureter, 3—Bladder, 4—Anterior corner suture connecting the anterior corner of the ureter with the anterior corner of the urinary bladder anastomosis, 5—Suture connecting the posterior corner of the ureter and urinary bladder before tying

(j)  The next step is to withdraw the guidewire from the JJ catheter placed through the ureter in the renal pelvis and to insert it into one of the lower side openings of the distal part of the JJ catheter and then to insert it into the urinary bladder. Hold the JJ catheter with two forceps and pull the guidewire out of the distal end of the JJ catheter and from the urinary bladder. Lift the previously applied sutures on the ureter and bladder slightly upwards and check if the edges of the bladder and ureter fit and adhere to each other without any tension. Check the position of the inserted JJ catheter (Figs. 4.61 and 4.62).

**Warning!**

After inserting the catheter into the ureter, the renal pelvis and the urinary bladder, you should see its position. It is important to see if the catheter lies in the renal pelvis and has not gone outside through the wall of the ureter, renal pelvis, kidney

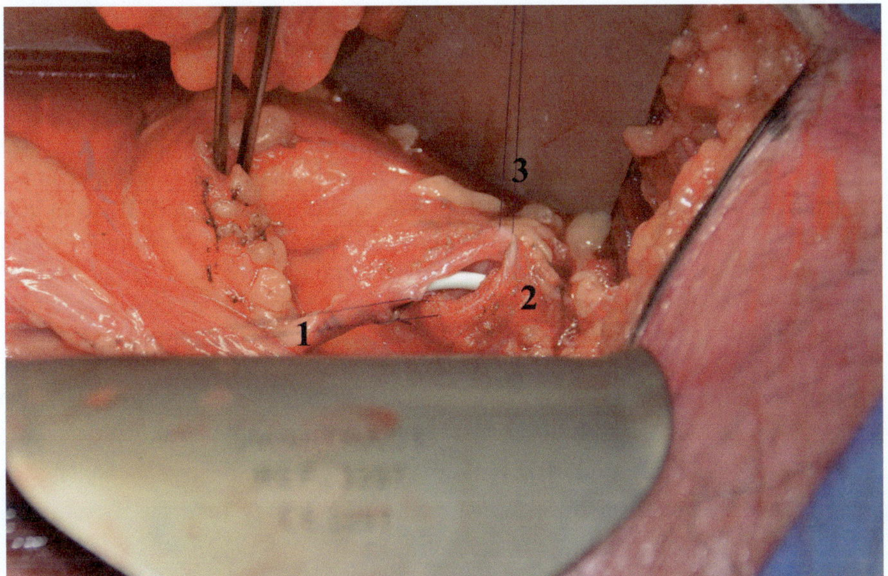

**Fig. 4.62** The beginning of the uretero-urinary bladder anastomosis. 1—The posterior corner suture will be tied first, 2—Bladder, 3—The anterior suture will be tied at the end of the anastomosis or not at all

parenchyma or urinary bladder wall. It is also important to check if the end of the catheter is in the ureter, if the catheter does not close the ureter and if the catheter does not fold. Remember that when the catheter is badly positioned, it must be repositioned, even if this would cause us to break down the vesicoureteral anastomosis and perform a second one.

Renal pelvis puncture or parenchyma occurs quite often in the kidneys of small and young donors when there is no resistance when inserting a JJ catheter.

If you are confronted with this type of complication during kidney transplantation, your first reaction should be as follows:

– always pull the catheter back and place it in a good position (in the renal pelvis).
– check the possibility of bleeding outside the kidney and into the renal pelvis. To control bleeding, use a suture, an Argon Beamer and coagulation topical hemostatic agents to break down the ureter-bladder anastomosis in the ureter lumen. Insert a small thin drain and move it very gently towards the renal pelvis. Close the lumen of the ureter with your fingers and flush very slowly and gently the warm Ringer's solution or 0.9% NaCl physiological solution into the renal pelvis and check for a leakage and/or bleeding. If there is a leakage through a small hole in the ureter, renal pelvis wall or renal parenchyma, suture it. If the bleeding comes back after flushing, you have to compress the renal pelvis for approximately 10–15 min or break down the anastomosis between the ureter and the urinary bladder and flush the ureter and renal pelvis with warm Ringer's

solution or physiological saline solution to check if there is still bleeding. If the above mentioned fail, ask a consultant of the Urology Department to perform a ureteroscopy and to stop the bleeding. The passage of the ureteroscope may result in a swelling in the ureter. Therefore, it may be necessary to temporarily leave a JJ, called a ureteral stent, inside the ureter temporarily to ensure that the kidney drains urine well. Another option is to perform the transplantation and to ask the interventional radiologist afterwards to perform an angio-CT and to treat the bleeding (coiling). In an extraordnary situation, if the bleeding is under control, accept the thrombi or even a big thrombus in the renal pelvis and the ureter. If the kidney starts to produce urine (which consists of urokinase which will dissolve all the clots over time) it will thus restore the normal route of the urine outflow from the kidney to the urinary bladder.

– remember that every time the JJ slides out of the renal pelvis into the ureter, it may perforate, bend or completely close its lumen.

After checking the position of the JJ catheter at the site of anastomosis, the posterior suture is released from the vascular clamp and tied. At the same as the

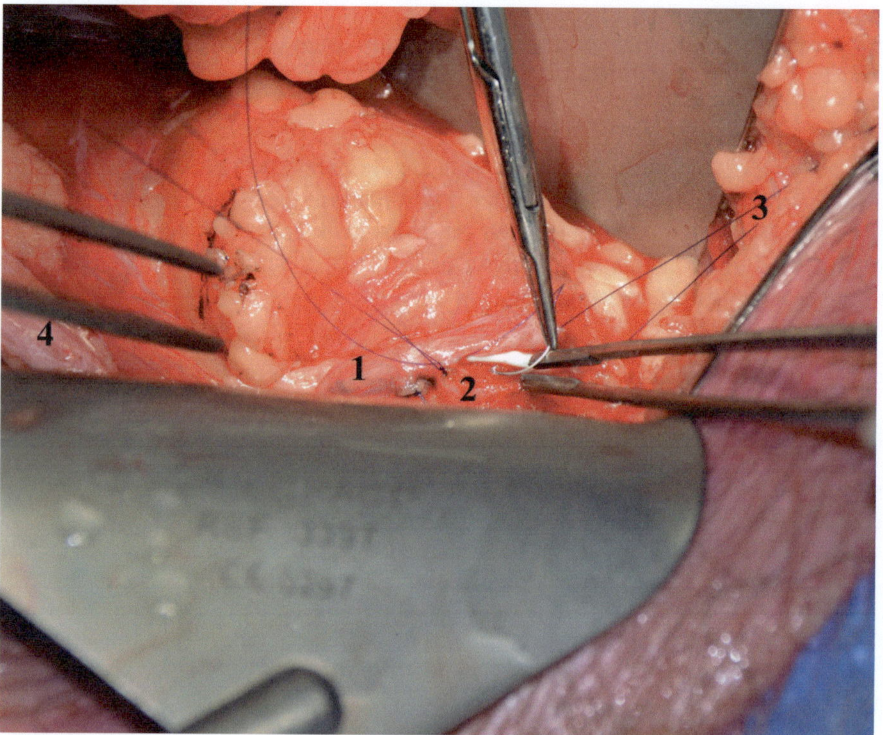

**Fig. 4.63** Anastomosis of the transplanted kidney ureter with the recipient's bladder. 1—Ureter, 2—Bladder, 3—Anterior corner suture connecting ureter to the bladder. 4—Spermatic cord

assistant lifts the ureter up with a gentle tension, he or she must pay attention during the tying to avoid alien tissues (fat tissue or the peritoneum) between the mucosa of the ureter and the urinary bladder. After tying, the left half of the suture is placed under the ureter and pulled towards the left side of the recipient and fixed with a small vascular clamp. The distal suture is not tied, but gently stretched (by the scrub nurse or assistant) under small tension in such a way that the edges of the ureter and bladder walls adhere perfectly to each other. Start to perform the anastomosis first from the posterior corner (proximal suture) and insert the needle from the outside into the ureter lumen and then from the inside of the bladder to the outside puncture of the bladder mucosa (Fig. 4.63). In most cases anastomosis is done with a running suture from the right and left side of the ureter with an absorbable monofilament 5/0 or 4/0. The ureter and the urinary bladder mucosa are mostly sutured 2–3 mm from their edges and the distance between the sutures is about 2–3 mm. The right and left running suture is finished about 4–5 mm before the distal suture and is located in the distal corner. The distal suture is then cut and removed. Both sutures are stretched by the assistant in such a way that they form a straight horizontal line with the ureter and the mucosa of the urinary bladder. The right suture is fixed with a small vascular clamp and the anastomosis is now performed by using the left suture —from the left to the right side. Finally, when the anastomosis is finished the sutures are tied and cut (Fig. 4.64).

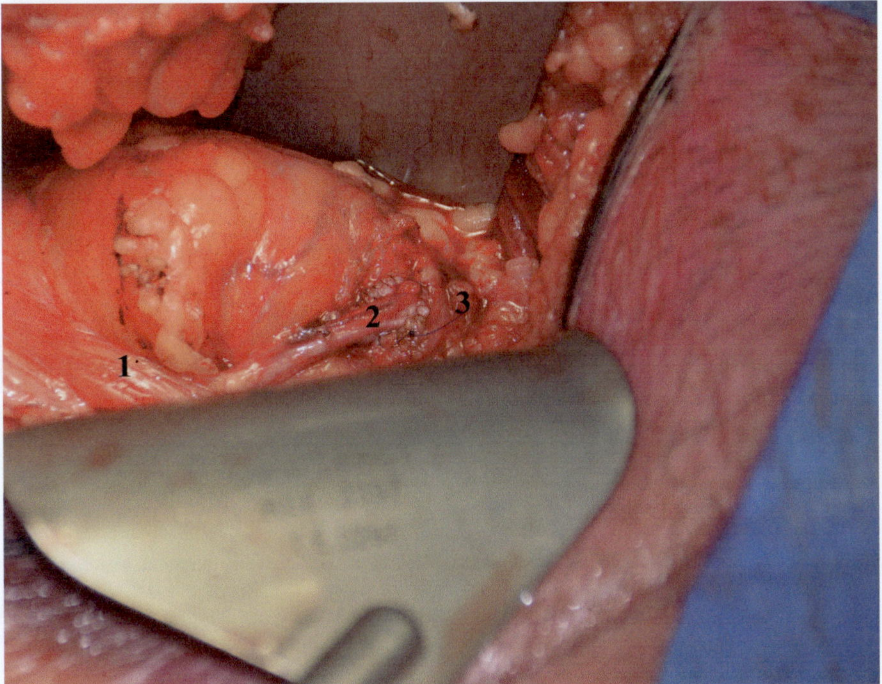

**Fig. 4.64** Completed urinary bladder–ureter anastomosis. 1—Spermatic cord, 2—Transplanted kidney's ureter, 3—Urinary bladder wall

**Warning! (The anastomosis between the ureter and urinary bladder must be tight without any leakage of urine)**

The vesicoureteral anastomosis must be tight and impervious to urine, therefore, when connecting the ureter with the bladder, in order for the anastomosis to be tight, it is necessary to take the suture together with the bladder mucosa and submucosa up to 30–50% of the urinary bladder muscle (layer of detrusor muscle). This maneuver will greatly strengthen and seal the entire anastomosis, especially when the bladder mucosa is very thin or fragile, for example in the event of repeated ureteral implantation into the bladder, in multiple bladder operations, or when the intestine is used to expand the bladder. If the ureter's wall is of a poor quality, a mucosa plus submucosa plus ureter's wall anastomosis can be performed.

(k) The last stage of the vesicoureteral anastomosis is to bring the edges of the bladder closer together above the anastomosis. We place two separate superficial transverse sutures in the bladder wall covering the anastomosis (Figs. 4.65 and 4.66). The stitches are tied loosely over the uretero-bladder anastomosis in order not to cause ureteral ischemia, so that the tissues above the anastomosis are slightly close to each other (Fig. 4.67).

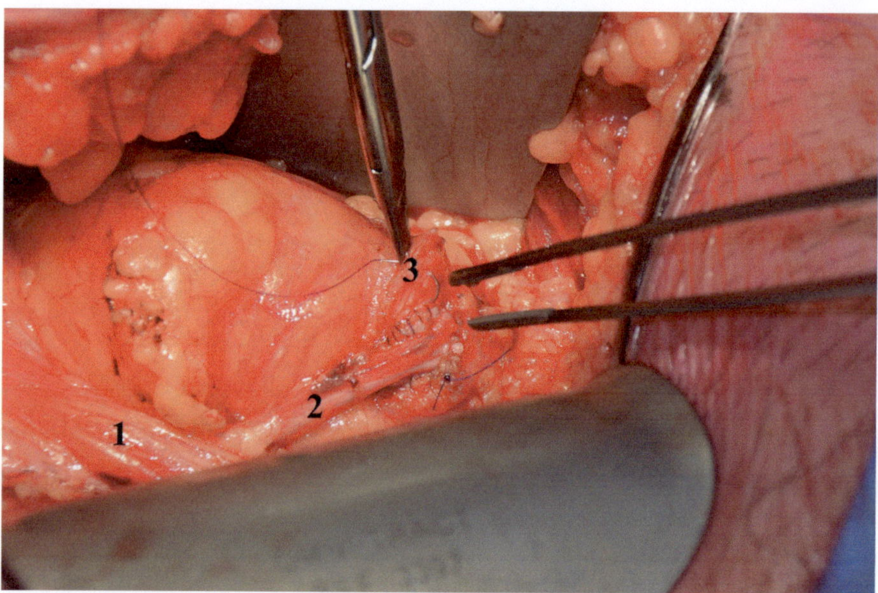

**Fig. 4.65** Ureter-bladder anastomosis: anti-reflux urinary bladder wall treatment which consists of bringing the previously cut bladder muscle tissue closer together above the anastomosis. 1—Spermatic cord, 2—Ureter, 3—First suture anti-reflux treatment closing the muscles above the anastomosis (which can be closed with an interrupted or continuous suture)

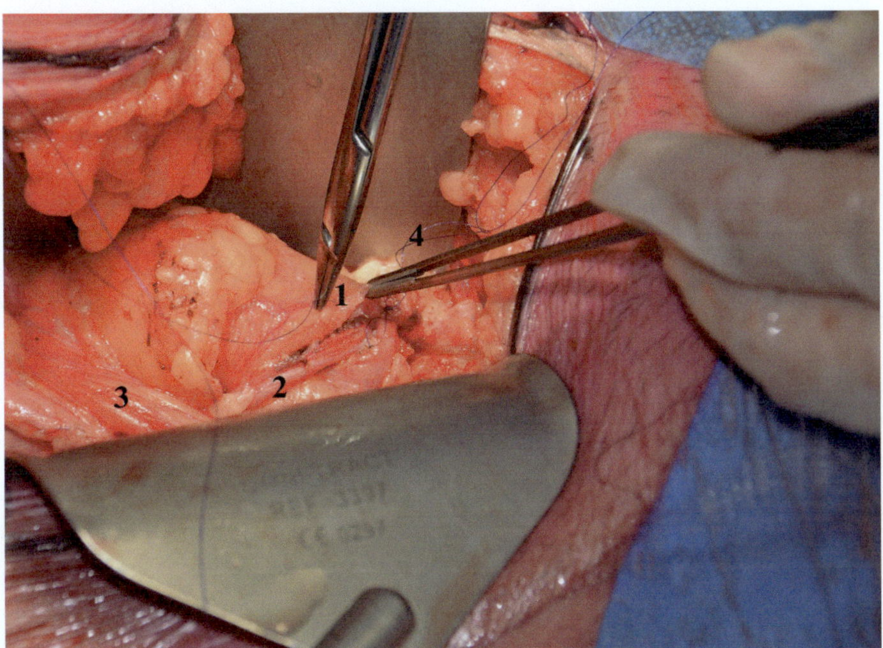

**Fig. 4.66** Anti-reflux surgical treatment of the ureter-bladder anastomosis by bringing the previously cut bladder muscle tissues closer together over the anastomosis. 1—Cut bladder muscles that are sewn together above the anastomosis: the second suture, 2—Ureter, 3—Spermatic cord, 4—The first suture applied and tied from the side of the anterior corner of the vesicoureteral anastomosis

(l) Uretero-bladder anastomosis can be completed with an anastomotic leak test by administering warm physiologic natrium saline chloride or Ringer's solution into the bladder. Administer the sterile fluids very slowly under eye observation, palpate the bladder and constantly check the degree of the bladder filling, while checking the tightness of the uretero-bladder anastomosis.

**Warning! (Do not fill the urinary bladder without closely monitoring the degree of filling)**
Remember that excessive bladder filling can lead to bladder damage, e.g. transitional epithelium, lamina propria, submucosa and/or muscle cracking and bleeding from the damaged bladder wall. Consequently, the bladder even requires sometimes to be opened or an intervention by a urologist. Filling the urinary bladder, before the kidney transplantation, may be a mistake because of the significant reduction of

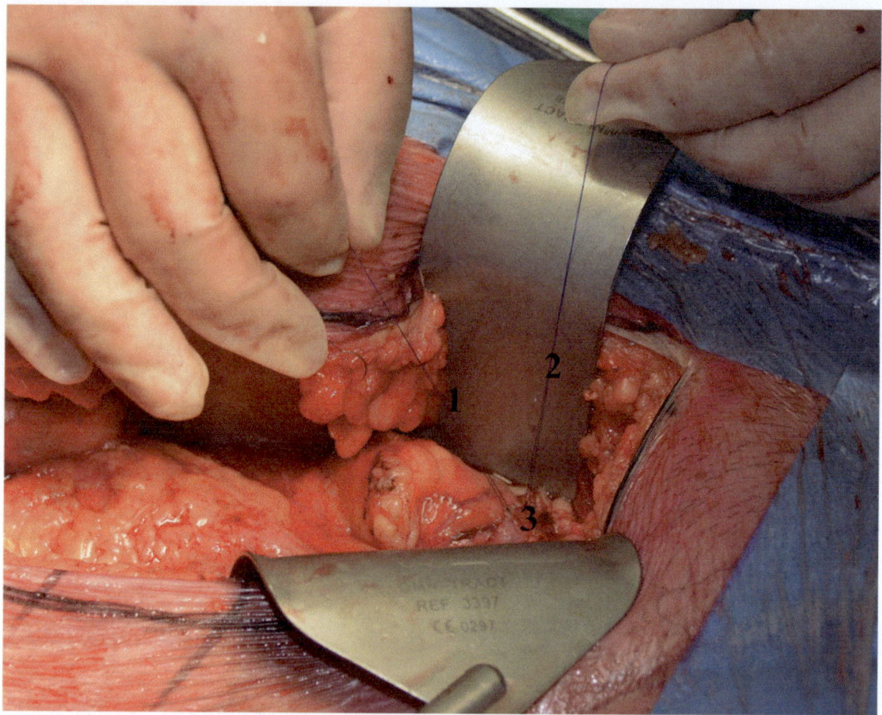

**Fig. 4.67**  1 and 2—Two sutures bringing the bladder muscle tissue closer to above the ureter urinary bladder anastomosis, 3—Completion of uretero-vesical anastomosis

access to the iliac arteries and due to the small and long unused bladder. Additionaly, it can be very dangerous for the urinary bladder mucosa and in some cases lead to bleeding or even rupture of the urinary bladder.

### 4.9.5.3   Ureterovesical Anastomosis and Urinary System Decompression With or Without Decompression (Splint)?

The European Association of Urology recommends universal usage of stents in renal transplant recipients due to strong evidence of preventing postoperative complications. The benefits of stenting the ureter are especially associated with facilitating the healing process of the performed anastomosis, which is often the source of postoperative complications. Stenting protects the ureter also from urinary leak. Moreover, ureteral obstruction as a result of postoperative swelling of the mucosa or external compression can be prevented. However, even though the benefits of an inserted stent during implantation are indisputable, possible complications should not be underestimated and should be taken into consideration. The most common and important complications associated with stents are urinary tract infections (UTIs). Stented patients have higher rates of UTIs even after their removal. Besides UTIs, stent migration, encrustation, pain and bladder discomfort may also occur. Stents may also be forgotten in situ, which may lead to further complications as reported by Friedersdorff et al. [53] and Bardapure et al. [54]. Additionally, Siparsky et al. demonstrated a higher risk for BK virus in stented renal transplant recipients. The BK virus may cause BK nephropathy, resulting in graft impairment and even graft loss [54].

In general, stent-related complications are especially seen in patients when the stent is left for a longer period in situ. Patel et al. [58] also demonstrated a better quality of life in patients with early stent removal. However, there is no consensus about the optimal time of stent removal. In most centers, stents are removed between two and six weeks after the transplantation. Since a later stent removal shows a higher risk for stent-related complications, some authors advocate an early removal of the stent after three weeks. Although stent-related complications may be reduced by an early removal, there still is some concern about higher rates of urinary leak and ureteral obstruction when they are removed too early. However, there is no doubt that a transplant ureteral stent reduces the incidence of major urologic complications, even when placed for a short period of time and removed after only five to seven  days. More research is needed in order to define and determine an optimal stent removal time.

The issue of decompressing the vesicoureteral anastomosis with the JJ catheter is still an international debate. Of course, those who do not use this method believe that it is not necessary, and those who use it have the opposite opinion. My personal experience can be divided into two stages: 15 years without and 15 years with a JJ catheter. Well, my personal opinion is very positive and in any case I recommend decompression of the vesicoureteral anastomosis with the JJ catheter. For how long you should keep the JJ catheter for decompression of the urinary system and anastomosis depends on many factors, including whether it is a first, second or third kidney transplant, the type and number of surgeries performed on the bladder in the past, excision of the bladder wall or if the patient had bladder enlargement surgery with one of the intestines. The results of the systematic review from the Imperial College Renal and Transplant Centre clearly point favorably towards an earlier stent removal around three weeks as opposed to the six weeks that is currently used in most transplant centers. An early removal, earlier than three weeks after the operation, results in fewer urinary tract infections without negatively affecting the anastomosis between the ureter and urinary bladder. There is also information in the literature that the JJ catheter can be removed from the bladder after seven days together with the urinary bladder catheter. Some centers create therefore special constructions to take out the JJ catheter in the period less than two weeks after the operation. These constructions consist for example of suturing the end of the JJ catheter with the end of the urinary bladder catheter. In my experience, removing the JJ catheter about two weeks after the surgery gives the best results, promotes healing of the anastomosis and prevents stenosis and urine leakage. Of course, the use of the catheter never protects the patient 100% against urine leakage, constriction or ureter necrosis. Let us remember that the kidney transplant is performed not only by experienced surgeons, but also by surgeons who are just learning this difficult art. Their technique of connecting the ureter to the bladder is not always ideal, they often work without magnifying glasses, sufficient supervision and at night or in the morning when the whole team is already very tired. In our clinic, 15 years after the introduction of the JJ catheter the number of diagnosed leaks in 160–170 transplanted kidneys per year has decreased from 8–10 to 0–3 cases. Of course, the incidence of UTIs increased and some JJ catheters had to be removed by the urologist earlier than assumed. Remember that a UTI in a patient after kidney transplantation with a JJ catheter placed in the urinary system before its removal is an indication to start antibiotic treatment. Only when the antibiotic therapy becomes ineffective as a result of the development of strains of bacteria which are resistant to treatment, should the JJ catheter be removed as soon as possible.

### 4.9.5.4 Urinary Diversion in Kidney Transplantation

#### 4.9.5.4.1 Introduction

The earliest attempt to divert the urine flow from the ureters to the intestine was performed in 1851 by John Simon. In the absence of antibiotics, ureterosigmoidostomy and its modifications during the 19th and early 20th century have been associated with a high rate of surgical and metabolic complications. In 1910, Robert Coffey demonstrated a new method for ureterointestinal anastomosis, which renovated the primary enthusiasm in ureterosigmoidostomy and gained broad popularity during the next 40 years. In 1950, Ferris and Odel reported an 80% incidence of hyperchloremic metabolic acidosis following ureterosigmoidostomy. Based on further investigations by Lapides in 1951, Parsons, Powel and Pyrah in 1952, and Stamey in 1956, which clearly demonstrated that hyperchloremic metabolic acidosis is an inevitable complication of the ureterosigmoidostomy, this urinary diversion lost its popularity. In the 1950s the ileal conduit, popularized by Bricker, became the gold standard for the procedure. Early attempts at continent urinary diversion occurred from 1888, by Guido Tizzoni and Alfonso Poggi, while the first reservoir-type ileal loop urinary diversion was performed by Cuneo in 1911. By better understanding of the principles of detubularization, based on the work of Kock, and the principles of clean intermittent catheterization, established by Lapides, interest in continent urinary diversion has increased. Up to date, various continent cutaneous stomal reservoirs, sigmoidal-rectal pouches and orthotopic bladder substitutes have been described. Regarding the encouraging improvements in biocompatible materials, alloplastic bladder replacement could be the next step for the future in bladder replacement surgery [56, 87].

### 4.9.5.4.2   Surgical Performance Techniques of Ileal Conduit and Ureter Conduit Connections

There are variations in approach to the formation of an ileal conduit; however, the main principles of the operation are described here. It can be performed open via a laparotomy, laparoscopically or robotically assisted. The first stage consists of isolating the ileal loop of approximately 15 cm long and situated 15 cm from the ileocecal junction [57]. This segment of the ileum is then inspected for its suitability as a conduit; for example, no evidence of inflammatory bowel disease. Next, it is important to ensure that the identified ileum will reach the stoma site tension free before dividing it and that the vascular arcade within the mesentery is not disturbed. In obese patients, the length of ileum needs to be longer to avoid tension on the stoma. The mesentery to the selected ileal segment must be divided with care to preserve the blood supply to both the conduit and the ileo-ileal anastomosis; a Kelly clamp and ties can be used or an energy device. When dividing the bowel, it is important to mark the distal end that will form the stoma. A GIA (Endovascular Gastrointestinal Stapler) stapler or non-crushing clamps and scalpel can be used to divide the bowel. The remaining two ends of the ileum are anastomosed using a stapled or hand-sewn technique to restore the bowel continuity, and the mesenteric window is closed with Vicryl sutures. Upon completing the anastomosis, the ileal segment for the conduit should be below that of the ileal anastomosis [56, 87]. The second stage involves mobilizing the patient's own ureters or performing a ureteral connection of the transplanted kidney with an early performed ileal conduit. The anastomosis of the patient's own ureter without a kidney transplant is essentially the same as the implantation of the transplanted kidney's ureter into the conduit. A number of surgical techniques for connecting the patient's own ureter or the ureter into the ileal conduit will now be described. This operation should be performed from the lateral side of the ureters as much as possible to preserve their blood supply. The distal ends of the ureters should be handled as little as possible to avoid traumatizing the tissue that is required for the anastomosis. The left ureter is moved to the right side of the abdomen through a window created in the mesentery behind the sigmoid colon. It is important that the blood supply to the sigmoid colon is not compromised and that the window is wide enough to avoid any constriction or tension on the left ureter. The distal ends of the ureters can be cut and sent for analysis to see if there is an extension of cancer.

The third stage is the uretero-enteric anastomosis; this can be an end-to-side anastomosis (Bricker technique) where the two ureters are anastomosed to the proximal end of the conduit at slightly different locations to avoid any compromise in blood supply. A full-thickness enterotomy is created on the side of the conduit; the ureter is spatulated and then anastomosed to the conduit taking interrupted full-thickness bites of both the ureter and bowel using 4/0 or 5/0 PDS (p-dioxanone absorbable monofilament suture). The adventitia of the ureter is sutured to the serosa of the bowel. A small full-thickness serosal and mucosal plug is removed. Interrupted 5/0 PDS sutures approximate the ureter to the full thickness of the mucosa and serosa. The anterior layer is completed by the interrupted sutures placed through the adventitia of the ureter and the serosa of the small bowel [88]. A ureteric stent can be placed across the anastomosis and securely fixed to the conduit. The Wallace technique is another popular uretero-enteric anastomosis that requires the proximal end of the conduit to be left open initially and then closed with the two ureters anastomosed over the end. The ureters are spatulated and laid adjacent to each other to be stitched together using PDS, both apexes are aligned together, and the distal ends of the ureters are combined. The free edges of the ureters are then anastomosed to the open end of the conduit sealing it off. One potential downside to the Wallace technique is that a recurrence in one ureter may compromise the other ureter. No matter which technique is used, several surgical principles apply to both techniques, including maintenance of an adequate distal ureteral blood supply, a tension-free anastomosis, and avoidance of ureteral kinking or twisting. The fourth stage is creating the stoma via a trephine incision where a circular piece of skin is removed at the pre-marked stoma site, followed by the dissection down to the anterior rectus sheath where a cruciate incision is made. Below the anterior sheath, the rectus muscles are split, and then entry into the peritoneal cavity is gained. The hole in the fascia should be able to admit two fingers. Once this has occurred, the distal end of the conduit is delivered through to the skin using a Babcock, ensuring there is no twist in the conduit. The stoma is then matured and spouted to prevent excoriation of the skin around the stoma site. The difference between the anastomosis of the patient's own ureter and the ileal conduit is that the ileal conduit in kidney transplantation patients is created much earlier for this purpose by the urologist and in order to mature for transplantation. It is usually created on the right side of the abdominal cavity at different heights, so it is important to assess before transplantation the position of the kidney in relation to its ureter [56, 89–91].

### 4.9.5.4.3 Complications

Early complications (less than 90 days) include those involving the bowel, such as obstruction, anastomotic leak and ileus. Ileus can occur in up to 20% of cases and is often the reason for prolonged hospital admission. The urinary leak is also important to consider and accounts for about 7% of complications [56, 89]. This often occurs due to tension at the anastomosis.

Delayed complications (more than 90 days) include those involving the newly formed stoma, such as parastomal hernia, retraction or stenosis and bleeding. Frequent UTIs can often be a problem for patients, and up to 6% end up dying from end-stage renal failure. These patients are also predisposed to develop renal stones; ultrasound (USS) imaging can detect this. Metabolic complications can be of significant consequence; hence regular follow-up is needed to ensure if the electrolytes are normal, and if the patient is not acidotic [89].

### 4.9.5.4.4   The Most Important Steps in Kidney Transplantation

A patient with urinary deviation who needs a kidney transplant is a complex patient and the creation of an ileal conduit usually takes place before the kidney transplant operation. First, the type of incision must be adjusted to the position of the ileal conduit on the abdominal surface. After making the incision and dissecting the iliac vessels, we must dissect the peritoneum along the entire length of the incision to locate the ileal conduit. I personally help myself in finding the conduit with different probes of an intra- and extrahepatic biliary tree. After cutting the peritoneum and performing adhesiolysis in order to locate the conduit, I insert my left hand into the abdominal cavity from the outside and from the surface of abdominal wall I insert through the ileostomy skin opening a thick metal curved biliary probe into the ileal conduit. Moving the probe in the ileostomy and palpating from inside makes it possible to locate the conduit. After finding it, its ileum part should be carefully and precisely dissected from the surrounding tissues taking care not to damage the mesentery of the vascular conduit and therefore does not cause any damage to the blood supply. The most important steps of this operation are that before the transplantation everything must be completely dissected, so the iliac vessels should be dissected, the ileal conduit should be located and dissected so that the ureter can be anastomosed to it immediately after the kidney transplantation. Never transplant a kidney and then search for the ileal conduit because firstly it will be difficult to

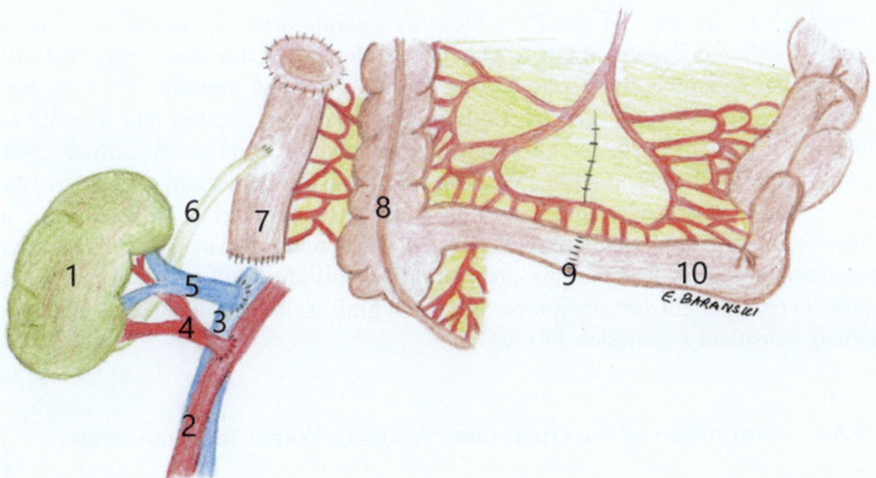


**Fig. 4.68** Urinary diversion in kidney transplantation. Transplanted kidney with ureter pointing upwards upwards and anastomosis of the transplanted kidney to the ureter with an ileal conduit. (Bricker technique). 1—Transplanted kidney, 2—Iliac artery, 3—Iliac vein, 4—Renal artery, 5—Renal vein, 6—Upward facing ureter of the transplanted kidney, 7—Ileal conduit, 8—Ascending colon, 9—Ileo–ileal end-to-end anastomosis, 10—Ileum

find and secondly the ureter will fold and then you will not be able to find its best position. Again I repeat, the safest technique is the one where everything is dissected. Now you can take care of measuring the kidney and the ureter, so that the vessels do not fold and are not twisted and so that the ureter by turning a gentle hatch can be anastomosed to the ileal conduit without tension and of course so that it does not fold either. To sum up, in order to obtain an optimal position of the kidney and the ureter, often the kidney must be grafted upside down with the ureter facing upwards. Of course, the whole ureteral anastomosis must or should be drained with one or two JJ drains. The operation is completed with the application of a ureterocutaneostomy catheter followed by the whole ileostomy and catheter which are inserted into the stoma bag. In the Sect. 4.9.5.4.1.2 the surgical technique of anastomosis between the ureter of the transplanted kidney and the ileal conduit was described in detail (Fig. 4.68).

### 4.9.5.4.5   Results

Surange et al. [90] investigated 59 renal transplants which were drained into an ileal conduit. There were 12 living related and 47 cadaveric kidneys transplanted. Spina bifida, the most common cause of end stage renal disease, was seen in 22 patients (41%). Actuarial graft survival was 90% at 1 year, 63% at 5 years, 52% at 10 years and 52% at 15 years. Actuarial patient survival was 95% at 1 year, 83% at 5 years, 69% at 10 years and 69% at 15 years. Graft and patient survival was statistically similar to the outcome of the 2579 other transplants done at our center between January 1980 and December 2001. At a mean follow up of 4.6 years (range 0.1–20) mean serum creatinine was in the 39 functioning grafts 156 mmol/l. Of the surgical complications 21% were directly attributable to the ileal conduit and it could be considered a risk factor contributing to the complication in a further 39%. Symptomatic UTI was noted in 65% of the patients, although it did not lead to graft loss. Kidney transplant drainage into an ileal conduit for urinary diversion is an effective treatment for patients with an end stage renal disease due to abnormal lower urinary tracts. Despite the preexisting comorbidity and the increased complication rate, patient survival of the long-term graft is comparable to the one in the normal transplant population [90, 91].

### 4.9.5.5   Completion of the Operation (Which Is Worth Remembering)

#### 4.9.5.5.1   Perfect Hemostasis

After the uretero-bladder anastomosis is completed, we draw our attention to the transplanted kidney: I personally use the automatic abdominal retractor to reveal the whole transplanted kidney once more. As many times as needed, rinse the kidney and its surroundings with warm physiologic natrium chloride solution or lactate Ringer's solution. Pay particular attention to the hemostasis. Use for example an

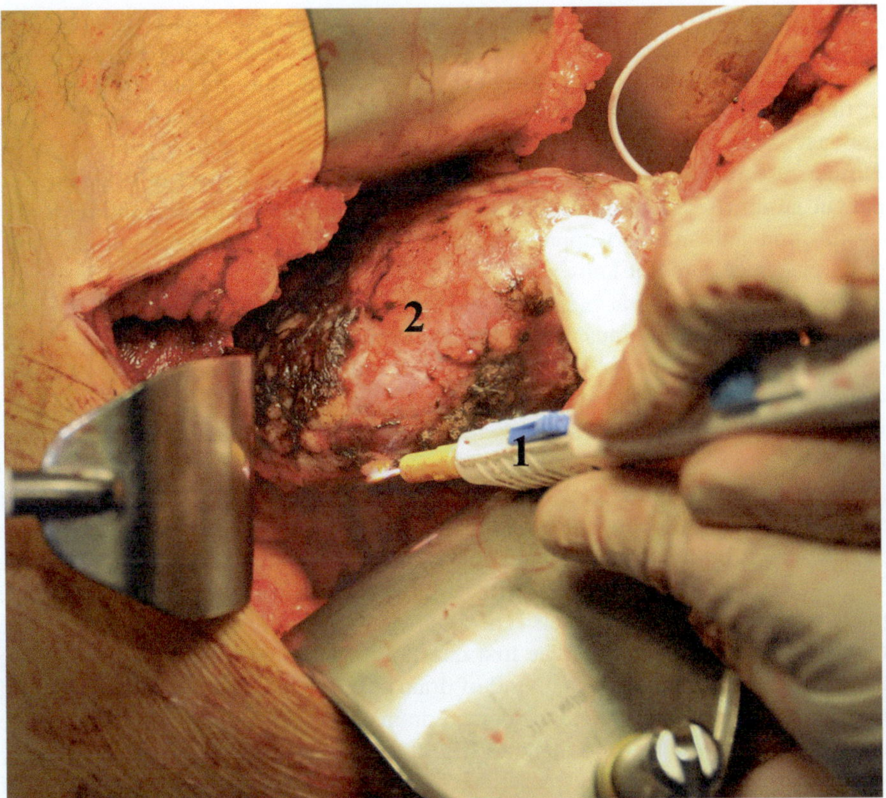

**Fig. 4.69** Last stage of kidney transplantation: exact hemostasis. 1—Argon beamer in action for perfect hemostasis, 2—Transplanted kidney

Argon Beamer and/or coagulation for it (Fig. 4.69). If necessary, use different topical hemostatic agents, especially around the renal pelvis and ureter, then check the vascular anastomosis for tightness (a too loosely tied suture, injury of vessel wall, too large a distance between the sutures). Finally, pay attention to subcapsular bleedings, the position of the kidney in relation to the renal vessels, and its blood supply.

### 4.9.5.5.2   Drains

Peri-graft collections and wound complications are common after transplantation. Drain placement is not associated with a significant reduction in wound complications kidney transplant and does not reduce the risk of clinically significant peri-graft collections. Since it is associated with a reduced need for imaging to diagnose collections, it has the potential to reduce transplant costs. Adult kidney transplantation is most commonly made into an extraperitoneal potential space, and surgically placed drains are used routinely in many centers. There is limited evidence of clinical benefit for prophylactic drainage in other major abdominal and vascular surgery. These data associate a higher rate of more frequent accumulation of fluid around the transplanted kidney collections with omission of prophylactic drainage, without a difference in the incidence of wound-related complications. Further research is required to definitively determine the impact of drains in this patient group [57]. Transplantation is, however, a unique setting combining organ dysfunction and immunosuppression, and the risks and benefits of prophylactic drain placement are not known [61].

The next problem that is always widely discussed is the drain or drains placement in the area of the transplanted kidney. Personally, I leave after transplantation one or two vacuum drains. The arguments that are given by the opponents of drains against the draining of the area of the transplanted kidney are that leaving the drain in the area of the kidney does not always prevent the accumulation of fluid and that the drains are a source of "infection" or a foreign organism whose colonization "only awaits" bacteria, fungi and viruses. Fluids that may collect around your transplanted kidney include blood, lymph, urine, dialysis fluid or peritoneal exudate (ascites). A build-up of fluid around your transplanted kidney can become infected. The infected and uninfected fluid collection may compress the parenchyma, renal pelvis, ureter and/or renal vessels. The renal vein and ureter are especially sensitive to pressure from the outside. The first question that arises, of course when we are the supporters of drains, is what kind of drains can we use to drain the area around the transplanted kidney? Silicone surgical drains (without a vacuum)—I do not use them immediately after transplantation, but often after each reoperation, especially when the fluid collection is/was infected or there is a need to rinse the site of infection. I also use them when I surgically drain lymphocele. The advantages of vacuum drain(s) include the creation of negative pressure in the retroperitoneal space which in turn promotes faster sticking of the peritoneum to the kidney, ureter, vessels and other structures of the retroperitoneal space because they cause elimination by suction of the air and fluid collection forming in the area of the transplanted kidney. The disadvantage of Redon drains is their stiffness and ease of clogging. The rigidity and hardness of these drains do not allow them to be kept for long close to the vessels or vascular anastomoses and the area of the ureter. Another drain that I have never used, but have seen other surgeons use, is the Blake drain. This drain differs from the Redon drain in that it has longitudinal grooves instead of side holes. Drainage occurs over a larger area, and the phenomenon of orifice occluding is rare in this type of drain. Blake drains come in a variety of configurations in length, thickness and groove distribution, and according to the literature are much less rigid than Redon tubes. JP drains I have been using for several years: the Jackson-Pratt silicone vacuum drains. The JP is a soft drain, has a cuboidal cross-section and a large number of holes. It can be kept in the transplanted kidney area for longer without fear of causing injury. After each transplantation, I place one or two JP drain(s) and put them around and behind the kidney in order to drain all the space around it, including the vascular and ureter anastomosis. How long do I keep a drain or removes in the extraperitoneal space? Firstly, you have to answer the question how many milliliters of fluid a drain drains per day, and secondly, what kind of fluid drained: urine or lymph? The results of aboratory measurements in the fluid of creatinine or triglyceride are very important here. If the drain does not remove either urine or lymph, I take it out when it has "produced" less than 20–30 ml of fluid over the last two days [46]—with no evidence of fluid collection by ultrasound examination. If the drain "produced" or "produces" more than 30 ml of liquid, I leave it.

It should also be asked how many drains should we use: one, two or maybe three? How are the drains located? drain is attached to a needle and pierced through the side wall (side flank) of the abdomen from the inside to the outside of the abdominal wall (right or left flank) and pulled out along with the needle. In the case of an IP, the drain is passed from the extraperitoneal space through the lateral flank of the abdominal cavity at half the distance between the lower and upper poles of the kidney. Sucking part of the drain is placed behind the upper pole of the kidney and then descends along the iliac vessels, behind the ureter towards the urinary bladder.

In the case of using two drains, both are led out through the side wall (side flank) of the abdominal wall. The upper drain is located behind the upper pole of the kidney, turns downwards and travels along the iliac vessels towards the bladder. A second drain extends downstream from the side flank of the abdominal wall and runs behind the lower pole, along the ureter, towards the bladder, where it then returns upwards along the iliac vessels.

### 4.9.5.5.3   Wound Closing

If the incision covers the posterior sheath of the rectus abdominal (above the arcuate line), we sew it with a continuous absorbable suture, preferably 2/0 monofilament. Sew the anterior sheath of the rectus abdominal with the same, but thicker suture—1/0 or 0/0. The question how to deal with the subcutaneous tissue: to suture it with a continuous suture or single stitches or not to suture? I stitch the entire thickness of the subcutaneous tissue with a continuous suture. Especially in obese patients, I try to leave a few dead spaces. In very obese people, I drain the subcutaneous tissue with the JP drain and suture the subcutaneous tissue tightly over it and use PREVENA (incision management system). The sewing must be tight, and channel must fit tightly to it, so that it works and does not suck the air in from the outside. The skin is usually sewn with an intracutaneous suture (Fig. 4.70) or closed with titanium staples. The operation ends with a dressing or very often with PREVENA. This system uses negative pressure—like a vacuum—to help to protect and heal your incision at the skin surface as well as below. The PREVENA system can be used on different incision types. PREVENA protects the incision from external

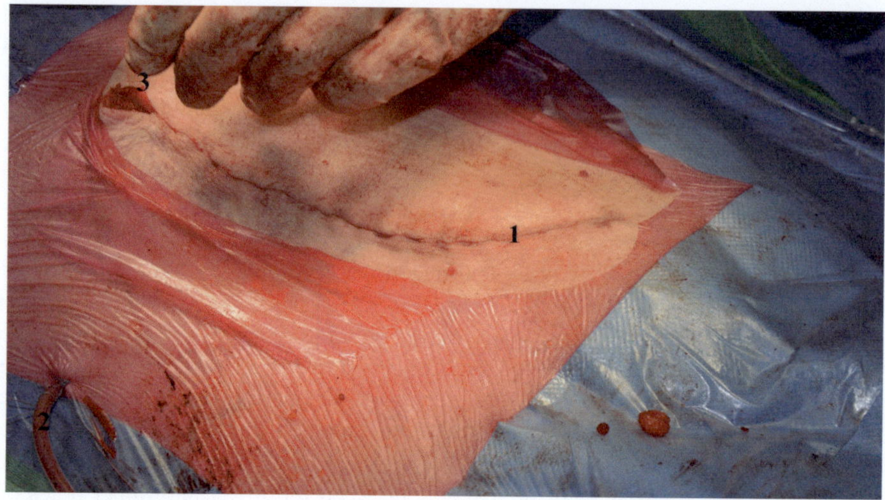

**Fig. 4.70** Completion of the operation. 1—The wound is closed with an intracutaneous suture, 2—JP drain has been placed behind the lower pole of the kidney, behind the ureter in the medial direction from the pelvic vessels to the bifurcation of the abdominal aorta, 3—Final wound closure

contamination, helps hold incision edges together, removes fluid and infection materials, and delivers continuous negative pressure at -125 mmHg for up to seven days. If the patient cannot tolerate a negative pressure of 125 mmHg after surgery and complains of pain in the wound, the pressure should be reduced to 80 mmHg [61].

Examples of kidneys transplanted to the right side are shown in Figs. 4.71, 4.72 and 4.73.

**Warning!**

After the vascular anastomosis is complete and the vascular clamps are released, not all kidneys will have a beautiful pink color, and also not all of them will start producing urine immediately. Some kidneys have spots, others will turn purple or be soft or hard under normal arterial blood pressure and also with normal blood inflow and outflow from the transplanted kidney. Nothing should be done with this type of kidney in the sense that, after completing the transplant, it is always worth the position of the kidney and to measure the flows in the renal and iliac vessels. If the flows are normal, and there is no arterial dissection, the kidney must be given a chance to regenerate and heal. Such kidneys require constant daily monitoring in the form of a blood flow test, such as a color Duplex Doppler sonography of the renal and iliac vessels and the renal's parenchyma, a MAG3 renal scan and/or a renal normal or dynamic scintigraphy.

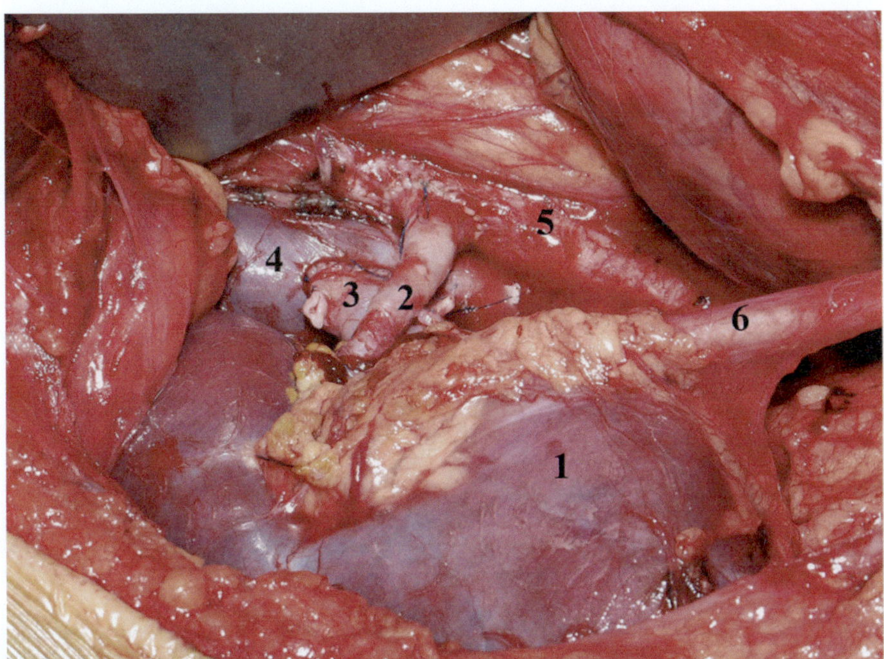

**Fig. 4.71** Example of a kidney transplanted to the right side of the body. 1—Kidney, 2—Renal artery with aorta patch, 3—Renal vein, 4—Common iliac vein, 5—Common iliac artery, 6—Through the ureteral wall visible JJ catheter located from the pelvis of the kidney through the anastomosis of the ureter with the urinary bladder, the end of which is located in the urinary bladder

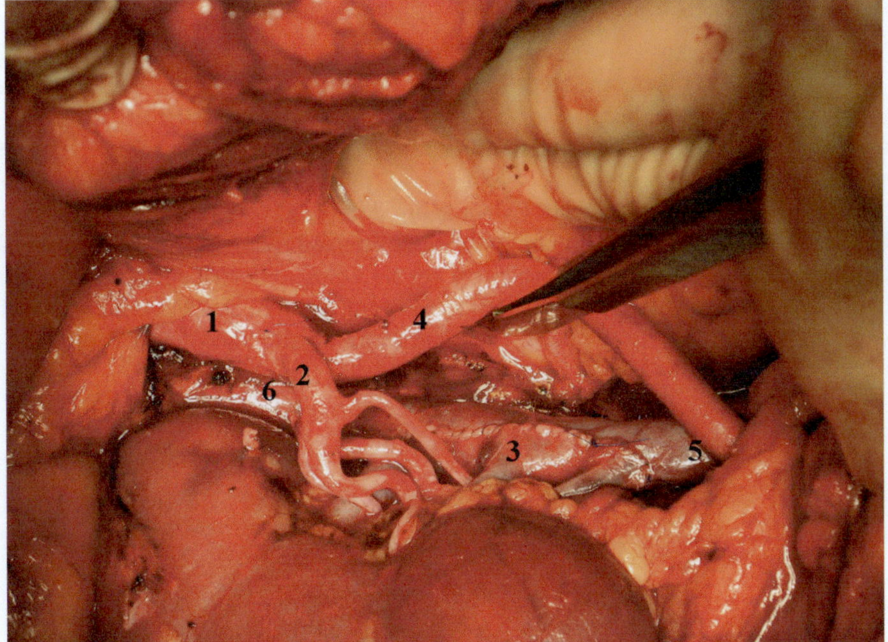

**Fig. 4.72** Example of a kidney transplanted to the right side of the body. 1—Right common iliac artery, 2—Renal artery, 3—Patch from the IVC with three renal veins, 4—Right external iliac artery, 5—External iliac vein, 6—Common iliac vein

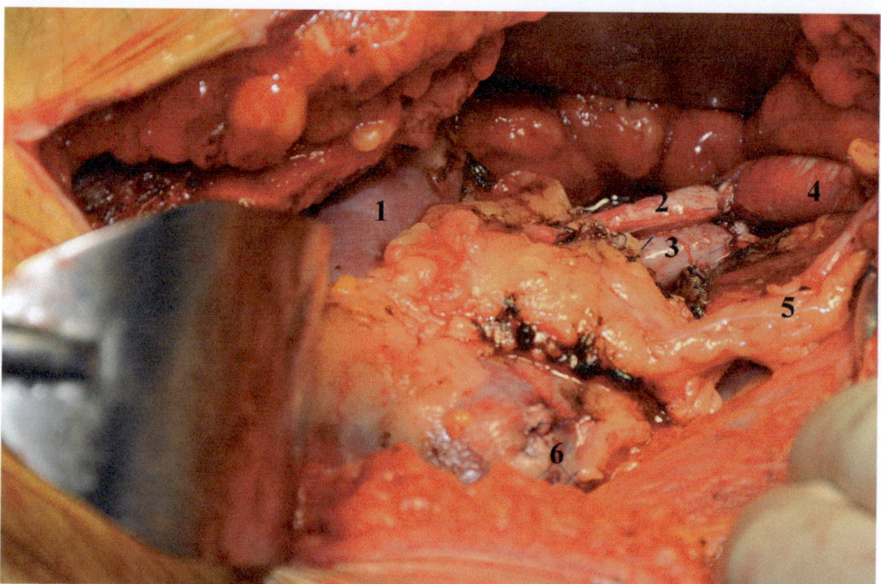

**Fig. 4.73** Example of a kidney transplanted to the right side of the body. 1—Kidney, 2—Renal artery, 3—Renal vein, 4—External iliac artery, 5—Ureter, 6—Open biopsy site, the sample was taken from the lower pole of the kidney

## 4.10	Kidney Transplantation on the Left Side

### 4.10.1	Introduction

You could say that there are no differences in the transplantation of the kidney on the right and left side, because on both sides the operation consists of performing renal anastomoses with the recipient's iliac vessels and bladder. However, the surgeon who has been involved in kidney transplantation for many years will say that this is not true because there are some big differences. As I have said before, it is easier for a surgeon to transplant to the right side and more difficult sometimes to transplant to the left side. In this section I am not going to describe the stages of the transplantation process that is common to the right and left kidneys again. Rather I will focus on describing the anatomical and technical differences in kidney transplantation to the left side.

## 4.10.2   Differences in the Position of the Iliac Vessels on the Right and Left

The left side iliac vessels are located differently than on right side and the surgical access to the common or external iliac vein is more difficult. The iliac veins on the left are located deeper and at a greater distance from the lumbar muscle than the same vessels on the right. The external iliac veins start at the level of the inguinal ligaments and at the level of the sacroiliac joints which they join with the internal iliac veins, forming the common iliac vein. On the right, the distal segment of the external iliac vein runs medially to the artery (Fig. 4.74), and when directed in the cranial direction, the external iliac vein moves backwards and runs on the right side of the artery, so that the right common iliac vein lies laterally from a single-named artery (Fig. 4.75). On the left side, the external iliac vein and the common iliac vein lie medially in relation to the mono-named arteries. The left common iliac vein passes beyond the initial segment of the right common iliac artery and is longer than the vein at the other side (Fig. 4.76).

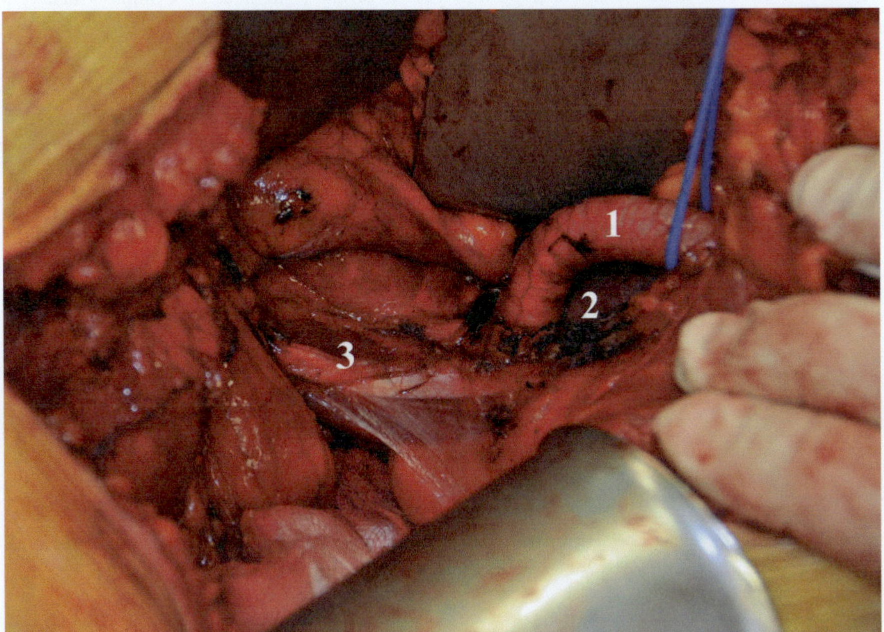

**Fig. 4.74** Iliac vessels on the right side. 1—Distal segment of the common iliac artery, 2—Proximal segment of the external iliac vein, the vein in this segment runs medially in relation to the common iliac artery, 3—Psoas major muscle

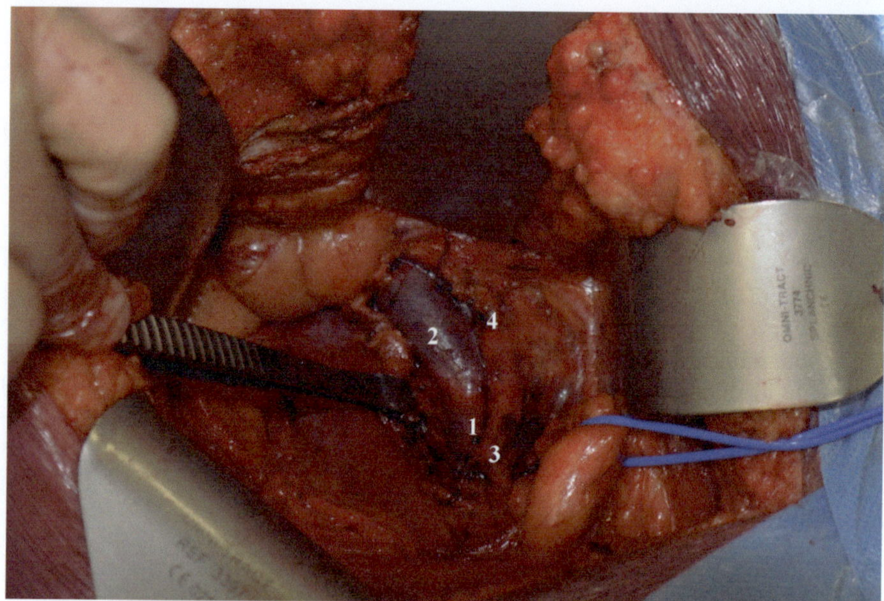

**Fig. 4.75** Reminder of the position of the iliac vessels on the right side. 1—Common iliac vein, 2—IVC, 3—External iliac artery, 4—Common iliac artery

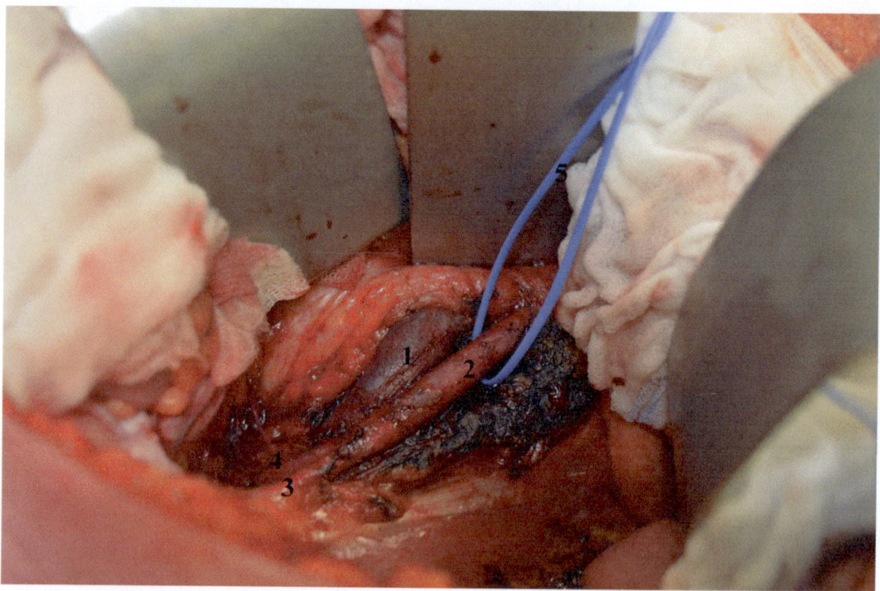

**Fig. 4.76** Position of the iliac vessels on the left side. 1—Common iliac vein, 2—Common iliac artery, 3—External iliac artery, 4—Internal iliac artery, 5—Vascular loop

### 4.10.3   *Method of Shortening the Distance Between the Short Renal Vein and the Iliac Veins*

The first and easiest method of renal vein elongation on the back table is the dissection of the vein from the renal hilum. Such a deep dissection of the renal vein towards the renal hilum will extend the former by about 1.5–2.5 cm. To get the renal vein longer, the small venous branches in the renal hilum have to be ligated. If the right kidney has been procured without the IVC, and you want to elongate it, you have to do the same maneuver as written before and first mobilize it well towards the hilum and then if necessary perform the vein elongation by using material other than the IVC. The source of other material for right renal vein reconstruction can come from an organ donor, a recipient or it can also be used as material for lengthening a vascular prosthesis.

Each right kidney with a short renal vein, which is transplanted to the left iliac fossa without elongating the right renal vein, is technically more difficult to transplant than to the right side. The transplantation of the right kidney into the left iliac fossa, especially in very obese recipients, without the possibility of elongation of the renal vein by means of the IVC or another vein, quite often requires extensive mobilization of the iliac vessels, including ligation and cutting of the iliac internal artery and vein. Sometimes the lateral part of the left common iliac vein runs behind the left common iliac artery. In such a case, after a complete mobilization from the extraperitoneal space of the common, internal and external iliac artery from the inguinal ligament to the aortic bifurcation, all these arteries can be gently pulled up, to the right and towards the midline with the renal vein blade retractor. After this maneuver the iliac venous system on the left side is visualized and shows the common, internal, external iliac veins, thus greatly shortening the distance between the renal vein and one of the iliac veins (Fig. 4.77). The end-to -side anastomosis

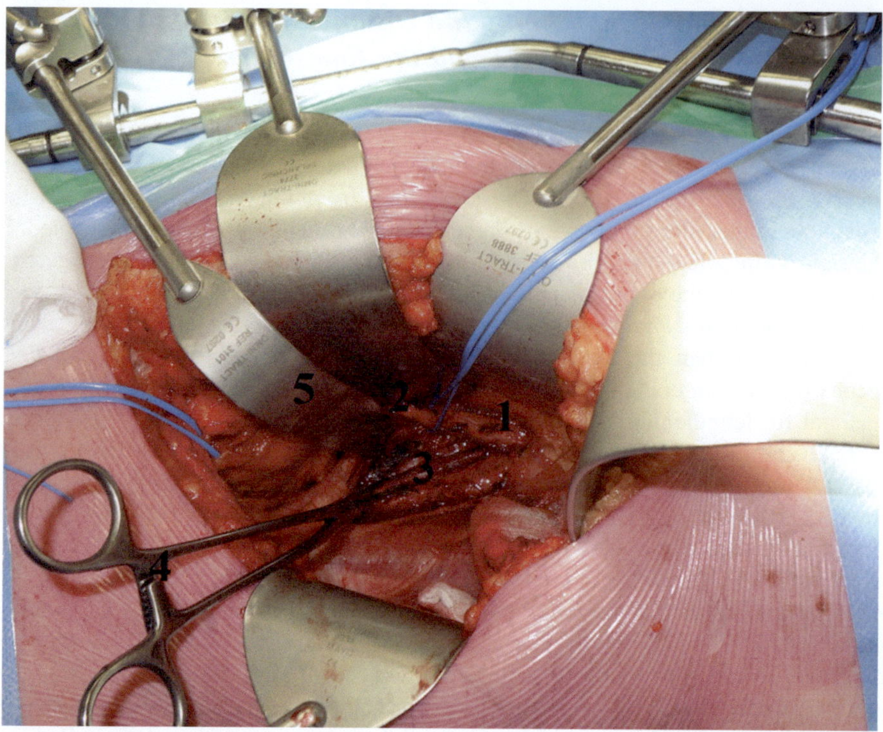

**Fig. 4.77** Left side, left iliac fossa. An example of mobilization of iliac arteries. The picture shows gentle pulling of the common, internal and external iliac artery by the renal vein blade of the retractor towards the midline. The end-to-side anastomosis of the renal vein was made with the common iliac vein behind the common iliac artery. 1—Common iliac artery, 2—External iliac artery, 3—Left common iliac vein, 4—Satinsky vascular clamp, 5—Dissected from the surrounding tissues common, internal and external iliac arteries. To ensure safe venous anastomosis, the mobilized iliac arteries are gently pulled in the medial direction of the body using the renal vein blade which is included in the equipotent the professional abdominal retractor.

between the renal vein and common iliac vein in this is case situated behind the common iliac artery. Examples of kidneys transplanted to the left side are shown in Figs. 4.78, 4.79 and 4.80.

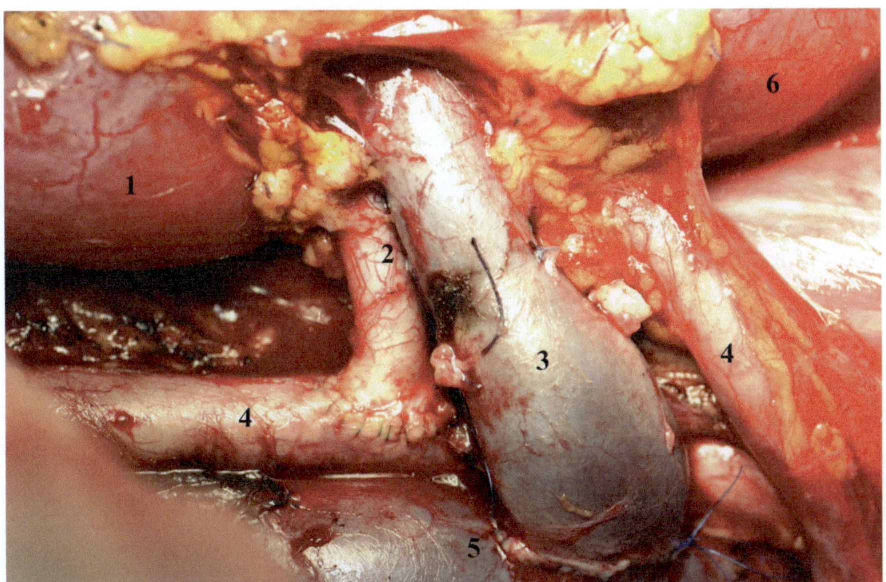

**Fig. 4.78** Left kidney transplanted to the left side. 1—Kidney, 2—Renal artery, 3—Renal vein, 4—Ureter decompressed with JJ catheter, 5—Common iliac vein, 6—Lower pole of the kidney (picture has been taken from the right side)

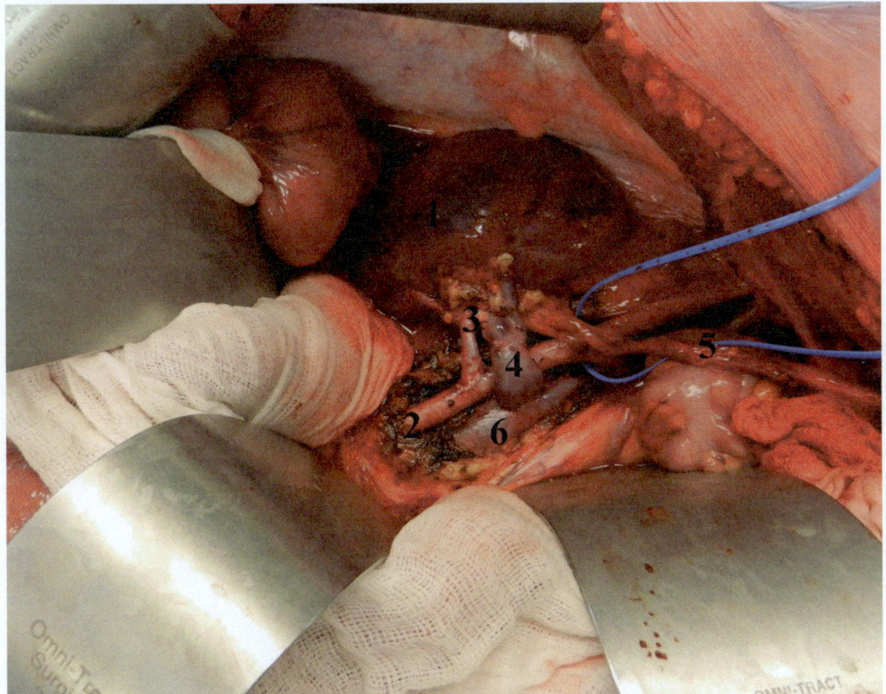

**Fig. 4.79** Left kidney transplanted to the left side during pancreas and kidney transplantation: intraperitoneal access from midline incision. 1—Kidney, 2—Common iliac artery, 3—Renal artery, 4—Renal vein, 5—Ureter, 6—Common iliac vein

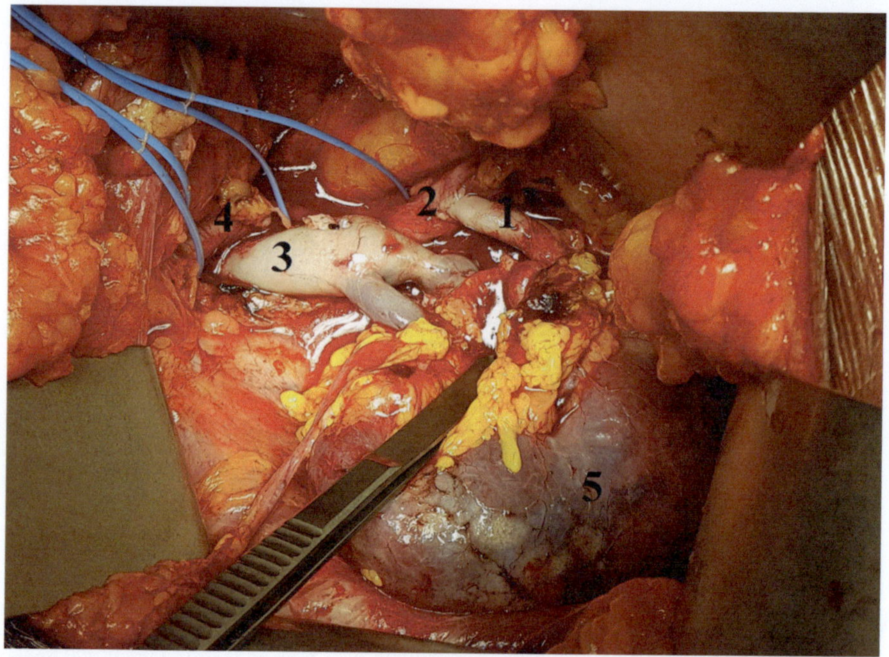

**Fig. 4.80** Transplanted right kidney to left side. Elongation of the two renal veins with the IVC. The IVC is placed behind the external iliac artery and anastomosed end-to-the side with the external iliac vein. 1—Renal artery, 2—Common iliac artery, 3—IVC as elongation material for two renal veins, 4—Left external iliac artery, 5—Kidney

## 4.11  Author's Own Experiences: Difficult Cases of Kidney Transplantation

### *4.11.1  Introduction*

I would like to describe some of the situations which I have encountered in my career. I know that the description of a case can be inspiring and provoke much thought and instruction, because we always ask ourselves: Would I also solve this problem in this way? I think that the cases I have chosen will be so inspiring that most readers will find a better and more creative solution to the problem than the one we have chosen—which I sincerely wish for.

## *4.11.2    First Case: Third Kidney Transplantation With the Simultaneous Removal of One of the Previously Transplanted, Failing Kidneys*

### 4.11.2.1    Introduction

There is controversy about the results of a second and third kidney transplantation. Generally, the outcomes and graft survival of the retransplantation have been reported to be inferior compared to the first transplant [59–61], but similar results have also been reported [59–61] [62–64]. In order to make a decision about retransplantation the following factors should be taken into account: the duration of the previous allograft function, the interval between transplants, previous transplant nephrectomy, the age of the recipient, his or her race, the presence of diabetes mellitus, histocompatibility leukocyte antigen (HLA) mismatch and donor source [57, 64–67]. If we look at the results of third kidney transplants made 20 years ago they were disappointing, so in 2006, Mazzucchi [71] described the results of third transplants in 21 patients. Note that third and subsequent transplants performed extraperitoneally are more time-consuming (more than 300 min) and require more transfusions in the perioperative period. A higher but acceptable incidence of arterial thrombosis and urinary obstruction were observed. One-year graft survival was 57.1% (75% for live and 46% for cadaver donors) for retransplants and 86% for first transplant patients (P < 0.0001). At that time the one-year graft survival was better with live donor grafts, but was still lower when compared with the first transplants using the same surgical technique [69].

With the passing of years, thanks to improvements in surgical technique and better preparation of the patient for the operation, good surgical results and survival of both the graft and the kidney recipient have finally been achieved. Friedersdorff [70] presented a total number of 16 kidney transplantations in which he demonstrated that 13 of them underwent a third and three of them a fourth kidney transplantation. The patient survival was 92.3% after one year and 76.9% after five years (third graft). One-year censored graft survival was 100% and a five-year graft survival was 74.1% (third graft), respectively. In the cases of the fourth transplantation, the graft survivals of 33.3% at one and two years were noted among three patients. All fourth graft recipients survived during the observation time. The overall rate of postoperative surgical complications among third graft recipients was 46.2 and 66.7% among patients after a fourth transplantation. Finally, the results of the third kidney transplantation showed satisfactory patient and graft survival with acceptable outcomes.

As far as the choice of incision is concerned, most authors preferred a medial incision with the possibility of choosing a suitable place in the abdominal cavity for the transplantation. As far as the treatment of the old graft is concerned, if it is small and does not interfere with the recipient and there is enough space to place the new kidney graft under or above it, the old graft should be left alone. Another group of surgeons strives to remove the graft by all means before the third transplantation. I am a member of another school of thought which advocates not removing grafts before the third transplantation unless there are clear indications to do so, and I am an advocate of removing a graft if necessary during the transplantation operation.

Preoperative three-phase CT and Duplex Doppler allow an accurate assessment not only of the recipient's iliac vessels but also of the condition and quality of the renal veins and arteries. The preparation of the iliac vessels and actually cutting them with scissors in the area of the completely fibrosed tissues around the iliac vessels which are as hard as a stone can lead to many unpleasant and irreversible complications in the recipient of a kidney. In my personal opinion, the removal of the graft before the third transplant only exacerbates the iliac vascular in fibrosis around the iliac vessels making the third kidney transplantation difficult and almost an impossible long-lasting operation.

### 4.11.2.2  Case Raport

This is the case of a 68-year-old female patient following two transplantations of a kidney, who was very highly immunized, and without the possibility of creating a vascular access for hemodialysis. For two years, the woman was on dialysis using a catheter inserted into the right subclavian vein. Both grafts, located on the right and left side, were insufficient and did not produce urine for many years. The transplanted kidneys were not removed because there was no indication that it was necessary to remove one or both kidneys until the third transplant. The patient was obese and suffered regularly in the last few weeks from biliary colic attacks because of the gallstones which before the transplantation manifested once or twice a week. In the performed CT screening without contrast, the iliac vessels on both sides showed slight calcifications and atherosclerotic changes.

The patient had been waiting for a suitable kidney for two years, but finally the Eurotransplant Programmed Framework found and offered her a matching right kidney. The donor was a young brain death organ donor who died because of craniocerebral injuries. Our centre received a right kidney with two renal arteries from the abdominal aorta on the aorta patch and two renal veins procured together with the inferior vena cava (IVC). Moving down the abdominal aorta from the top to the bottom, we first encounter the main renal artery of about 8–9 mm in diameter, which divides about 1 cm from the aorta patch into two renal arteries; the superior renal artery of 3–4 mm in diameter, which enters the upper pole of the kidney, and the main renal artery of 6–7 mm in diameter, which enters the renal hilum. 1 cm below the first renal artery is an additional renal artery that runs directly from the aorta to the lower pole of the kidney. There are two renal veins leading from the kidney to the IVC: the superior and inferior veins, which were obtained with the IVC (Fig. 4.81). The diameter of the lower renal vein was 6–7 mm and the upper vein was 20 mm. Taking the vessels of the transplant recipient into account, we tried to prepare the kidney for transplantation in such a way that the number of vascular anastomoses in the recipient's body was reduced to a minimum.

These are the general questions that I think every surgeon should ask himself or herself in such a situation before deciding to transplant:

– Which kidney, right or left, and from what kind of donor should be accepted for a third transplant?

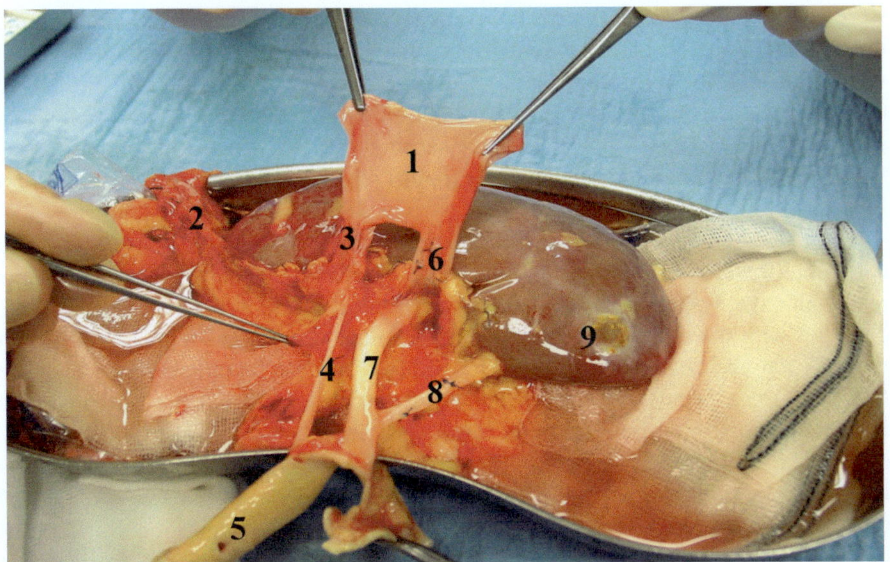

**Fig. 4.81**   Right kidney accepted. 1—IVC, 2—Ureter, 3—Aberrant renal vein going out from the lower pole, 4—Aberrant renal artery going to the lower pole, 5—Aortic patch, 6—Renal major vein, 7—Renal main artery, 8—Early branch of the renal artery to the upper pole, 9—Upper pole of the kidney

- Will each accepted kidney be technically feasible for transplantation? If not, what criteria does the kidney have to meet in order to be transplanted reasonably safely?
- To what extent are there atherosclerotic lesions in the recipient's vessels? Which side is "better" and which side is "worse" in terms of the severity of atherosclerotic lesions?
- What is the best place for the transplantation: the right or left side?
- What is the best surgical access to keep the risk of surgery as low as possible?
- Do you remove the gallbladder before the transplantation or do you leave it? Or maybe you should first perform a cholecystectomy or give up the offered kidney and wait for the next one?
- Have previous transplants been removed or not? If not, do you have to remove them during the transplantation? Can a new kidney be transplanted next to an old one? How do you deal with this difficult decision and finally difficult operation?
- Is it worth taking the risk, and if so, how great it is? How can you reduce the risk of the transplantation and how far can you go to transplant a third kidney?

The main aim of the inspection of this rather richly vascularized kidney was to reconstruct its vessels during the preparation for transplantation (benching) to limit the number of anastomoses to two or three in order to achieve the shortest possible time of warm ischemia during transplantation. After the renal vessels and ureter were prepared, fresh preservative fluid was injected into the main renal vein and the injected fluid was observed to come out of the smaller (lower pole) diameter renal vein (from the aberrant renal vein). Also very slowly, 50 ml of cold, fresh UW (University of Wisconsin) preservation solution was injected into the renal vein of a smaller diameter (lower pole); without sensing any resistance, the organ preservation solution passed into the superior (main) renal vein and then the preservation fluid came out of this main renal vein.

On this basis, a very good contact between the two veins was found. The additional lower renal vein was found to be a vein that did not play a role in the renal drainage system and due to its small diameter and excellent contact of its branches with the main trunk branches of the renal vein this vein was ligated with two 2/0 non-absorbable sutures. The lower artery, due to its diameter and distance from the main renal artery, was cut off from the aortic patch, shortened and implanted end to side into the main trunk of the renal artery as part of the plan to reduce the time of warm ischemia to a minimum. The lower pole artery was implanted in end-to-side fashion which was made on the catheter with a 7/0 non-absorbable running suture (Figs. 4.82 and 4.83). The whole renal artery, including the anastomosis place, was flushed with heparinized cold preservation solution and its tightness was checked. The ureter was also checked. The kidney was repacked and put in the transport box on ice.

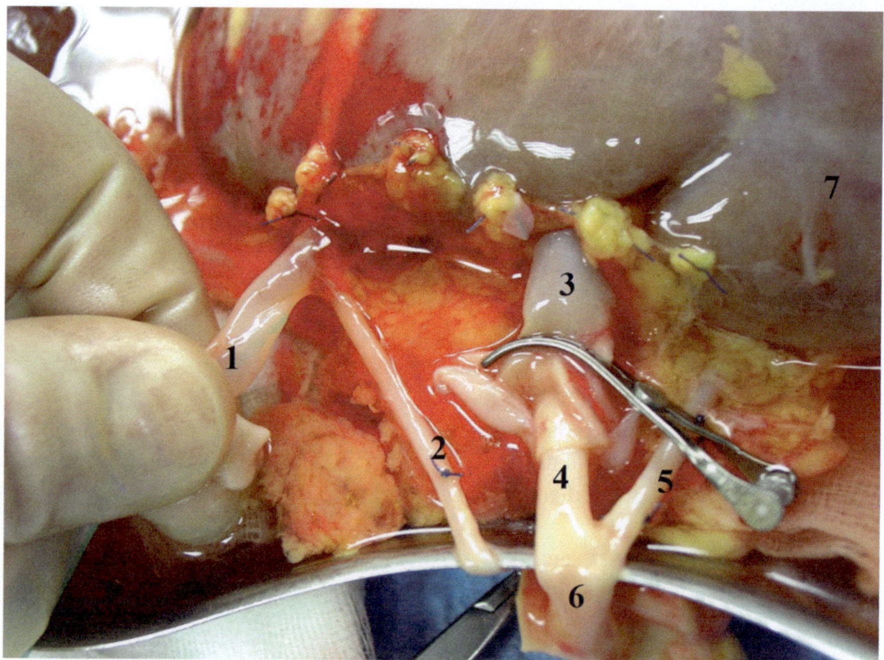

**Fig. 4.82**  1—Aberrant renal vein to the lower pole of the kidney, 2—Aberrant renal artery to the lower pole of the kidney, 3—Main renal vein, 4—Main renal artery, 5—Early branch of the renal artery to the upper pole (aberrant to the upper pole renal artery), 6—Main trunk of the renal artery, 7—Upper renal pole

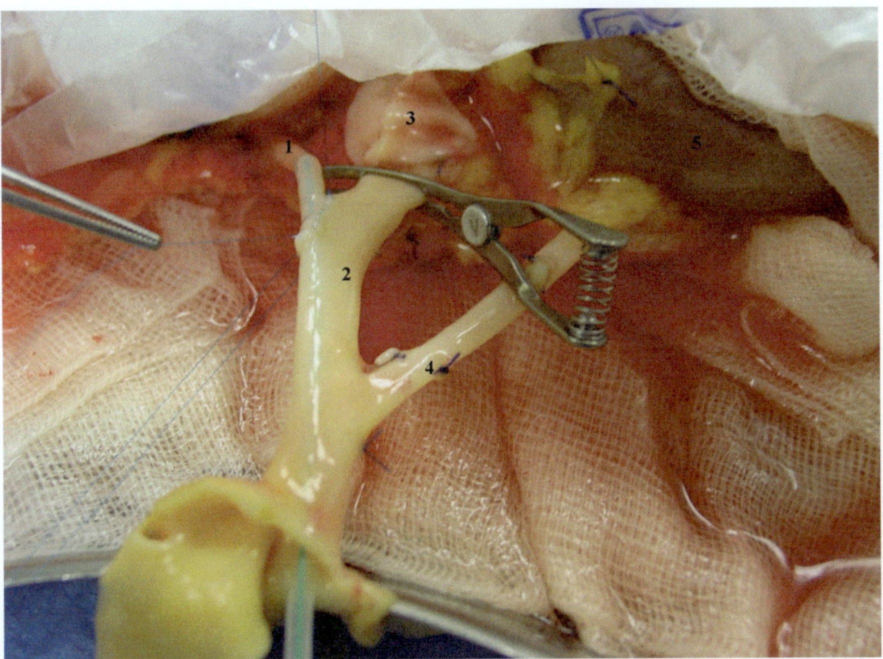

**Fig. 4.83** An aberrant renal vein going out from the lower pole was irrigated after examination. The aortic patch was too long for the recipient without severe arteriosclerosis. An aberrant renal artery to the lower pole was cut and sewn end-to-side to the main stem of the renal artery. 1—Aberrant renal artery to the lower pole of the kidney during suturing on the silicone tube, 2—The main stem of the renal artery, 3—Renal vein, 4—Early branch of the renal artery to the upper pole, 5—Upper pole of the kidney

The kidney transplantation was performed by a midline incision (Fig. 4.84). Examination of the abdominal organs did not reveal any significant lesions except gallbladder stones and a condition after two kidney transplants to the right and left iliac fossa. Both transplanted kidneys were in situ. The operation started with a classical gallbladder excision (Fig. 4.85), followed by the release of many massive adhesions, mainly between the intestines, different organs and abdominal wall, particularly at the sites of the transplanted kidneys. Due to better access to the kidney vessels decided to transplant the kidney to the right side. In the right side the old transplant was quite large and technically impossible to transplant a new kidney above or below the old one. It was decided to remove the old kidney in the first stage of the operation, keeping its vessels as long as possible and then transplant the new one. After repositioning the professional abdominal retractor to the lower abdomen, a stable operating field was obtained and the removal of the long ago transplanted kidney was started.

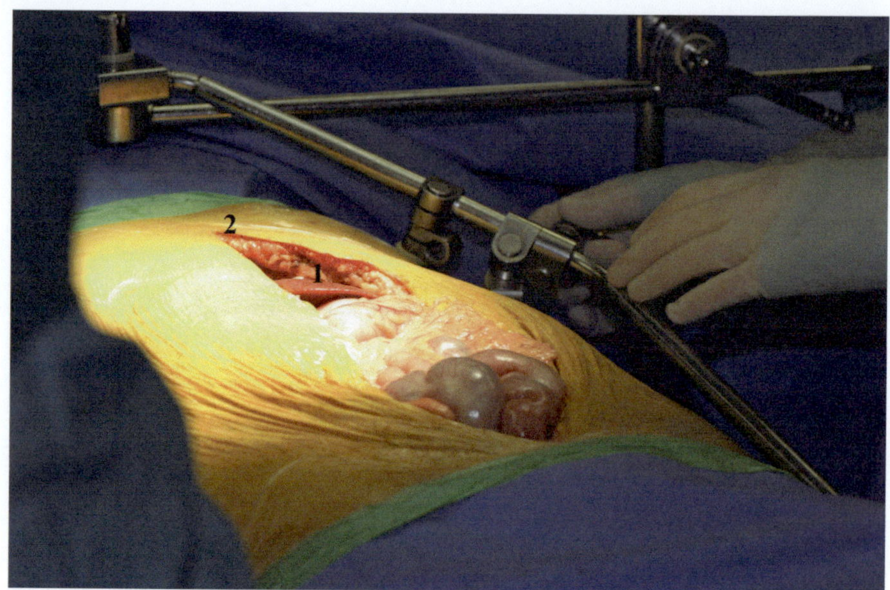

**Fig. 4.84** 1—Liver, 2—Middle line incision

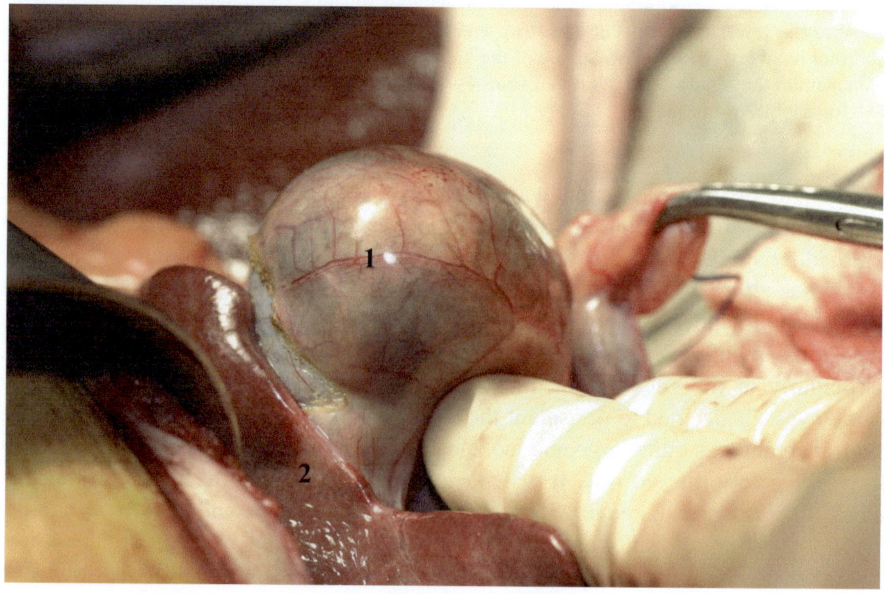

**Fig. 4.85** Operation started with cholecystectomy, 1—Gallbladder, 2—Liver

Surgical steps to remove the old kidney transplant and replace it with a new one:

1. Fill the bladder with warm Ringer's solution or physiologic saline chloride.
2. Localize the old ureter-urinary bladder anastomosis and ureter.
3. Ligate the ureter with two ligatures near the anastomosis and cut it.
4. Dissect the ureter of the transplanted kidney from the surrounding tissues towards the kidney's hilum. This kind of mobilization of the ureter from the bladder towards the renal hilum gives us access to the external iliac and renal vessels and to the posterior surface of the kidney (Fig. 4.86).
5. Mobilize the kidney from the retroperitoneal space: it is usually quite a difficult procedure. Mobilization of the old transplanted kidney should be continued along the posterior side of the kidney towards the upper pole, renal pelvis, and up and down the iliac vessels, where the vascular anastomoses are (very sharp scissors, an Argon Beamer and coagulation in this case become indispensable when cutting and dissecting fibrous tissues which very often resemble stone or rock hardness).
6. Free the old renal vessels as much as possible towards the renal hilum, then ligate and cut them. The renal vessels have to be prepared in such a way that they always have to be kept as long as possible and not damaged during the preparation—especially in patients with severe calcifications in the iliac vessels, where sometimes the old vessels are the only place to perform anastomoses between the kidney and the recipient's vessels.

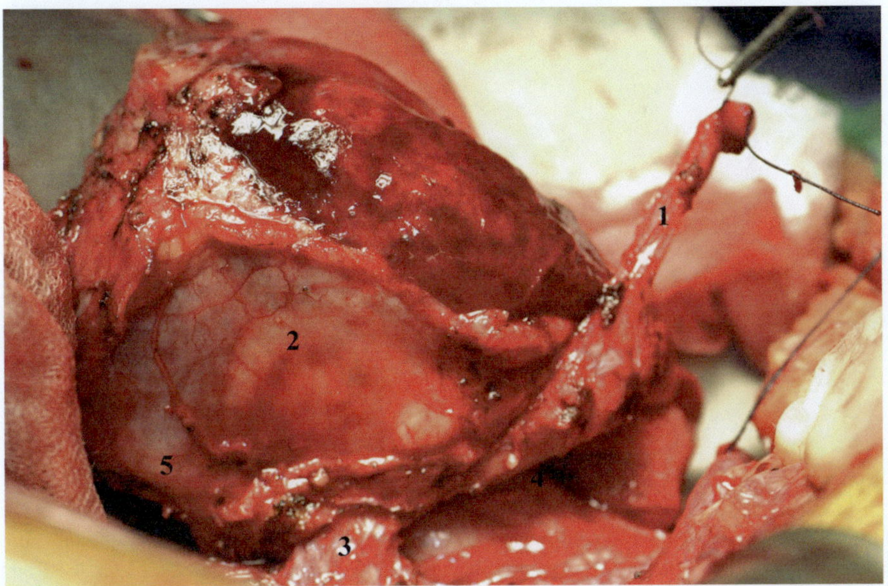

**Fig. 4.86** 1—Tied and cut off close to the urinary bladder—the ureter of the transplanted kidney, 2—Kidney, 3—Prepared renal vein of old kidney transplant, 4—Lower pole of the kidney released from retroperitoneal space. This is also the easiest place to access the recipient's pelvic vessels, as well as the vessels of the previous kidney that will be removed for transplantation of the next kidney. 5—Released posterior side of the kidney from retroperitoneal space

7. At this stage, remove the previously inspected transplantation kidney from the transport box. Take an open biopsy from the upper pole and briefly insert the kidney wrapped in cold gauze into the retroperitoneal space of the recipient in order to determine the best position of the kidney, the best places for the vascular anastomoses and the best length of the renal vessels. If the iliac vessels are in a good condition, then we decide to use them and perform the vascular anastomoses in the new places. If it is impossible or the vessels are in a bad condition, you can use the old vessels of the resected kidney. The renal vessel stumps, if they are not used, have to be shortened, ligated and sewn (Fig. 4.87).

8. In this case, since the iliac artery was only slightly atherosclerotic, I decided to perform new vascular anastomoses in completely different places than the previous ones. The renal vein and artery stumps (in this case, each vessel) were tied twice with 2/0 non-absorbable sutures and shortened.

9. The first venous anastomosis was performed, an end-to-side anastomosis of the renal vein to the right common iliac vein with a 5/0 non-absorbable monofilament suture. The anastomosis of the renal artery was performed end-to-side with the common iliac artery of the recipient with a 6/0 non-absorbable monofilament suture (Fig. 4.88).

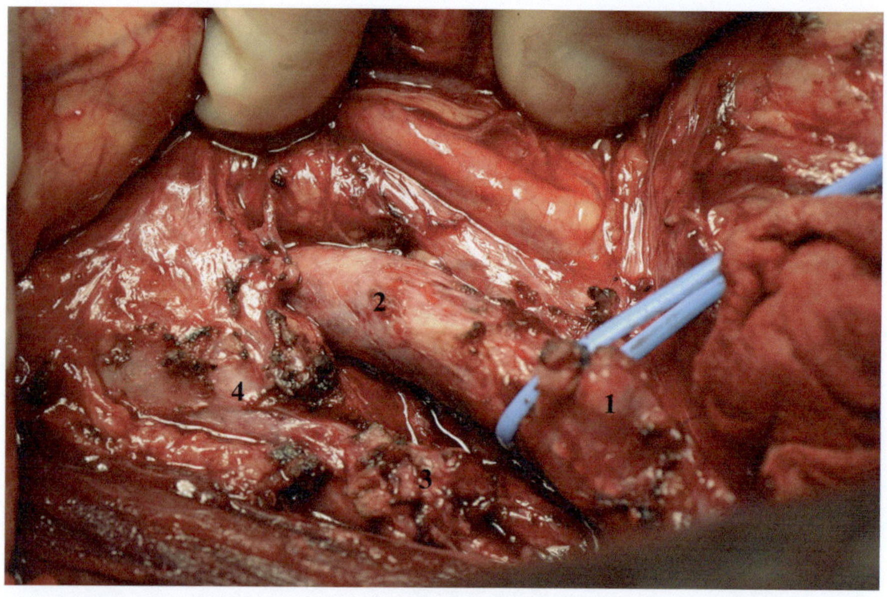

**Fig. 4.87** The very difficult operating field after the kidney was removed on the right side. 1—Stump of the old renal artery, 2—Common iliac artery, 3—Stump of an old renal vein, 4—Right common iliac vein

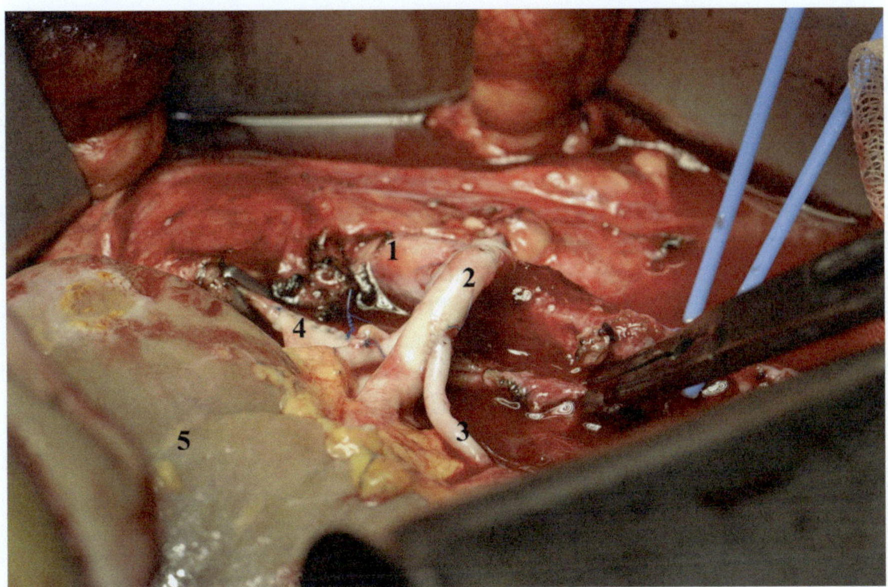

**Fig. 4.88** Picture of the second kidney transplant, before releasing the vascular clamps. 1—Common iliac artery, 2—Main stem of renal artery, 3—Renal aberrant artery, end-to-side anastomosis with the main renal artery, 4—End-to-side anastomosis of the renal vein with the common iliac vein, 5—Kidney

10. After the vascular clamps were released, the kidney immediately began to produce a small amount of urine (Fig. 4.89).
11. The ureter-bladder anastomosis was performed in the same place as the first one. The first ureter-urinary bladder anastomosis was completely excised, the new anastomosis was decompressed with the JJ catheter.
12. The kidney was partially covered with the peritoneum, which was led over the kidney and sutured to the abdominal wall, ensuring the permanent position of the kidney and preventing its possible movement within the abdominal cavity.
13. The space around the kidney was drained with two 27CH silicone surgical drains.
14. The abdomen was closed and the postoperative course was without any complications.

**Warning! (When one kidney is replaced by another kidney, try to keep the vessels of the old kidney as long as possible before retransplantation during the dissection)**

For the preparation of the renal and iliac vessels of the old kidney I recommend very sharp and pointed preparation scissors. Very often the tissues around the kidney and vessels are fibrotic, hard and cannot be processed by any other methods of preparation than cutting. The renal vessels of the transplanted old kidney should be prepared deeply in the hilum, systematically ligated or sutured so that after removing the kidney, the stumps of the "old" kidney vessels are not injured and are as long as possible. Vessel stumps can always be shortened, if they are in a good condition. If the iliac vessels of the recipient are not atherosclerotic, the renal vessels of the new kidney can be anastomosed at other sites in the iliac arteries and veins rather than the previously anastomosed old renal vessels (Fig. 4.89).

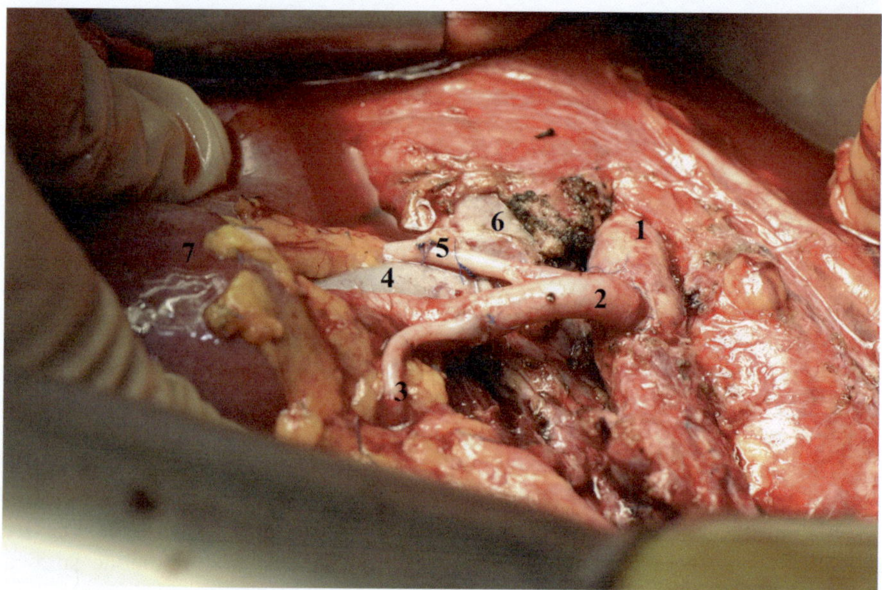

**Fig. 4.89** Second transplanted kidney; the following anastomoses were performed; end of the renal vein on the side of the common iliac vein and main stem of the renal artery "end to side" of the common iliac artery, 1—The right common iliac artery, 2—The main trunk of the renal artery, 3—The accessory renal artery, which runs to the lower pole of the kidney and is anastomosed at the end to the side of the main trunk of the renal artery. 4—Renal vein, 5—Renal artery branch to the upper pole of the kidney, 6—Border between the IVC and iliac vein, 7—Retraansplanted kidney

## *4.11.3   Second Case: Kidney Retransplantation With End-to-end Anastomosis Between the New Renal Artery and Old Renal Artery*

### 4.11.3.1   Introduction

I am a member of another school of thought which advocates not removing the grafts before the third transplantation unless there are clear indications to do so; and I am an advocate of removing a graft if necessary during the transplantation operation. In patients who have undergone a pancreas-kidney transplant the replacement of the kidney is challenging and sometimes a very complicated operation.

It is well known that early and late graft survival of the third or fourth transplants are inferior compared with the first or second transplants. Surgical problems—such as difficult access and dissection of an old organ, or hyperimmunization—and therefore a high rate of acute rejection and comorbidities, such as severe atherosclerosis (for example coronary diseases, severe atherosclerosis and calcification in aortoiliac vessels) or a long time on dialysis, make the third transplantation of a kidney a difficult operation which still gives many non-surgical complications: lymphocele (23%), vascular thrombosis (3.3–14%), ureter obstruction (7–10%), different fistulas (6–8%), and 30% of patients had episodes of acute rejection in the first month after retransplantation. The third kidney transplant has a high-risk recipient population. However, the results regarding the graft and patient survivals and complications encourage us to continue with this procedure; finally, it should also be remembered that worse results should be expected among the patients who lost previous grafts early or are highly hyperimmunized [71].

### 4.11.3.2   Case Report

This case concerns a second kidney transplant with the simultaneous removal of an insufficient kidney graft and replacing it with a new one in a patient with very advanced atherosclerotic lesions in the left iliac arterial traject.

A short history of the patient's disease: a man aged 55 years, who received a simultaneous pancreas and kidney transplantation seven years ago. The pancreas functioned well, but after a few years after grafting the kidney failed completely. The quality of the old grafted renal artery was good: no calcification, atherosclerotic changes and/or strictures. The computed tomography, performed without contrast, informed us about the severe bilateral atherosclerotic lesions localized from the aorta's bifurcation up to the inguinal ligament. The arterial vessels consisted of very advanced 2 mm thick closed calcium rings which were located at a small distance from each other in the lumen of the iliac vessels. Vascular access for dialysis was surgically impossible to perform. For several months the patient had been undergoing dialysis using a catheter inserted into the left subclavian vein. This possibility of dialysis due to partial subclavian vein thrombosis was also slowly coming to an end. The only chance to keep the patient alive was a second kidney transplant with arterial anastomosis to the unchanged renal artery of the transplanted kidney with simultaneous removal of the graft situated on the left side (the second, new kidney came from a living family donor, from whom the left kidney with one artery, one vein and one ureter was procured). The iliac veins on both sides were unchanged. The renal vein and anastomosis of the first graft were patent, without any obstruction. If necessary, the end of the renal vein of the new kidney can be anastomosed to the end of the renal vein of the transplanted kidney.

In short it was a very high risk operation. The living donor and the recipient and their families were informed about the possible intra- and post-operative complications and they agreed to the operation.

Surgical access was achieved by a midline incision. The justification for this choice is that the midline incision gives safe access to the graft and the iliac vessels on both sides and by using a professional abdominal retractor you obtain a stable surgical field. In the case of a difficult-to-control hemorrhage, the iliac vessels can, at the beginning of the bleeding, be brought under control and quickly closed. In the case of irreversible damage to one of the iliac arteries, an aorto-iliac or aorto-femoral by-pass can be performed. The midline incision also gives very good access to the urinary bladder during the operation.

**Operation Description**

After the midline incision was performed and the abdominal organs were inspected, numerous adhesions in the abdominal cavity were released. The descending colon and the sigmoid were mobilized halfway, revealing an insufficient graft on the left side. The intestines were wrapped in a wet gauze, moved towards the midline, and stabilized using professional abdominal retractor blades. The urinary bladder was filed with warm Ringer's solution and the ureter-bladder anastomosis was found. The ureter of the transplanted kidney was ligated close to the bladder and completely cut. By pulling the ureter of the transplanted kidney upwards and to the left, with very sharp scissors, it was slowly freed from the surrounding tissues and iliac vessels to the lower pole of the transplanted kidney. The left common iliac artery was dissected just next to the bifurcation of the aorta and the left external iliac artery close to the inguinal ligament. One vessel loop was placed around each dissected artery, the ends of vessel loops were fixed with the small clamps. The internal iliac artery was not mobilized (not dissected) because it was completely closed with atherosclerotic plaques. The next stage is the complete mobilization of the kidney from the retroperitoneal space, the posterior side kidney dissection and the ligation of all small branches of the renal artery and the vein deep in the hilum of the transplanted kidney. After cutting them deep in the hilum of the transplanted kidney, the graft was removed from the retroperitoneal space (Fig. 4.90). The postoperative course was uncomplicated and the patient went home in a good condition after three weeks.

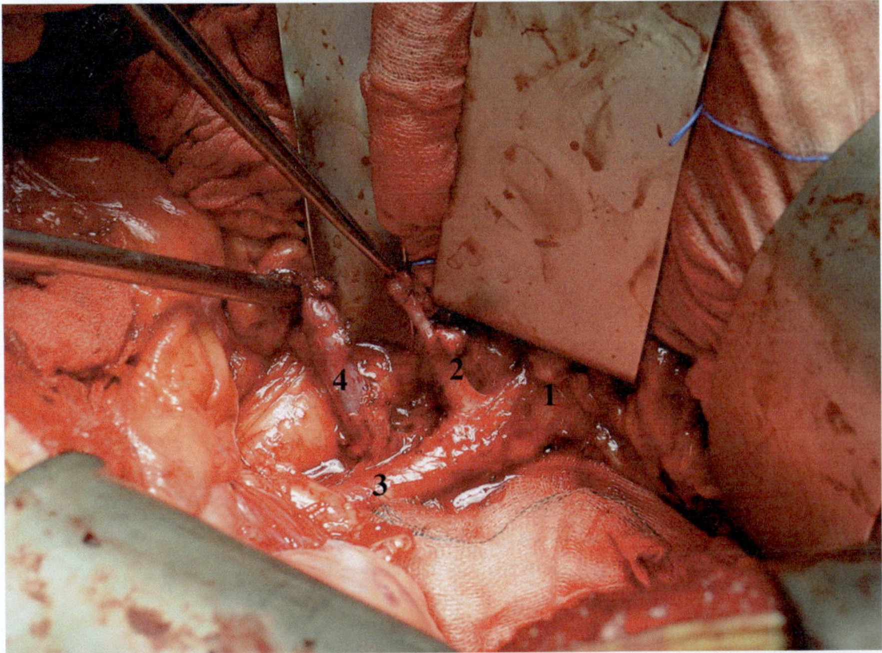

**Fig. 4.90** Left side. Graftectomy and kidney retransplantation performed at the same time. Left iliac vessels. 1—Common iliac artery, 2—Stump of the old renal artery of the removed kidney, 3—Common iliac artery below the anastomotic site, 4—Stump of the old kidney renal vein

**Attention!**

The mobilization of a large sized old kidney graft from the retroperitoneal space is difficult and requires surgical experience and sensitivity. The tissues around the transplanted kidney are very hard and fibrous. With one careless move, the graft vessels or iliac vessels can be irreversibly damaged. Such a hemorrhage is very difficult and sometimes impossible to control and repair because of fibrosis and the lack of any plasticity, i.e. stiffness of the vessels and tissues. When the kidney is large and has very strongly grown into the retroperitoneal muscle with its posterior surface, it is necessary to remember not to damage the nerves and its branches (such as the lateral femoral cutaneous nerve which is responsible for the innervation of the lateral tight and the genitofemoral and femoral nerve) during the posterior surface dissection. To prevent the above mentioned nerve injuries, the posterior surface of the kidney can be removed without the capsule. If during the kidney dissection it is impossible or dangerous to free its posterior surface together with the kidney capsule, the best solution is to separate the kidney capsule from the kidney parenchyma and to leave the capsule in the retroperitoneal space in the recipient's body intact. After complete mobilization of the kidney, its vessels are prepared as high as possible in the hilum and are ligated. The renal vessels have to be obtained as long as possible, undamaged and well preserved along the whole length from the place of their ligation in the renal hilum up to the anastomoses with the iliac vessels.

After complete separation from the surrounding tissues, the common iliac vein was closed with a Satinsky vascular clamp. The vein contained in the clamp and was incised along its long axis, and an end-to-side venous anastomosis was performed with a non-absorbable 5/0 continuous suture. Before completion of the venous anastomosis, both veins were regularly flushed with a heparinized solution of physiologic saline chloride. After making about 3 mm lateral incisions on the opposite sides of the donor's and recipient's renal arteries a spatulated anastomosis end-to-end was performed with a monofilament non-absorbable 6/0 suture. During the anastomosis of both renal arteries, the lumens were regularly rinsed with heparinized physiological natrium chloride solution. Immediately after removing all vascular clamps, the transplanted kidney was warmed with 1.5–2.0 L of warm Ringer's solution. All bleeding vessels were then thoroughly coagulated, ligated and sewn. Try to achieve a perfect hemostasis in all cases, especially around the ureter and in the kidney hilum (Fig. 4.91). Sew the ureter into the bladder using the previously described modified Linch–Gregoir method with the JJ catheter decompression. Depending on the situation and the technical possibilities, suture the

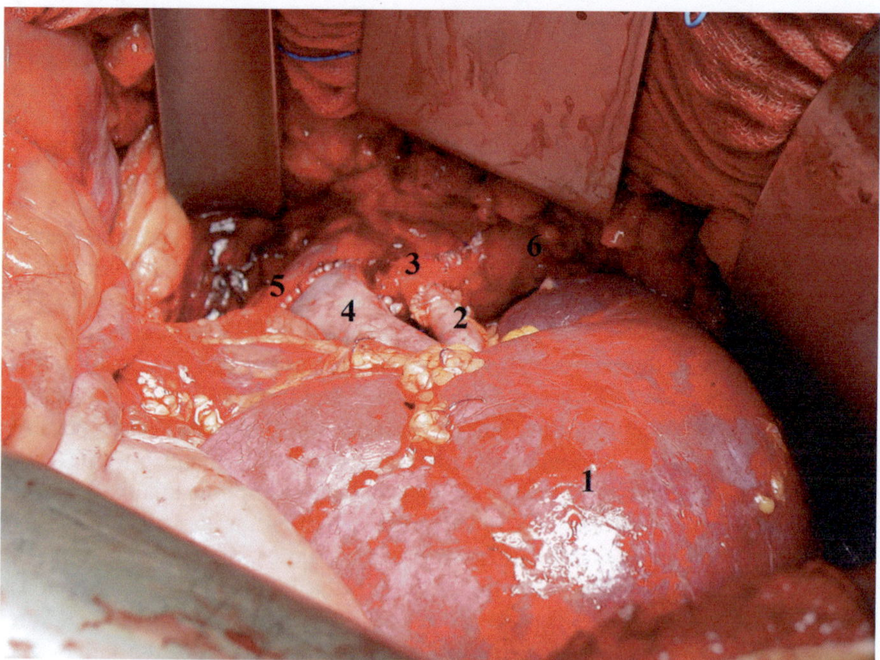

**Fig. 4.91**  1—Left side of the retransplanted kidney, 2—New kidney renal artery, 3—Old renal artery anastomosed end to end with a new kidney renal artery, 4—Renal vein of new kidney was anastomosed end to side to another (new) place on the common iliac vein, 5—Common iliac vein, 6—Common iliac artery

peritoneum over the transplanted kidney and drain the peritoneum with one or two JP drains. If the peritoneum cannot be sutured over the graft and the ureter, I usually drain the area of the kidney with two silicone surgical drains (without vacuum): one is left in the area of the upper pole behind the kidney, and the other close to the bladder in the deeper punt of the abdominal cavity.

**Warning! (Techniques for a third and fourth kidney transplantation)**
**Several techniques are described** [72]:

1. Trans-peritoneal kidney retransplantation.
2. Retro-peritoneal heterotopic kidney retransplantation.
3. Retroperitoneal heterotopic kidney retransplantation using the vessels of the previously transplanted kidney—this technique was described by Nghiem [72].
4. Orthotopic kidney transplantation (OKT). This technique is used for selected patients when the iliac vessels are deemed unsuitable for vascular anastomosis. It was first described by Gil-Vernet et al. [74] in 139 patients. Musquera et al. [74] from Barcelona published the largest series of 223 patients who had OKT. Patient survival was 92.23, 78.3 and 62.5% at 1, 10 and 20 years, respectively. Graft survival was 87.7, 59.3 and 34.5% at 1, 10 and 20 years, respectively. There was no difference in the 20-year patient and graft survival between orthotopic and heterotopic kidney transplantation performed during the same period [72].

**Warning! (If possible during retransplantation do not damage the old vascular anastomoses)**
Remember to prepare the renal and iliac vessels very carefully in order not to damage the old vessels of the transplanted kidney. The renal vessels should be dissected as long as possible, i.e. ligated and cut as deep as possible in the kidney hilum. In case of damage to the iliac recipient vessels or the old renal vessels, the kidney recipient can be at high risk of a large operation, combined with a huge blood loss, vascular surgeon intraoperative consultation, loss of the new kidney transplant and even—in more complicated cases—the loss oflimb and/or death.

**Warning! (Unsatisfactory blood flow from the lumen of the stump)**
In the case of unsatisfactory blood flow from the lumen of the stump we have the following ways to correct this.

– Covering the external wall with cellulose (Surgicel—Johnson & Johnson, Ethicon) soaked with papaverine (papaverine HCl, 40 mg/2 ml or papaverine HCl, 100 mg/3 ml) and injecting into the lumen of the renal artery and/or in the old renal artery stump (100 ml, 0.9% sodium chloride + 40 mg papaverine), e.g. heparin solution, with the old renal artery closed 5 mm from the anastomosis with a small gentle vascular clamp. Fur this purpose, we use a syringe with a special bent needle with which the drug is administered under a slight pressure, watching the entire renal artery stump slightly distend. After this kind of procedure, we always check the blood flow from the renal artery stump.

- The second method is to use the first method and combine it with using a Fogarty catheter with a capacity of 0.3–0.5 cc. In this case, you can limit yourself to enlarging the diameter of the artery stump and if there is an insufficient blood flow, you can use the catheter to enlarge (distend) the diameter of the iliac artery above the anastomosis, the anastomosis itself and the stump of the renal artery of the removed kidney—look and palpate or perform a Duplex Doppler for another site on one of the iliac arteries or on the aorta without atheromatous changes where renal artery bypass grafting can be safely performed.
- If the above methods did not help, you can close the artery and the vein with sutures or clips, and ask an intervention radiologist to stent both or one of the anastomoses with a very short stent(s).
- Ask a vascular surgeon to perform an acute aorto-femoral or aorto-iliac graft and implant the kidney with end-to-side anastomosis between the graft and the renal artery after it.

## 4.11.4   Case 3: Kidney Transplantation. Renal Artery Anastomosis with a Vascular Prosthesis (Patient with Renal Failure after Aorto-bifemoral Vascular Reconstruction)

### 4.11.4.1   Introduction

Due to a very calcified aorto-iliac axis, renal transplantation with implantation of the artery on a vascular prosthesis can be proposed. An aorto-bifemoral vascular reconstruction with prothesis, as a preparation for kidney transplantation in patients with renal failure, is a procedure with many complications and is usually associated with a higher mortality rate in kidney recipients than a normal kidney transplant but it offers on selected patients a much better alternative to dialysis [76]. Several techniques for renal allograft implantation on a prosthetic vascular graft according to the timing of the vascular intervention in relation to the transplantation are described as follows.

1. An aortic bifurcated prosthesis is implanted before kidney transplantation [76, 77].
2. Prosthetic iliac artery replacement and kidney transplantation is performed simultaneously [80]. This means that during the same operation a vascular prosthesis is first implanted and then the kidney, whose end of the renal artery is sewn into the side of the prosthesis. The simultaneous implantation of a vascular prosthesis with a kidney transplantation can, according to various authors, lead to a slightly increased graft infection and a prolongation of warm renal ischemia [76, 79]. The best solution in such a case is to use a fresh graft which consists of the donor's aorta and/or iliac vessels from the kidney or another donor [79].

Grafting of the renal artery to a vascular prosthesis is feasible and yields good results, despite the technical difficulties involved. The five-year patient and graft survival rates were 85.2 and 74%, respectively [77].

In my opinion the presence of a vascular prosthesis means that kidney transplantation requires a lot of experience and surgical skill. In short the operation is, as I have said, difficult and consists of very hard and difficult to dissect tissues growing around the wall of the prosthesis [77]. If you have no experience in vascular surgery, it is worth doing it together with a vascular surgeon.

Personally, I prefer the two-stage technique. If the post-operative period is without complications and the prosthesis wall has properly grown into the surrounding tissues and there are no signs of infection of the prosthesis, then only following a few months following the implantation of the prosthesis do we decide to perform a kidney transplant with an end-to-side anastomosis of the renal artery of the previously implanted prosthesis (Fig. 4.91). By contrast, the one-stage procedure involves vascular repair and transplantation at the same time which is the only advantage of this one-stage treatment.

### 4.11.4.2 Transplantation Procedure

Access to the extraperitoneal space is done by a hockey-stick incision. The difficulty of this procedure is to locate the iliac vessels and the prosthesis. It should be remembered that after the first operation, the branches of the vascular prosthesis are strongly connected with the recipient's iliac vessels and also with the surrounding very hard fibrotic tissues. As I wrote earlier, the preparation of the iliac vessels can begin as close to the inguinal ligament as possible. For the preparation of 5 cm of the ingrown prosthesis and one of the iliac veins during the kidney transplant, I recommend the use of sharp ended scissors, a surgical scalpel and the sterile head of the Duplex Doppler apparatus, which after exposing the extraperitoneal space will help us to locate the prosthesis leg itself.

The dissection of the vessels and the prosthesis must be carried out carefully in order not to damage the prosthesis and the recipient's vessels. After reaching the extraperitoneal space, the entire vascular prosthesis should be dissected at a distance of 5 cm which is sufficient to close it with two clamps, to cut a hole in it with a scalpel and/or with scissors and to flush it with heparin solution and properly perform the arterial anastomosis.

After the succesful preparation of the vascular prosthesis, the following stages of the operation are the most important.

– Before the prosthesis itself or its leg is closed, a patient should receive intravenous heparin adequate to her/his body weight. After the administration of heparin, do not close the clamps too quickly, wait 5 min—heparin starts to work in the human body 3–4 min after its intravenous administration.
– The vascular prosthesis should be closed after thorough palpation examination to locate atherosclerotic changes (when you have to deal with severe arteriosclerosis inside the prosthesis with plaques on its back wall, close the

prosthesis then use a vascular clamp horizontally). If the prosthesis is normal, so without atherosclerosis plaques and severe calcification, you can vertically close the prosthesis with two vascular clamps. Horizontal closing of vascular grafts may lead to sticking of the prosthesis walls together and it may make it technically very difficult to perform an end-to-side anastomosis between the renal artery and/or aortic patch and the vascular prosthesis.

–  The earlier implanted vascular prosthesis should be closed with a clamp first distally and then proximally—it is about filling the graft with blood, which makes it much easier to make a hole in it by cutting out a piece of wall.

–  After the transplantation, the kidney area should be well drained and the patient should be given heparin in such a dose that the APTT (Activated Partial Thromboplastin Time) does not exceed 60–70 s. Patients with a well-functioning kidney may receive Fraxiparin in the first phase, but in case of an insufficient kidney graft with delayed graft function, Fraxiparin may accumulate, which can lead to bleeding.

–  When the kidney (renal artery) is implanted in a vascular prosthesis and if it does not produce urine (Fig. 4.92), it should be subjected to regular examinations, such as 99mTc-MAG 3 and ultrasound (Duplex Doppler). In the postoperative period the patient should receive anticoagulants and platelet aggregation inhibitors.

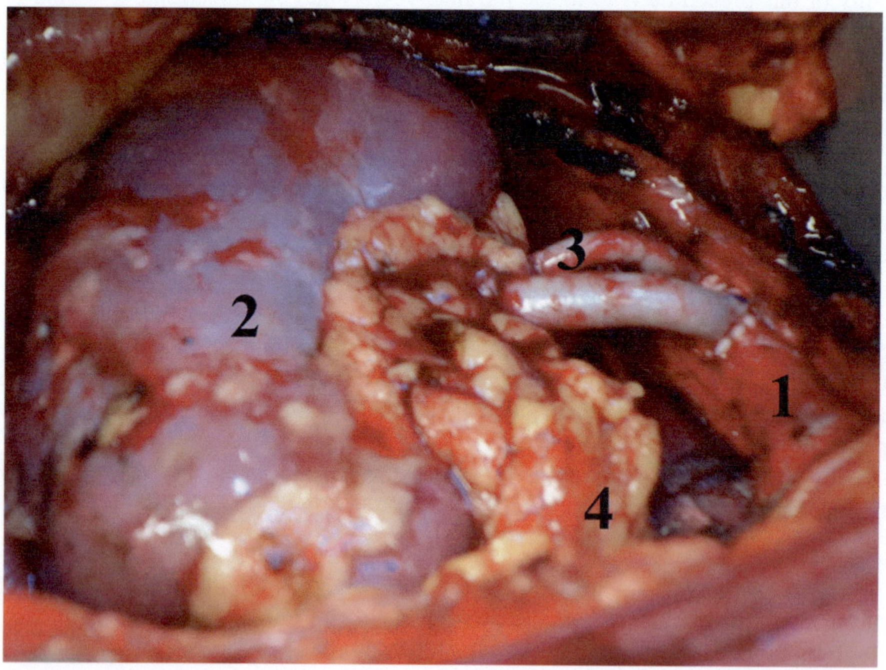


**Fig. 4.92** Transplanted kidney with two arteries on the aortic patch sewn end-to-side of the right leg of the aortic bifurcation graft. 1—Right leg of the aortic bifurcation graft, 2—Kidney, 3—Renal arteries on the aortic patch, 4—Area of the renal pelvic and ureter of the transplanted kidney running towards the bladder

**Warning! (For everybody older than 55, use CT without contrast)**
Atherosclerotic plaques and severe calcifications of the arterial vessels are best detected by means of computed tomography made without contrast. During Doppler ultrasonography, only rapid flows and hardening of the vessel wall are detected. Some atherosclerotic plaques do not form lime rings, but their volume increases systematically from the posterior wall to the anterior one, which in turn manifests itself in the slow closing of the arterial vessels and the slow development of claudication is intermittent. In our protocol, the compulsory examinations of iliac vessels in every potential recipient of a kidney over 55 years of age use computed tomography without contrast and Doppler ultrasonography.

## *4.11.5   Kidney Transplantation with Two Ureters*

### 4.11.5.1   Introduction

During the organ procurement procedure, a surgeon is often confronted with anatomical anomalies. These changes may put the success of the transplant into question. Despite the thorough diagnosis of the potential donor, these anomalies are often diagnosed during organ donation. Taking into consideration the well-being of the recipient, organs with anatomic abnormalities should be carefully considered for transplantation. This is especially important when there is a constant shortage of organs for transplantation [80].

A double ureter is an anomaly consisting of two independent ureters departing from the kidney. The double ureters have separate openings in the bladder. This defect occurs in 10% of people, more often in women, bilaterally in 20% of cases. The ureters from the doubled pelvis sometimes fuse before reaching the bladder to form a single bifurcated ureter. A bifurcated ureter is an anomaly in the structure of the ureter, consisting of its dilation in a certain section, with the presence of a single bladder opening. In kidneys with a double and bifurcated ureter, there is a duplication and separation of the calico-pelvic system. When procured kidneys from a deceased obese donor have such an anatomical anomaly as the double ureter, it may be difficult to diagnose during the abdominal organ procurement procedure. In such cases, it should be remembered that a person may have two ureters, of different course and diameter, in different places leading to the bladder, which may merge into one ureter in front of the bladder. Therefore, the kidneys together with the ureters, and especially the ureters, should be procured with as much surrounding tissue as possible. Of course, the best thing to do would be to identify the double ureters and any abnormalities before organ procurement, but we know that such detailed diagnostics is difficult in many hospitals, and sometimes even impossible. It should be remembered at this point that the left gonadal vein is often confused with the second ureter on the left side. Without magnifying surgical loupes, it is often very difficult to find the difference between the ureter and the blood vessel or any other structure in the abdominal cavity that may appear to resemble the ureter. In magnifying surgical loupes, you will immediately see a star shape on the cross-section, which will indicate that it is a ureter. In case of doubt (as I have already described and suggested in the previous chapters), it remains to fill the suspect structure with cold preservative fluid or to dissect the gonadal vein in the kidney on the left side of the renal vein or IVC. When making the diagnosis of two ureters, we must be 100% sure. The question is whether one or two catheters should be used for splinting a double ureter with a JJ catheter. If you have two separate renal pelvic systems, two ureters and two uretero-bladder anastomoses, you should always drain them separately. In the case of a bifurcated ureter with a common bladder section, two very thin JJ catheters can be used. When splinting the common bladder segment with two catheters, it should be borne in mind that very often the bladder segment of the ureter is not wide enough to accommodate two JJ catheters. If the diameter of the bladder ureter is too small, the entire system can be drained with one JJ catheter. In preparing the kidney for transplantation, one can easily check for any of the above-mentioned situations by cannulating and flushing one ureter with a thin catheter connected to a syringe filled with cold preservative fluid.

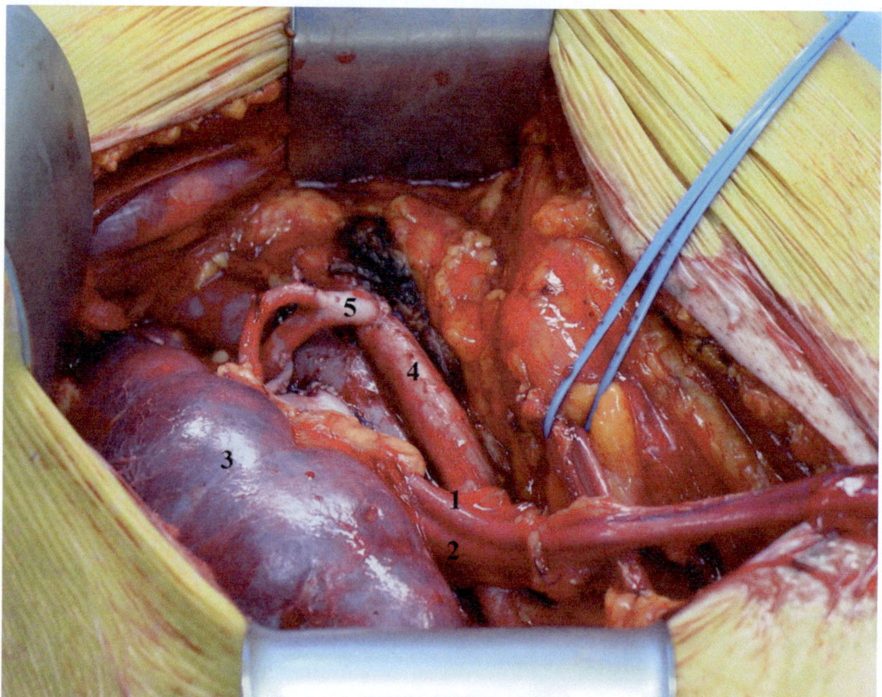

**Fig. 4.93** Transplanted kidney with two ureters. 1 and 2—Ureters, 3—Transplanted kidney, 4—Common iliac artery, 5—Renal artery

### 4.11.5.2  Surgical Technique

There are two methods of implanting a double ureter into the bladder. The first one involves cutting the sides of the walls of both ureters 0.8–1.5 cm long and joining their medial edges with a soluble monofilament suture, and then implanting the ureters sewn together into one hole which was previously made in the bladder. Another method, which in my opinion is safer (I personally have transplanted a kidney with a double ureter three times), consists of separating them from each other, with complete preservation of their blood supply, and implanting them separately, from separate incisions, into the bladder using the Lich-Gregoir method. In each case of transplanting a kidney with two ureters, I splinted the ureter, the pelvis of the transplanted kidney and the uretero-vesicular anastomosis with the JJ catheter. As already noted, I personally prefer to implant each ureter into the bladder separately, as it seems to me to be a more logical method, giving the ureters a better ability to heal with the urinary bladder reducing the risk of urinary leakage (Figs. 4.94 and 4.95). The fusion of the two sides of the cut and sewn ureters

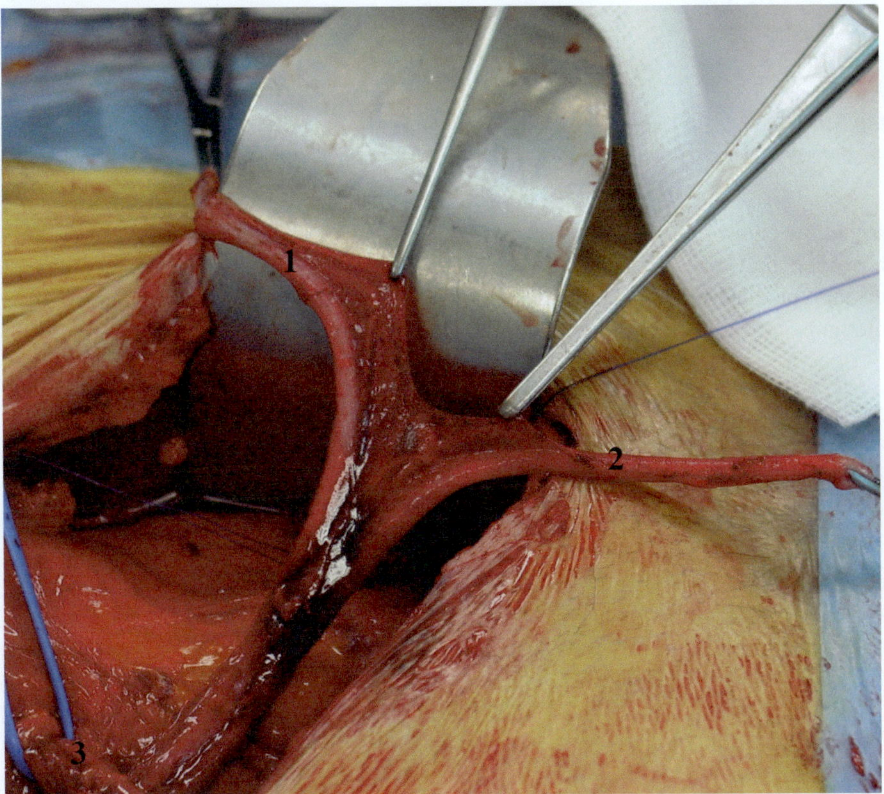

**Fig. 4.94**  1 and 2—Separated ureters before their shortening and separated implantation into the urinary bladder, 3—Spermatic cord

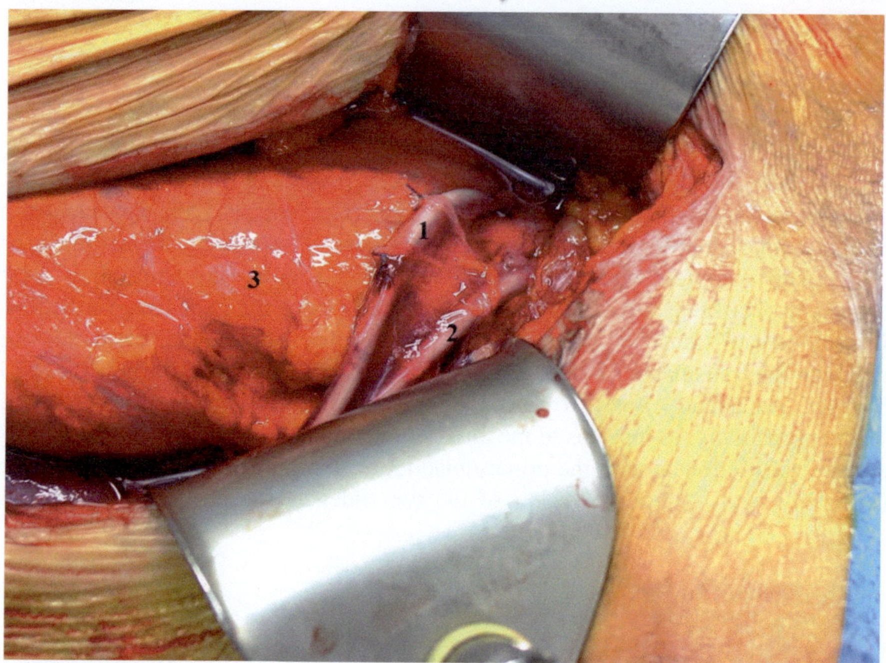

**Fig. 4.95** 1 and 2—Ureters separately sewn into the urinary bladder. Each uretero-bladder anastomosis has been decompressed with the JJ catheter, 3—Peritoneum, 4—Transplanted kidney

somehow cannot convince me of the reliability of this method. It should be added, however, that research on both methods of transplanting a double ureter into the urinary bladder has not statistically demonstrated the superiority of one of these methods over another [81].

## *4.11.6   Transplantation of Two Kidneys from One Donor*

### 4.11.6.1   Introduction

Double kidney transplantation is an accepted strategy to increase the donor pool. Regarding older donor kidneys, protocols for deciding to perform a dual or a single transplantation are mainly based on preimplantation biopsies. Taking into account the kidney shortage, Cruzado showed [83] the excellent transplant outcomes with dual kidney transplantation (DKT). Of the 182 kidney transplantations in the "old for old" program, 79 were dual kidney transplantations; 15 of 79 patients lost one of their kidney grafts during one year, but the renal function was lower and the proteinuria greater among the one kidney patients than the DKT group. Patient survival was similar in both groups. However, death-censored graft survival was lower in the one kidney group than the DKT patients. The five-year graft survival rate was 70% in the one kidney group versus 93% in the DKT cohorts.

A transplant program was initiated to transplant kidneys from donors of over 60 years performing a single or dual transplantation. DKT was performed with donors of more than 75 years, and with donors between 60 and 74 years of age and glomerulosclerosis of >15%. The kidneys of donors between 60 and 74 years of age and with glomerulosclerosis of <15% were used for the single kidney transplantation (SKT) [87].

The main disadvantage of this method is the use of kidneys taken from elderly people and in many cases with impaired function for transplantation. One kidney transplanted by a recipient from this type of donor is usually not enough to free him from dialysis, and thus improve his quality of life and survival. To become dialysis independent, patients need more nephrons and therefore a transplantation of two kidneys. It should be emphasized here that not every two kidneys transplanted from a deceased donor guarantee the patient freedom from dialysis. In order for the transplant patient to leave the dialysis unit, the transplanted organs must come from a kidney donor with an appropriate number of relatively healthy and secretionally active nephrons, ensuring adequate blood filtration. An elderly donor kidney usually does not have enough nephrons to make a patient independent of dialysis, and so the idea arose to use two kidneys or to transplant two kidneys for one patient.

Transplanting two kidneys from one donor to one recipient is associated with another inconvenience, namely, prior to transplantation of the kidneys, an open biopsy is required and a very careful assessment of the condition of nephrons (artherosclerosis) in both kidneys, often performed at night by an experienced anatomopathologist.


### 4.11.6.2   Surgical Techniques

When transplanting two kidneys to one recipient, different surgical techniques are used, which can be divided into intraperitoneal and retroperitoneal, unilateral and bilateral. Some centers transplant two kidneys intraperitoneally, fusing the kidneys to the right and left iliac vessels (Fig. 4.96), and some centers prefer retroperitoneal transplantation from two separate incisions. Other centers have changed the technique of the surgical transplantation of two kidneys: instead of a midline incision or two incisions on each side of the abdominal cavity, one incision is made on the right side and two kidneys are transplanted retroperitoneally to the right side of the recipient. Such an operation was carried out for the first time in the world by Douglas Mason from the Virginia Mason Medical Center in Seattle, USA [84]. The technique consists of transplanting both kidneys extraperitoneally in the same iliac fossa (Fig. 4.97a, b). The procedure begins with the classic Gibson incision, preferably on the right side. After creating an adequate extraperitoneal space, the

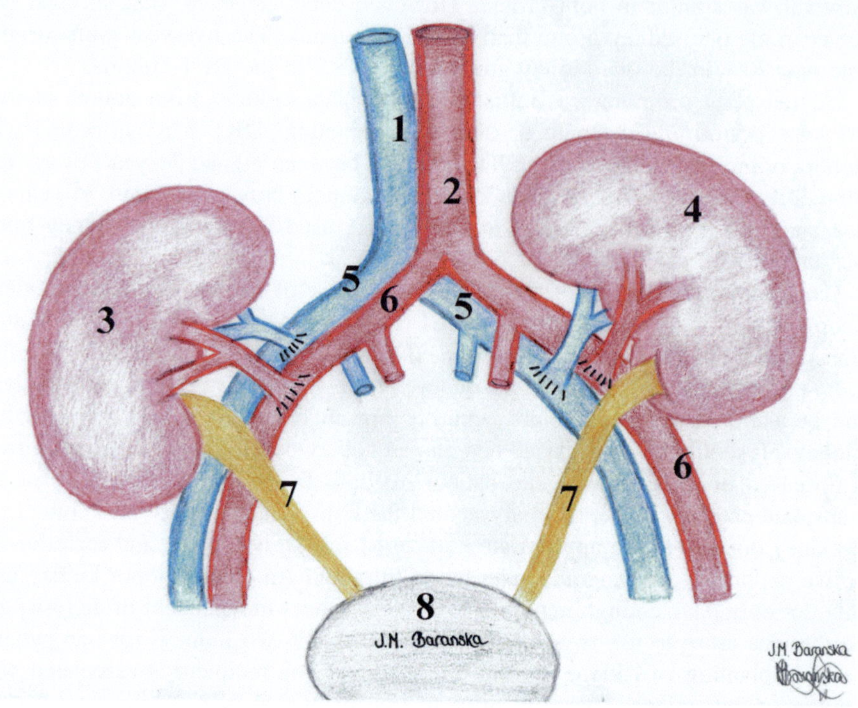



**Fig. 4.96** Surgical technique for the transplantation of two kidneys on both sides of the abdominal cavity from an intra- or extraperitoneal access. 1—Lower IVC, 2—Aorta, 3—Right side kidney, 4—Left side kidney, 5—Right common iliac vein, 6—Left external iliac artery, 7—Ureters, 8—Bladder

right donor kidney is preferably placed superiorly because its renal vein can be lengthened by a segment of the IVC, with mechanical stapling of both (upper and lower) openings of the IVC segment. Occasionally, the division of the IVC at its upper opening, associated with procurement of the liver, does not allow the use of a mechanical stapler. In such cases, we suture the upper IVC opening manually. Another reason to position the right kidney super-laterally in the right flank is that the right kidney has a longer artery. If necessary, the internal iliac (hypogastric) vein is dissected to mobilize the external iliac vein and thus facilitates the renal vein anastomoses to the external iliac vein of the recipient. The extended renal vein and renal artery of the right kidney are anastomosed end-to-side to the iliac vessels of the recipient; these anastomoses are often performed to the external iliac vessels. After revascularization of the right kidney, vascular clamps are placed immediately below the venous and arterial anastomoses. The left donor kidney is transplanted distally, allowing the transplanted right kidney to continue to be perfused. The left kidney is positioned inferomedially to the right kidney. The renal artery and the vein of the left kidney are anastomosed end-to-side to the external iliac vessels.

(a)

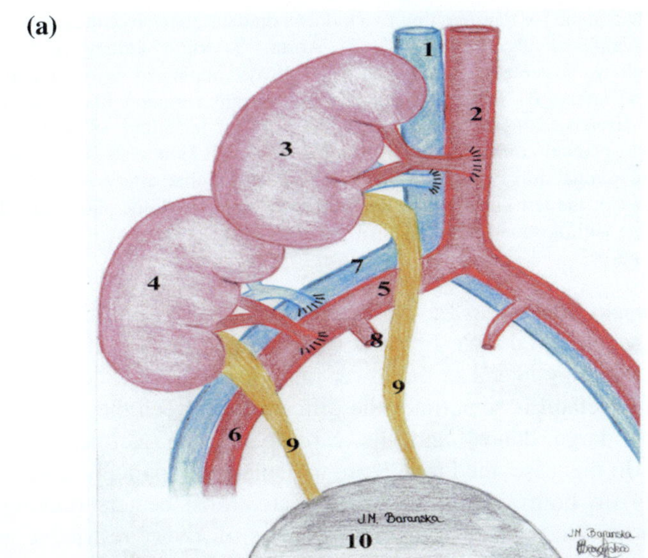

(b)

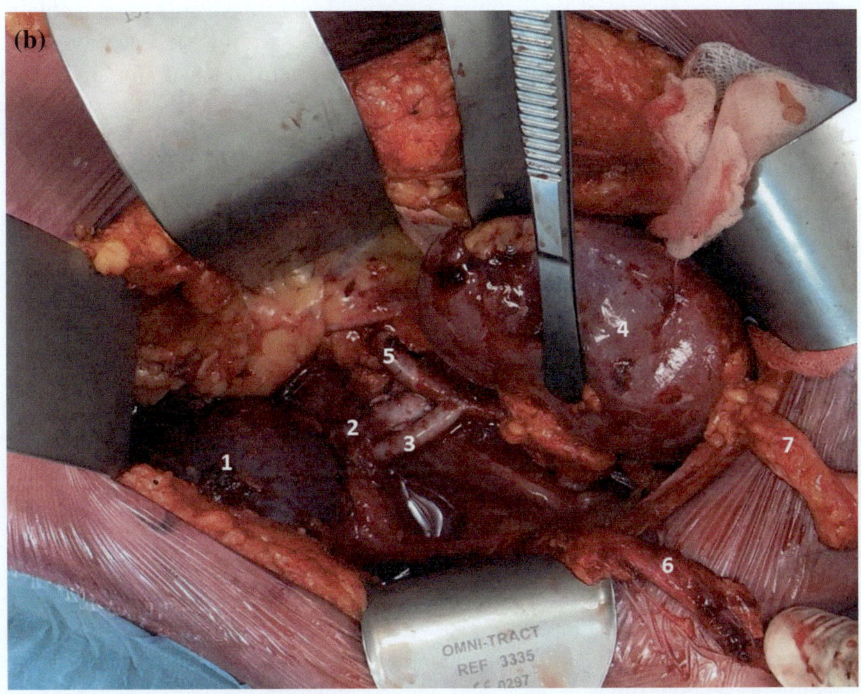

◀**Fig. 4.97** (**a**) A surgical technique for transplanting two kidneys on the right side of the iliac fossa: retroperitoneal or intraperitoneal access. 1—IVC, 2—Aorta, 3—Right kidney is always transplanted first, as high as possible, 4—Left kidney is always implanted below the right kidney, 5—Common iliac artery, 6—External iliac artery, 7—Right common iliac vein, 8—Internal iliac artery, 9—Ureters, 10—Urinary bladder. (**b**) Surgical technique of unilaterally positioned dual kidney transplantation into the right iliac fossa. 1—Right kidney, 2—Right kidney renal vein, 3—Right kidney renal artery, 4—Left kidney, 5—Common iliac artery, 6—Ureter of the right kidney, 7—Ureter of the left kidney. (The operation was performed, the photograph has been made available to me with the kind permission of prof. dr. I.P.J. Alwayn)

Extravesical ureteroneocystostomies are performed separately, according to the Lich–Gregoir technique, with a double J stent for each ureter, leaving the ureter of the upper transplanted kidney lateral to the lower one [86].

A limitation of this method is sometimes the difference between the size of the two kidneys (from a large donor) and the capacity of the recipient's right retroperitoneal space. In this case, the kidneys are transplanted separately from two cuts, retroperitoneally on both sides of the iliac plate. Most centers running a two-kidney transplant to one recipient program, in cases of a very restrictive and selective policy of accepting and transplanting two kidneys to one recipient, were able to achieve the results of the recipient's survival and transplants comparable to the results obtained in recipients who were transplanted with a good quality single kidney. In centers where two kidney transplant programs from one donor are carried out, an anatomopathologist is usually employed, who is able to assess the suitability of the kidneys for transplantation 24 hours a day, seven days a week by means of an emergency pathological examination [83–86].

**Warning! (Where can you find an experienced pathologist available 24 hours a day and seven days a week?)**
Most people who die after the age of 70 years have a lifetime kidney disease or systemic disease that is directly or indirectly responsible for the damage to their kidney parenchyma during their lifetime. The small number of this type of transplant results from the fact that often these types of kidneys, after their procurement, even if they are offered to one recipient, are assessed by an anatomopathologist and are in most cases not suitable for transplantation. The next point is that there are very few university medical hospitals in the world where an experienced anatomopathologist is available 24 hours a day and seven days a week. University transplant hospitals, where kidney transplant departments have a two-kidney transplant program, generally accept kidneys based on their function in the donor's body only, and the approval of the kidneys for transplantation takes place without a prior evaluation by an anatomopathologist. At my Department of Abdominal Organ Transplantation at the University of Leiden, two kidneys are also transplanted to one recipient several times a year and indeed without the participation of an anatomopathologist (Fig. 4.97a, b).

### 4.11.6.3  Stimulation of Diuresis after Kidney Transplantation

**Living-donor Kidney Transplantation**

*Before revascularization*

Maintain central venous pressure (CVP) 5–10 cm $H_2O$, maintain mean arterial pressure (MAP) $\geq$ 60 mm Hg and maintain systemic blood pressure (SBP) $\geq$ 90 mm Hg; mannitol, 0.20 g/kg, intravenous over 1 h, start with the first vascular anastomosis; furosemide, 0.20 mg/kg, intravenous during second half of vascular anastomosis; consider giving albumin in case of hypoalbuminaemia.

**Cadaveric Kidney Transplantation**

Before revascularization

Maintain the CVP at 5–10 cm $H_2O$, maintain MAP $\geq$ 60 mm Hg, maintain SBP $\geq$ 90 mm Hg. Increase the mannitol dose to 1 g/kg (maximum 50 g) intravenous; increase furosemide dose to 1 mg/kg intravenous; albumin, 1 g/kg (to 50 g), intravenous, over 2–3 h Verapamil, 0–10 mg, into renal artery based on blood pressure and weight, [1–4, 24, 43, 93–94].

From the European Renal Best Practice (ERBP) Transplantation Guidelines I will quote some important and interesting statements.

1. There is no evidence to prefer one type of solution (crystalloids versus colloids, normal saline versus Ringer's) for intravenous volume management of the recipient during kidney transplant surgery. In view of the available data in the literature, and in line with the ERBP position on prevention of acute kidney injury, we suggest being cautious with the use of starches in the kidney transplant recipient during the perioperative period, although specific data in this setting are lacking. They recommend monitoring for metabolic acidosis when normal saline is used as the only intravenous fluid in the perioperative and post-operative period [92–94].
2. There is no evidence to support the claim that low-dose dopamine can improve graft outcome in terms of relevant outcomes; as a delayed graft function (DGF), or in the mid and reduction of creatinine levels in the mid- or long term after transplantation. The use of low-dose dopamine might induce arrhythmias. They do not recommend the use of "renal doses" of dopaminergic agents in the early post-operative period, since it does not improve the graft function or survival. The ERBP states that the guideline development group judged that the use of low dose dopamine could not be recommended [92–94].
3. They do not recommend routinely using low-molecular weight heparin, un-fractionated heparin or aspirin before transplantation to prevent graft thrombosis [92–94].

4. In kidney transplant recipients, what are the effects of using a JJ stent at the time of operation on outcomes? The ERBP recommend the placement of a prophylatctic JJ stent as a routine surgical practice in adult kidney transplantation. They suggest that if a JJ stent is in place, cotrimoxazole is given as an antibiotic prophylaxis. The ERBP suggest removing the JJ stent within four to six weeks [92–94].

5. They suggest removing the urinary bladder catheter as soon as possible after the transplantation, balancing the risk of urinary leak against that of urinary tract infection. They recommend monitoring adverse event rates (urinary tract infection, urinary leakage) in each center, to inform the decision over when to remove the indwelling bladder catheter [92–94].

# References


1. Barry JM. Technical aspects of renal transplantation. In: Henrich WL, Bennet WM, editors. Atlas of kidney disease. Tom V. 2001. https://www.kidneyatlas.org/book5/adk5-14.ccc.QXD. pdf.

2. Morris P, Knechte S. 7th Edition Kidney Transplantation. Principles and Practice, Chapter 11-Watson Ch. J. E, Friend P, Surgical Techniques of Kidney Transplantation, 2014, Elsevier–Saunders, p. 161–175. ISBN 978455740963.

3. Humar A, Sturdevant ML. Atlas of organ transplantation, 2nd ed. Chapter 5. In: Gunabushanam V, Matas A, Humar A, editors. Kidney transplantation. Springer, p. 109–54. ISBN-9781447147749.

4. Englesbe MJ, Mulholland MW. Operative techniques in transplantation surgery, Section III, kidney transplantation surgical procedures, Chapters 7–13; 45–94. Wolters Kluwer Health; 2015. ISBN—9781451188745.

5. Berlinger N, Dietz E. Time-out: the professional and organizational ethics of speaking up in the OR. AMA J Ethics. 2016;18(9):925–32. https://doi.org/10.1001/journalofethics.2016.18.9. stas1-1609

6. Thompson Surgical Instruments Inc.— www.thompsonsurgical.com.

7. Omni—Trac Surgical—www.omni-tract.com.

8. https://www.surgicalholdings.co.uk/bookwalter-retractor.html.

9. Zomorrodi A, Kakei F, Bagheri A, Zomorrodi S, Mohammadrahimi M. 1.Does early removal of Foley's catheter have any influence on infection of recipient post renal transplantation? Is it safe? A randomized clinical trial, Journal of Nephropathology. J Nephropathol. 2018;7(3):122–6.

10. Sussman M, Russell RB. Infection after cadaver renal transplantation. Proc R Soc Med. 1972;65:471–3.

11. Lorenz EC, Cosio FG. The impact of urinary tract infections in renal transplant recipients. Kidney Int. 2010;78:719–21. https://doi.org/10.1038/ki.2010.219.

12. Barbouch S, Cherif M, Ounissi M, Karoui C, Mzoughi S, Hamida FB, et al. Urinary tract infections following renal transplantation: a single-center experience. Saudi J Kidney Dis Transpl. 2012;23:1311–4. https://doi.org/10.4103/13192442.103586.

13. 3MTM IobanTM 2 Antimicrobial Incise Drapes EZ from 3M internet side.

14. Guideline for Prevention of Surgical Site Infection. Center for Disease Control, U.S. Public Health Service, Revision 1999 Vol. 20 N. 4.

15. Nanni G, Tondolo V, Citterio F, Romagnoli J, Borgetti M, Boldrini G, Castagneto M. Comparison of oblique versus hockey-stick surgical incision for kidney transplantation.

Transplant Proc. 2005;37(6):2479–81. https://doi.org/10.1016/j.transproceed. **2005.06.055. PMID: 16182716.**

16. Amirzargar MA, Babolhavaeji H, Hosseini SA, Bahar H, Gholyaf M, Dadras F, Khoshjoo F, Yavangi M, Amirzargar N. The new technique of using the epigastric arteries in renal transplantation with multiple renal arteries. Saudi J Kidney Dis Transpl. 2013;24(2):247–53. https://doi.org/10.4103/1319-2442.109565 PMID: 23538346.

17. El-Sherbiny M, Abou-Elela A, Morsy A, Salah M, Foda A. The use of the inferior epigastric artery for accessory lower polar artery revascularization in live donor renal transplantation. Int Urol Nephrol. 2008;40(2):283–7. https://doi.org/10.1007/s11255-007-9257-z PMID: 17721826.

18. Malinka T, Banz VM, Wagner J, Candinas D, Inderbitzin D. Incision length for kidney transplantation does not influence short- or long-term outcome: a prospective randomized controlled trial. Clin Transplant. 2013;27(5):E538–45. https://doi.org/10.1111/ctr.12209. **Epub 2013 Aug 8. PMID: 23924205.**

19. Zorgdrager M, Lange JF, Krikke C, Nieuwenhuijs GJ, Hofker SH, Leuvenink HG, Pol RA. Chronic inguinal pain after kidney transplantation, a common and underexposed problem. World J Surg. 2017;41(2):630–8. https://doi.org/10.1007/s00268-016-3713-9.

20. Bhanot SM, Gopalakrishanan R. Smiley incision: a direct surgical approach for retropubic radical prostatectomy. Urology. 2002;60:149–51.

21. Grantcharot TP, Rosenberg J. Vertical compared with transverse incisions in abdominal surgery. Eur J Surg. 2001;167:260–7.

22. Manoharan M, Gomez P, Sved P, Soloway MS. Modified Pfannenstiel approach for radical retropubic prostatectomy. Urology. 2004;64:369–71.

23. Kishore TA, Shetty A, Tharun BK, John EV, Bhat S. Renal transplantation through a modified non-muscle-cutting Pfannenstiel incision. Int Urol Nephrol. 2014;46(5):901–4. https://doi.org/10.1007/s11255-013-0608-7 Epub 2013 Nov 28 PMID: 24287884.

24. Barry JM. Surgery Ilustrated, renal transplant—recipient surgery ©2007 the author journal compilation. BJU internatl. 2007;99:701–17. https://doi.org/10.1111/j.1464-410X.2007. 06785.

25. Mac Ginley R, Champion De Crespigny PJ, Gutman T, et al. KHA-CARI guideline recommendations for renal biopsy. Nephrology (Carlton). 2019;24(12):1205–13. Guideline.

26. Williams WW, Taheri D, Tolkoff-Rubin N, Colvin RB. Clinical role of the renal transplant biopsy. Nature Rev Nephrol. 2012;8(2):110–21. https://doi.org/10.1038/nrneph.2011.213.

27. Paripović D, Kostić M, Kruščić D, et al. Indications and results of renal biopsy in children: a 10-year review from a single center in Serbia. J Nephrol. 2012;25(6):1054–9.

28. Printza N, Bosdou J, Pantzaki A, et al. Percutaneous ultrasound-guided renal biopsy in children: a single centre experience. Hippokratia. 2011;15(3):258–61.

29. Bakdash K, Schramm KM, Annam A, Brown M, Kondo K, Lindquist JD. Complications of percutaneous renal biopsy. Semin Intervent Radiol. 2019.

30. Mehta R, Cherikh W, Sood P, Hariharan S. Kidney allograft surveillance biopsy practices across US transplant centers: a UNOS survey. Clin Transplant. 2017;31(5):[Medline].

31. Bakdash K, Schramm KM, Annam A, Brown M, Kondo K, Lindquist JD. Complications of percutaneous renal biopsy. Semin Intervent Radiol. 2019;36(2):97–103.

32. Han Y, Guo H, Cai M, Xiao L, Wang Q, Xu X, Huang H, Shi B. Renal graft biopsy assists diagnosis and treatment of renal allograft dysfunction after kidney transplantation: a report of 106 cases. Internatl J Clin Exp Med. 2015;8(3):4703–7.

33. Ahmad I. Biopsy of the transplanted kidney. Semin Intervent Radiol. 2004;21(4):275–81. https://doi.org/10.1055/s-2004-861562.PMID:21331139;PMCID:PMC3036241.

34. Van den Berg TAJ, Minnee RC, Lisman T, Nieuwenhuijs-Moeke GJ, van de Wetering J, Bakker SJL, Pol RA. Perioperative antithrombotic therapy does not increase the incidence of early postoperative thromboembolic complications and bleeding in kidney transplantation—a retrospective study. Transpl Int. 2019;32(4):418–30. https://doi.org/10.1111/tri.13387. Epub 2019 Jan 2. PMID: 30536448; PMCID: PMC6850661.

35. Bakir N, Sluiter WJ, Ploeg RJ, van Son WJ, Tegzess AM. Primary renal graft thrombosis. Nephrol Dial Transplant. 1996;11(1):140–7 PMID: 8649623.

36. Buder K, Zirngibl M, Bapistella S, Nadalin S, Tönshoff B, Weitz M. Members of the "Transplantation Working Group" of the European Society for Paediatric Nephrology (ESPN). Current practice of antithrombotic prophylaxis in pediatric kidney transplantation-Results of an international survey on behalf of the European Society for Pediatric Nephrology. Pediatric Transplant. 2020;24(7):e13799. https://doi.org/10.1111/petr.13799. Epub 2020 Aug 18.

37. Prince M, Wenham T. Heparin-induced thrombocytopaenia. Postgrad Med J. 2018;94(1114):453–7. https://doi.org/10.1136/postgradmedj-2018-135702 Epub 2018 Aug 20 PMID: 30126928.

38. Riedel R, Schmieder A, Koster A, Kim S, Baumgarten G, Schewe JC. Die heparininduzierte Thrombozytopenie (HIT II) : Eine medizinökonomische Betrachtung [Heparin-induced thrombocytopenia type II (HIT II): a medical-economic view]. Med Klin Intensivmed Notfmed. 2017;112(4):334–46. German. https://doi.org/10.1007/s00063-016-0237-x. Epub 2016 Dec 22.

39. Gäckler A, Rohn H, Lisman T, Benkö T, Witzke O, Kribben A, et al. Evaluation of hemostasis in patients with end-stage renal disease. PLoS ONE 2019;14(2):e0212237. https://doi.org/10.1371/journal.pone.0212237.

40. Abularrage CJ, Neville RF. Chapter 60—Infrainguinal revascularization, Editor(s): Stephen R.T. Evans, Surgical pitfalls

41. Saunders WB. 2009;613–30. ISBN 9781416029519.

42. Simforoosh N, Gharaati MR, Moslemi MK, Feizzadeh B. One-suture, 1-knot technique in renal vascular transplant. Exp Clin Transplant. 2010;8(3):224–7.

43. Jofré R, López-Gómez JM, Moreno F, Sanz-Guajardo D, Valderrábano F. Changes in quality of life after renal transplantation. Am J Kidney Dis. 1998;32(1):93–100.

44. Barry JM, Morris PJ. Surgical techniques of renal transplantation. In: Morris PJ, Knechte SJ, editors. Kidney transplantation. Philadelphia, PA: Saunders; 2008. p. 161.

45. Haberal M, Karakayali H, Bilgin N, Moray G, Arslan G, Büyükpamukçu N. Four-quadrant running-suture arterial anastomosis technique in renal transplantation: a preliminary report. Transplant Proc. 1996;28(4):2334–5.

46. Haberal M, Moray G, Sevmis S, et al. Corner-saving renal artery anastomosis for renal transplantation. Transplant Proc. 2008;40(1):145–7.

47. Ye G, Mo HG, Wang ZH, Yi SH, Wang XW, Zhang YF. Arterial anastomosis without sutures using ring pin stapler for clinical renal transplantation: comparison with suture anastomosis. J Urol. 2006;175(2):636–40; discussion 640.

48. Mital D, Foster PF, Jensik SC, et al. Renal transplantation without sutures using the vascular clipping system for renal artery and vein anastomosis–a new technique. Transplantation. 1996;62(8):1171–3.

49. Dalal R, Bruss ZS, Sehdev JS. Physiology, renal blood flow and filtration. [Updated 2020 Aug 11]. In: Stat Pearls [Internet]. Treasure Island (FL): StatPearls Publishing; 2020. https://www.ncbi.nlm.nih.gov/books/NBK482248/.

50. Zomorrodi A, Bohluli A, Tarzamany MK. Evaluation of blood flow in allograft renal arteries anastomosed with two different techniques. Saudi J Kidney Dis Transpl. 2008;19(1):26–31 PMID: 18087119.

51. Hakim NS, Papalois VE, Romagnoli J. Arteriotomy using the aortic punch in kidney transplantation. Transplant Proc. 1998;30(5):1800. https://doi.org/10.1016/s0041-1345(98)00438-2 PMID: 9723289.

52. Alberts VP, Idu MM, Legemate DA, Laguna Pes MP, Minnee RC. Ureterovesical anastomotic techniques for kidney transplantation: a systematic review and meta-analysis. Transpl Int. 2014;27(6):593–605. https://doi.org/10.1111/tri.12301 Epub 2014 Apr 8 PMID: 24606191.

53. Friedersdorff F, Weinberger S, Biernath N, et al. The ureter in the kidney transplant setting: ureteroneocystostomy surgical options, double-j stent considerations and management of related complications. Curr Urol Rep. 2020;21:3. https://doi.org/10.1007/s11934-020-0956-7.

54. Bardapure M, Sharma A, Hammad A. Forgotten ureteric stents in renal transplant recipients: three case reports. Saudi J Kidney Dis Transpl. 2014;25(1):109–12.
55. Siparsky NF, Kushnir LF, Gallichio MH, Conti DJ. Ureteral stents: a risk factor for polyomavirus BK viremia in kidney transplant recipients undergoing protocol screening. Transplant Proc. 2011;43(7):2641–4.
56. Patel P, Rebollo-Mesa I, Ryan E, Sinha MD, Marks SD, Banga N, Macdougall IC, Webb MC, Koffman G, Olsburgh J. Prophylactic ureteric stents in renal transplant recipients: a multicenter randomized controlled trial of early versus late removal. Am J Transplant. 2017;17(8):2129–38.
57. Basic DT, Hadzi-Djokic J, Ignjatovic I. The history of urinary diversion. Acta Chir Iugosl. 2007;54(4):9–17. https://doi.org/10.2298/aci0704009b PMID: 18595222.
58. Cimen S, Guler S, Tennankore K, Imamoglu A, Alwayn I. Surgical drains do not decrease complication rates but are associated with a reduced need for imaging after kidney transplant surgery. Ann Transplant. 2016;14(21):216–21. https://doi.org/10.12659/aot.898260 PMID: 27074868.
59. D'Souza K, Crowley SP, Hameed A, Lam S, Pleass HC, Pulitano C, Laurence JM. Prophylactic wound drainage in renal transplantation: a systematic review. Transplant Direct. 2019 27;5(7):e468. https://doi.org/10.1097/TXD.0000000000000908.PMID: 31334342; PMCID:PMC6616136.
60. https://www.mykci.com/patients/prevena-therapy-for-patients.
61. Park SC, Moon IS, Koh YB. Second and third kidney transplantations. Transplant Proc. 2006;38(7):1995–7. https://doi.org/10.1016/j.transproceed.2006.06.018 PMID: 16979976.
62. Gutierrez Banos JL, Rodrigo Calabia E, Rebollo Rodrigo MH, et al. Surgical aspects in the third and fourth kidney retransplant. Actas Urol Esp. 2005;29:212–6.
63. Etienne T, Ruedin P, Goumaz C, Spiliopoulos A, Leski M, Mégevand R. Retransplantation rénale: résultats et facteurs de pronostic [Kidney retransplantation: results and prognostic factors]. Helv Chir Acta. 1992;58(6):899–904. French. PMID: 164461
64. Tejani A, Sullivan EK. Factors that impact on the outcome of second renal transplants in children. Transplantation. 1996;62(5):606–11. https://doi.org/10.1097/00007890-199609150-00011 PMID: 8830823.
65. Delmonico FL, Tolkoff-Rubin N, Auchincloss H Jr, Farrell ML, Fitzpatrick DM, Saidman S, Herrin JT, Cosimi AB. Second renal transplantations. Ethical issues clarified by outcome; outcome enhanced by a reliable crossmatch. Arch Surg. 1994;129(4):354–60. https://doi.org/ 10.1001/archsurg.1994.01420280024003. PMID: 8154961.
66. Ossareh S, Ghods AJ. Results of second renal transplants. Transplant Proc. 1999;31(8):3122–3. https://doi.org/10.1016/s0041-1345(99)00744-7 PMID: 10616402.
67. Ahn HJ, Kim YS, Rha KH, Kim JH. Technical refinement for third kidney transplantation. Urology. 2006;68(1):189–92. https://doi.org/10.1016/j.urology.2006.01.049 Epub 2006 Jun 27 PMID: 16806427.
68. Hagan C, Hickey DP, Little DM. A single centre study of the technical aspects and outcome of third and subsequent renal transplants. Transplantation. 2003;75:1687–91.
69. Izquierdo L, Peri L, Piqueras M, et al. Third and fourth kidney transplant: still a reasonable option. Transp Proc. 2010;42:2498–502.
70. Mazzucchi E, Danilovic A, Antonopoulos IM, Piovesan AC, Nahas WC, Lucon AM, Srougi M. Surgical aspects of third and subsequent renal transplants performed by the extraperitoneal access. Transplantation. 2006;81(6):840–4. https://doi.org/10.1097/01.tp. 0000203559.57088.f6 PMID: 16570005.
71. Friedersdorff F, Patabendhi S, Busch J, Kempkensteffen C, Halleck F, Fuller TF, Miller K, Peters R. Outcome of patients after third and fourth kidney transplantation. Urol Int. 2016;97 (4):445–9. https://doi.org/10.1159/000445216 Epub 2016 Jun 17 PMID: 27310597.
72. Blanco M, Medina J, Gonzalez E, Dominguez M, Rodriguez A, Pamplona M, Andres A, Leiva O, Morales JM. Third kidney transplantation: a permanent medical-surgical challenge. Transplant Proc. 2009;41(6):2366–9. https://doi.org/10.1016/j.transproceed.2009.06.105. PMID: 19715921.

73. Halawa A. The third and fourth renal transplant; technically challenging, but still a valid option. Ann Transplant. 2012;17(4):125–32. https://doi.org/10.12659/aot.883703 PMID: 23274333.

74. Nghiem D. Orthotopic kidney retransplantation in simultaneous pancreas kidney transplant patients with renal failure. Transplant Proc. 2008;40(10):3609–10.

75. Gil-Vernet JM, Gil-Vernet A, Caralps A, et al. Orthotopic renal transplant and results in 139 consecutive cases. J Urol. 1989;142:248–52.

76. Musquera M, Peri LL, Alvarez-Vijande R, et al. Orthotopic kidney transplantation: an alternative survival technique in selected patients. Eur Urol. 2010;58(6):927–33.

77. Nédélec M, Glémain P, Rigaud J, Karam G, Thuret R, Badet L, Kleinclauss F, Timsit MO, Branchereau J. Transplantation rénale sur prothèse vasculaire [Renal transplantation on vascular prosthesis]. Prog Urol. 2019;29(12):603–11. French. https://doi.org/10.1016/j.purol. 2019.06.005. Epub 2019 Aug 22. PMID: 31447181.

78. Patrono D, Verhelst R, Buemi A, Goffette P, De Pauw L, Kanaan N, Goffin E, De Meyer M, Mourad M. Renal allograft implantation on prosthetic vascular grafts: short- and long-term results. World J Surg. 2013;37(7):1727–34. https://doi.org/10.1007/s00268-013-2028-3 PMID: 23604302.

79. Ozçelik A, Treckmann J, Paul A, Witzke O, Sotiropoulos G, Nadalin S, Malago M, Broelsch CE. Results of kidney transplantation with simultaneous implantation of vascular graft. Transplant Proc. 2007;39(2):509–10. https://doi.org/10.1016/j.transproceed.2006.12. 017 PMID: 17362769.

80. Galazka Z, Grochowiecki T, Jakimowicz T, Kowalczewski M, Szmidt J. Is severe atherosclerosis in the aortoiliac region a contraindication for kidney transplantation? Transplant Proc. 2011;43(8):2908–10. https://doi.org/10.1016/j.transproceed.2011.08.023 PMID: 21996186.

81. Matia I, Adamec M, Varga M, Janousek L, Lipar K, Viklicky O. Aortoiliac reconstruction with allograft and kidney transplantation as a one-stage procedure: long term results. Eur J Vasc Endovasc Surg. 2008;35(3):353–7. https://doi.org/10.1016/j.ejvs.2007.09.022 Epub 2007 Dec 11 PMID: 18065247.

82. Pilichowska E, Ostrowski P, Kotowski MJ, Tejchman K, Ostrowska-Clark K, Ostrowski M, Sieńko J. Transplantation of a kidney with duplicated ureter harvested from a donor with vascular anomaly in the form of double inferior vena cava: a case report. Transplant Proc. 2020;52(8):2533–5. https://doi.org/10.1016/j.transproceed.2020.02.089 Epub 2020 Apr 17 PMID: 32307140.

83. Sulikowski T, Zietek Z, Ostrowski M, Kamiński M, Sieńko J, Romanowski M, Majewski W, Ostrowska-Clarck K, Domański L, Różański J, Ciechanowski K. Experiences in kidney transplantation with duplicated ureters. Transplant Proc. 2005;37(5):2096–9. https://doi.org/ 10.1016/j.transproceed.2005.03.041 PMID: 15964349.

84. Cruzado JM, Fernandez L, Riera L, Bestard O, Carrera M, Torras J, Gil Vernet S, Melilli E, Ngango L, Grinyó JM. Revisiting double kidney transplantation: two kidneys provide better graft survival than one. Transplant Proc. 2011;43(6):2165–7. https://doi.org/10.1016/j. transproceed.2011.05.018. **PMID: 21839222.**

85. Medina-Polo J, Pamplona-Casamayor M, Miranda-Utrera N, González-Monte E, Passas-Martínez JB, Andrés BA. Dual kidney transplantation involving organs from expanded criteria donors: a review of our series and an update on current indications. Transplant Proc. 2014;46(10):3412–5. https://doi.org/10.1016/j.transproceed.2014.10.025 PMID: 25498062.

86. Masson D, Hefty T. A technique for the transplantation of 2 adult cadaver kidney grafts into 1 recipient. J Urol. 1998;160(5):1779–80 PMID: 9783951.

87. Ekser B, Furian L, Broggiato A, Silvestre C, Pierobon ES, Baldan N, Rigotti P. Technical aspects of unilateral dual kidney transplantation from expanded criteria donors: experience of 100 patients. Am J Transplant. 2010;10(9):2000–7. https://doi.org/10.1111/j.1600-6143.2010. 03188.x Epub 2010 Jul 15 PMID: 20636454.

88. Bricker EM. Bladder substitution after pelvic evisceration. Surg Clin North Am. 1950;30 (5):1511–21.
89. Lee DJ, Tyson MD, Chang SS. Conduit urinary diversion. Urol Clin North Am. 2018;45 (1):25–36.
90. Farnham SB, Cookson MS. Surgical complications of urinary diversion. World J Urol. 2004;22(3):157–67.
91. Surange RS, Johnson RW, Tavakoli A, Parrott NR, Riad HN, Campbell BA, Augustine T. Kidney transplantation into an ileal conduit: a single center experience of 59 cases. J Urol. 2003;170(5):1727–30. https://doi.org/10.1097/01.ju.0000092023.39043.67 PMID: 14532763.
92. Tanna RJ, Powell J, Mambu LA. Ileal Conduit. [Updated 2020 Dec 5]. In: StatPearls [Internet]. Treasure Island (FL): StatPearls Publishing;2020. https://www.ncbi.nlm.nih.gov/books/NBK565859/.
93. Abramowicz D, Cochat P, Claas FH, Heemann U, Pascual J, Dudley C, Harden P, Hourmant M, Maggiore U, Salvadori M, Spasovski G, Squifflet JP, Steiger J, Torres A, Viklicky O, Zeier M, Vanholder R, Van Biesen W, Nagler E. European Renal Best Practice Guideline on kidney donor and recipient evaluation and perioperative care. Nephrol Dial Transplant. 2015 Nov;30(11):1790–7. https://doi.org/10.1093/ndt/gfu216. Epub 2014 Jul 9. PMID:
94. Davidson IJA, Ar'Rajab. Perioperative fluid and drug therapy During cadaver kidney transplantation. In: Terasaki PI, Secka JM, editors. Clinical transplants 1992. Los Angeles: UCLA Tissue Typing Laboratory; 1993:267–84.

# Chapter 5
# Methods of Treatment of Surgical Complications After Kidney Transplantation

## 5.1 Bleeding: Surgical Side Bleeding

Postoperative surgical bleeding in the area of the transplanted kidney may lead to compression of the renal vessels and/or kidney transplant. Massive hemorrhaging, if not treated promptly, can lead to severe shock with consequences which can lead to graft loss and finally patient death. In most cases, bleeding after kidney transplantation occurs in the early postoperative period and generally within the first hours and/or days after surgery. Postoperative surgical-site hemorrhage which has occurred days after surgery was defined as a drop in hemoglobin $\geq 20$ g/l over a 24-hour period within three days of transplantation, followed by an ultrasound indicating a significant hematoma/collection [1, 2]. Bleeding may occur from vascular anastomoses, vessels in the renal hilum which dilate following reperfusion, or retroperitoneal tissues surrounding the graft which were traumatized during the exposure of the iliac fossa and mobilization of the iliac vessels. The donor type had a strong effect on the postoperative surgical side hemorrhage (SSH) as the living donor kidney transplants had a lower risk of bleeding by 70% versus the deceased donor kidney transplants. Bleeding is often captured late into the postoperative period (up to two weeks), but a few studies have focused on bleeds occurring within 24–48 h after the kidney transplantation [3–5]. It is important to distinguish early and late postoperative bleeds, because the latter type are not common due to the surgery but are instead characterized by distinct risk factors including biopsy procedures or therapeutic systemic anticoagulation [5].

Though perioperative anticoagulant therapy has been associated with an increased risk of bleeding [6, 7], a thorough investigation of other potential risk factors for SSH has yet to be conducted in the kidney transplant population. Furthermore, the effect of postoperative SSH on the long-term clinical outcomes, including graft loss or death, requires investigation.

Although the incidence of postoperative surgical-site hemorrhage in kidney transplantation is fairly low, it is associated with an increased risk of graft loss and/or death. Deceased donor transplants may be the strongest predictor of surgical-site hemorrhage;

© The Author(s), under exclusive license to Springer Nature Switzerland AG 2023

A. Baranski, *Kidney Transplantation*,
https://doi.org/10.1007/978-3-030-75886-8_5

however, lower recipient BMI may also be considered a significant risk factor. These findings can aid in identifying high-risk patients for postoperative hemorrhage to optimize their care during the perioperative period. Future studies are warranted to determine the underlying mechanisms by which the postoperative hemorrhage in kidney transplant patients leads to worse long-term clinical outcomes [1].

## *5.1.1   Indications for Emergency Surgery*

- A bleeding leading to hemodynamic instability of the patient after renal replacement without clotting disorders should be operated on an emergency basis.
- A bleeding leading to hemodynamic instability in the patient after renal transplantation, caused by severe coagulation disorders, should be operated on an emergency basis after correcting the coagulation before or during surgery.

## *5.1.2   Indications for Intensive Monitoring of a Patient with Suspected Bleeding into the Transplanted Kidney Area or into the Abdomen*

**5.1.2.1. A bleeding that has stopped spontaneously**, leaving only a large hematoma in the area of the transplanted kidney, may obstruct the drainage of blood or urine from the transplanted kidney, resulting in a renal vein thrombosis, ureteral stenosis and/or necrosis, kidney edema or a severe reduction in the arterial blood flow to the kidney. A prolonged compression of the hematoma on the renal vein and/or artery may contribute to a decrease in diuresis, an increase in arterial pressure, elevated creatinine values and can be responsible for not only renal vein thrombosis but also for renal artery thrombosis.

**5.1.2.2. A chronic bleeding, leading to a decreasing of hemoglobin value**, resulting in the build-up of a hematoma around the transplanted kidney, should be monitored by the rate and amount of blood loss or drop in the hematocrit or enlargement of the hematoma around the affected kidney monitored several times a day with Duplex Doppler ultrasound. An increasing of the hematoma volume in the retroperitoneal space is responsible for an increase in the pressure on the iliac vessels, the vessels of the transplanted kidney, the renal pelvis and/or the ureter. A compression of the renal pelvis or ureter may result in difficulties in the flow of urine from the renal pelvis to the urinary bladder. On the ultrasound we will see a significant widening of the renal pelvis. A hematoma in the retroperitoneal space, affecting the blood inflow and/or only outflow disorders through the kidney or ureter, should be treated as needed by a radiologist (puncture and drainage) and/or a surgeon.

**5.1.2.3. Any hematoma which is formed in the upper pole** of the transplanted kidney or around it, for example after an open biopsy, does not expand if it is stable and therefore it does not include the iliac and renal vessels and the ureter and may

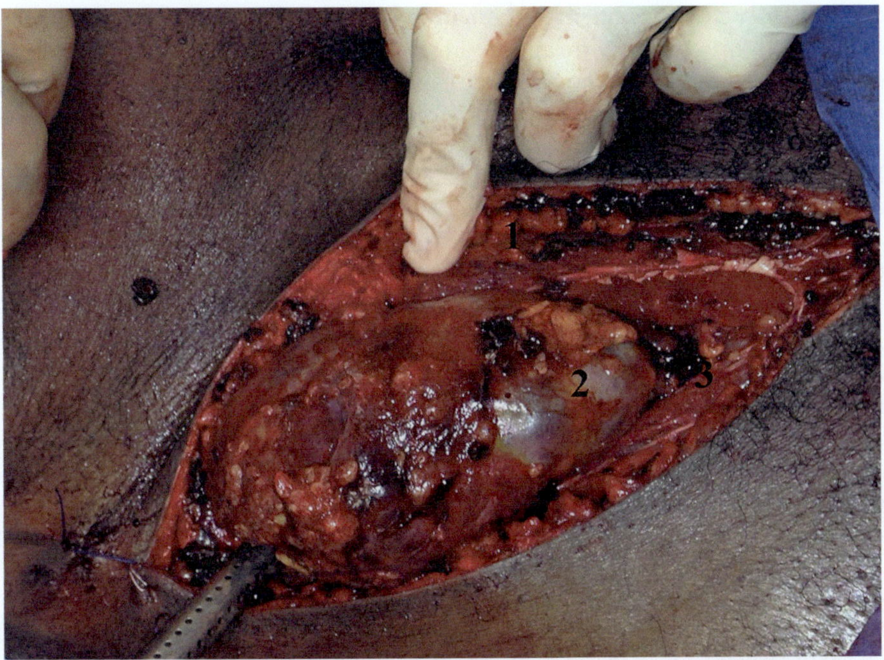


**Fig. 5.1** Infected, treated surgically, poorly drained hematoma in the area of the transplanted kidney. 1—Subcutaneous tissue, 2—Kidney, 3—Infected hematoma in liquid-solid form

be treated conservatively. At a later stage, when the hematoma has liquefied or the patient has a complaint or the hematoma becomes infected, it can be drained by the radiologist or surgically (Fig. 5.1).

**5.1.2.4. Any hematoma around the transplanted kidney suspected of being infected** (fever, pain, infection of the urinary tract, tenderness or peritoneal symptoms when palpating the area of the transplanted kidney) should first be punctured with a needle under ultrasound guidance and its contents aspirated into a syringe to obtain material for bacteriological examination. In case of the presence of bacteria, intravenous administration of an antibiotic should be initiated and as a first step the hematoma should be drained with a thick radiographic drain. If this is not possible, for example because it is close to the renal vessels or the ureter runs through it, the infected hematoma should be immediately surgically drained. During drainage, material of the infected hematoma should be collected for further cultures. The infected side should be surgically well drained or using radiological drains.

**5.1.2.5. Small hematomas or large hematomas**, for example in the area of the upper pole, which do not compress any important structures of the transplanted kidney and are painless and not infected, can be treated conservatively using the "wait and see" method.

**5.1.2.6. Operative treatment of hematomas around the transplanted kidney**: Indications for operative treatment are usually large hematomas pressing on essential structures of a kidney such as a vein, artery, ureter, or urinary bladder and infected and non-infected small hematomas which have been drained by a radiologist with radiological drains, but this type of treatment has not been successful. Evacuation of a hematoma in the operating theatre takes place with complete anesthesia of a patient, administration of antibiotics, and insertion of a catheter into a urinary bladder. The operation is carried out under sterile conditions and here are the most critical steps.

a)   opening the wound and reaching the hematoma
b)   taking a sample of the hematoma for culture
c)   evacuation of the hematoma and attempt to stop the bleeding
d)   washing the hematoma itself and the transplanted kidney area with hot Ringer's solution or physiological saline
e)   performing accurate hemostasis
f)   leaving silicone drains or Jackson-Pratt-type drains around the transplanted kidney
g)   closure of the wound
h)   suturing the skin and subcutaneous tissue with or without covering the wound with Prevena or, in the case of massive infection, not suturing the skin, cover the entire wound with wet gauze soaked in warm sterile physiologic saline, or use a sterile sponge with negative pressure for this type of wound treatment, postponing suturing until the wound is free of infection and, once the skin is sutured until it heals quickly without complications.

**5.1.2.7. Handling of the radiological drain**: we define the daily "production" and content of the drain in milliliters, depending on the density of the drained environment. The content may include lymph, urine, pus, fluid and remnants of a hematoma. A drain with poor drainage after radiologic control of position can always be flushed (passive rinse to keep openings in drain holes: $2 \times 5{-}10$ ml, active rinse: 500–600 ml of warm Ringer's solution, warm sterile saline or betadine water solution—use very careful irrigation). After cleaning the drain, if the drainage is still poor, ask the intervention radiologist to try to replace the thin drain with a thicker one or to move the drain to a place that was not drained by it. Always check that everything is well drained (ultrasound, CT) before removing a drain. Always discuss the removal or correcting the position of the radiological drain with the radiologist.

### 5.1.3   Management of Early Sub-renal Capsule Hemorrhage Occurring Immediately During or Sometimes Shortly After Renal Reperfusion. May Occur After any Form of Kidney Donation by Both Deceased and Living Donors

Perform a quick opening of the kidney capsule at the site of the bleeding. It is usually a vessel that is bleeding under the kidney capsule, because of the earlier contact with the retroperitoneal space in the donor's body. A small vessel under the kidney capsule may not have been ligated or coagulated during or after retrieval and kidney benching. In many cases this small vessel has moved under the kidney capsule. A bleeding vessel can be very dangerous because, after a kidney reperfusion, it can bleed very intensely under the kidney capsule and detach it and cause a giant subcapsular hematoma which finally can destroy the kidney. If you are confronted with a subcapsular bleeding during kidney retrieval, procure the kidney and preserve it with cold preservation solution. Then open the renal capsule, find the bleeding vessel and sew up or ligate it and—if possible—suture the kidney capsule. In some cases, one of the contact hemostatic agents may be left under and/ or on the kidney capsule before suturing it, and then the capsule may be sutured over it. In the event of subcapsular bleeding after kidney transplantation, the capsule should be opened, the vessel sewn up or coagulated, and then one of the hemostatic agents should be applied and the capsule should be sutured (if possible).

A procured and flushed kidney reduces its volume. This means that the kidney parenchyma surface becomes smaller compared to the surface of the kidney capsule. The suturing of the kidney capsule is performed after the kidney has been flushed and before the implantation when the volume of the parenchyma is smaller than the volume of the capsule. After transplantation the volume of the kidney parenchyma increases rapidly. If the defect of the kidney capsule is very big, we do not sew it up but we coagulate the parenchyma of the transplanted kidney capsule which usually bleeds.

### 5.1.4   Delayed Hemorrhage in Kidney Transplantation: A Life-threatening Condition

One of the most catastrophic complications of kidney transplantation is the non-traumatic delayed bleeding caused by an arterial dissection and pseudoaneurysm, which endanger the survival of the graft. Delayed bleeding caused by the dissection of the arterial anastomosis is a life threatening event following kidney transplantation. Renal artery dissection and pseudoaneurysms in the absence of endovascular procedures have been reported after renal transplantation and may occur due to adjacent pelvic infections. Although this is a rare complication, its importance cannot be overemphasized considering the catastrophic consequences, including sudden death. An early recognition of this entity based on a high index of suspicion and subsequently employing the most appropriate treatment are vital for its successful management [7].

These cases show that non-traumatic hemorrhage after renal transplantation is a hazardous event that may occur repeatedly. Hemoglobin decline and hematoma around the transplanted kidney—which were present in all our cases before the arterial dissection—were associated with a significant risk of infection. In our cases, we encountered pus and necrotic tissue before the nephrectomy and the surgical field was obviously infected. We think that the infection of the artery at or around the site of the arterial anastomosis may lead to an anastomotic leak or local dissolution of the arterial wall and, consequently, carry the potential of rupture with catastrophic consequences. We therefore believe that hematoma and pus should be drained early to prevent morbidity and mortality. The choice of treatment strategy is still a subject of debate. Some authors have recommended immediate graft nephrectomy as the treatment of choice of the extra-renal arterial dissection after renal transplant [8]. On the other hand, re-suturing or re-anastomosis is contraindicated in a contaminated field. Endovascular placement of drug-eluting stent (DES) grafts is a valuable therapeutic option in cases of renal artery dissection and pseudoaneurysms after renal transplantation. It is relatively safe and easy to perform, with good early and long-term results and it allows the graft nephrectomy to be performed in a safer manner. The placement of DES grafts overcomes the risk of bleeding and allows the graft nephrectomy to be performed more easily and safely [9]. To prevent non-traumatic massive hemorrhage after renal transplantation due to arterial dissection or pseudoaneurysm, it is necessary to notice post-operative hematomas and surgical field infections. We prescribe longer courses of perioperative antibiotics in susceptible patients with diabetes mellitus and perirenal hematoma. Massive perirenal hematomas should be evacuated as soon as possible to prevent superimposed infection. *S. aureus* was found in two patients and *C. albicans* in one patient. Prophylaxis with a broad-spectrum antibiotic which is active against staphylococcus given at the induction of the anesthesia has been recommended to be of benefit in peripheral vascular surgery [10, 11]. We recommend this approach in diabetic patients too. When nephrectomy is indicated, stent placement in the common iliac and external iliac artery is recommended followed by graft nephrectomy. In conclusion, delayed bleeding after kidney transplantation is a catastrophic complication that can occur repeatedly and hence requires aggressive treatment [8–11].

## 5.2   Renal Allograft Rupture and Surgical Treatment

### 5.2.1   Introduction

Rupture of a transplanted kidney was first described by Murray et al. in 1968 [12]. The cause of rupture of the transplanted kidney is virtually unknown, and its incidence is 0.3–9.6%. Rupture of a transplanted kidney usually occurs in two to three weeks. Spontaneous renal allograft rupture is one of the most dangerous complications of kidney transplantation, which can result in graft loss. This condition needs immediate surgical intervention. Conservative management has dismal results. Predisposing factors for graft rupture are acute rejection, acute tubular necrosis (ATN) and renal vein thrombosis. The most common causes of kidney rupture is acute rejection followed by ATN, venous anastomotic obstruction or severe narrowing at the anastomosis site, thrombosis or torsion of the renal vein or ureter obstruction (in this case the most common one is rupture of the renal pelvis) [11]. The mechanism of kidney rupture is most likely a growing kidney and an increase in the volume that no longer can be accommodated by the kidney capsule [13]. Tulatz et al. measured in 58 patients that the volume of the kidneys was established by continuous sonographies of the grafts during the first 25 days after the operation. In non-rejecting patients it increased on average by 20%, in rejecting and rupturing patients by 35%. The transplants with rupture of the parenchyma revealed the greatest increase to the volume maximum per time unit. Sonography is a suitable screening method for the purpose of rejection diagnostics and can give prognostic statements concerning the threatening rupture of the parenchyma. A rapid increase of kidney volume and a constantly high blood pressure indicate a threatening rupture of the transplant [13]. In rare cases the kidney allograft rupture might present itself as a hematuria; it frequently occurs with the sudden onset of pain, bulging and tenderness over the site of the grafted kidney associated with hemodynamic alterations and shock. Recently there have been numerous reports suggesting that these kidneys may be saved with appropriate management. Success rates above 80% have been reported for preservation of these grafted kidneys resulting in normally functioning kidneys after repair [11–15].

### *5.2.2   Treatment*

The surgical procedure consists of patient exploration in the operating room and reaching the ruptured kidney, its vessel(s) and iliac vessel(s) as quickly as possible. If the bleeding is massive from the site of the kidney rupture, the first reaction of the surgeon should be to reduce the blood flow to the kidney and in the meantime apply pressure to the bleeding kidney rupture. The first vessel that should be taken under control is the renal artery by temporary clamping. If this is inadequate or even impossible, try to control next the bleeding of the iliac vessels on both sides of the arterial anastomosis. Once the bleeding is controlled, the renal vein is assessed for its patency. If the renal and/or iliac vein is free of thrombus and the bleeding is under control, we can concentrate on deciding whether to repair the kidney or perform a nephrectomy. The kidney repair consists of the following options: when we are dealing with a kidney rupture we are often confronted with one to several kidney fractures which is/are relatively shallow and does/do not extend into the renal pelvis. I twist the rolls of the 100% oxidized regenerated cellulose (Surgicel, Ethicon), insert them into every rupture in the kidney parenchyma and then I put a 2/0 Catgut or 2/0 PDS suture 5–8 mm from the edge of the rupture [11, 14]. The

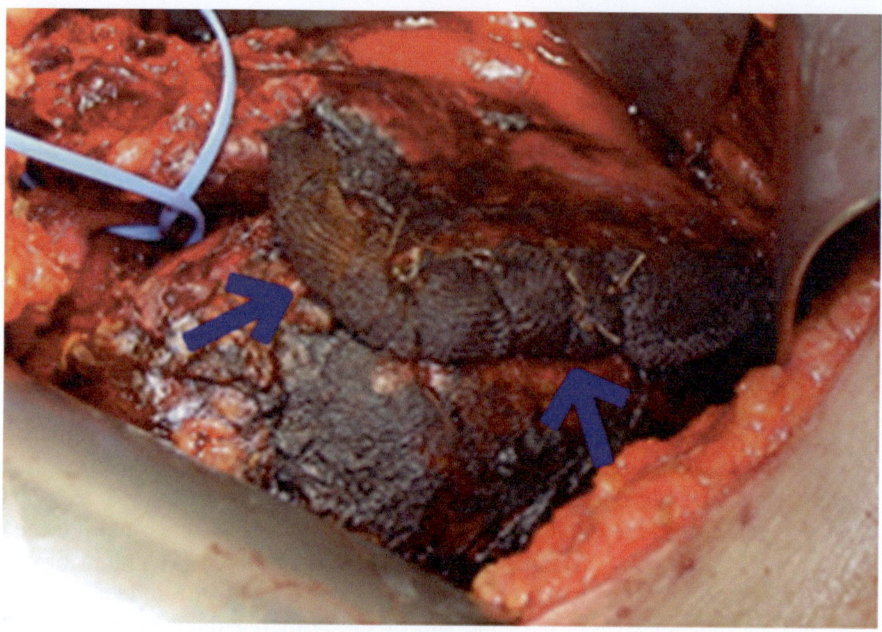

**Fig. 5.2** Ruptured kidney. The blue arrows indicate the stopping of bleeding by forming a roll of 100% oxidized regenerated cellulose (absorbable), then inserting it into the kidney rupture followed by suturing it for complete hemostasis. The material used for hemostasis has bactericidal and bacteriostatic properties

sutures I put on quite densely, 5–7 mm apart, deeply pass under the bottom of the rupture. The ends of the sutures are then tied on the soluble cellulose rollers inserted into the rapture gap. We tie the sutures on the rollers very slowly and with high sensitivity, so we do not cut the kidney parenchyma during tying. Remember that a ruptured kidney is large, swollen and its parenchyma is very fragile and easily damaged during sewing. If the tying is too tight, parenchyma may be severed, injured and torn, leading to even more bleeding and more blood loss (Fig. 5.2). Other surgical methods of treating a kidney rupture that are described in modern literature include temporary clamping of the renal artery, similar to the method used in partial nephrectomy. Second, at the time of temporary clamping of the renal and/ or iliac artery, a hemostatic matrix (FLOSEAL; Baxter International) could be sprayed on the surface of the renal graft. The third possibility mentioned above, consists of compressing the whole renal parenchyma with both and applying a dry pad for five minutes on the whole surface. Finally, remove the pad and wrap the graft with oxidized cellulose (SURGICEL; Ethicon). Other methods for repairing kidney rupture are: large mattress Dexon absorbable sutures tied over Teflon pledgets and applying prolonged pressure on the exposed kidney [2]; large mattress Dexon absorbable sutures tied over a piece of external oblique aponeurosis; and [3] 2/0 Dexon sutures tied over a piece of Surgicell or autologous fat. All surgeons used all the above mentioned methods with quite a good success rate [11, 14, 15].

Any kidney rupture that comes into contact with the renal pelvis, a second rupture and any subsequent kidney rupture within a short period of time, followed by acute rejection, are all indications to remove the transplanted kidney without attempting any repair.


## 5.3  Renal Artery Thrombosis

Renal graft survival has improved over recent years, mainly owing to better immunosuppression. The incidence of arterial thrombosis was reported to be 0.2–7.5% with the highest incidence among children and infants, and the lowest in living donor reports. The most significant risk factors for developing thrombosis were the donor-age below 6 or above 60 years, or the recipient-age below 5–6 years, pre- or postoperative hemodynamic instability, peritoneal dialysis, diabetic nephropathy, a history of thrombosis, deceased donor, or >24 h cold ischemia. Multiple arteries were not a risk factor [16]. Despite meticulous attention to reduce thrombotic risk factors, thrombosis cannot be entirely prevented, which means that an early detection of this complication is desirable in order to save the kidneys through prompt reoperation. The cause of renal artery thrombosis is multifactorial and thus can be found in various circumstances, such as: (usually) a bad position (twisting, bending, kinking—technical factors), a hypercoagulable state, acute rejection, poor cardiac output, delayed graft function, a history of previous thrombosis, renal artery intima injury, atherosclerotic plaque separation from the renal artery wall of the transplanted kidney, the recipient's iliac artery at the anastomosis site and/or any type of damage caused by the clamp used to close the atherosclerotic altered iliac artery above or below the anastomosis site—in this case, not only the transplanted kidney but also the recipient's lower limb is at risk. As I mentioned earlier, prevention is the best treatment, so in cases of poor pulsation of the renal artery and insufficient blood supply to the kidney, using a direct flowmeter and measuring the speed of blood flow through the renal artery and the iliac arteries before closing the surgical wound appears to be the treatment of choice. Of course, in many hospitals it is not possible to measure the blood flow directly but we have our own finger, experience and the possibility of aggressive monitoring after the operation (Doppler ultrasound, angiography directly from the femoral artery puncture or computer or magnetic angiography). CTA (computed tomography angiography) remains useful as a diagnostic tool in the assessment of the transplant arterial anatomy; particularly when there is a significant tortuosity of the donor's or recipient's artery or if the patient's factors, such as body habitus, limit a satisfactory sonographic evaluation [17].

If, after transplantation, the kidney does not urinate, the patient's arterial pressure should be continuously monitored, a Doppler ultrasound should be performed twice a day to monitor the correct blood supply to the transplanted kidney and the correct flow through the transplanted kidney vessels. In case of doubt about the blood supply or outflow, the next examination to be performed is the direct computer angiography (angio-CT).

If, after a kidney transplant, the kidney secretes urine correctly and then suddenly stops or slowly starts to decrease, the first step to be performed is a Doppler ultrasound of the transplanted kidney, especially the renal vessels, including an examination of the iliac vessels on the transplanted kidney side. If there is any doubt as to the blood flow in and from the kidney, computer angiography or classical angiography should be performed to show the normal or abnormal arterial blood supply to the transplanted kidney and the flow through the iliac arteries.

Early detection of an incomplete renal artery thrombosis can be attempted by administering intravenous heparin in a continuous infusion of heparin and/or by trying to dissolve the clot locally with clot-dissolving drugs like urokinase. Surgical treatment is not indicated when the single intrarenal arterial branch or branches are involved in thrombosis. In any case, it is best to consult a vascular surgeon and an interventional radiologist who can attempt to aspirate the clot during direct angiography, e.g. from the lumen of the renal artery or branches. Another method of treating renal artery obstruction by the radiologist may be to leave a thin drain near or at the beginning of the thrombus. Urokinase will be injected very slowly over 24 hours through a drain placed in this way to dissolve the clot closing the renal artery.

A very important factor preventing the occurrence of renal artery thrombosis is the state of surgeon training in vascular anastomoses and microsurgery. A wrong approach, wrong vascular reconstruction of a renal artery and then wrong technical anastomoses are a frequent cause of renal artery thrombosis. Repeated execution of vascular anastomoses eventually leads to a longer time of warm ischemia, destruction of a vessel wall (intima damage) and thrombosis. All these are iatrogenic injuries of vessels caused by wrong or insufficient training of a surgeon in vascular surgery and vascular anastomoses. Let us remember that a thrombosis of the renal artery can appear in a few minutes after the execution of the anastomoses and the restoration of blood circulation through a kidney.

During a thrombosis of the renal artery there is one thing to remember: if the clot covers only the trunk of the renal artery and does not penetrate into the kidney, if we act quickly we can try to save the kidney by submitting it to treatment by an interventional radiologist or by a vascular and/or transplant surgeon. If a thrombosis of the small arterioles inside the parenchyma has taken place, then the chance of saving the kidney is almost zero.

As a rule, a total thrombosis of the renal artery ends in irreversible changes in the parenchyma of the kidney. It should be remembered that a kidney and its ureter are very sensitive to ischemia and in the absence of blood flow they easily undergo very serious injuries. Let us not delude ourselves that everything can be repaired—this complication in most cases, unfortunately, ends with the removal of the kidney.

## 5.4   Transplant Renal Artery Stenosis or Renal Artery Stenosis of the Transplanted Kidney

### 5.4.1   Introduction

Transplant renal artery stenosis (TRAS) is the most common vascular complication of renal grafts with incidences ranging from 1 to 23%. It occurs most frequently in the first six months, but it can present itself at any time after transplantation. TRAS usually manifests itself several years after a kidney transplantation. In slim patients with a large narrowing of the renal artery, a vascular murmur can be heard over the transplanted kidney. Renal hypoperfusion occurring in the TRAS results in activation of the renin–angiotensin–aldosterone system; in these patients, the usual form of renal artery stenosis manifests itself in the form of difficult to control hypertension with worsening after almost every treatment, fluid retention (foot oedema), congestive heart failure and often allograft dysfunction. All these symptoms may occur in patients whose intraluminal diameter of the renal artery is narrowed by more than 50–70% [18–36].

### 5.4.2   Etiology

Several risk factors for the TRAS have been reported, including: older recipient's age, retrieval damage caused to the renal artery, intimal damage at the time of retrieval and benching perfusion, atheroma at the site of anastomosis, [19] faulty suture technique, disparity in the diameters of the donor's and recipient's arteries in end-to-end anastomosis, [20] prolonged cold ischemia time, acute rejection, [21] and cytomegalovirus infection [22]. Some authors have reported a higher incidence of the TRAS in cadaveric donors (13.2–17.7%) than in living donor renal transplants [23–26]. In this study, the incidence of the TRAS in deceased donors was 11.5%. The following factors can be responsible for renal transplant artery stenosis after kidney transplantation over different periods of time, such as: an inexperienced surgeon, bad surgical technique, more than one renal artery, kinking of the renal vessels, cytomegalovirus, BK virus, severe atherosclerosis, infection and rejection [20–26].

### 5.4.3   Diagnostics

Stenosis diagnostics include Doppler ultrasonography, classical angiography with pressure measurement before and after stenosis, computer angiography and magnetic resonance angiography (MRA) [18, 25].

### 5.4.4  Treatment

PTA is the gold standard and treatment of choice. The most popular operation is to excise the stenosis with an end-to-side or end-to-end re-anastomosis of the renal artery with the previously prepared renal and/or internal iliac artery. Other surgical methods consist of releasing the kinking, local endarterectomy, or a bypass with a vascular conduit from the saphenous vein, hypogastric artery and/or donor vessels. Revision open surgery which is considered a rescue therapy is reserved for patients with unsuccessful angioplasty or with complicated stenosis [26, 27]. The success rate ranges from 63 to 92%, and the recurrence rate is around 12%. The surgery has high complication rates such as ureteral injury (14%), graft loss (15–20%), reoperation (13%) and mortality (5%) [36, 37]. PTA with stenting is now recognized as the treatment of choice. The technical success rate of the endovascular treatment is reported as between 89 and 100% [29–34] while clinical success is around 65.5–94% [19, 31, 33]. PTA alone carries a higher risk of restenosis with an incidence ranging from 16 to 62% [33]. However, restenosis following by a PTA and stenting are low, varying from 5.5 to 20% of cases [35, 36].

## 5.5  Renal Vein Thrombosis

### 5.5.1  Introduction

Complete renal vein thrombosis (RVT) after renal transplantation has an incidence of 0.55–3.4% and accounts for up to one-third of early allograft losses. Transplant renal vein thrombosis (TRVT) of an allograft has a dramatic clinical presentation and is one of the main causes of early graft dysfunction after renal transplant, with a reported prevalence of 0.1–4.2% of all transplants. When an early post-transplant RVT occurs, prior to the development of the collaterals (no venous outflow), it may be catastrophic and cause kidney rupture, loss of the allograft and may even lead in very complex cases to the recipient's death. Early diagnosis and urgent treatment are necessary but often unsuccessful. The prevalence of TRVT is higher in kidneys derived from deceased-donor as opposed to living-donor transplant. This may be because in kidneys derived from living-donor transplants procedures are usually done under more favorable conditions and are not usually subjected to ischemic injury. We must take into account, also, patients with an end stage kidney insufficiency who are hypercoagulable, for example, patients with systemic lupus erythematosus (SLE). In a large series, 73% were detected with a median delay of eight days suggesting that RVT develops gradually, presumably beginning as partial vein thrombosis. There may thus be a narrow but important window for early diagnosis of partial RVT, which would allow for timely intervention, e.g. starting anticoagulants [37–43].

## 5.5.2   *Manifestation, Detection and Thrombolytic Therapy*

Clinical manifestation of chronic or partial renal vein thrombosis after kidney transplantation is usually asymptomatic. Conventional ultrasonography with color and spectral Duplex Doppler is used for early detection of complications and evaluation of the renal allograft. The diagnostic capability of ultrasonography is influenced by the patient's body habitus and the radiologist's skills. Although angiography or CT angiography remains the standard for the diagnosis of renal vascular pathology, it is invasive and associated with significant nephrotoxicity. Other investigations, such as nuclear medicine scintigraphy or magnetic resonance angiography, offer excellent alternatives to the criterion standard with no nephrotoxicity and a greater sensitivity than ultrasonography. Partial renal vein thrombosis can be treated at the beginning conservatively by the implementation of thrombolytic therapy, which is the administration of drugs whose task is to dissolve in our case the thrombus in the renal vein. There are two ways as to how thrombolytic agents can be given: peripheral intravenously (IV) (systemic thrombolysis) or percutaneously through a catheter (thin tube) that has been navigated to the site of the clot. The length of a treatment session varies depending on the underlying cause. A session can take from 60 minutes to 48 hours. Systemic thrombolytic treatment can cause life-threatening hemorrhage, especially in the perioperative period. A catheter directed thrombolysis is more suitable for the treatment of complete and partial renal vein thrombosis especially later after kidney transplantation when surgical access could be difficult and a danger to the graft. Catheter directed thrombolysis can be sometimes combined with suction of the thrombus [40].

## 5.5.3   *Surgical Treatment*

### 5.5.3.1   Introduction

The surgical management of renal vein thrombosis, in particular early post-transplantation, must include surgical exploration of the allograft. Operative interventions can facilitate a better evaluation of the cause of thrombosis and can allow for the correction of technical complications. The most important in surgical treatment of renal vein thrombosis is not only the thrombectomy, but first of all it is the repair of the cause of the thrombosis: in the case of stenosis of the venous anastomosis, its surgical revision and re-anastomosis; in the case of vein bending, shortening it and re-anastomosis with the iliac vein or the stump of the renal vein; in the case of its twisting, new anastomosis; and in the case of acute rejection as the cause of thrombosis, introduction of aggressive antirejection therapy.

Surgical thrombectomy should be attempted whenever we hope to restore normal blood flow from the kidney. It is only likely to be successful if the thrombus is located in the main stem of the renal vein and/or in the iliac vein and there is no thrombosis of the small intrarenal veins yet.

A total massive renal vein thrombosis is dramatic. The kidney slowly decreases the urine production (from oliguria to anuria) with a rapid onset of hematuria. The transplanted kidney systematically increases its volume which causes tension in the renal capsule and peritoneum. The patients feels therefore more and more pain at the place of the transplanted kidney. Rapid closure of the renal vein may lead to kidney rupture, hemorrhage and finally to hemorrhagic shock and even death in a very short time. In this case, the patient requires immediate surgical or radiological intervention and massive and rapid blood transfusion.

### 5.5.3.2  Surgical Thrombectomy of the Complete Thrombosed Renal Vein Soon After Transplantation: The Most Important Surgical Steps

1. Good diagnosis: use color Doppler, angiography, CT or MRI angiography for:

    (a)  thrombosis of the renal vein with restriction only to the main renal vein;
    (b)  thrombosis of the renal vein with thrombus elongation, protruding into the iliac vein above and/or/only below into the iliac vein(s).

2. In the operating room: open the old incision and install a professional abdominal retractor.

3. Evaluate the kidney in terms of survival: Is it a blue, swollen, enlarged organ with very good pulsation in the renal artery (open) or is it swollen, black, with very bad or no flow through the renal artery?

4. Think during surgery about the indications for intravenous heparin and give it if needed.

5. Palpate the renal and iliac veins delicately in order to find the end of the clot below and/or above the anastomosis of the renal vein with one of the iliac veins. Place soft vascular clamps below and above the thrombus anastomosis. When thrombosis is found with extensions to the common and external iliac vein, do not place vascular clamps on the thrombus. Very slowly try to feel with your finger where it ends and where it begins. The clamped veins should be completely free of clot.

    (a)  There is no stenosis of the anastomosis but a thrombus extending from the renal vein to one of the iliac veins or the IVC: Cut transversely 30% of the circumference of the renal vein at a distance of about 2 cm from the renal hilum. Use the Fogarty embolectomy catheter or your fingers to move the clots outside the renal vein and rinse copiously the lumen of the renal and iliac vein(s) with heparinized physiologic saline solution chloride.
    (b)  The second possibility is that there is no stenosis in the place of anastomosis between the anastomosis of the renal vein which is anastomoses "end to side" with one of the iliac veins, there is no thrombus or thrombus extension, so there is no risk that by placing a clamp on one of the iliac veins you will break up a clot that could cause a pulmonary embolism in a kidney recipient. You

can use only one Satinsky clamp and use it for closing the iliac vein below the anastomosis then cut transversely 30% of the circumference of the renal vein at a distance of about 2 cm from the renal hilum.

(c)   If it is very difficult to perform an embolectomy via one opening in the renal vein's wall then you can make two or three incisions in the renal and/or iliac veins to clean the clots properly.

6.   After a successful thrombectomy operation, if you think that the operated kidney has a chance of survival, close the renal and/or iliac vein without any stenosis, place one or 2 JP drains around the kidney, close the patient and send him or her to the ICU or medium care unit (MC), prescribe heparin IV and warfarin to obtain an international normalized ratio of 2.0–3.0 in a period of eight weeks. The dosage of anticoagulant tablets must not exceed an INR (International Normalized Ratio) value of 2.5–3.5.

7.   If the kidney is swollen and black with a renal vein thrombus and there is very poor or even no pulsation on the renal artery, perfom a graftectomy and/or if necessary a thrombectomy of the iliac vein(s). Perform after that a good hemostatis, leave the JP drains, close the patient and send him/her for observation to ICU or the MC.

**Warning! (Shortly after transplantation)**
Pain in the area of the transplanted kidney, a decreased amount of urine secreted and an increased concentration of creatinine in the blood are indications for immediate ultrasound examination by Duplex Doppler.

**Warning! (Black kidney: do not be afraid to perform a graftectomy)**
Remember that an ischemic, dead organ kept in the recipient's body for too long may lead to shock or even the death of the recipient in a very short time. In such cases, always save the recipient, not the organ, at all costs! If the recipient survives all this, has good vessels and is young, he/she will still have a chance to get a new kidney.

**Warning! (Avoid an air embolism)**
After the complete closure of a large section of the iliac vein and the removal of the kidney, the inside of the vein should be filled with a saline solution with heparin before completing the suturing of the iliac vein or stump of the renal vein to prevent air embolism. Then release the first clamp located closer to the inguinal ligament and when the whole closed section is filled with blood, close it with a suture and release the clamp which was placed closer to the IVC.

**Summary Based on the Literature**
Renal vein thrombosis can not only lead to the loss of the graft itself but may also result in a high mortality rate due to graft rupture and embolic complications [38]. Successful revascularization with thrombolytic therapy, thrombus-aspiration or direct surgical thrombectomy have been reported [39–41]. Interestingly, one case series demonstrated a significant reduction in renal vein thrombosis following kidney transplant in patients receiving a low-dose of Aspirin [42, 43].

## 5.6   Urine Fistula/Urinary Leakage

### *5.6.1   Introduction*

A post-transplant urinary leakage is the so-called Achilles heel in kidney transplant surgery. Urinary leaks can be divided into early and late leaks and those producing (draining) small and large amounts of urine. The surgeon is responsible for early leaks up to the fourth or fifth day after the transplant and for the technical mistakes that probably were made during the kidney harvest, preparation of the ureter and making a new anastomosis between the ureter and the bladder. Fistulas formed after the fifth day and later after kidney transplantation are usually caused by insufficient blood supply or other types of damage to the ureter leading initially to its ischemia and later to its necrosis. Fluid collection during the postoperative period can be caused by urine leak or lymph leak of seroma. Urine fistula/leakage is the most common early complication, occurring in 1.2–8.9% of renal transplant patients. Urinary fistulas occur usually during the first four weeks after surgery and represent more than 50% of all urological complications [44]. The type of ureter-urinary bladder anastomosis with the lowest risk of fistulas is the method of extra urinary ureter bladder anastomosis, i.e. the Lich-Gregoir method. Urine leak is considered to be less common in patients whose ureterovesical anastomosis has been conducted with the use of an indwelling double J ureteric stent. Biochemical analysis of the drained liquid is essential and should be compared with a concomitant serum sample [44]. Urinoma can manifest itself in the form of increased drainage, delayed graft function or even sometimes wound leakage [45]. In most cases the drained liquid will show high creatinine and potassium levels in the drained or aspirated fluid. The place of the urine leakage may be the renal parenchyma with a minor or major calyx, the renal pelvis, the ureter and bladder, or ureter-bladder anastomosis, but the most common postoperative site of the urine leakage is the anastomosis of the ureter with the urinary bladder [44]. As far as the ureter and the renal pelvis are concerned, urine leakage occurs when the wall of the ureter or renal pelvis is somehow damaged. It is mainly mechanical damage—an incision, perforation or rupture as a result of a complete blockage of the urine drain from the pelvis or the ureter to the urinary bladder or thermal damage caused during kidney procurement or transplantation. If the incision of the ureter or pelvis is very small and the kidney is transplanted with a JJ catheter in the urinary tract, the incision usually heals spontaneously. Within a few days, the coagulated wall of the renal pelvis or ureter wall becomes necrotic and starts to pass urine outside, causing it to leak into the extraperitoneal space. It should be remembered that sometimes the stenosis of the ureter-bladder anastomosis is caused directly by its edema (for example a massive swelling of the ureter which has not been drained by a JJ catheter). Severe edema of the ureter-urinary bladder anastomosis may lead to a complete or partial closure of its lumen and thus impede the outflow of urine from the renal pelvis and a significant distension of the ureter followed by a urinary tract infection (UTI), pyelonephritis, ureter and/or renal pelvis necrosis, and/or rupture.

## 5.6.2   Unusual Description of Two Cases with Urinary Leakage (Author's Own Experience)

### 5.6.2.1   First Patient

I describe here a rather rare case of urine leakage after kidney transplant. One week after transplantation, the transplant function was good. After two weeks, the amount of urine suddenly decreased, there was almost a double increase in creatinine concentration in the blood, and the patient started to complain about increasing abdominal pain in the area of the transplanted kidney. The ultrasound showed a small amount of fluid around the kidney and the kidney scintigraphy (99mTc-MAG 3) showed a clear leak of urine into the retroperitoneal space. A small amount of fluid around the transplanted kidney was drained with a radiological drain, and a fluid sample was taken to determine the concentration of creatinine and to perform a culture. Very high creatinine values were found in the examined fluid. The patient was operated on and in the extraperitoneal space a small amount of fluid was found,

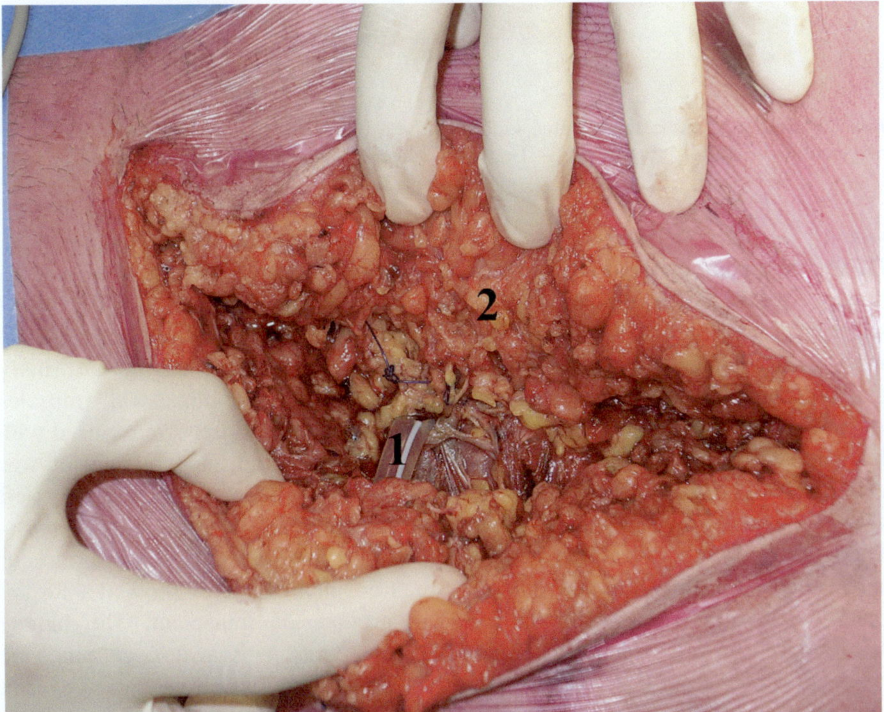

**Fig. 5.3**  1—Silicone drain with protruding holes left after the previous operation. The lateral holes of the drain removed urine from the extraperitoneal space to the area of subcutaneous tissue, which then escaped through the wound, 2—Subcutaneous tissue

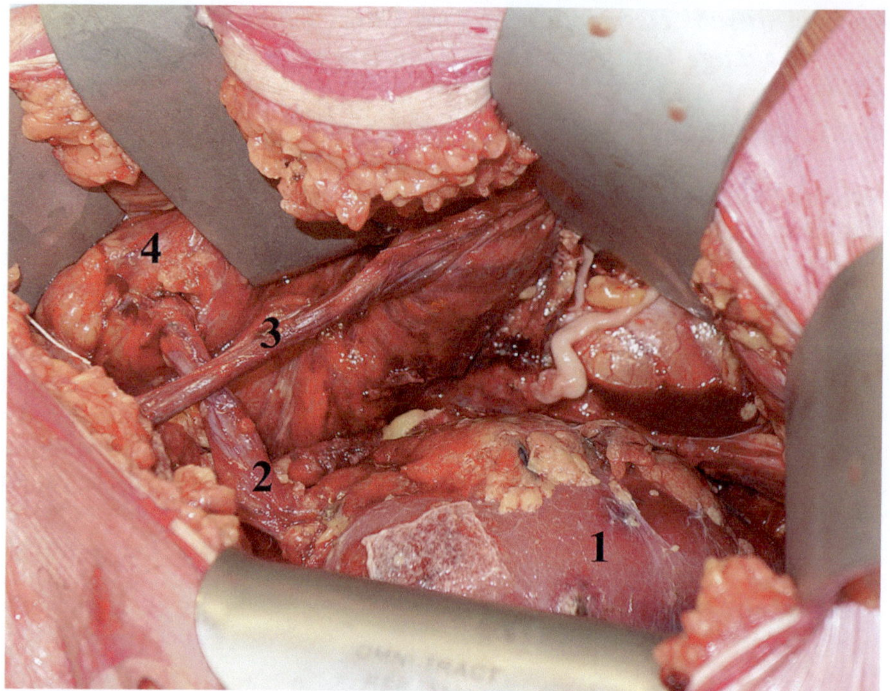

**Fig. 5.4** The area of the transplanted kidney without obvious signs of urinary leakage. Third reoperation. 1—Kidney transplant, 2—Ureter, 3—Spermatic cord, 4—Urinary bladder

which was taken into the syringe, again to perform bacteriological examination. During the operation the ureter-urinary bladder anastomosis and renal pelvis of the transplanted kidney were checked: no abnormalities were found in their blood supply and no mechanical damage was detected. Next the urinary bladder was filled with warm Ringer's solution and there were no leaks from the ureter-urinary bladder anastomosis. The cultures were taken from the abdominal wall (muscles and subcutis tissues). The surroundings of the transplanted kidney were rinsed with a few liters of warm Ringer's solution, drained with two drains and the incision was closed. From the second day after the operation the "production" of the drain left around the transplanted kidney started to increase and diuresis started to decrease. The concentration of creatinine in the fluid removed by the drains was again to our surprise very high. An ultrasonography of the transplanted kidney showed a normal renal pelvis and a small amount of fluid around the transplant. The kidney scintigraphy showed even greater urine leak into the retroperitoneal space. Since the production of the drain did not decrease but increase and the urine started to leak through the wound, we decided to reoperate the patient. As you can see in Fig. 5.3, the lateral hole of the silicone surgical drain was situated in the subcutaneous tissue, which explains the leakage of urine through the wound. The use of a professional abdominal retractor gave us a very stable surgical field (Fig. 5.4). The area around

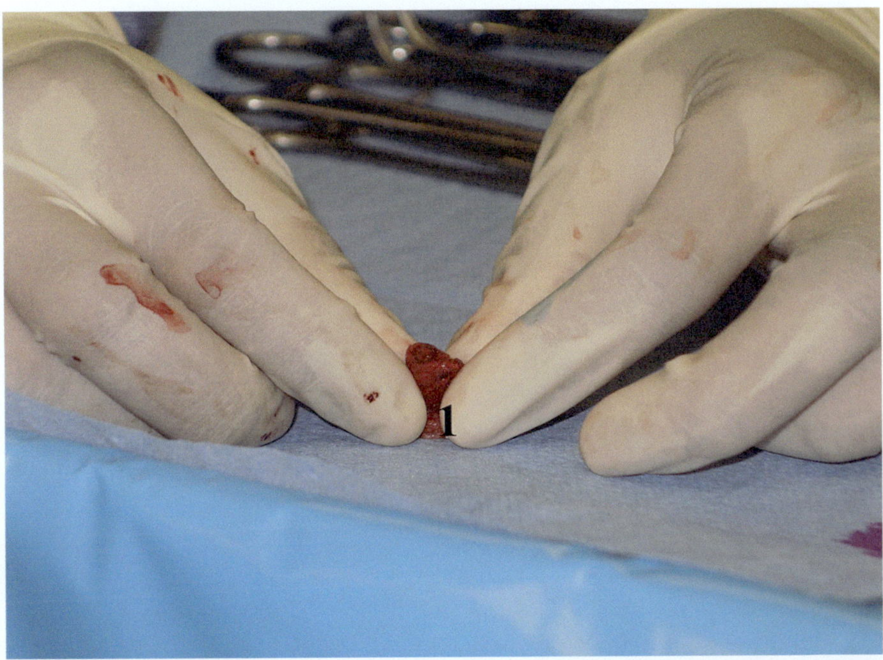

Fig. 5.5  1—An excised distal ureter closed by a swollen mucosa with a thrombus completely occluding its lumen

the transplanted kidney was one more time very carefully examined, the fluid around the kidney was taken for culture and then the entire extraperitoneal space around the kidney was rinsed with a warm Ringer's solution. The bladder was filled up under tension with warm saline solution. Unfortunately, the ureter-urinary bladder anastomosis was tight. The urine with the renal pelvis was examined very carefully, but no source of leakage was found anywhere. How to check where the leak is located? There is an option for the patient, i.e. intravenous administration of sterile methylene blue and waiting for about one to two hours until a green urine leakage site appears somewhere. We chose the short version consisting of cutting off the ureter-urinary bladder anastomosis with, under slight pressure, direct injection of a small amount of methylene blue dissolved in saline into the ureter and renal pelvis. This patient had already been operated on several times with poor results; this time during the operation we decided to choose such a method of treatment that would provide a 100% solution to the problem in the shortest possible time. The ureter-urine bladder anastomosis was cut off. The ureter and urinary bladder mucosa were very swollen. The ureter-urinary bladder anastomosis was open but 1 cm before it a thrombus was visible in the lumen of the ureter, which completely closed its lumen (Fig. 5.5). We shortened the ureter twice, the first time the ureter was shortened by 2 cm but its lumen closed and did not look normal. The second time we shortened the ureter by 1 cm, we saw a healthy open lumen of the

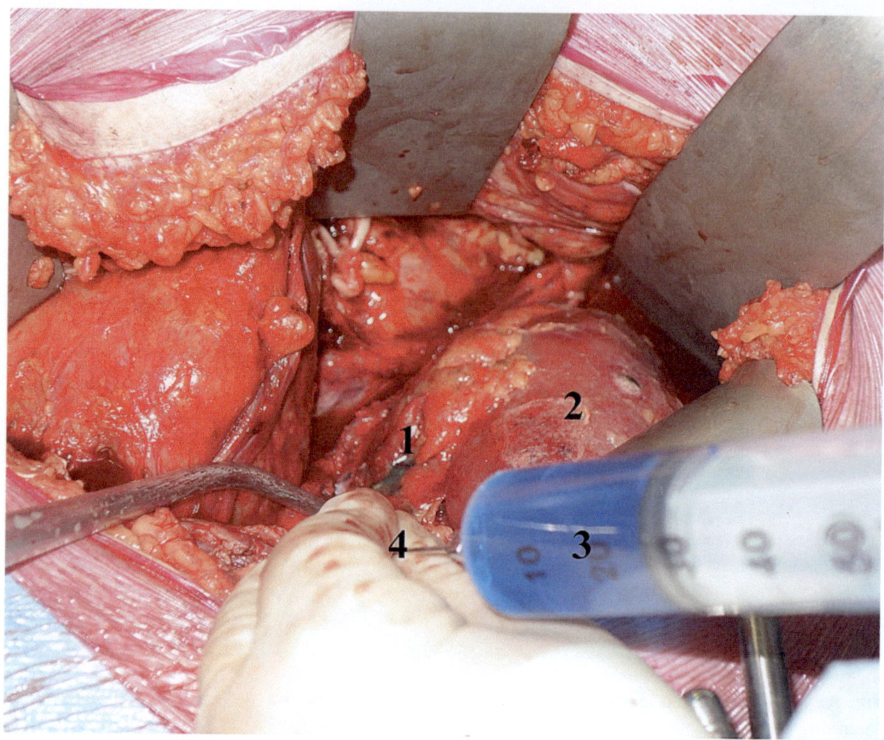

**Fig. 5.6** The ureter-urinary bladder anastomosis was completely detached from the urinary bladder. 1—Injection of methylene blue into the lumen of the detached ureter picture shows leakage from the anterior renal pelvic wall of the transplanted kidney, 2—Transplanted kidney, 3 —Syringe filled with diluted saline and methylene blue, 4—A special curved and thin cannula inserted into the ureter, which was closed around the cannula surgeon's fingers to prevent the leakage of dye administered into the ureter and renal pelvis

ureter with a healthy-looking mucous membrane. At this point, I decided to place a thin tube in the lumen of the ureter and to inject with a syringe under slight pressure methylene blue into the ureter and renal pelvis. A few seconds after administration, the urine stained with methylene blue began to flow out of the medial surface of the renal pelvis (Fig. 5.6). The site of damage to the renal pelvis (the rupture was about 5 mm) was found and sutured, the kidney was slightly mobilized and a new ureter-urinary bladder anastomosis was made in the same place with decompression with a JJ catheter (Fig. 5.7). The further postoperative course was uneventful.

I have described a rare case of rupture of the renal pelvis due to the narrowing of the uretero-bladder anastomosis caused by an anastomotic edema and, additionally, the closure of the ureter outflow by a thrombus (which most probably formed during the bleeding from the anastomosis of the ureter with the urinary bladder of the transplanted kidney, or renal pelvis), which resulted in complete closure of the

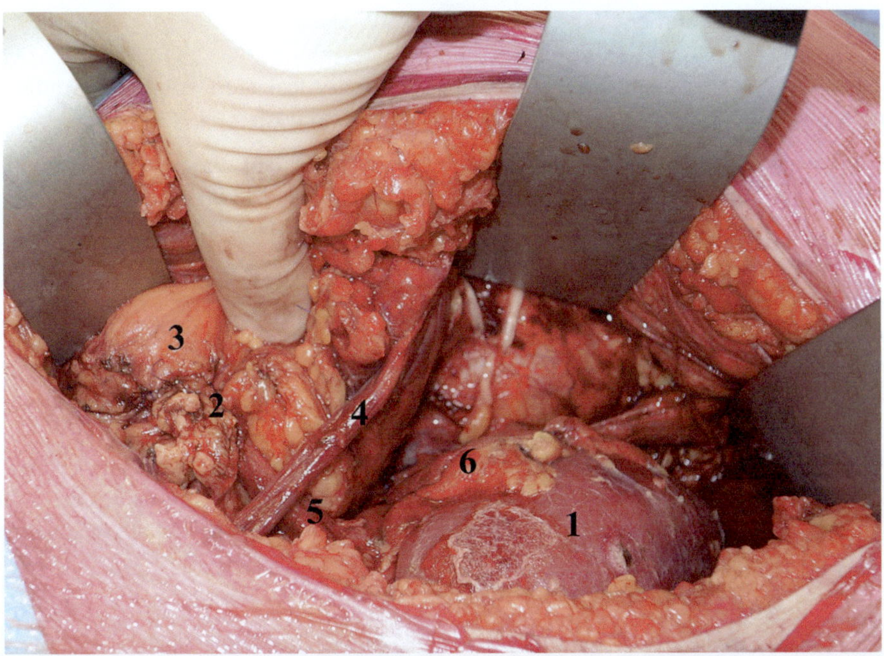

**Fig. 5.7** Once the leak has been localized, the renal pelvis is sutured and the ureter is implanted in the same place in the urinary bladder with which it was previously anastomosed. 1—Transplanted kidney, 2—Ureter implanted in the same place as before, 3—Urinary bladder, 4—Spermatic cord, 5—Ureter, 6—Renal pelvis sewn with two PDS 4/0 stitches

ureter and ureter-urinary bladder anastomosis which in effect led to the rupture of the renal pelvis and a leak of urine.

As mentioned before, the most common site of urinary leakage is the ureter-urinary bladder anastomosis. The causes of anastomotic leakage are all types of ureteral blood supply disorders, which include: anatomical anomalies; external pressure; technical errors in the procurement and preparation of the ureter and renal arteries leading the blood mainly to the lower pole of the kidney and/or during kidney transplantation, for example long warm ischemia time, low blood pressure during kidney revascularization and/or low pressure in the post-operative period.

Please never forget that the insufficient blood supply to the ureter after transplantation will always lead to poor healing, urine leakage, infection, fibrosis or even necrosis of the transplanted ureter. Also do not forget about the influence of other factors on the ureter, such as BK virus infection [45] and rejection.

### 5.6.2.2   Second Patient

This is a typical example of a patient with a urinary leakage resulting from ureter necrosis at the site of a ureter-urinary bladder anastomosis.

**Clinical presentation**: six days after the kidney transplant, the patient developed severe and increasing pain in the area of the transplanted kidney.

**Actions taken**:

- ultrasound—fluid collection around the kidney graft;
- scintigraphy—to show a urine leakage;
- percutaneous drainage of the fluid by the intervention radiologist;
- fluid collection for biochemical and bacteriological examination (high creatinine value in the drained fluid and/or a urine infection);
- first attempt at conservative treatment by antibiotic therapy IV and reinserting a catheter into the urinary bladder, placing nephroureterostomy catheter by an interventional radiologist both treatments failed after a few days due to

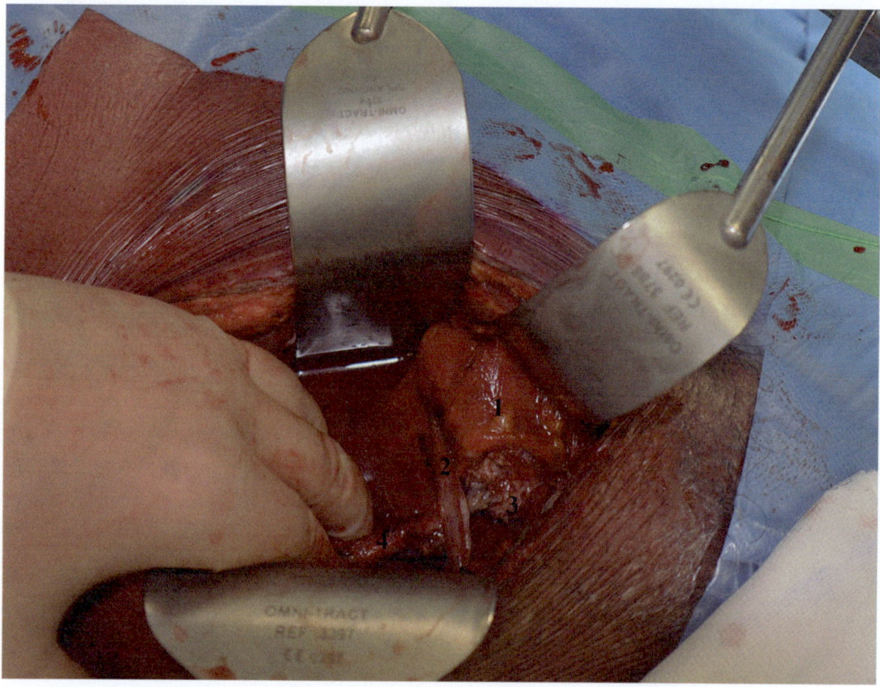

**Fig. 5.8** Transplanted kidney: distal ureter necrosis. 1—Urinary bladder, 2—Spermatic cord, 3—Necrosis of the ureter and urine leak, 4—Well arterial blood supply ureter of the kidney transplanted is seen above the level of the spermatic cord

increasing urine leakage, icreatinine, pain in the transplanted kidney area and fever

- no improvement—first reoperation with attempt to repair the ureter.

**Operation stages:**

- explore the transplanted kidney;
- culture all the fluid collection around the kidney graft, ureter and urinary bladder;
- rinse the area of the kidney and urinary bladder with warm Ringer's solution;
- carefully inspect the renal pelvis, ureter and vesico-ureteral anastomosis (Fig. 5.8);
- assess the complications arising and a plan for their surgical treatment.

Treatment of this type of complication usually consists of removing the necrotic end of the ureter and reattaching it to the bladder or native ipsilateral ureter at the same or a different place (Fig. 5.9). Due to the shortening of the ureter, the uretero-bladder anastomosis cannot be performed under tension. Sometimes the ureter—despite its shortening—is long enough and the ureter-urinary bladder anastomosis can be performed without tension. If the ureter, after being cut off,

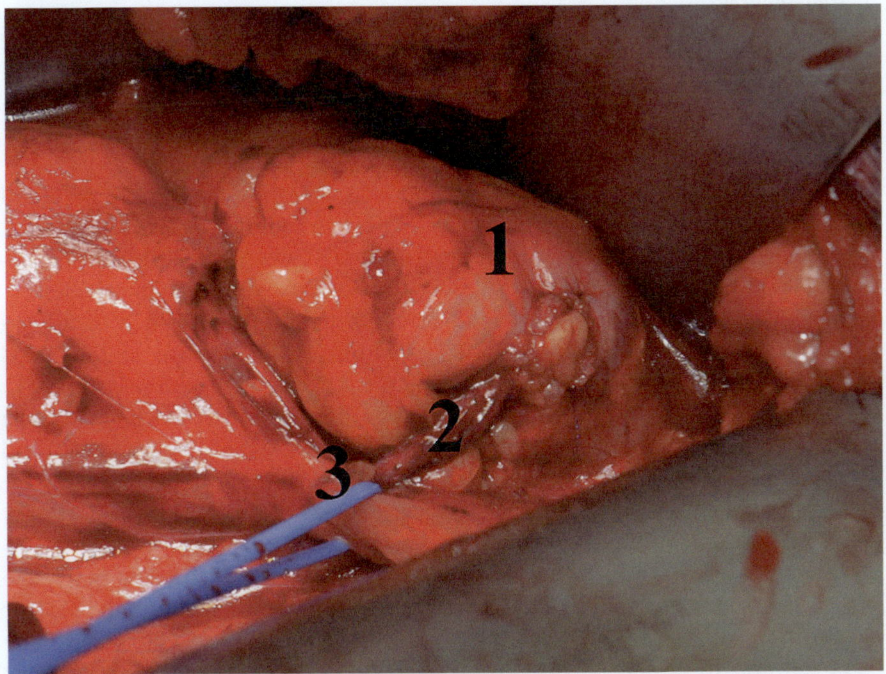

**Fig. 5.9** New uretero-bladder anastomosis. 1—Urinary bladder, 2—Ureter, 3—Spermatic cord

with a good blood supply, is not long enough, then this is an indication to mobilize the urinary bladder or the kidney, or both, in such a way that the new uretero-bladder anastomosis is not under tension. In case of the complete necrosis of the ureter, after excision of the necrosis, the end of the ureter or the renal pelvis can be anastomosed with the recipient's ureter by decompressing the anastomosis with a JJ catheter and if necessary a psoas hitch. Urinary bladder mobilization and fixation to the psoas muscle, called a psoas bladder hitch (PBH), is a surgical technique of first choice for the reconstruction of the ureter after partial resection. Psoas hitch ureteral reimplantation can be successfully used for bridging defects of the lower ureter up to 10 cm in length in difficult clinical situations [46] (Fig. 5.10).

### 5.6.2.3  The Most Common Causes of Pathological Changes Occurring During Organ Procurement, Benching and After Transplantation in the Ureter of the Transplanted Kidney [46–50]

1. Injury to the renal artery or small accessory renal artery running to the lower pole of the kidney during the kidney procurement or inspection before transplantation.
2. Procurement of the ureter with too little tissue and/or excision of too much perirenal tissue.
3. Acute kidney rejection.
4. Infection with BK virus (polio virus) or cytomegalovirus (CMV).
5. All kinds of injuries caused by the insertion of the bladder catheter.
6. All kinds of ureteral mechanical injuries due to wrong positioning of the JJ catheter including ureter or renal pelvis perforation during JJ insertion.
7. Compression of the ureter of the transplanted kidney from the outside (hematoma, urinoma, spermatic cord, inferior epigastric vessels, lymphocele).
8. In kidneys with multiple renal arteries, more frequent appearance of urinary fistulae was observed, most probably resulting from damage to the blood supply to the ureter during organ procurement and/or preparation.
9. Leaving the ureter too long may also lead to disorders of its blood supply (the longer the ureter, the greater the risk of its ischemia, especially at the end) and kinking; chronic ischemia can lead to ureteral strictures.
10. Donor age, recipient age, delayed kidney function [44–50].
11. Type of donor: DBD, DCD, living, euthanasia.
12. Other causes: slight rupture of the bladder during uncontrolled filling before the operation, sudden closure of the lumen of the catheter inserted into the bladder with clots or other material, prostatic hyperplasia, torsion of the ureter, swelling of the uretero-bladder anastomosis and finally a technical error, i.e. incorrect anastomosis, e.g. with peritoneum or with colon.

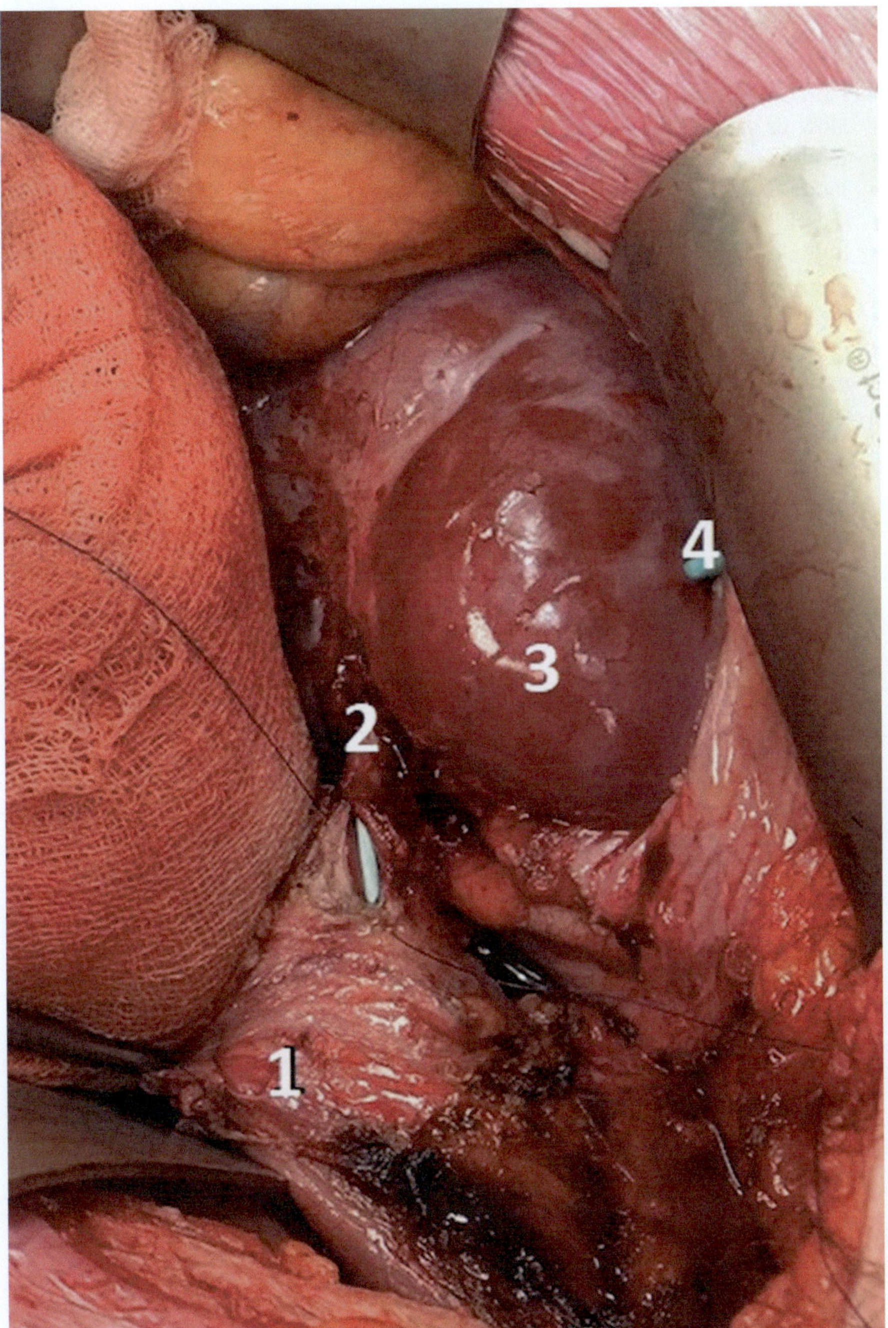

**Fig. 5.10** Ureter necrosis, almost to the renal pelvis. Excision of necrotic ureter. 1—Mobilized urinary bladder, 2—Rest of the ureter at the border of the renal pelvis long anastomosis between the rest of the ureter and urinary bladder, 3—Transplanted kidney, 4—A Nephrostomy catheter inserted through the skin into the kidney pelvis was inserted into the pelvis at the start of treatment together with the insertion of the bladder catheter

### 5.6.3  *Symptoms of Urinary Leakage*

- pain or discomfort in the area of the transplanted kidney and/or lower abdomen;
- slow or sudden deterioration of the graft function;
- reduction in urine production;
- increasing drain output;
- increase in blood creatinine levels;
- high levels of creatinine in drained fluid from the area of the transplanted kidney;
- swelling of the labia on the side of a transplanted kidney in women;
- in men, pain in the testicle on the side of a transplanted kidney;
- redness and pain in the wound
- sometimes leakage of urine through the wound (Fig. 5.11) [44–50].

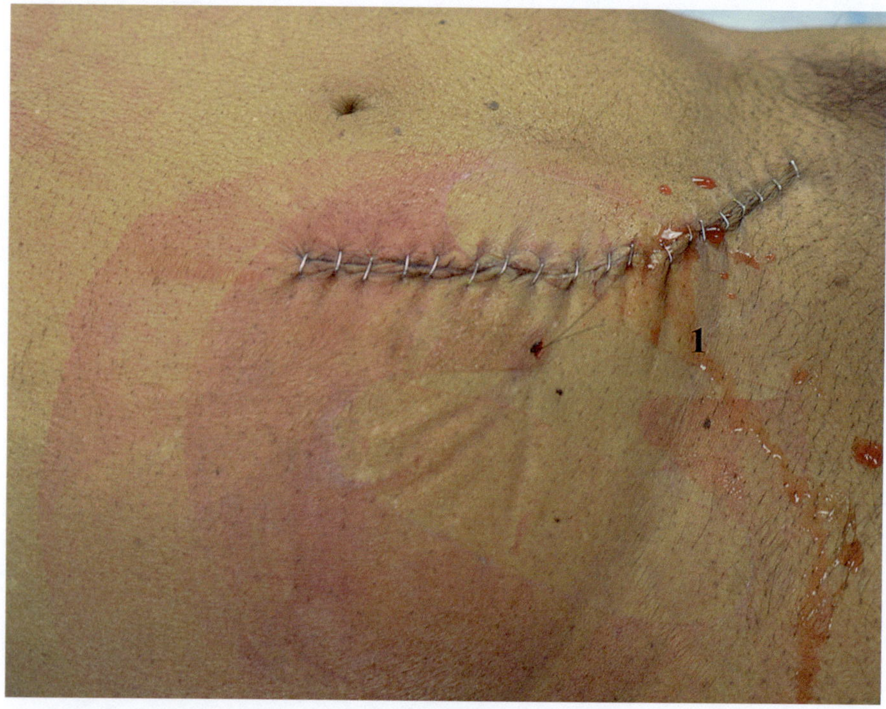


**Fig. 5.11**  1—Leakage of urine through the wound: urinary leakage

## 5.6.4  *Treatment of Urinary Leakage*

### 5.6.4.1  Conservative

Conservative treatment consists of maximal decompression of the whole system by drainage of the renal pelvis with an external drain (to reverse the flow of urine), drainage of urine around the kidney with a radiological drain, decompression of the bladder by means of a transurethral bladder catheter into the bladder, decompression of the anastomosis of the urinary bladder and the ureter by means of a JJ drain, which is inserted by the radiologist from above (via renal pyelum drain). The transurethral bladder catheter is changed if blocked and removed after two weeks in a high-risk case. A blocked JJ stent can be changed cystoscopically over a guide wire. If a JJ stent is not present, it is placed either as I mentioned above retrograde cystoscopically, which is technically challenging, or antegrade through a nephrostomy, which is more accessible and safer, although owing to lack of backpressure, fixation of a nephrostomy tube may be difficult, warranting the expertise of an experienced radiologist or endo-urologist. Conservative management is effective in approximately 60% of cases, especially for small, distal, late leaks [46–50]; Fig. 5.12.

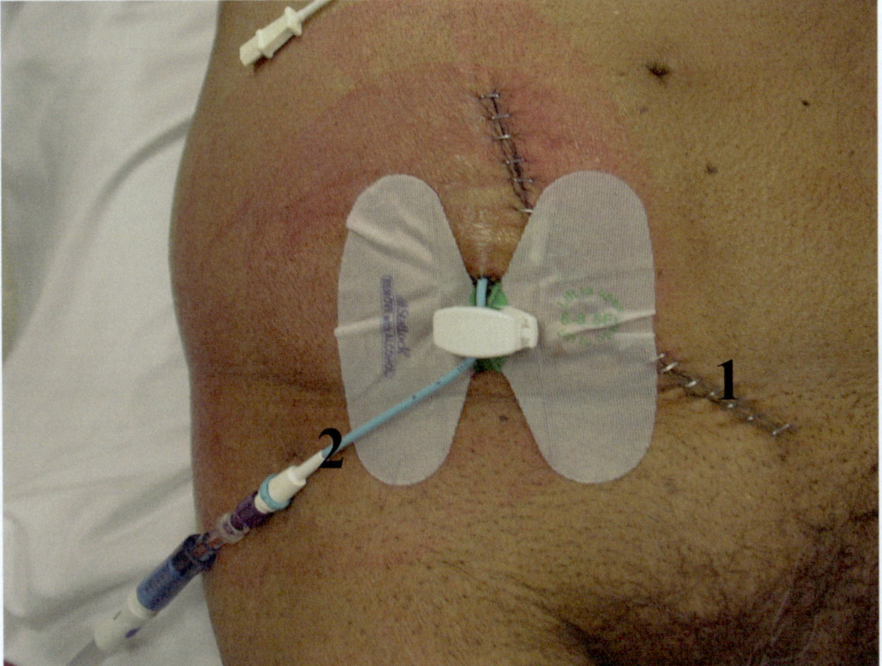

**Fig. 5.12** Drained by the interventional radiologist with a radiological drainage tube of the fluid that accumulated around the kidney after its transplantation. 1—Wound, 2—Radiological drain connected with urine bag

### 5.6.4.2 Surgical Treatment

Large-volume or proximal leaks which do not respond to conservative management require surgery with resection of the necrosed ureter and tension-free reimplantation of a well-vascularized ureter over a JJ stent, closure of a perforated bladder, or other procedures. In complex cases, a replacement for the ureter can be performed with the appendix, the wall of the bladder (Boari flap) or the small intestine. In some cases, after mobilizing the bladder, the vesicoureteral anastomosis remains under tension. Then the solution is to sew the posterior upper wall of the bladder to the greater lumbar muscle, executing the so-called psoas hitch maneuver or bladder psoas hitch technique. This will cause our ureter-urinary bladder anastomosis to be made without tension and to heal well [45–51].

## 5.7 Ureteral Stricture After Kidney Transplantation

### 5.7.1 Introduction

The incidence of urological complications, of which ureteral stricture is the most common, varies in contemporary reports from 0.9 to 34% [52–54]. The male gender of the recipient, delayed graft function and donor age were found to be significant risk factors for urological complications after kidney transplantation [52].

### 5.7.2 Causes of Obstruction or Complete Closure of the Ureter in a Renal Transplant Patient

Multiple risk factors have been investigated, of which patient gender, age, diabetes, marginal donor characteristics, anatomical graft variations, rejection and the BK virus appear to contribute most significantly [55–58].

**5.7.2.1. Non ureteral obstructions**, mostly caused by external compression of the ureter (lymphocele, urinoma, hematoma, urinary tract, seminal cord, uterine ligament, inflammatory appendix, and adhesions between the ureter, peritoneum and other retroperitoneal structures).

**5.7.2.2. Ureteral obstruction** and/or caused by pathological changes in its wall torsion, bending, twisting, stenosis due to chronic ischemia-fibrosis of the ureter; rejection of the transplant may lead to irreversible changes in the ureter, its acute or chronic ischemia, which may later cause constrictions, UTIs or even ureter necrosis.

**5.7.2.3. An inguinal hernia** incarcerated when the ureter of the transplanted kidney protrudes through the spot in the abdominal muscles. The bulging can be painful especially when the patient coughs, bends over or lifts a heavy object.

**5.7.2.4. Mucosa swelling ischemia**, fibrosis and stenosis of the ureter are quite often observed as a result of an infection by the BK virus.

**5.7.2.5. The occurrence of small thermo-injuries** of the ureter during kidney procurement and/or transplantation.

**5.7.2.6. Ureter and renal pelvis lumen:** urolithiasis; exfoliated epithelium of the renal pelvis, for example inflamed or necrotic renal papillae during interstitial kidney inflammation; fungi infection.

### 5.7.3   Symptoms

Usually an increase in creatinine concentration in the blood, a decrease in the amount of urine production, sometimes discomfort and even pain in the area of the transplanted kidney and in the abdomen; recurrent UTIs may occur [56–58].

### 5.7.4   Diagnostics

Ultrasonography, CT of the transplanted kidney (image of the inflated and dilated renal pelvis) and determination of the BK virus titer in the blood—in this case the most sensitive is the polymerase chain reaction test (PCR).

### 5.7.5   Treatment

**5.7.5.1. Hydronephrosis** [59, 60] initial treatment: The first step is to insert a urinary catheter into the bladder and the second step is to decompress the rest of the system, for example the renal pelvis. In the next step is the nephrostomy tube is inserted under local anesthesia and ultrasound control and guidance are performed. Steps: the catheter is inserted through the skin, abdominal wall, and kidney parenchyma into the renal pelvis of the transplanted kidney. The next step is to perform an antegrade pyelography and/or sometimes urethrography (administration of contrast through the drain located in the renal pelvis), in order to investigate and diagnose abnormalities, such as any kind of stricture of the ureter, ureter-urinary bladder anastomosis or uretero-pelvic junction. Retrograde pyelography is rarely used for diagnosis to visualize the ureter or ureters and renal pelvis. In more complicated cases, the patient must be diagnosed under general anaesthesia via a rigid cystoscope to cannulate the ureter with the special catheter. If the catheter is in a good position, inject then 5–8 ml of contrast to examine the ureter and renal pelvis.

**5.7.5.2. Radiological treatment**: consists of a regular widening of the site of the renal ureter stenosis using a specially designed balloon, with or without leaving a stent. The role of the stent is to prevent the formation of a new stenosis in the previously constricted and later dilated site of the ureter. In some centers a yttrium aluminum garnet (YAG) laser is used to treat the narrowing of the ureter of the transplanted kidney—in particular the resistant constrictions are cut from the middle with special tiny blades designed for this purpose; after the incision, the constrictions are usually slightly widened without or with a stent left in place [61, 62].

**5.7.5.3. Surgical treatment** [63]: depends on the place and extent of the ureter necrosis or stenosis or ureter-bladder anastomosis. It consists of:

(a) A new anastomosis of the ureter with the urinary bladder after the excision of the stenosis without the mobilization of the kidney and bladder.

(b) A ureter-urine bladder anastomosis with the excision of the narrowing section of the ureter with the mobilization of the urinary bladder. In some cases, the urinary bladder may be attached with a suture to the psoas muscle in order to avoid tension at the site of their anastomosis between the ureter and urinary bladder (psoas bladder hitch) (Fig. 5.10).

(c) After the excision of the stenotic or necrotic part of the ureter with the new anastomosis of a graft ureter or renal pelvis with the recipient's urinary bladder and/or own ureter; always use anastomosis always use the double J stent placement to decompress the anastomosis of the ureter or pelvis of the transplanted kidney with the urinary bladder of the kidney recipient.

(d) The new anastomosis of the ureter or renal pelvis with the bladder using a Boari flap, which is taken from the anterior wall of the bladder, sutured around the JJ catheter with urinary bladder mobilization and a psoas bladder hitch to relieve the anastomosis.

(e) A rarely used technique is the anastomosis of a short ureter with the bladder using a small intestine or appendix insertion in between.

(f) Bricker ileal conduit for urinary diversion named after its inventor, Eugene M. Bricker, who invented it in 1940. Uretero-enteric anastomosis is made so that after separating a piece of small bowel from the ileum (approx. 25 cm). The piece of ileum is closed loosely at one end, and the other end is led out through a previously made hole in the abdominal wall. Bricker procedure. The Bricker operation is performed when a urinary bladder ureter anastomosis is not advisable now because of infection or is not possible for example in case of bladder excision.

(g) Ileal ureter replacement: this is end-to-end anastomosis between the rest of the ureter and the urinary bladder. Despite the difficult and risky process of the ileal ureter, the procedure can be carried out effectively and safely by skilled surgeons after careful patient selection.

### 5.7.6   An Unusual Patient as an Example of Ureteral Stenosis (Author's Own Experience) [64]

I have decided to describe here an interesting and very difficult and seldom case of ureter stenosis, which I encountered during my medical career. I hope that you will learn a lot from this case and that this knowledge will help you decide how to treat the narrowing of your transplanted kidney ureter.

A 22-year-old man was admitted to the hospital for a third transplant due to end-stage renal failure. His medical history included premature birth with perinatal asphyxia, spastic tetraplegia, mild mental retardation and severe vertebral column scoliosis (Fig. 5.13). He developed end-stage renal failure by the perinatal asphyxia and dysplasia of the kidneys and a neuropathic bladder by tetraplegia. As a result of continuous infectious diseases, he received a nephrectomy of both kidneys, without the removal of both ureters. In 2001, he started on peritoneal dialysis, which was replaced by hemodialysis one year later. In 2006 and 2008, he received renal transplants in the right and the left iliac fossa, which were both rejected but not

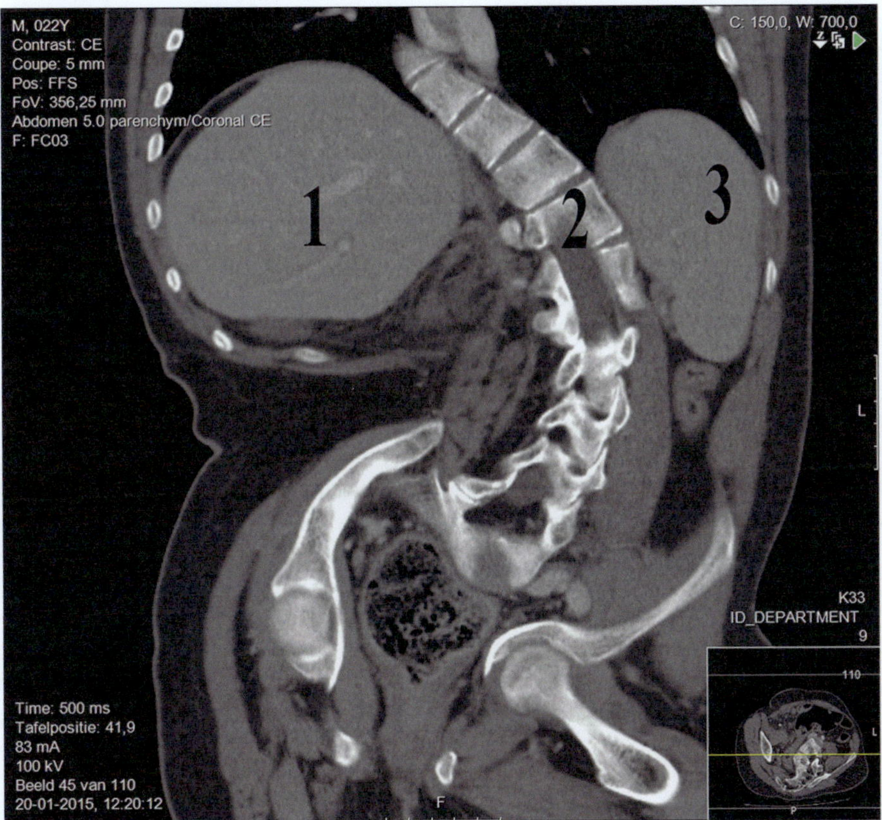


**Fig. 5.13** Computed thomography revealed severe vertebral column scoliosis. 1—Liver, 2—Spine, 3—Spleen

removed. The patient returned to hemodialysis, but preferred to receive a third transplant. In November 2014, the patient received a renal transplant from a donor after cardiac death, which had an acceptable mismatch of panel reactive antibody of 99%, mismatch 0-1-0 (Cytomegalovirus test negative, Epstein-Barr virus test negative). The donor's left kidney was placed high at the right side of the recipient's abdominal cavity because the left side was not feasible due to deterioration of the kyphosis through aging. The old right transplant incision was extended to the upper side of the abdomen. This, however, was done using an intraperitoneal approach because the retroperitoneal approach had been impossible due to severe adhesions after peritoneal dialysis and the first transplant. In addition, the ureter was placed partially intra- and retroperitoneally due to these adhesions. The distal part was anastomosed with the urinary bladder by means of the Lich-Gregoir technique, and a ureteral stent (J stent) was placed. The vascular anastomoses of the kidney were done end to side to the IVC and in the lower part of the abdominal aorta (Fig. 5.14). Because the kidney was placed high in the abdominal cavity, the distance from the kidney to the urinary bladder was longer than average. However, after kidney reperfusion, vascularization of the distal ureter was good without any signs of insufficient blood supply.

Immediately after surgery the kidney functioned properly. However, two weeks later, the patient developed increasing abdominal pain at the side of the renal transplant. Additional investigations revealed a mild to moderate hydronephrosis with stenosis of the distal ureter. The hydronephrosis was treated by an insertion nephrostomy, dilatation of the ureteral stricture and retrograde placement of a JJ stent (Figs. 5.15, 5.16, 5.17). Because of recurrent dilation of the collecting system after the removal of the nephrostomy drain and stent, a reconstruction of the ureteric stenosis using the native ureter was considered. A uretero-cystoscopy measurement was performed to assess the length and integrity of the native ureters by the insertion of a catheter from the urinary bladder. This measurement revealed 11-cm right and 25-cm left native ureter lengths. On the basis of these results, it was agreed to anastomose the transplanted ureter with the left (contra-lateral) native ureter. A median laparotomy was performed. The sigmoid and the descending colon were mobilized and freed from the retroperitoneum. The whole longer portion of the left native ureter was mobilized from the urinary bladder up to the colon's splenic flexure. The mobilized portion of the left native ureter was vital and well vascularized (Fig. 5.18). During the next step, the freed portion of the left ureter was tunneled under the sigmoid close to the proximal part of the ureter of the transplanted kidney. The ureter of the transplanted kidney was dissected from the retroperitoneum up to the stenosis, and was subsequently ligated and cut close to the renal pelvis of the transplanted kidney and cut. An end-to-end anastomosis was made between the ureter of the transplanted kidney and the left remaining native ureter using a polydioxanone 4/0 suture and placement of a J stent (Fig. 5.19). The anastomosis was tested with sterile 0.9% NaCl for leakage and good passage into the urinary bladder. The test revealed no leakage and good passage to the urinary

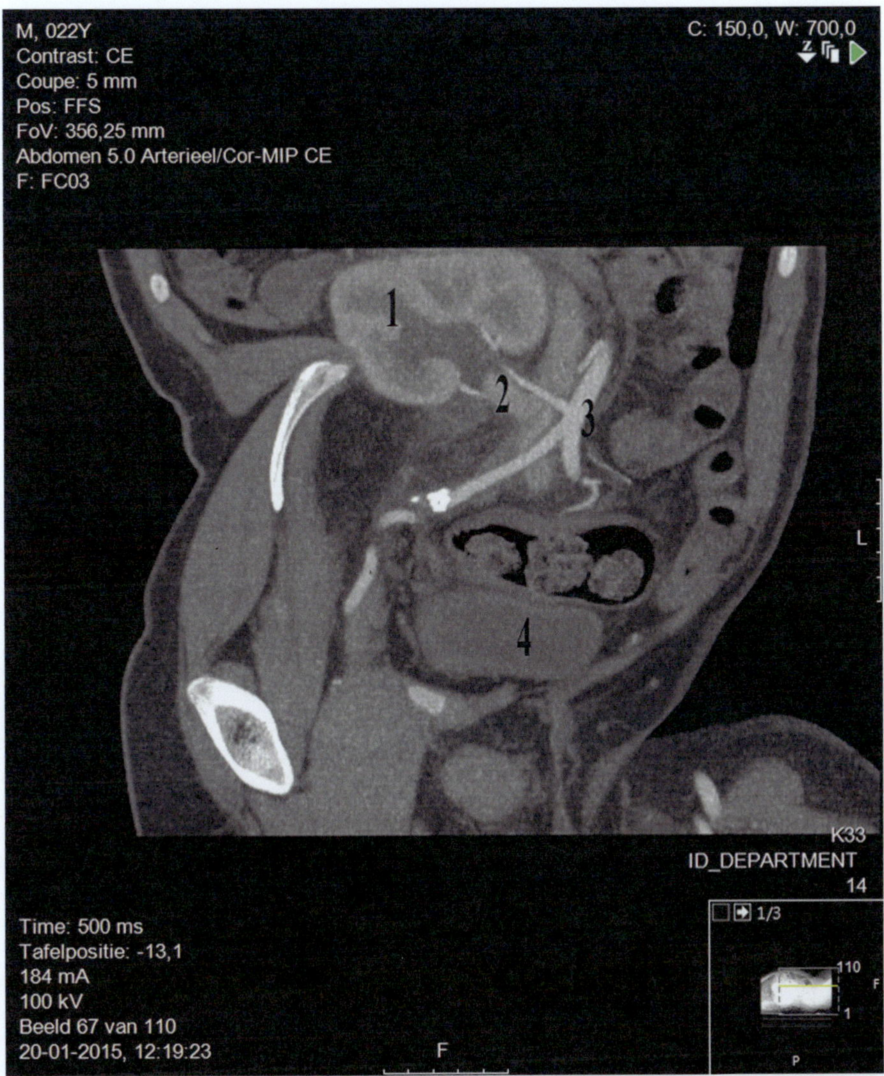

**Fig. 5.14** Computed tomography performed to assess the patency of vascular anastomoses. 1—Transplanted kidney located under the liver, 2—Renal vein, 3—Aorta: normal anastomosis with the renal artery visible. The anastomosis is patent and non-constricted, 4—Urinary bladder

bladder. The peritoneal cavity was drained with one drain placed close to the ureter-ureter anastomosis, and the abdomen was closed. The postoperative course was without severe complications. Two days later, antegrade pyelography revealed good passage to the urine bladder (Fig. 5.20). The peritoneal drain was successfully removed after 8 days, the J stent after 14 days, and the nephrostomy drain after

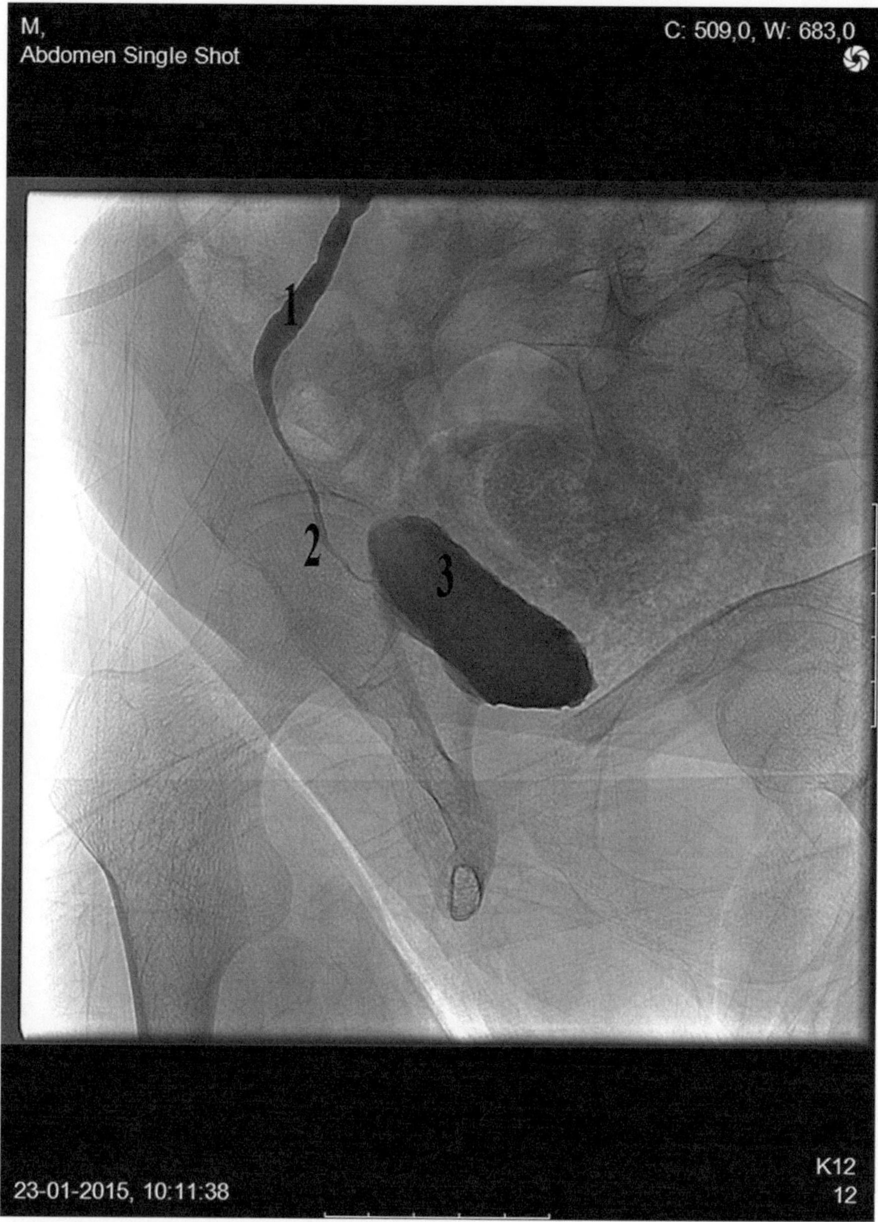


**Fig. 5.15** Anterograde uretero-cystography imaging: contrast applied to the drain located in the renal pelvis of the transplanted kidney. The above examination revealed stenosis of the distal ureter of a transplanted kidney. 1—Normal ureter, 2—Stenosis of the distal ureter, 3—Urinary bladder

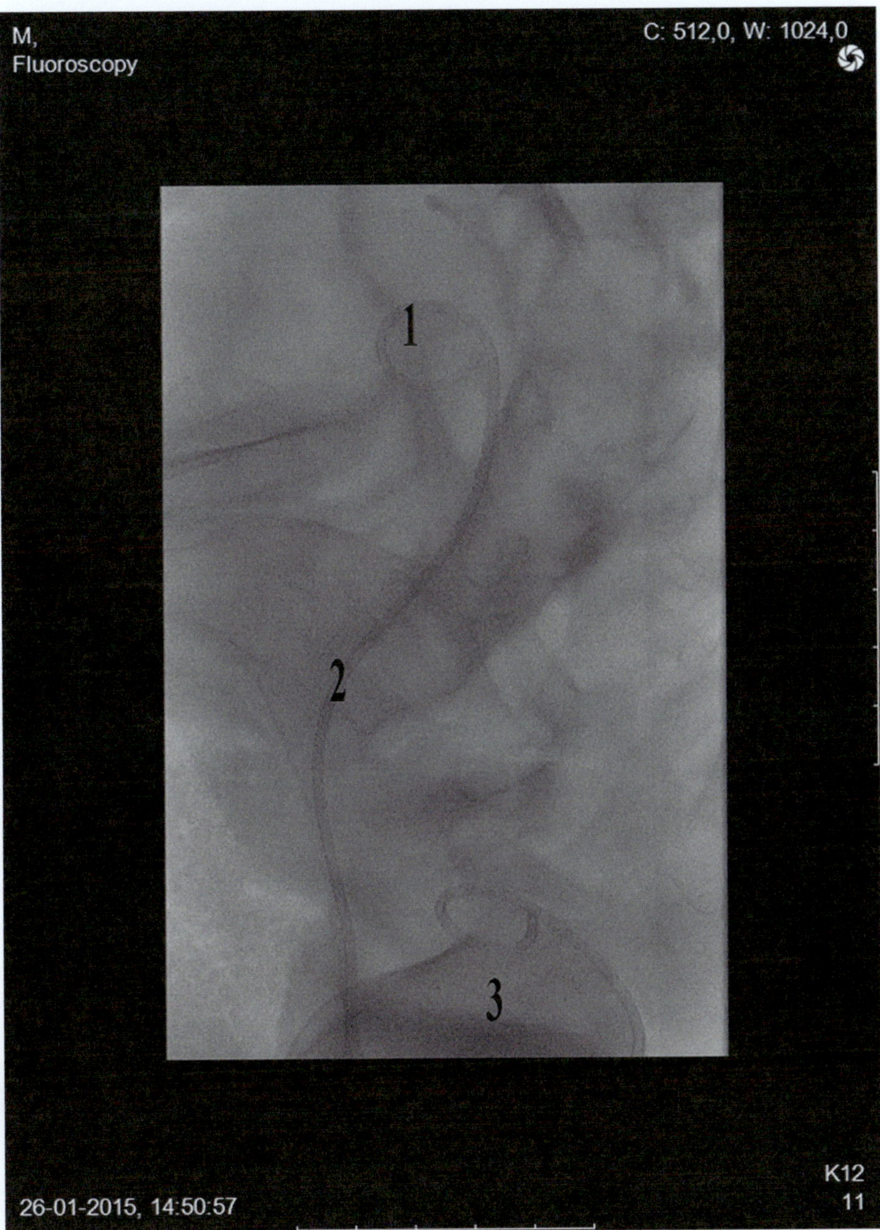

Fig. 5.16 Anterograde uretero-cystography: contrast applied to the drain located in the pelvis of the transplanted kidney. 1—Renal pelvis transplanted with a correctly positioned JJ catheter, 2—Ureter, 3—Urinary bladder with the other end of the JJ catheter placed in it. Normal outflow of urine from the renal pelvis into the urinary bladder

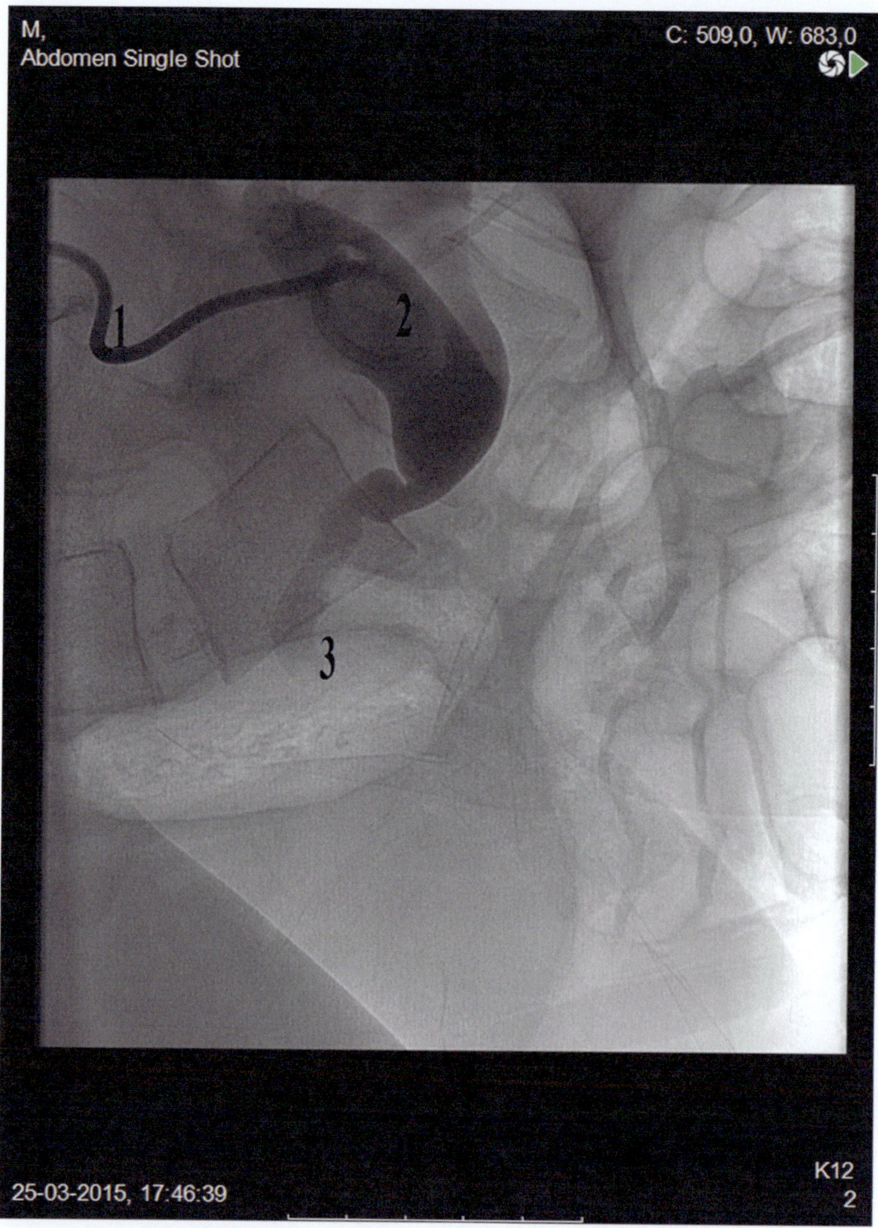


**Fig. 5.17** Anterograde uretero-cystography: contrast applied to the drain located in the pelvis of the transplanted kidney. Complete stop of contrast flow to the bladder, critical stenosis, even closure of the distal ureter. 1—Percutaneous radiological catheter inserted into the renal pelvis of the transplanted kidney, 2—Renal pelvis, 3—Beginning of ureter of the transplanted kidney

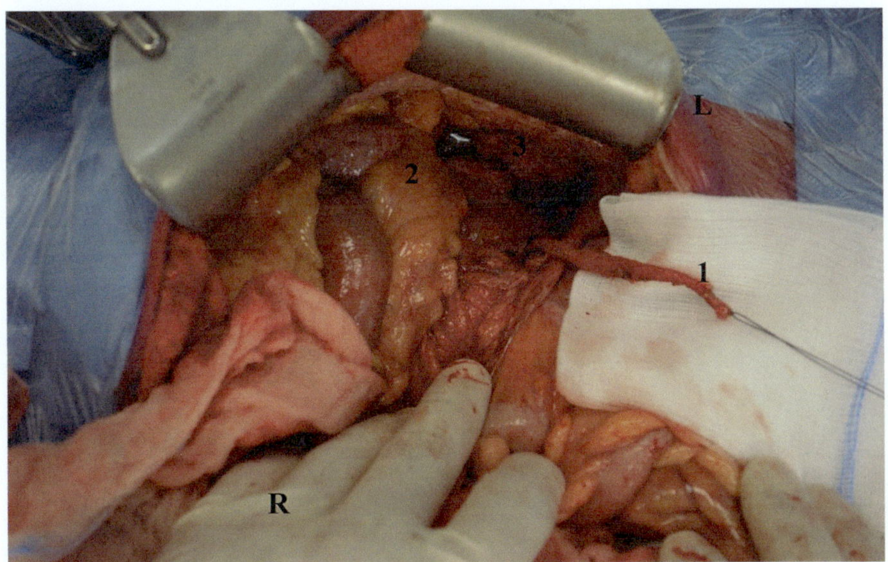

**Fig. 5.18**  1—The dissected stump of own left ureter from extraperitoneal space (we remember that the left kidney was removed a long time ago), 2—Descending colon, 3—Left side of the extraperitoneal space, R—Right side, L—Left side

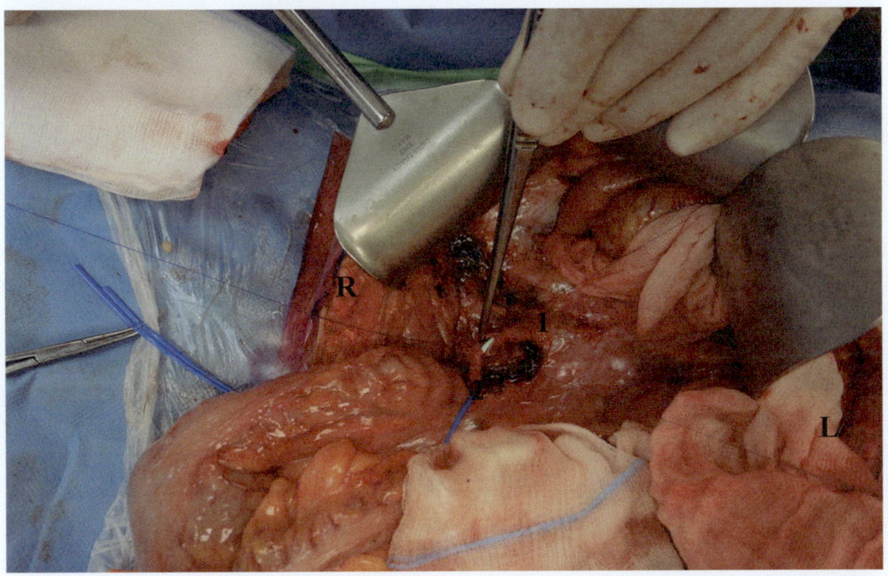

**Fig. 5.19**  1—The rest of the healthy ureter of the transplanted kidney below the liver, 2—Dissected left own ureter replaced retroperitoneally to the right side close to the renal pelvis of the transplanted kidney end-to-end anastomosis on the JJ catheter brought inside and positioned from the renal pelvis to the urinary bladder, R—Right side of the kidney recipient, L—Left side of the kidney recipient

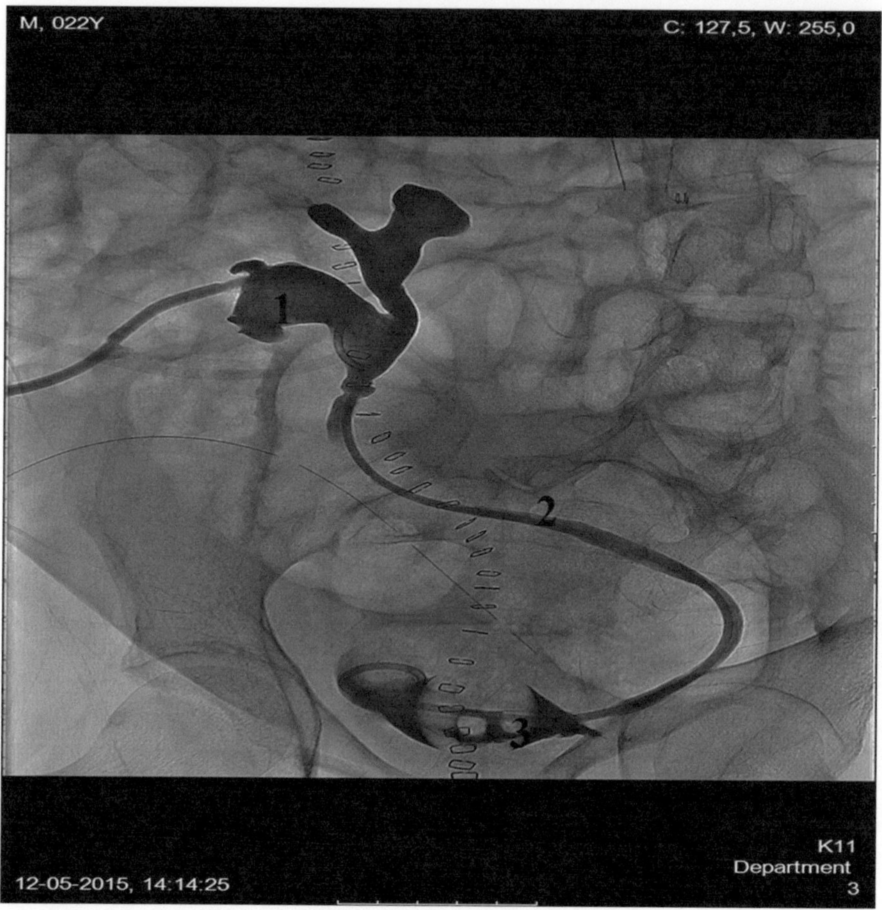


**Fig. 5.20** Anterograde uretero-cystography: contrast applied into the drain located in the pelvis of the transplanted kidney. Correct passage of contrast to the bladder. 1—Renal pelvis, 2—Patient's own ureter with a JJ catheter inserted into its lumen, 3—Urinary bladder

25 days. On day 29, the patient was discharged from the hospital. Four months after the transplantation the ultrasonography revealed a normal kidney graft (Fig. 5.21). After 13 months, the third transplanted kidney developed a chronic rejection; despite medical treatment, this resulted in a graftectomy.

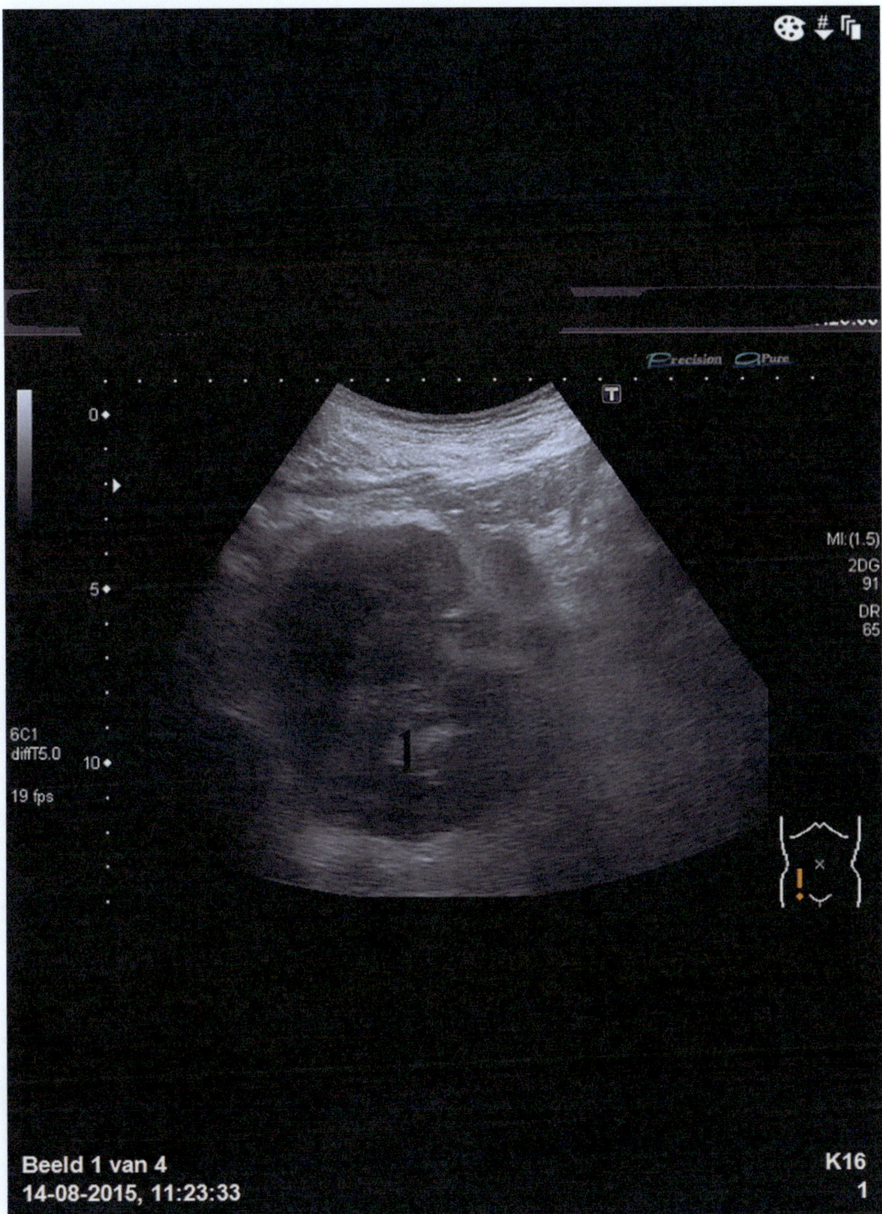

**Fig. 5.21** Normal ultrasonography of the transplanted kidney after reconstruction: four months after ureter reconstruction. 1—Normal outline of the transplanted kidney and its renal calyces

### 5.7.6.1   Discussion

In cases unsuitable for heterotopic renal transplant, an orthotopic renal transplant is worth considering. Two recent studies have recommended this technique for patients with advanced atherosclerosis disease of the iliac arteries, bilaterally retained iliac fossae from previous kidney transplants, pelvic malformations, venous thrombosis, and obesity [65, 66]. The studies additionally described the orthotopic technique as challenging, with a slightly higher complication rate. Nevertheless, the present case reveals that an almost orthotopic position between the right common iliac artery and the patient's liver is feasible.

The complication rate of ureteric stenosis after orthotopic transplant is slightly higher than the rate of ureteric stenosis in heterotopic renal transplants.

It remains arguable whether this is caused by poor vascularization due to an above-average length of the transplanted ureter. Two retrospective studies stated that the length of the transplanted ureter does not affect postoperative urologic complications, but these studies do not mention a ureter length exceeding 12 cm [67–69].

Most common ureter reconstruction methods are not feasible in patients with an extensive medical history. An anastomosis to the native ureter can be an appropriate method. However, Pike and associates stated that this method was not appropriate as the dissection of the native ureter is often difficult in the presence of a transplanted kidney and the integrity of a native ureter is mostly not known or investigated [69]. Here, however, we showed that the assessment of the integrity of the ureters can be done properly by urologists using a urethra cystoscopy during the preoperative period. Moreover, this method provides the opportunity to directly measure the length of the rest of the ureter and to place into the lumen of the ureter one of the stents to make it easier to find the ureter during the operation.

Use of the contralateral native ureter in graft ureter reconstruction has, to the authors' knowledge, only been described in detail in the study of Orlando and associates [70]. Their technique entailed retroperitoneoscopic preparation of the native ureter contralateral to the renal graft, followed by an open anastomosis to the transplant ureter through the Retzius space. Retroperitoneoscopic preparation allows for surgery with high precision; however, in our case, an open approach with tunneling under the sigmoid was preferred because of the patient's complex anatomy.

In conclusion, renal transplant with a high abdominal position is an appropriate alternative in cases unsuitable for heterotopic transplant, even in patients with severe comorbidities. In addition, ureter reconstruction by use of the native ureter contralateral to the graft through tunneling under the sigmoid is a recommended and safe surgical approach for a ureteric stricture when treatments with stenting and primary surgical reparation are not feasible.

### Warning!

For the best possible decompression of the renal pelvic-ureter-urinary bladder system, all new urethral anastomoses should be decompressed with a JJ catheter.

**Warning!**
Conservative treatment should be applied in case of a polyomavirus (BK) infection. This consists of percutaneous drainage of the transplanted kidney's renal pelvis and stopping the administration of tacrolimus and mycophenolate mofetil (MMF). Tacrolimus or MMF should be substituted with cyclosporine, or everolimus, and/or an antiviral treatment could be started by an intravenous administration of one of the antiviral drugs. Modest et al. reported beneficial effects of drugs, such as cidofovir, leflunomide, IV immunoglobulin (IVIG) and fluoroquinolone therapy. Under the influence of immunosuppressive drugs, the BK virus multiplies in the transplanted kidney and is responsible for BK nephropathy, which, if not treated in time, often causes the loss of the transplanted kidney. The BK virus is also responsible for swelling and narrowing of the ureter, and hemorrhagic bladder inflammation [71]. When the infection with the BK virus has been successfully eradicated, a descending pyelography must be made through the drain inserted percutaneously into the pelvis. If this examination finds no narrowing of the ureter, no impaired passage of contrast to the urinary bladder and the absence of the virus in the blood, the patient is to be considered healed. If the stenosis persists, the patient should be treated with radiological or surgical treatment. A patient should never be operated on during the period of active infection with the BK virus, but only after it has been completely eliminated from the blood which is confirmed by very thorough blood and urine tests. There are no specific antiviral agents that are available for the treatment of BKV infection. Multiple agents have been evaluated for its treatment with mixed results in human studies. Cell-based therapies have shown some encouraging results in limited studies [72].

## 5.8   Lymphocele

### 5.8.1   Introduction

Lymphocele—a fluid reservoir, or lymph accumulation or, as some people call it, a lymphatic cyst—is one of the complications after a kidney transplant. The frequency of this complication varies from 0.6 to 33.9% [73, 74]. Most lymphocele appear between the sixth to twelfth week after the transplant. In most cases it is less than 3 cm, does not give clinical symptoms and is absorbed spontaneously in the extraperitoneal space, and therefore does not require any treatment. If it starts to show symptoms, as any reservoir of fluid, a difference must be made between a urinoma (urine leakage) and an abscess. The creatinine, urea and potassium concentrations in the lymphocele are the same as those in the blood serum, in contrast to the urinary tract, where the creatinine and urea concentrations are much higher than their serum concentrations; only the sodium concentrations are lower. The cause of lymphocele formation is not exactly known. It is believed that it is caused by a build-up of lymph, which comes from the lymphatic vessels which have been damaged during the surgery running around the recipient's iliac vessels and open lymphatic vessel which are located in the kidney hilum and are not recognized and ligated during the kidney inspection. In order to reduce the incidence of lymphocele, it is necessary to prepare the recipient's iliac vessels very gently and to ligate each of the lymphatic vessels precisely in the kidney hilum. All articles on lymphocele prevention emphasize the special importance of a very careful and gentle preparation of the iliac vessels with special attention to lymphatic vessel ligation in the case of cutting [75–79].

## 5.8.2   Incidence, Risk Factors, Prevention

The incidence of lymphocele in patients in whom the kidney's vessels have been connected with external iliac vessels was four times higher than in patients in whom the kidney's vessels have been anastomosed with the common iliac vessels. This is due to a much smaller range of surgical injury of the lymphatic vessels during the kidney transplantation with renal vessel anastomosis to the common iliac vessels [79].

The factors that favor the formation of lymphocele after the operation include: high doses of steroids, sirolimus, everolimus, mycophenolic acid derivatives, heparin, prior radiotherapy, hypoalbuminemia, repeated transplants, autosomal dominant polycystic disease and diuretics.

Postoperative lymphocele risk factors include: obesity, diabetes, advanced age of the organ recipient, long warm ischemia time, delayed kidney graft function, frequent episodes of rejection and acute cellular rejection.

Lymphocele prevention consists of a gentle preparation of the iliac vessels, the ligation of the lymphatic vessels which lie along and around the iliac vessels, the ligation of the lymphatic vessels which lie in the kidney hilum during the back table and the performance of vascular anastomoses with the common iliac vessels [73–80].

## 5.8.3   Symptoms

In most cases, when it the lymphocele small, it gives no symptoms. If it is enlarged or large, you can feel that the coating lift or a tumor by palpation around the transplanted kidney. The lymphocele may press on the kidney, ureter, kidney vessels, bladder and hip vessels, which in turn may manifest in worsening kidney function, increased creatinine concentration, hypertension, lower limb lymphatic oedema on the kidney transplant side, thrombotic vein inflammation, and in case of infection: fever, pain, urinary retention, UTI and lymphatic fistula.

## 5.8.4  *Diagnostics*

Ultrasonography; other methods, for example, CT or MRI are less important.


## 5.8.5  *Treatment*

External drainage (fine needle aspiration) has an efficacy of 50% and a recurrence rate of 80%; there is a high infection rate [80, 81].

Percutaneous aspiration and external drainage combined with sclerotherapy (alcohol, iodine solution [81], tetracycline, fibrin glue, bleomycin) are the most popular treatments of lymphoceles. As a rule it takes 20–30 days to stop the lymph leakage, though it fails in 10–15% of cases. The lymphocele recurrence after sclerotherapy remains high at around 30–60% [70, 73–81].


### 5.8.5.1  Drainage with the Use of a Tenckhoff Catheter [82]

Occasionally, lymphoceles recur after renal transplantation in relatively inaccessible pelvic locations, usually in the setting of a transversely oriented allograft that separates the lymphocele from the peritoneal cavity. Such lymphoceles do not share a common wall with the peritoneal cavity and, therefore, are not manageable by conventional open surgical or laparoscopic drainage techniques. These use an internalized Tenckhoff catheter to drain the recurrent lymphocele into the peritoneal cavity. After local anesthesia and after skin incision, one end of the catheter is introduced into the lymphocele, and from the second incision the other end of the catheter is carried under the skin and introduced into the peritoneal cavity. The authors of this idea have not observed a single relapse of lymphocele during the year.


### 5.8.5.2  Laparoscopic Fenestration [76]

The laparoscopic excision of a hole in the peritoneum allows us to direct the lymphocyte content into the abdominal cavity. The inconvenience of this method is the possibility of damaging the ureter, kidney parenchyma, renal or iliac vessels during surgery. The contraindications for this type of surgery are the numerous abdominal surgeries, the expected large number of adhesions, very difficult access (for example access to the fluid collection localized on the right or left side of the vessels' anastomoses), injury to the adjacent structure requiring repair and a pre-existing hernia.

### 5.8.5.3   Surgical Fenestration

A method very similar to the previous one. In the surgical treatment of lymphocele, as a rule, the incision is carried out through a permanent scar in order to access and drain the reservoir of accumulated lymph. This is the method of choice in the case of an expected large number of incisions after abdominal surgery, numerous lymphoceles or lymphocele consisting of many chambers. It is an invasive method, with a higher risk of infection and associated with a longer stay in hospital [76].

Lymphocele is one of the most common complications after kidney transplantation. It is usually asymptomatic, but can cause pressure on the kidney transplant, ureter, bladder and adjacent vessels with deterioration of graft function, ipsilateral leg edema and external iliac vein thrombosis. A very interesting observation is that in the symptomatic lymphocele requiring treatment (LRT), acute rejection episodes (ARE) and delayed graft function (DGF) were more frequent. ARE and age were independent risk factors for the LRT in the multivariate analysis [83].

### 5.8.5.4   Personal Experience of the Author

Lymphocele is very rare in our population—on average out of 170 transplantations (taking into account the population of our patients) five to ten years ago we met three to four cases per year. Maybe it is because most of the kidneys at that time were transplanted to the common iliac vessels, and each kidney was very carefully prepared before the transplantation, including the ligation of the lymphatic vessels in the renal hilum. Lymphatic vessels running along and around the veins and arteries are carefully tied and/or closed with an Argon Beamer or coagulation during the preparation of the iliac vessels. In the case of a simple lymphocele, in our clinic the first stage of treatment consists of its drainage by means of a drain inserted percutaneously into the lymphocele. Then we apply all the above described treatment methods. The only difference is that during the laparoscopic fenestration of the lymphocele after aspiration, we administer into the lymphocele sterile methylene blue dissolved in a solution of physiological saline via the drain. Filling up the lymphocele with an additional amount of methylene blue colored fluid makes it easier to find from the abdominal cavity and shortens the operation considerably. During the operation, the connections with the abdomen consist of the hole or holes which are made by the surgeon in the peritoneum wall to connect the lymphoceles with the abdomen. Into the place where the lymphocele is located, we always put one or two thick surgical drains with the side holes of each drain located in the lymphocele and preritoneal cavity and lead them through the lymphocele and abdominal wall outside the abdominal cavity. The drain or drains are removed after 10–14 days depending on their "production" and the results of the radiological examination (echo or CT)—there should be no fluid collection and no lymphocele in the transplanted kidney area.

## 5.9  Wound Infection in Renal Transplant Patients

### 5.9.1  Introduction

Transplant wound infection (1.8 to 56%) deserves particular attention because of the special patient conditions, such as: the uremic state at the time of surgery and sometimes in the immediate post-transplant period (acute tubular necrosis, delayed graft function), diabetes (incidence of infection is twice as high as in non-diabetic patients), acute graft rejection, recipient's age (a higher incidence in the third and fourth decades), nutritional status, smoking, obesity (BMI more than 30–35), colonization with microorganisms, length of pre- and postoperative stay, graft infection (small renal and perinephric abscesses $\leq 5$ cm may be treated with antibiotics alone, targeting enterobacteriaceae and enterococci, but larger abscesses usually require drainage), immunosuppression, cadaver kidney or living-related (recipient of cadaver kidney has a three times greater chance of infecting the wound) [84–89].

The factors contributing to wound infection in patients after kidney transplantation are: uremia, immunosuppression and hemodialysis.

The main complications resulting in wound infection are: septicemia, mycotic aneurysm of the abdominal aorta or iliac or renal arterial vessels as a complication from the deep wound infection, and graftectomy due to kidney infections (peri- and intra-nephric infections) [84–89].

Wound infection is defined by the US Centre for Disease Control and Prevention (CDC) as a surgical site infection (SSI). This is further defined as [85, 86]:

A. Superficial incisional SSI—infection involves only skin and subcutaneous tissue of incision.
B. Deep incisional SSI—infection involves deep tissues, such as facial and muscle layers.
C. Organ/space SSI—infection involves any part of the anatomy in organs and spaces other than the incision, which was opened or manipulated during the operation.

SSI is a common postoperative complication that leads to significant morbidity, increased antibiotic use and length of hospital stay, additional costs, and a decline in patients "quality of life" [89, 90].

### 5.9.2  Signs and Symptoms of Wound Infection

A. Primary: rubor—erythema, dolor—pain, calor—warmth, edema—swelling, fever.
B. Secondary: delayed healing, hyper granulation, increased odor and wound purulence, production.

### 5.9.2.1   Superficial Incisional SSI Wound Infection: Treatment [84–90]

An infected wound requires intensive treatment such as: opening, taking bacteriological specimen, regular irrigation, removal of necrotic tissue and frequent dressing changes. The use of an antibiotic in this case is debatable and depends on the speed of improvement in the appearance of the wound, the patient's condition and the culture result. We always leave the decision to administer antibiotics to the infectious disease specialist. In mild forms of infection antibiotic therapy is not always advisable.

### 5.9.2.2   Deep Incisional SSI Wound Infection: Treatment [84–90]

Infection of a deep wound involves deeper structures of the surgical wound, which include the fascia and muscles of the abdominal wall. In addition to the above-mentioned symptoms, infection usually leads to a sudden rupture of the abdominal muscle fascia and the edges of the infected wound split apart. In most cases, the patient must be treated surgically. Under general anesthesia, the wound is thoroughly cleaned of necrotic tissues, infected fluid collections and abscesses. A culture or several cultures should be taken (also necrotic tissues are cultured), the wound should be wide opened, flushed and very well drained. We should remember that in the case of a wound infection in a patient after transplantation, the material delivered to the Bacteriology Department must be analyzed by sowing it on the appropriate nutrient not only to confirm the presence of bacteria but also fungi. Changing the dressings and irrigating the wound must be done at least twice a day. The use of broad-spectrum antibiotics should always be discussed with an infection disease specialist.

In only a small percentage of cases, a single deep abscess can be treated with percutaneous drainage by an interventional radiologist who introduces a drain into the abscess cavity under ultrasound or computed tomography guidance. We control the progress of abscess drainage by recording the "production" of the drained fluid collection once a day and measuring the temperature at least twice a day. In the event of a sudden increase in temperature, immediately check the patency and position of the drain. If the drain no longer removes fluid collection secretions, ultrasound or computerized tomography should be performed prior to removal to confirm complete drainage of the abscess cavity. In case of an incomplete abscess drainage, the position of the drain should be replaced or repositioned using ultrasound or, if necessary, computed tomography. If the drain is or was not positioned correctly, it should be moved and placed in the center of the abscess or fluid content. In some cases, a second abscess drain may be requested to better drain it and/or to create a continuous irrigation system. In the case of a blocked drain or its incorrect position, you can try to flush it or replace it with a new, thicker drain.

Let us not forget about fixing the drain well, so that it does not fall or slip out of the abscess cavity, which may be responsible for the lack of drainage and increased temperature. Multi-chambered abscesses, difficult to drain even under ultrasound and/or computed tomography control, should be surgically drained by opening them wide, culturing for the presence of bacteria, rinsing and ensuring a perfect drainage of the wound after surgery.

If possible, reduce the dose of immunosuppressive drugs taken by the patient or replace them with immunosuppressive drugs that prevent the recipient from fighting the infection as little as possible.

In both cases, the use of negative pressure therapy can bring about good results and speed up the wound healing. The therapeutic benefits of this method are: removal of necrotic tissue, inhibition of bacterial growth, reduction of edema, improvement of blood flow through the wound area and promotion of granulation tissue production.

Various types of special sterile foam dressings are used for this therapy, selected according to the size and depth of the wound and the composition of the wound secretion [91]. The suction pressure of the suction device is programmed depending on the type of wound, type of discharge and the patient's pain tolerance.

In both cases, the use of vacuum therapy can bring good results and accelerate the healing of the wound [92]. The therapeutic benefits of this method are: removal of necrotic tissues, inhibition of bacterial growth, reduction of swelling, improvement of blood flow through the wound area and stimulation of granulation production, less pain, improvement of breathing ability and reduction of respiratory insufficiencies.

## 5.10   Infection or Recurrent Infection of the Urinary Tract After Kidney Transplantation Due to Urethra-Bladder Anastomosis Decompression with a JJ Catheter

As I have already mentioned, kidney transplant patients who have had a JJ catheter inserted after transplantation or surgical reintervention are much more likely to have single or chronic UTIs. In general, any UTI after kidney transplantation should be treated with a targeted antibiotic, selected according to the result of the urine culture. Patients with prostate hypertrophy should be treated by inserting a bladder catheter and administering an antibiotic and urological consultation. A double J stent inserted after kidney transplantation in many cases does not prevent complications, but reduces the need for reoperation. In addition, the use of a double J stent is not always associated with increased urinary tract infections in renal transplant recipients [93].

In the case of the failure of antibiotic treatment of UTIs in patients with a JJ catheter, the only right decision is to remove the catheter and continue the antibiotic treatment.

## 5.11   Wound Dehiscence

### 5.11.1   Introduction

Surgical incisions are entry sites sutured or held together by a margin approximation dressing or device after an operative procedure. Dehisced surgical wounds are defined by the separation of the incision line prior to complete healing resulting in an open wound. The most common complications for surgical wounds are infection and dehiscence.

### 5.11.2   Symptoms of Dehisced Surgical Wounds

A.  Partial dehiscence of a surgical wound will present as superficial layers or a small amount of tissue layers being reopened.
B.  Complete dehiscence, however, will present as all layers being separated with underlying tissue and organs being exposed and sometimes protruding through the wound opening.
C.  Other symptoms of dehiscence include visibly broken sutures before the wound has healed completely, as well as renewed pain, bleeding and drainage from the surgical wound site [94, 95].

### 5.11.3   Risk Factors of Dehisced Surgical Wounds

Dehiscence can also be caused by infections or poor wound healing. Common risk factors for abnormal healing include the presence of necrotic tissue, infection, ischemia, smoking, diabetes, malnutrition, glucocorticoid use, and patients undergoing immune-, chemo- or radiotherapy [96].

### 5.11.4   Treatment of Dehisced Surgical Wounds

For a dehisced wound, a patient should return for medical care immediately. This may include debridement, antibiotic therapy and resuturing or use of another type of wound closure device. Following this treatment, the wound will need to be monitored extremely closely for signs of recurring dehiscence. Small wound cavities, without the presence of infection, should be stitched or treated conservatively —depending on the patient's condition. Surgical wounds of significant length should be treated with primary suturing with or without mesh reinforcement. In this type of case when a sutured wound needs reinforcement, I recommend using the meshes that dissolve after a few years or collagen meshes that are replaced by the patient's own collagen after a few years. These meshes are probably the only ones that can be sewn into the wounds of patients taking immunosuppressive medicines. In addition to their long absorption time, they are characterized by high bacterial clearance—that is to say, they can be used in infected wounds, where they perfectly cope with the infection, and they do not need to be removed at any time during the sewing of the wound, maintaining their structure and strength [94–97].

# References


1. Hachem LD, Ghanekar A, Selzner M, Famure O, Li Y, Kim SJ. Postoperative surgical-site hemorrhage after kidney transplantation: incidence, risk factors, and outcomes. Transplant Int. 2017;30(5):474–483. https://doi.org/10.1111/tri.12926. Epub 2017 Mar PMID: 28120465.
2. Hernández D, Rufino M, Armas S, González A, Gutiérrez P, Barbero P, Vivancos S, Rodríguez C, de Vera JR, Torres A. Retrospective analysis of surgical complications following cadaveric kidney transplantation in the modern transplant era. Nephrol Dial Transplant. 2006;21(10):2908–15. https://doi.org/10.1093/ndt/gfl338.
3. Salehipour M, Salahi H, Jalaeian H, et al. Vascular complications following 1500 consecutive living and cadaveric donor renal transplantations: a single center study. Saudi J Kidney Dis Transpl. 2009;20:570.
4. Yablon Z, Recupero P, McKenna J, Vella J, Parker MG. Kidney allograft biopsy: timing to complications. Clin Nephrol. 2010;74:39.
5. Eng M, Brock G, Li X, et al. Perioperative anticoagulation and antiplatelet therapy in renal transplant: is there an increase in bleeding complication? Clin Transplant. 2011;25:292.
6. Mathis AS, Dave N, Shah NK, Friedman GS. Bleeding and thrombosis in high-risk renal transplantation candidates using heparin. Ann Pharmacother. 2004;38:537.
7. Gooran S, Javid A, Pourmand G. Delayed hemorrhage in kidney transplantation: a life-threatening condition. Int J Organ Transplant Med. 2018;9(1):46–49. Epub 2018 Feb 1. PMID: 29531647; PMCID: PMC5839630.
8. Bracale UM, Santangelo M, Carbone F, et al. Anastomotic pseudoaneurysm complicating renal transplantation: treatment options. Eur J Vasc Endovasc Surg. 2010;39:565–8.
9. Delles C, Wittmann M, Renders L, et al. Restoration of renal allograft function by endovascular stenting of an iliac artery dissection. Nephrol Dial Transplant. 2002;17:1116–8.
10. Kaiser AB, Clayson KR, Mulherin JI, et al. Antibiotic prophylaxis in vascular surgery. Ann Surg. 1978;188:283–9.
11. Shahrokh H, Rasouli H, Zargar MA, Karimi K, Zargar K. Spontaneous kidney allograft rupture. Transplant Proc. 2005;37(7):3079–80. https://doi.org/10.1016/j.transproceed.2005.07.054 PMID: 16213311.
12. Murray JE et al. In Annals of Surgery in 1968 Sep;168(3):416–35.
13. Yadav RV, Sinha R. Graft repair: the treatment of choice for renal allograft rupture. J Urol. 1994;151(6):1498–9. https://doi.org/10.1016/s0022-5347(17)35285-0 PMID: 8189555.
14. Tulatz A, Seeger W, Müller P. Transplantationsvolumenzunahme—ein prognostisches Zeichen der drohenden Nierenruptur? [Increase in transplant volume—a prognostic sign of threatened kidney rupture?]. Z Urol Nephrol. 1985;78(5):259–65. German. PMID: 3898646.
15. Ko K, Jeong HC, Jeon HJ, Ko K, Lee S. Temporary renal artery clamping with hemostatic materials in diffuse type of spontaneous renal allograft rupture: a case report. Transplant Proc. 2019;51(8):2845–7. https://doi.org/10.1016/j.transproceed.2019.03.057 Epub 2019 Aug 27 PMID: 31471013.

16. Keller AK, Jorgensen TM, Jespersen B. Identification of risk factors for vascular thrombosis may reduce early renal graft loss: a review of recent literature. J Transplant. 2012;2012:793461. https://doi.org/10.1155/2012/793461. Epub 2012 May 31. PMID: 22701162; PMCID: PMC3369524.

17. Sugi MD, Albadawi H, Knuttinen G, Naidu SG, Mathur AK, Moss AA, Oklu R. Transplant artery thrombosis and outcomes. Cardiovasc Diagn Ther. 2017;7(Suppl 3):S219–27. https://doi.org/10.21037/cdt.2017.10.13. PMID: 29399525; PMCID: PMC5778523.

18. Patil AB, Ramesh D, Desai SC, Mylarappa P, Guttikonda SH, Puvvada S. Transplant renal artery stenosis: The impact of endovascular management and their outcomes. Indian J Urol. 2016;32(4):288–92. https://doi.org/10.4103/0970-1591.189707. PMID: 27843211; PMCID: PMC5054659.

19. Sutherland RS, Spees EK, Jones JW, Fink DW. Renal artery stenosis after renal transplantation: the impact of the hypogastric artery anastomosis. J Urol. 1993;149:980–5.

20. Rijksen JF, Koolen MI, Walaszewski JE, Terpstra JL, Vink M. Vascular complications in 400 consecutive renal allotransplants. J Cardiovasc Surg (Torino). 1982;23:91–8.

21. Wong W, Fynn SP, Higgins RM, Walters H, Evans S, Deane C, et al. Transplant renal artery stenosis in 77 patients—does it have an immunological cause? Transplantation. 1996;61:215–9.

22. Ardalan MR, Shoja MM, Tubbs RS, Ghabili K. Transplant renal artery stenosis associated with acute cytomegalovirus infection: Resolution following ganciclovir administration. Ren Fail. 2009;31(10):982–4. https://doi.org/10.3109/08860220903288526. PMID: 20030536

23. Pouria S, State OI, Wong W, Hendry BM. CMV infection is associated with transplant renal artery stenosis. QJM. 1998;91:185–9.

24. Sankari BR, Geisinger M, Zelch M, Brouhard B, Cunningham R, Novick AC. Post-transplant renal artery stenosis: Impact of therapy on long-term kidney function and blood pressure control. J Urol. 1996;155:1860–4. [PubMed] [Google Scholar].

25. Halimi JM, Al-Najjar A, Buchler M, Birmelé B, Tranquart F, Alison D, et al. Transplant renal artery stenosis: Potential role of ischemia/reperfusion injury and long-term outcome following angioplasty. J Urol. 1999;161:28–32.

26. Lacombe M. Arterial stenosis complicating renal allotransplantation in man: A study of 38 cases. Ann Surg. 1975;181:283–8.

27. Merkus JW, Huysmans FT, Hoitsma AJ, Buskens FG, Skotnicki SH, Koene RA. Renal allograft artery stenosis: Results of medical treatment and intervention. A retrospective analysis. Transpl Int. 1993;6:111–5.

28. Roberts JP, Ascher NL, Fryd DS, Hunter DW, Dunn DL, Payne WD, et al. Transplant renal artery stenosis. Transplantation. 1989;48:580–3.

29. Benoit G, Moukarzel M, Hiesse C, Verdelli G, Charpentier B, Fries D. Transplant renal artery stenosis: experience and comparative results between surgery and angioplasty. Transpl Int. 1990;3:137–40.

30. Peregrin JH, Stríbrná J, Lácha J, Skibová J. Long-term follow-up of renal transplant patients with renal artery stenosis treated by percutaneous angioplasty. Eur J Radiol. 2008;66:512–8.

31. Patel NH, Jindal RM, Wilkin T, Rose S, Johnson MS, Shah H, et al. Renal arterial stenosis in renal allografts: Retrospective study of predisposing factors and outcome after percutaneous transluminal angioplasty. Radiology. 2001;219:663–7.

32. Pappas P, Zavos G, Kaza S, Leonardou P, Theodoropoulou E, Bokos J, et al. Angioplasty and stenting of arterial stenosis affecting renal transplant function. Transplant Proc. 2008;40:1391–6.

33. Ghazanfar A, Tavakoli A, Augustine T, Pararajasingam R, Riad H, Chalmers N. Management of transplant renal artery stenosis and its impact on long-term allograft survival: a single-centre experience. Nephrol Dial Transplant. 2011;26:336–43.

34. Beecroft JR, Rajan DK, Clark TW, Robinette M, Stavropoulos SW. Transplant renal artery stenosis: Outcome after percutaneous intervention. J Vasc Interv Radiol. 2004;15:1407–13.

35. Audard V, Matignon M, Hemery F, Snanoudj R, Desgranges P, Anglade MC, et al. Risk factors and long-term outcome of transplant renal artery stenosis in adult recipients after treatment by percutaneous transluminal angioplasty. Am J Transplant. 2006;6:95–9.

36. Su CH, Lian JD, Chang HR, Wu SW, Chen SC, Tsai CF, et al. Long-term outcomes of patients treated with primary stenting for transplant renal artery stenosis: a 10-year case cohort study. World J Surg. 2012;36:222–8.

37. Voiculescu A, Schmitz M, Hollenbeck M, Braasch S, Luther B, Sandmann W, et al. Management of arterial stenosis affecting kidney graft perfusion: a single-centre study in 53 patients. Am J Transplant. 2005;5:1731–8.

38. Lerman M, Mulloy M, Gooden C, Khan S, Khalil A, Patel L, Zhou XJ. Post- transplant renal vein thrombosis, with successful thrombectomy and review of the literature. Int J Surg Case Rep. 2019;61:291–3.

39. Nerstrom B, Ladefoged J, Lund FL. Vascular complications in the 155 consecutive kidney transplantations. Scand J Urol Nephrol. 1972;6(suppl 15):S65–74.

40. Chiu AS, Landsberg DN. Successful treatment of acute transplant renal vein thrombosis with selective streptokinase infusion. Transplant Proc. 1991;23(4):2297–300 PMID: 1871875.

41. Modrall JG, Teitelbaum GP, Diaz-Luna H, Berne T. Local thrombolysis in a renal allograft threatened by renal vein thrombosis. Transplantation. 1993;56:1011–3.

42. Renoult E, Cormier L, Claudon M, Cao-Huu T, Frimat L, Gaucher O, Hubert J, Kessler M. Successful surgical thrombectomy of renal allograft vein thrombosis in the early postoperative period. Am J Kidney Dis. 2000;35(5):E21. https://doi.org/10.1016/s0272-6386(00)70286-1 PMID: 10793050.

43. Robertson AJ, Nargund V, Gray DW, Morris PJ. Low-dose Aspirin as prophylaxis against renal vein thrombosis and renal transplant recipients. Nephrol. Dial. Transplant. 2000;15:1865–8.

44. Stecman MJ, Charlwood N, Gray DW, Handa A. Administration of 75 mg of Aspirin daily for 28 days is sufficient prophylaxis against renal transplant vein thrombosis. Phlebiology. 2007;22(2):83–5.

45. Hamouda M, Sharma A, Halawa A. Urine leak after kidney transplant: a review of the literature. Exp Clin Transplant. 2018;16(1):90–5 PMID: 29409437.

46. Muhsin SA, Wojciechowski D, Review, BK virus in transplant recipients: current perspectives. Transpl Res Risk Manag. 2019:11.

47. Englesbe MJ, Dubay DA, Gillespie BW, et al. Risk factors for urinary complications after renal transplantation. Am J Transplant. 2007;7(6):1536–41.

48. van den Heijkant F, Vermeer TA, Vrijhof EJEJ, Nieuwenhuijzen GAP, Koldewijn EL, Rutten HJT. Psoas hitch ureteral reimplantation after surgery for locally advanced and locally recurrent colorectal cancer: complications and oncological outcome. Eur J Surg Oncol. 2017;43(10):1869–75. https://doi.org/10.1016/j.ejso.2017.05.018 Epub 2017 May 26 PMID: 28732671.

49. Kumar S, Ameli-Renani S, Hakim A, Jeon JH, Shrivastava S, Patel U. Ureteral obstruction following renal transplantation: causes, diagnosis and management. Br J Radiol. 2014;87 (1044):20140169.

50. Duty BD, Barry JM. Diagnosis and management of ureteral complications following renal transplantation. Asian J Urol. 2015;2:202–7.

51. Duty BD, Conlin MJ, Fuchs EF, Barry JM. The current role of endourologic management of renal transplantation complications. Adv Urol. 2013;2013:

52. Saini DK, Sinha RJ, Sokhal AK, Singh V. Boari flap reconstruction in a male infant with solitary kidney and associated megaureter. BMJ Case Rep. 2016;2016:bcr2016217577. https://doi.org/10.1136/bcr-2016-217577. PMID: 27979846; PMCID: PMC5174856.

53. Arpali E, Al-Qaoud T, Martinez E, Redfield RR III, Leverson GE, Kaufman DB, Odorico JS, Sollinger HW. Impact of ureteral stricture and treatment choice on long-term graft survival in kidney transplantation. Am J Transplant. 2018;18(8):1977–85. https://doi.org/10.1111/ajt. 14696 Epub 2018 Mar 31 PMID: 29446225.

54. Streeter EH, Little DM, Cranston DW, Morris PJ. The urological complications of renal transplantation: a series of 1535 patients. BJU Int. 2002;90(7):627–34.

55. Luna E, Cerezo I, Abengozar A, et al. Urologic complications after kidney transplantation: involvement of the double-J stent and the urologic suture. Transplant Proc. 2010;42(8): 3143–5.

56. Shivde SR, Date J, Dighe TA, Joshi PM. Unusual causes of obstruction to transplant ureter. Saudi J Kidney Dis Transpl. 2010;21(2):310–3. PMID: 20228519.

57. Whang M, Yballe M, Geffner S, Fletcher HS, Palekar S, Mulgaonkar S. Urologic complications in more than 2500 kidney transplantations performed at the Saint Barnabas healthcare system. Transplant Proc. 2011;43(5):1619–22.

58. Emiroglu R, Karakayall H, Sevmis S, Akkoc H, Bilgin N, Haberal M. Urologic complications in 1275 consecutive renal transplantations. Transplant Proc. 2001;33(1–2):2016–7.

59. Crossref CAS PubMed Web of Science®Google ScholarGetIt@Leiden Keller H, Noldge G, Wilms H, Kirste G. Incidence, diagnosis, and treatment of ureteric stenosis in 1298 renal transplant patients. Transpl Int. 1994;7(4):253–7.

60. Shoskes DA, Hanbury D, Cranston D, Morris PJ. Urological complications in 1,000 consecutive renal transplant recipients. J Urol. 1995;153(1):18–21.

61. Patel K, Batura D. An overview of hydronephrosis in adults. Br J Hosp Med (Lond). 2020;81 (1):1–8. https://doi.org/10.12968/hmed.2019.0274 Epub 2020 Jan 28 PMID: 32003628.

62. Datta PK. Hydronephrosis. Nurs Times. 1982;78(33):1393–5. PMID: 6922484.

63. Gdor Y, Gabr AH, Faerber GJ, Wolf JS Jr. Holmium:yttrium-aluminum-garnet laser endoureterotomy for the treatment of transplant kidney ureteral strictures. Transplantation. 2008;85(9):1318–21. https://doi.org/10.1097/TP.0b013e31816c7f19 PMID: 18475190.

64. Xiong SW, Yang KL, Ding GP, Hao H, Li XS, Zhou LQ, Guo YL. [Advances in surgical repair of ureteral injury]. Beijing Da Xue Xue Bao Yi Xue Ban. 2019. 18;51(4):783–789. Chinese. https://doi.org/10.19723/j.issn.1671-167x.2019.04.034. PMID: 31420641; PMCID: PMC7433491.

65. van den Dool WM, Baranski AG. High position of the third renal transplant and alternative urinary tract reconstruction in a complicated case. Exp Clin Transplant. 2019;17(4):546–9. https://doi.org/10.6002/ect.2016.0265 Epub 2017 Jul 11 PMID: 28697719.

66. Musquera M, Peri LL, Alvarez-Vijande R, Oppenheimer F, Gil-Vernet JM, Alcaraz A. Orthotopic kidney transplantation: an alternative surgical technique in selected patients. Eur Urol. 2010;58(6):927–93.

67. Hevia V, Gomez V, Alvarez S, Diez-Nicolas V, Fernandez A, Burgos FJ. Orthotopic kidney transplant: a valid surgical alternative for complex patients. Curr Urol Rep. 2015;16(1):470.

68. Ooms LS, Slagt IK, Dor FJ, et al. Ureteral length in live donor kidney transplantation; Does size matter? Transpl Int. 2015;28(11):1326–31.

69. Pike TW, Pandanaboyana S, Hope-Johnson T, Hostert L, Ahmad N. Ureteric reconstruction for the management of transplant ureteric stricture: a decade of experience from a single centre. Transpl Int. 2015;28(5):529–34.

70. Orlando, G., Di Clemente, L., Gravante, G., Overton, J., Di Cocco, P., Rizza, V., D'Angelo, M., Famulari, A. and Pisani, F. (2008), Urinary tract reconstruction using the controlateral native ureter and a combined open-retroperitoneoscopic approach after renal transplantation. Clinical Transplantation, 22: 842–846. https://doi.org/10.1111/j.1399-0012.2008.00883.x

71. Aldiwani M, Tharakan T, Al-Hassani A, Gibbons N, Pavlu J, Hrouda D. BK Virus Associated Haemorrhagic Cystitis. A systematic review of current prevention and treatment strategies. Int J Surg. 2019 Mar;63:34–42. https://doi.org/10.1016/j.ijsu.2019.01.019. Epub 2019 Feb 1. PMID: 30711618.

72. Sharma R, Tzetzo S, Patel S, Zachariah M, Sharma S, Melendy T. BK virus in kidney transplant: current concepts, recent advances, and future directions. Exp Clin Transplant. 2016;14(4):377–84. https://doi.org/10.6002/ect.2016.0030 Epub 2016 Jun 3 PMID: 27267780.

73. Khauli RB, Stoff JS, Lovewell T, Ghavamian R, Baker S. Post-transplant lymphoceles: a critical look into the risk factors, pathophysiology and management. J Urol. 1993;150(22):3.

74. Howard RJ, Simmons RL, Najarian JS. Prevention of lymphoceles following renal transplantation. Ann Surg. 1976;184:166–8.

75. Braun WE Banowsky LH Straffon RA et al. Lymphocytes associated with renal transplantation. Report of 15 cases and review of the literature. Am J Med 1974; 57:714–29.

76. Ebadzadeh MR, Tavakkoli M. Lymphocele after kidney transplantation: where are we standing now? Urol J. 2008;5:144. 4. Atray NK, Moore F, Zaman F, et al. Post transplant lymphocele: a single centre experience. Clin Transplant 2004;18(Suppl. 12):46.5.

77. Lucewicz A, Wong G, Lam VWT, et al. Management of primary symptomatic lymphocele after kidney transplantation: a systematic review. Transplantation. 2011;92(663):6.

78. Adani GL, Baccarani U, Bresadola V, et al. Graft loss due to percutaneous sclerotherapy of a lymphocele using acetic acid after renal transplantation. Cardiovasc Intervent Radiol. 2005;28:836.

79. Joosten M, d'Ancona FC, van der Meijden WA, Poyck PP. Predictors of symptomatic lymphocele after kidney transplantation. Int Urol Nephrol. 2019;51(12):2161–7. https://doi.org/10.1007/s11255-019-02269-0. Epub 2019 Sep 5. PMID: 31486950; PMCID: PMC6848241.

80. Inoue Saito, Narita, et al. Evaluation of persistent lymphatic fluid leakage using a strategy of placing a drain after kidney transplantation: a statistical analysis to assess its origin. Transplant Proc. 2017;49(8):1786–90. https://doi.org/10.1016/j.transproceed.2017.06.021.

81. Metcalf KS, Peel KR. Lymphocele. Ann R Coll Surg Engl. 1993;75(6):387–92. PMID: 8285540; PMCID: PMC2498000.

82. Gilliland JD, Spies JB, Brown SB, Yrizarry JM, Greenwood LH. Lymphoceles: percutaneous treatment with povidone-iodine sclerosis. Radiology. 1989;171(1):227–9. https://doi.org/10.1148/radiology.171.1.2648473 PMID: 2648473.

83. Lucas BA, Gill IS, Munch LC. Intraperitoneal drainage of recurrent lymphoceles using an internalized Tenckhoff catheter. J Urol. 1994;151(4):970–2. https://doi.org/10.1016/s0022-5347(17)35137-6 PMID: 8126839.

84. Bzoma B, Kostro J, Dębska-Ślizień A, Hellmann AR, Zadrożny D, Śledziński Z, Rutkowski B. Treatment of the lymphocele after kidney transplantation: a single-center experience. Transplant Proc. 2016;48(5):1637–40. https://doi.org/10.1016/j.transproceed.2016.03.025 PMID: 27496462.

85. Kyriakides GK, Simmons RL, Najarian JS. Wound infections in renal transplant wounds: pathogenetic and prognostic factors. Ann Surg. 1975;182(6):770–5. https://doi.org/10.1097/00000658-197512000-00021. PMID: 1106338; PMCID: PMC1343978.

86. Mangram AJC, Horan TC, Pearson ML, Silver LCh, BS, Jarvis WR. Vol. 20 No. 4 Infection control an hospital epidemiology. Guideline for prevention surgical site infection, 1999, 250–77, US Department of Health and Human Services Hospital Infection Control Practices Advisory Committee Membership List, January 1999.

87. Harris AD, Fleming B, Bromberg JS, Rock P, Nkonge G, Emerick M, Harris-Williams M, Thom KA. Surgical site infection after renal transplantation. Infect Control Hosp Epidemiol. 2015;36(4):417–23. https://doi.org/10.1017/ice.2014.77. PMID: 25782896; PMCID: PMC4367121.

88. Camara B, Mouzin M, Ribes D, et al. Perihepatitis and perinephric abscess due to Mycoplasma hominis in a kidney transplant patient. Exp Clin Transplant. 2007;5(2):708–9.

89. Ison MG, Grossi P, Practice ASTIDCo. Donor-derived infections in solid organ transplantation. Am J Transplant. 2013;13(Suppl 4):22–30.

90. Lee SH, Jung HJ, Mah SY, Chung BH. Renal abscesses measuring 5 cm or less: outcome of medical treatment without therapeutic drainage. Yonsei Med J. 2010;51(4):569–73.

91. Menezes FG, Wey SB, Peres CA, Medina-Pestana JO, Camargo LF. What is the impact of surgical site infection on graft function in kidney transplant recipients? Transpl Infect Dis. 2010;12(5):392–6. https://doi.org/10.1111/j.1399-3062.2010.00527.x. PMID: 20561302.

92. Dumville JC, Gray TA, Walter CJ, Sharp CA, Page T, Macefield R, Blencowe N, Milne TK, Reeves BC, Blazeby J. Dressings for the prevention of surgical site infection. Cochrane

Database Syst Rev. 2016;12(12):CD003091. https://doi.org/10.1002/14651858.cd003091. pub4. PMID: 27996083; PMCID: PMC6464019.

93. Chen X, Liu L, Nie W, Deng R, Li J, Fu Q, Fei J, Wang C. Vacuum sealing drainage therapy for refractory infectious wound on 16 renal transplant recipients. Transplant Proc. 2018;50 (8):2479–2484. https://doi.org/10.1016/j.transproceed.2018.04.014. Epub 2018 Apr 12. PMID: 30316382.

94. Kırnap M, Boyvat F, Torgay A, Moray G, Yıldırım S, Haberal M. incidence of urinary complications with double j stents in kidney transplantation. Exp Clin Transplant. 2019;17 (Suppl 1):148–52. https://doi.org/10.6002/ect.mesot2018.p14. PMID: 30777542.

95. https://teachmesurgery.com/perioperative/skin/wound-dehiscence/.

96. Gottrup F, Melling A, Hollander DA. An overview of surgical site infections: aetiology, incidence and risk factors. World Wide Wounds. 2005. http://www.worldwidewounds.com/2005/september/Gottrup/Surgical-Site-Infe. Accessed 30 Mar 2017.

97. Rosen RD, Manna B. Wound Dehiscence. [Updated 2020 Jul 10]. In: StatPearls. Treasure Island (FL): StatPearls Publishing; 2020. https://www.ncbi.nlm.nih.gov/books/NBK551712/.

# Chapter 6
# Surgical Technique to Remove a Transplanted Kidney: Graftectomy or Transplantectomy

## 6.1 Introduction

Approximately 4–10% of incident patients on dialysis have a non-functioning kidney graft, and referring to literature [1–13], as many as 32% patients require transplantectomy for a variety of reasons. We rarely talk about the 7% of people whose transplant failed within a year or the 17% of people who have lost their transplants within three years. It is hard to find any guides or brochures for patients and families about how to deal with a failed transplant—for the nearly 3000 people who lose their kidney transplants in the first year or the over 6000 people who lose their transplants within three years. At ten years, 54% of transplant kidneys are still working. In fact, over 20% of kidney transplants every year are retransplants [1–13]. The mortality in these patients is significantly higher than in those with a functioning graft or on renal replacement therapy without having received a graft. Indications for kidney graftectomy are graft intolerance syndrome, graft loss due to BK virus nephropathy and a high level of BK viraemia, severe proteinuria, chronic inflammation syndrome, vascular thrombosis, severe acute rejection, hyperacute rejection, recurrent urinary infections, sepsis or cancer [1–10].

When the cause of graft loss is due to primary non-function, arterial or venous thrombosis, hyperacute or early refractory acute rejection, most treating physicians advocate transplantectomy and immunosuppression cessation. In these circumstances, graft rupture or hemorrhage may occur if the graft is left in situ. However, when the allograft has been in place for more than one to two years, it is common practice to leave the failed allograft in situ. Nonetheless, a retained failed transplant has been suggested to be a source of chronic inflammatory states, potentially leading to unfavorable outcomes [3].

Chronic inflammation syndrome occurs in patients with high levels of inflammatory markers (C-reactive protein), who are anemia resistant to treatment with erythropoiesis stimulators, and malnutrition markers. This inflammatory state is provoked by the graft, and reverts when a transplantectomy is performed, as several

© The Author(s), under exclusive license to Springer Nature Switzerland AG 2023  453
A. Baranski, *Kidney Transplantation*,
https://doi.org/10.1007/978-3-030-75886-8_6

studies have shown [4]. Between 30 and 40% of patients that return to dialysis with a non-functioning graft develop immunological intolerance once the immunosuppressant therapy is reduced [3–6]. Immunosuppression management in such patients can be challenging, although the maintenance of the low dose immunosuppression may preserve the residual kidney function, circumvent graft intolerance syndrome, minimize allosensitization, prevent reactivation of systemic disease, prevent adrenal insufficiency syndrome, decrease incidence of graft intolerance syndrome and avoid overt acute rejection. On the other side, long-term maintenance immunosuppression is not without adverse effect, such as diabetes, hypertension, dyslipidemia, avascular necrosis, cardiovascular complication, infections, and malignancy (especially skin cancers, Kaposi's sarcoma, non-Hodgkin's lymphoma and lip cancers) [3, 4, 7].

Graft and recipient survival is influenced by the donor's age, kidney function, type of donation, ischemia time, underlying kidney disease, degree of recipient immunization, donation technique, preservation, preparation and the advancement of atherosclerotic lesions in the iliac blood vessel. According to a US report, the cumulative probability of transplantectomy at one week, three months, six months and one year after graft failure was 5.3, 17.6, 25.0 and 30.9, respectively [5]; 89.3% of all nephrectomies were performed in the first year after transplant failure [3, 6]. In patients who had zero, one, or two or more rejection episodes, transplantectomy was required in 30, 53 and 83% of cases, respectively. It is suggested that gradual immunosuppression weaning or indefinite low-dose maintenance immunosuppression may prevent the need for transplantectomy [3, 7]. Despite the undoubted success of medicine in the field of kidney procurement, preservation and transplantation, as well as advances in immunology and immunosuppressive pharmacotherapy, 7–10% of transplanted kidneys become insufficient after one year, and patients must undergo replacement therapy such as hemodialysis, peritoneal dialysis or second transplantation. According to the available literature [1–7], the cessation of the transplant function is not always an indication for its removal. In many patients, immunosuppression can be stopped and, without any side effects, the transplanted kidney becomes slowly fibrous and atrophied, shrinking to the size of a walnut. Some recipients complain of numerous trouble from the inoperative graft, which is an indication for its removal.

In one single-center study, patients with failed kidney transplants returning to hemodialysis were shown to exhibit worsened anemia, erythropoietin resistance and hypoalbuminemia, as well as worsened C reactive protein (CRP), erythrocyte sedimentation rate (ESR) and ferritin profiles compared with their transplant naïve hemodialysis counterparts. Furthermore, amelioration of both clinical and laboratory parameters of the chronic inflammatory state was observed following transplantectomy [2, 8].

Although symptomatic patients undergoing transplantectomy had lower baseline hemoglobin and higher CRP, ESR and ferritin compared with those with a retained graft, the former group of patients had a better hematologic and biochemical profile at six months after the transplantectomy compared with the latter [2, 8, 9].

The surgical removal of a transplanted kidney (graftectomy or transplantectomy) can be divided into early and late transplantectomy. An early transplantectomy (early graft loss) is usually performed within two to three weeks after the transplantation because of the following indications: irreversible renal vascular thrombosis, kidney rupture involving the renal pelvis, septic hemorrhage, contamination of the transplanted kidney area resistant to any kind of treatment when only increasing the diameter of the renal and/or iliac vessels of the patient (threat of septic hemorrhage), any bleeding from the kidney or vascular anastomoses leading to hemorrhagic shock unmanageable during reoperations, resistance to treatment of acute rejection, primary or secondary lack of function of the transplanted kidney poor or no tolerance of the non-functioning graft by the recipient's organism consisting of high body temperature of the recipient, enlargement and constant pain of the transplanted but non-functioning kidney, advanced haematuria and proteinuria) [1–10].

The extracapsular nephrectomy approach is generally used for early graft loss, whereas for late nephrectomies the approach is usually subcapsular, by intense fibrotic reaction to adjacent tissues, which makes it difficult to complete the nephrectomy. Even if the two methods are not comparable, some authors have reported that the subcapsular method was associated with a higher rate of bleeding in the operation. The subcapsular technique of the graftectomy is the technique of choice due to the low incidence of serious complications, although the extracapsular technique could be performed safely during the early post-transplantation period when fibrosis and adhesions have not been established yet [11, 12].


## 6.2  Early Graftectomy or Graft Loss During One Year

Early transplantation, especially emergency transplantation, is characterized by a higher blood loss and a higher incidence of mid- and post-operative complications and, consequently, higher mortality. Patients qualified for early transplantation usually do not die on the operating table, but during the postoperative period. The main cause of death is a septic shock or circulatory and respiratory failure. The surgical technique of the removal of the transplanted kidney is based on the fact that we usually reach the kidney by an old incision and then we slowly peel off the peritoneum from the anterior surface of the transplanted kidney; during graftectomy (transplantectomy) we take numerous cultures and rinse the kidney area with a warm Ringer's solution, which allows for a better mobilization (detachment) of the posterior surface of the kidney from the extraperitoneal space [11]. The process of detaching the peritoneum and mobilizing the kidney is done very gently in order not to damage the peritoneum. As a rule, the kidney can be removed with the capsule, and the surgical supply of the renal vessel stumps or iliac vessels and the ureter is easy and does not present a major surgical challenge. The technique of ligation of transplanted kidney vessels was described earlier. Putting the vascular glue on the vein and renal artery together or ligating the two renal vessels (vein and artery) together may lead to an arteriovenous fistula at a later stage. The ureter can be tied at a distance of 1–2 cm from the bladder or completely removed by cutting off the ureter-urinary bladder anastomosis, where the bladder can be sutured tightly. After suturing the opening in the bladder, the urinary bladder should be tested for tightness by filling it with warm saline solution or Ringer's solution with or without the addition of a small amount of sterile methylene blue in order to make the place of the possible leakage more visible. In my opinion, the place where the kidney is removed should always be drained with a surgical or vacuum Redon or JP type drain. Personally, I use vacuum drains which, by removing air from the removed kidney area, facilitate the peritoneum to adhere and quickly stick well to the wall of the abdominal cavity and the retroperitoneal space, and thus to quickly make contact with the mentioned structures.

## 6.3  Late Graftectomy or Graft Loss

### 6.3.1  *Introduction*

Late graftectomy is a complicated procedure that requires great surgical skills. This is mainly due to the fact that the kidney and the ureter are always strongly attached to the retroperitoneum and surrounding tissues (rejection episodes, fibrosis, infection, surgical reinterventions after transplantation). Sometimes the kidney to be removed is small and hard as stone; othertimes it is significantly enlarged, extremely well supplied with blood and with an easy self-disintegrating parenchyma. The indication for the removal of the graft is intolerance by the recipient, usually manifested by high temperature (rejection, recurrent infections, most often of the urinary tract), hematuria, pain in the area of the transplanted kidney, chronic kidney rejection, increased chronic proteinuria, graft infection, recurrent urinary tract infections, failure to respond to the treatment used to maintain the function of the transplant and inhibit rejection, and the patient's request. The surgical technique of the late removal of a transplanted kidney I will describe it very briefly using the previous incision after a kidney transplant with subcapsular removal of the graft. In some other cases, indications for graftectomy include an infected renal artery aneurysm, a ruptured aneurysm, and septic and hemorrhagic shock—in the above-mentioned examples quick abdominal access is indicated in the form of midline laparotomy [9–12]. As I mentioned, this operation is very complicated. I think it might be sometimes too difficult for a not-well-trained surgeon. This procedure is loaded with quite high mortality, reaching 10% and much more in some centers. Therefore, it seems that the percutaneous intra-arterial graft embolization can be an alternative and is reported to have less complications [13–16]. Vascular embolization is a less invasive technique for the management of graft intolerance syndrome. At present, embolization is mostly performed by an intra-arterial administration of inert microparticles, like microspheres of polyvinyl alcohol, causing occlusion of distal capillaries, leading to necrosis, followed by insertion of stainless steel coils in the renal artery [13–17]. Allograft percutaneous embolization is performed using local anesthesia at the puncture site, using the transfemoral approach to reach the midportion of the renal artery. To avoid reflux, a balloon occlusion catheter is positioned and inflated immediately before the ethanol injection. The amount of the absolute ethanol used was 10–12 cc. Finally, the positioning of coils in the main renal artery or its principal branches completed the procedure. No systematic prophylactic antibiotic or steroid treatment was administered. Success rates of the initial embolization for the resolution of the graft intolerance syndrome are 65–100% [16]. In some patients with persistent graft intolerance a second attempt with embolization was performed, but in most of these cases graft removal was finally required [14, 15]. After graft embolization a transient post-embolization syndrome frequently occurs, mainly characterized by fever and local pain. It only requires a symptomatic treatment and can eventually be prevented by a short course of steroids [13–17].

### 6.3.2   Surgical Preparation for Late Graftectomy in Steps:

Before surgery, if possible, read the description of the operation from a previous kidney transplant, try to avoid (the same) mistakes and obtain the following information:

A. How long ago was this kidney transplanted? How many arteries, veins and ureters does the kidney have?
B. How many arteries were there on the aortic patch: one, two or more? Did they have to be reconstructed during the preparation for transplantation, and if so, how was it done, to which iliac artery and how were they anastomosed?
C. How many renal veins have been involved in the veneus anastomosis: one, two or more? Did they have to be reconstructed during the preparation for transplantation, and if so, how was it done and to which iliac vein and how were they connected?
D. How many ureters were there and how and where were they implanted into the urinary bladder or ileum?
E. What was the position of the kidney after transplantation? What was the position of the kidney pelvis in relation to the iliac vessels (transverse, longitudinal, vertical)?
F. What complications occurred after surgery, especially surgical complications requiring surgical intervention or radiologist intervention (insertion of intra-arterial stents)? Into which artery, for what reason, and when? How many were there and how were they treated?

Provided with this information, we can thoroughly prepare for the surgery to remove the transplanted kidney, determine the tactics and safe technique of the operation and discuss it with the anesthesiologist and your assistant and prepare the patient for the procedure, explaining the surgical technique and its possible intra- and postoperative complications. In the case of poor general patient condition, the possibility of percutaneous intra-arterial embolization of the renal artery should be considered and discussed with an experienced interventional radiologist [14].

### 6.3.3  Author's Own Experience: How Dangerous Can Be?

During my work at Warsaw University our Department performed during two or three years graftectomies for three kidney transplant centers. More than 35 years ago, transplant surgeons from small volume transplant centers found transplantectomy too difficult to perform. I found out how dangerous this procedure can be when I was asked to help with the removal of a failing transplanted kidney. Here is my story.

Several years ago, I was asked to help perform a graftectomy where a major hemorrhage occurred and the surgeon blindly closed the kidney vessels with one vascular clamp and quickly excised the kidney. As he later claimed, the clamp which closed the kidney vessels was placed in the highest place in the kidney hilum, and the kidney was cut off at the pelvic level. The patient did not bleed, the clamp was well closed, but on further inspection of the operating field it turned out that 3 cm of the external iliac artery and 1 cm of the anterior surface of the vein were excised together with the kidney. The surgeon was saved by the attention of an experienced instrumentalist who, when examining the removed kidney, stated that "there are too many vessels near the cut kidney". After the dissection of the iliac vessels above and below the site of the anastomoses, the vessels were closed and thus control of the bleeding was achieved after the clamps were removed from the damaged vessels. The repair operation consisted in mobilizing the external iliac artery, refreshing its ends and performing a new end-to-end anastomosis with a 6/0 non-absorbable monofilament suture. The vein was reconstructed with a patch made of a renal vein of the removed kidney. The postoperative course was uneventful and the 28-year-old patient was discharged home in a generally good condition and with a normal flow in the right lower limb.

### 6.3.4  Own Modified Surgical Technique for Late Transplantectomy Step-by-step

(1)  Activities in the operating theatre prior to the start of surgery;
    a) prophylactic administration of antibiotics according to the last anybiogram.
    b) time out—involved nurses, surgeons, anaesthetists and all others involved in the patient's care. Immediately prior to incision, active communication is required between all relevant surgical team members. Until any questions or concerns have been addressed, the procedure

cannot begin. During the preincision timeout, activities are suspended as much as possible. This allows team members to focus on actively confirming the patient, site and procedure.

- c) anaesthetising the patient.
- d) maintain bladder sterility by inserting a catheter into the bladder.
- e) shaving, surgical site disinfection, sterile draping of surgical field.

(2) Review of anticipated critical events;

- a) the surgeon reviews critical and unexpected steps, duration of surgery and expected blood loss,
- b) anaesthetic staff review patient-specific concerns,
- c) nursing staff review confirmation of sterility, availability of equipment and other concerns.

(3) The first stage is the incision of the skin and subcutaneous tissue. In this case I use an old skin incision, which is sometimes extended downwards and upwards if necessary.

(4) After the incision of the skin and subcutaneous tissue, we come to the transplant scar (old wound) which is on the medial side of the scar to the anterior surface of the rectus abdominis muscle and on the lateral side aponeurosis of the external musculus obliques. The skin and subcutis are mobilized towards the middle auxiliary line 3–4 cm laterally from the scar. The first cut of the muscles is about 5–6 cm and is performed over the most protruding part of the graft after carefully palpating the cutting site. The incision is made vertically in the aponeurosis of the external oblique muscle. If you are too close to the middle line with your incision, you have almost a 100% chance of opening the peritoneum.

(5) Then through the internal oblique muscle we palpate and determine the position of the lower, upper pole and lateral border of the kidney in the retroperitoneal space. We estimate the distance from the scar to the lateral border of the kidney. Now we carry the incision of the internal oblique muscle at the side or 1 cm laterally from the renal border. Please remember that only the maximal lateral access to the kidney's capsule will prevent damage to the parietal peritoneum.

(6) The kidney capsule usually adheres directly to the internal oblique muscle (there is no peritoneum between the transplanted kidney capsule and the lateral side of the abdominal wall) and only here; after cutting the muscle and kidney capsule, we usually do not cut the peritoneum but reach the kidney capsule and kidney parenchyma. The incision length should be at least 15–20 cm, depending on the size of the transplanted kidney—in most cases the kidney is large (rejected and very swollen) (Fig. 6.1).

(7) After reaching the transplanted kidney capsule and parenchyma, we dissect and separate the kidney capsule from the parenchyma with our index finger. Bleeding from the renal parenchyma can be controlled with gauze or coagulation.

(8) During detachment of the kidney capsule, make slow movements with your index finger, detach the entire surface of the kidney capsule from the parenchyma, including its poles and as close as possible to the renal hilum. When

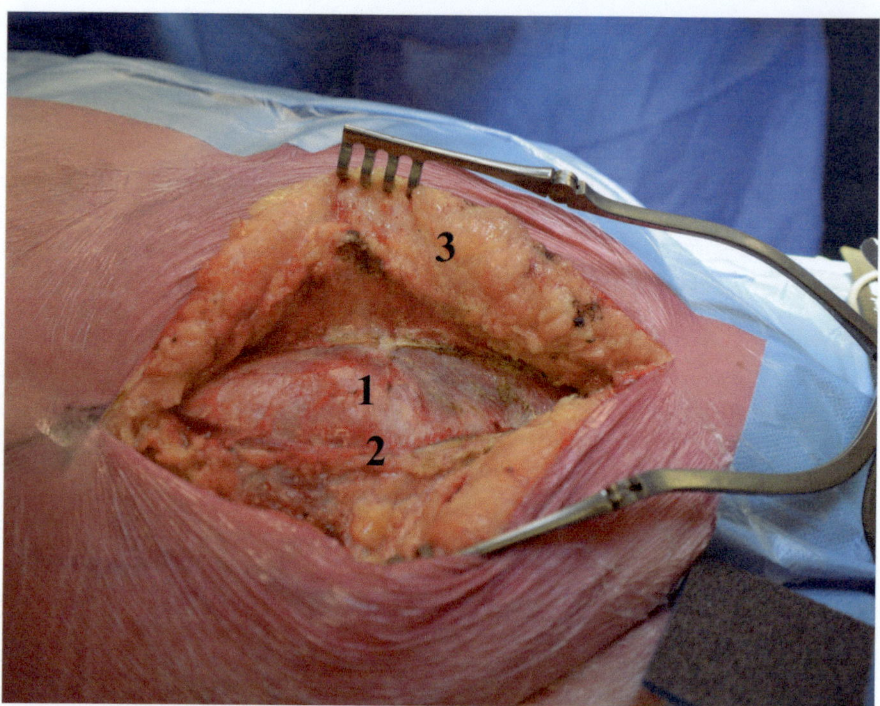

**Fig. 6.1** 1—Internal oblique muscle shows a clearly outlined posterior edge of the transplanted kidney, 2—Incised fascia of the rectus abdominis muscle with the external oblique muscle, 3—Subcutaneous tissue

you see the kidney's poles without the kidney capsule, try to very carefully move the kidney out of the freed capsule and out of the surgical field. In this way you have access to the renal hilum which means that the kidney capsule has been totally detached from the parenchyma (Fig. 6.2).

**Warning!**

Now you can put on a large clamp and cut out the kidney. But what if the renal artery was very short and the external iliac artery is very tortuous and has a slight aneurysm? At this stage, I would advise further dissection of the kidney.

(9)   The next step is to locate the ureter. Cut very carefully the capsule released from the lower pole of the transplanted kidney along the lateral edge of the kidney towards the lower pole and ureter, thereby opening the retroperitoneal space. When preparing the tissues towards the iliac vessels, if we dissect close to the lower pole and a bit downwards, the first structure which we encounter is the renal pelvis and a little downwards the beginning of the ureter.

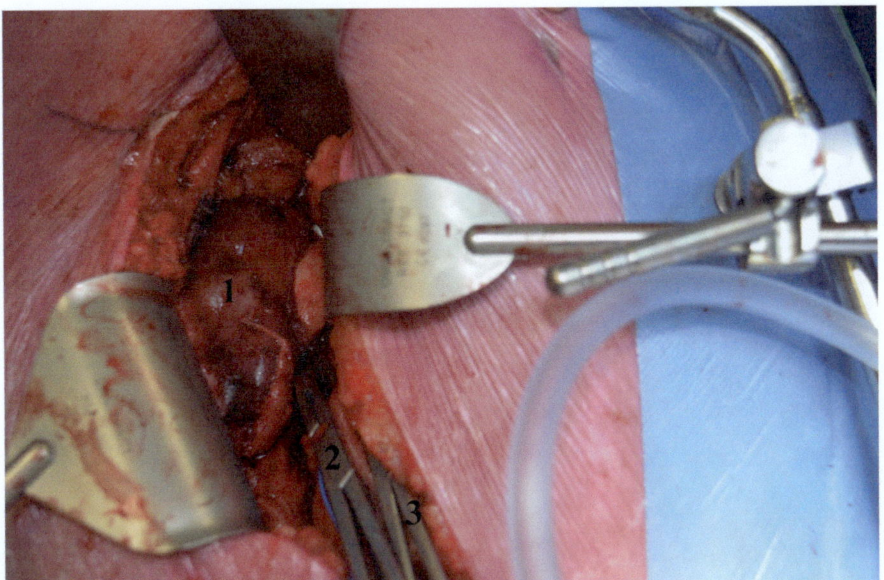

**Fig. 6.2**  1—Kidney without capsule, 2 and 3—Vascular clamps closing the kidney vessels very close to the renal hilum. Please remember this moment—it is extremely important for the patient and for you as a surgeon. After closing the renal vessels with the vascular clamps, before removing the kidney, check with your fingers or vascular Doppler for the presence of pulsatile flow, i.e. good blood flow, in the external iliac or common femoral artery below the vascular anastomoses. Remember that a moment's inattention with the clamps in place can cost the patient the excision of the iliac vessels, a major and then very difficult operation to restore the continuity of the vessels, or even the loss of a limb

(10)  Follow the ureter up to the urinary bladder, ligate it on both sides and cut it.

(11)  Pull up the ureter and free it together with the renal pelvis from the surrounding tissues. A mobilized renal pelvis will give you access to the iliac and renal vessels, vascular anastomoses and the posterior surface of the kidney and the renal hilum of the transplanted kidney. Dissect, ligate or suture and cut the renal vessels as high as possible in the renal hilum.

(12)  After the graftectomy, the internal surface of the kidney capsule is coagulated with an Argon Beamer or sprayed with an electro-coagulation device and drained with a surgical or JP drain. The drain is fixed and the abdominal wall, subcutaneous tissue and skin are sewn in layers (Fig. 6.3).

(13)  We maintain the drain for several days and remove it when the "production" is less than 20 ml per day for two consecutive days.

(14)  If there is no urine secretion, the catheter inserted into the bladder is removed the same day, immediately after the operation. The urinary bladder is flushed with warm Ringer's or saline solution before the removal of the catheter to remove blood and clots. The next day or a few days after the operation, remove the catheter depending on the quality of the recipient's bladder. As a

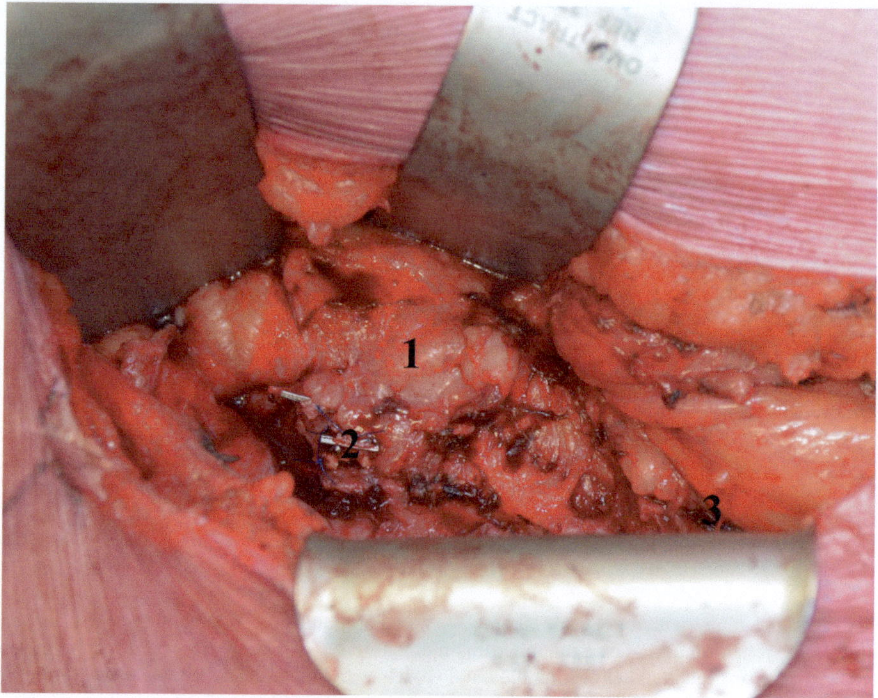

**Fig. 6.3**  1—The site after excision of the transplanted kidney, 2—Some of the vessels are double tied and some are double-sewn with nonabsorbable sutures, 3—The area of the urinary bladder

rule, we remove the bladder catheter under the cover of antibiotics in consultation with a hospital infection disease specialist.

Each kidney  is sent for an anatomopathological examination and, if there is an indication, also for a bacteriological culture (Fig. 6.4).

**Warning!**

Each opening in the peritoneum is left for stitching at the end of the operation. I believe that each small opening in the peritoneum has to be sutured at the end of the operation because, during this time, the stretching of the peritoneum will be minimal. If you are unable to close even the smallest hole in the peritoneum due to its bad quality, open it as far as you can and do not close it. This way you can prevent preperitoneal herniation.

**Warning!**

Now you can put on a large clamp and cut out the kidney. However, what happens if the renal artery is very short and the external iliac artery is very winding and has a slight aneurysm change? I would advise you at this stage to dissect the kidney further in order to be sure of a few anatomical details before you blindly clamp and remove the kidney.

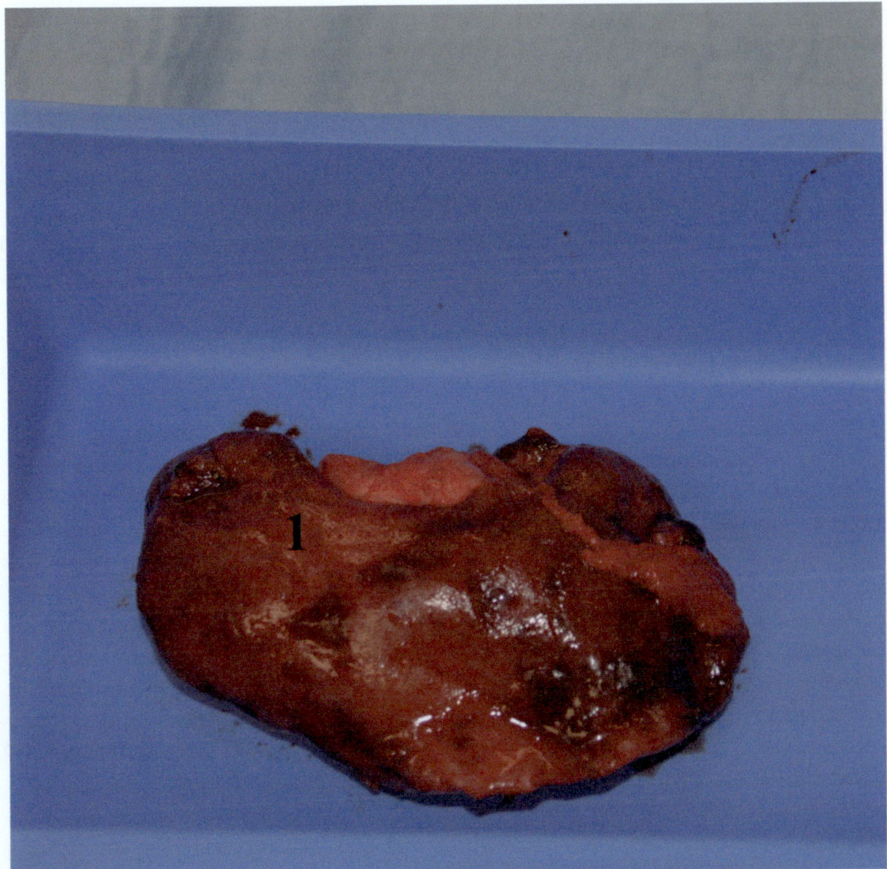

**Fig. 6.4**  1—Removed under the capsule: inactive and rejected kidney after transplantation

The next stage is to locate the ureter. You should very carefully cut the transplanted kidney capsule along the lateral edge of the kidney in the direction of the lower pole and thus open the extraperitoneal space. When preparing the tissues towards the iliac vessels, if we prepare near the lower pole and slightly downwards, we will come across the renal pelvis and the beginning of the ureter as the first structure.

The midline incision gives us a chance to quickly reach the vessel(s) above and below the kidney anastomosis site, and thus enable full bleeding control, which gives us therefore maximum patient safety on the operating table. If during a regular late graftectomy (access through an old incision) there is bleeding that cannot be controlled, do not try to blindly close everything with large vascular clamps, thinking that the bleeding will be stopped. My advice is when you are unable to control the bleeding with a clamp, try to control the hemorrhage with your finger(s) at the beginning. Be polite, do not shout. If you have stopped the bleeding, calm yourself down, your partner surgeon and the scrub nurse. Speak in a friendly way with the anesthesia team and the rest of the medical personnel present in the operating room. Do not let them know that you are afraid. Please politely call for the most experienced people who you trust, who are the best and who are most able to help the patient and stop/control the bleeding. Do not panic, let the anesthesiologist and the nurse know that the patient is still bleeding and you need as quickly as possible the cell saver and much more blood or that you already have managed to control the bleeding. Try to communicate in the operating room with everyone politely on the same level.

Let us list the necessary resources that you will need in the operating room to control the bleeding. If the patient has low blood pressure and is not bleeding, do not try to operate on him or her further, but wait for appropriate help and give time to the anesthesiologist to stabilize the patient's condition. After the arrival of new forces and completing all the necessary things in the operating room, make one more attempt to control the bleeding with the most experienced people who have come to your department to the operating room. If not, perform a midline laparotomy to quickly reach, control and clamp the iliac vessels above and below the anastomosis site.

At this point the following question arises: To remove or not to remove a transplanted kidney that is inactive and/or ineffective, and/or insufficient when the patient is not receiving immunosuppressive drugs and the kidney and the patient are not suffering from any symptoms? The opinions of transplant nephrology specialists on this subject are divided. Some centers remove almost every transplanted kidney immediately after it starts failing. The proponents of this approach (early graftectomy) argue that as a result of chronic rejection with or without immunosuppressive medications, patients with a failed transplant who are undergoing dialysis, often develop a variety of unsafe bacterial and non-bacterial infections, which increases the number of complications during dialysis, and may have a significant impact on the survival of patients awaiting another transplant. Other proponents of early transplantectomy (graftectomy) argue that after early removal of the kidney, the number of complications during dialysis is significantly reduced, resulting in a lower risk of contracting infectious diseases, longer survival and ultimately a bigger chance of receiving a second transplant. Other centers, on the other hand, believe that the removal of a transplanted kidney without any symptoms is not necessary, because the transplanted old kidney has a protective effect on the new kidney and immediately after transplantation it absorbs antibodies against the transplanted kidney from the recipient's body, which is supposed to protect the new kidney, and therefore be responsible for the longer survival of the transplanted kidney. Another theory is that removal of the transplanted kidney significantly increases the immunoreactivity proponents of the recipient, which will contribute to a faster onset of episodes of acute rejection of the second or subsequent kidney that has just been transplanted. For some recipients of a kidney that has been rejected, especially in those with a severe heart and peripheral arterial disease, surgery to remove an asymptomatic rejected kidney may be an operation that exceeds the capacity of their body. Therefore, I deeply believe that if you do not need to remove the rejected and inactive (producing little or no urine) kidney after transplantation, then stay away and leave it alone.

## 6.4   Conclusion

The surgical technique for the late removal of a transplanted kidney can be very difficult and often requires an experienced surgeon with good surgical skills. This procedure is burdened with a quite high mortality, reaching 10% and much more in less experienced centers. Therefore, it seems that the embolization of the renal artery of the transplanted kidney may be a good alternative for patients who were thoroughly selected for this procedure.

## References


1. https://www.kidney.org/transplantation/transaction/TC/summer09/TCsm09_TransplantFails and https://www.srtr.org/.
2. López-Gómez JM, Pérez-Flores I, Jofré R, Carretero D, Rodríguez-Benitez P, Villaverde M, Pérez-García R, Nassar GM, Niembro E, Ayus JC. Presence of a failed kidney transplant in patients who are on hemodialysis is associated with chronic inflammatory state and erythropoietin resistance. J Am Soc Nephrol. 2004;15:2494–501. [PubMed] [Google Scholar].
3. Pham PT, Everly M, Faravardeh A, Pham PC. Management of patients with a failed kidney transplant: dialysis re-initiation, immunosuppression weaning, and transplantectomy. World J Nephrol. 2015;4(2):148–59. https://doi.org/10.5527/wjn.v4.i2.148. PMID: 25949929; PMCID: PMC4419125.
4. Antón-Pérez G, Gallego-Samper R, Marrero-Robayna S, Henríquez-Palop F, Rodríguez-Pérez JC. Transplantectomy following renal graft failure. Nefrologia. 2012;32(5):573–8. English, Spanish. https://doi.org/10.3265/Nefrologia.pre2012.Jun.11100. PMID: 23013942.
5. United States Renal Data System. 2016 USRDS annual data report: epidemiology of kidney disease in the United States. National Institutes of Health, National Institute of Diabetes and Digestive and Kidney Disease, Bethesda, MD, 2016.
6. Johnston O, Rose C, Landsberg D, et al. Nephrectomy after transplant failure: current practice and outcomes. Am J Transplant. 2007;7:1961–7.
7. Saeb-Parsy K, Watson CJE. Kidney transplantation: surgical aspects. Medicine. 2011;39 (8):443–7. ISSN 1357-3039. https://doi.org/10.1016/j.mpmed.2011.05.013.
8. Ayus JC, Achinger SG. At the peril of dialysis patients: ignoring the failed transplant. Semin Dial. 2005;18:180–4.
9. Ayus JC, Achinger SG, Lee S, Sayegh MH, Go AS. Transplant nephrectomy improves survival following a failed renal allograft. J Am Soc Nephrol. 2010;21:374–80.
10. Fiorentino M, Gallo P, Giliberti M, Colucci V, Schena A, Stallone G, Gesualdo L, Castellano G. Management of patients with a failed kidney transplant: what should we do? Clin Kidney J. 2021;14(1):98–106. https://doi.org/10.1093/ckj/sfaa094.
11. Bonilla AJA, Alfaro AG, Henández JPC, Rubio JHG, Gómez EG, Valiente JC, García JMR, López JM, Tapia MJR. Review of a transplantectomy series. Transpl Proc. 2015;47(1):81–3.

12. Dinis P, Nunes P, Marconi L, Furriel F, Parada B, Moreira P, Figueiredo A, Bastos C, Roseiro A, Dias V, Rolo F, Macário F, Mota A. Kidney retransplantation: removal or persistence of the previous failed allograft? Transplant Proc. 2014;46(6):1730–4. https://doi.org/10.1016/j.transproceed.2014.05.029. PMID.
13. Takase HM, Contti MM, Nga HS, Bravin AM, Valiatti MF, El-Dib RP, Modelli de Andrade LG. Nephrectomy versus embolization of non-functioning renal graft: a systematic review with a proportional meta-analysis. Ann Transplant. 2018;23:207–17. https://doi.org/10.12659/AOT.907700. PMID: 29581414; PMCID: PMC6248024.
14. Delgado P, Diaz F, Gonzalez A, Sanchez E, Gutierrez P, Hernandez D, Torres A, Victor V. Intolerance syndrome in failed renal allografts: incidence and efficacy of percutaneous embolization. Am J Kidney Dis. 2005;46(2):339–44.
15. O'Sullivan DC, Murphy DM, McLean P, Donovan MG. Transplant nephrectomy over 20 years: factors involved in associated morbidity and mortality. J Urol. 1994;151(4):855–8.
16. Delgado P, Diaz F, Gonzalez A, Hernández E, Hidalgo R, Hernández D, Gutierrez P, Lorenzo V. Transvascular ethanol embolization: first option for the management of symptomatic nonfunctioning renal allografts left in situ. Transplant Proc. 2003;35(5):1684–5. ISSN 0041-1345.
17. Bunthof KLW, Hazzan M, Hilbrands LB. Review: management of patients with kidney allograft failure. Transplant Rev (Orlando). 2018;32(3):178–86. https://doi.org/10.1016/j.trre.2018.03.001 Epub 2018 Mar 29 PMID: 29628415.

# Chapter 7
# The Most Important Issues in Qualifying a Patient for a Kidney Transplant by a Surgeon

1. Body weight.

Increasing Body Mass Index (BMI), in the most recent large cohort analysis, is not associated with increased risk of death or graft loss but is associated with new-onset post-transplant diabetes mellitus (PTDM). Post-transplant diabetes mellitus affects approximately 10-40% of patients undergoing solid organ transplantation. The PTDM is associated with higher rates of graft loss and mortality compared to patients who do not develop the condition [1]. The data now suggest that a low BMI is the greater concern, with malnourished patients having higher mortality rates. The problem that both physician and patient face is the task of reducing weight in the very obese and increasing weight in the malnourished before the BMI exceeds 30. Various authors in the medical literature claim that in kidney recipients with a BMI over 30 there are more postoperative complications (wound infection, pneumonia). In our center, we try rather not to transplant kidneys to people with a BMI above 30. Of course, we also transplant very obese patients with kidneys, but only for vital signs, for example if they do not have access to dialysis or they do not have enough time for bariatric surgery, but they are all with a BMI above 30. The prevalence of class III obesity (body mass index [BMI] $\geq$ 40 kg/m$^2$) has increased dramatically in several countries and currently affects 6% of adults in the US, with uncertain implications for the risk of disease and death. Class III obesity is associated with substantially increased rates of all-cause mortality, with most of the excess deaths due to heart disease, cancer and diabetes, and with a substantial reduction in life expectancy compared with normal weight [2]. A BMI of 35–40 [4–6] will result in transplant team recommendation for the patient to enroll in a weight loss program. This must include established weight loss goals and BMI monitoring by the transplant team. On the other hand, candidates with morbid obesity do have poorer outcomes after transplantation than those with a normal weight. Although there is no evidence that weight reduction before transplantation improves survival afterwards, it seems reasonable to believe the cardiovascular risk profile would benefit from such an

© The Author(s), under exclusive license to Springer Nature Switzerland AG 2023
A. Baranski, *Kidney Transplantation*,
https://doi.org/10.1007/978-3-030-75886-8_7

intervention. How weight loss should be achieved is less clear. Although the benefits of dietary treatment will reasonably outweigh the harms, both pharmacological therapy and bariatric surgery will likely cause more adverse events, making the risk–benefit balance more problematic [5, 6]. We recommend that patients with a body mass index >30 kg/m$^2$, if it is possible, reduce weight before transplantation [6].

2. Duplex Doppler ultrasound examination.

Before kidney transplantation, each patient must have a Duplex Doppler examination of the iliac vessels, both venous and arterial. These are the questions we should usually ask a radiologist before the examination in order to order the examination; significance of the iliac vessels, calcification, thrombosis, stenosis and at least congenital malformations involving the arteries, iliac veins and abdominal aorta. The description of the examination should include the ankle pressure index (API) and not only the blood flow velocities in the examined arteries, but also if it is possible their diameters.

3. Indication for contrast enhanced computed tomography (CT).

Contrast-enhanced CT is performed on each potential kidney recipient who has intermittent claudication, in recipients of the second kidney after previous kidney transplantation, in patients after two kidney transplants, before the third transplant, if kidneys are present or if they have been removed before the transplant, in every patient who has lost a kidney transplant as a result of septic hemorrhage caused by bacteria or fungi, before kidney transplantation, in patients after an aorta bifurcation graft (we are looking for signs of infection or fluid around the prosthesis).

4. In every patient over 50 years of age, we perform CT without contrast to see the number, length and arrangement of atherosclerotic calcifications in the iliac vessels and in the aorta. I recommend this—it is a very good examination. You can see if the calcifications close and take the shape of a circle, calcifications of the iliac arteries that can be detected by CT without contrast may involve the posterior wall of the vessel (this is usually where calcium deposition begins). Intense deposition of calcium deposits in the vessel wall can lead to arterial stenosis and, in advanced cases, to intermittent claudication. The most dangerous situation is when calcium deposits are deposited in the vessel in the form of rings (360 degrees). This is a very dangerous situation since any attempt to be consulted by a vascular surgeon before being qualified for transplantation. In this case, there are two solutions: to perform a kidney transplant together with a vascular surgeon, or to prepare for transplantation by performing vascular surgery, replacing the diseased vessel with a prosthesis and then performing a kidney transplant with anastomosis of the renal artery with a previously implanted prosthesis. In this case, prior to the operation, a vascular surgeon's consultation is required and a bilateral or unilateral bifurcation prothesis should be performed, depending on the stage of atherosclerosis. In patients with chronic renal failure, this is a procedure with a relatively high risk of complications. The decision to perform a unilateral or bilateral kidney transplant should be discussed in great detail with the patient and his family, as well as with the vascular

surgeon. My experience is that there have always been and still are great problems convincing a vascular surgeon from a non-university hospital to perform a bifurcation graft in a patient without intermittent claudication. On the other hand, we are talking about patients with renal insufficiency who may sometimes require vascular surgery, such as bilateral or unilateral bypasses between the aorta and the iliac or femoral vessels, and/or the implementation of complex dialysis access. It must be said that these are the patients with the highest risk. To keep these patients alive, they must be dialysed continuously or three times a week, which means that due to low haemoglobin levels, low plasma protein and albumin, frequent use of anticoagulants, limited fluid intake and dietary restrictions, these patients are more prone to all kinds of complications, such as infection, bleeding, slow wound healing, infection and wound dehiscence.

5. Some people may also benefit from receiving a kidney transplant before needing to go on dialysis, a procedure known as preemptive kidney transplant. But for certain people with kidney failure, a transplant may be more risky than dialysis. Conditions that may prevent you from being eligible for a kidney transplant include: advanced age, severe heart and peripheral arterial disease, diagnosed or treated neoplastic disease, dementia or poorly controlled mental illness, alcohol or drug abuse. Other factors can influence the capacity to safely undergo transplantation and taking the medications honestly as needed after a transplant to prevent organ rejection.

6. We recommend native nephrectomy before transplantation (unilateral or bilateral) in patients with autosomal polycystic kidney disease (ADPKD) when there are severe, recurrent symptomatic complications (bleeding, infection, stones). We suggest unilateral nephrectomy of asymptomatic ADPKD kidneys when space for the transplant kidney is insufficient. We do not recommend routine native nephrectomy, unless in cases of recurrent upper urinary tract infections or when the underlying kidney disease predisposes to enhanced cancer risk in the urogenital tract [6]. The author's own experience is to recommend all of the above to patients, plus everyone with ADPKD kidneys reaching the iliac arteries who have qualified for a living donor kidney transplantation has bilateral nephrectomy to both their kidneys six weeks before transplantation.

7. Do not forget: Patients over 65 years old are the fastest growing age group among the population with end-stage renal disease worldwide. In the European Renal Association-European Dialysis and Transplant Association (ERA-EDTA) Registry Annual Report of 2012, patients aged 65 to 74 years and 75 years or older constitute 22 and 20%, respectively, of the prevalent renal replacement therapy population [5].

**Conclusion**

Currently, qualification of a patient for kidney transplantation by a surgeon and a nephrologist from a transplantation unit seems to be insufficient. To fully qualify and place a patient on a waiting list for a transplant we usually need to have the patient assessed by a lot of different specialists in which the surgeon plays a very important role.

# References


1. Chowdhury TA. Post-transplant diabetes mellitus. Clin Med (Lond). 2019 Sep;19(5):392–5. https://doi.org/10.7861/clinmed.2019-0195. PMID: 31530687; PMCID: PMC6771354.
2. Kitahara CM, Flint AJ, Berrington de Gonzalez A, Bernstein L, Brotzman M, MacInnis RJ, Moore SC, Robien K, Rosenberg PS, Singh PN, Weiderpass E, Adami HO, Anton-Culver H, Ballard-Barbash R, Buring JE, Freedman DM, Fraser GE, Beane Freeman LE, Gapstur SM, Gaziano JM, Giles GG, Håkansson N, Hoppin JA, Hu FB, Koenig K, Linet MS, Park Y, Patel AV, Purdue MP, Schairer C, Sesso HD, Visvanathan K, White E, Wolk A, Zeleniuch-Jacquotte A, Hartge P. Association between class III obesity (BMI of 40–59 kg/m$^2$) and mortality: a pooled analysis of 20 prospective studies. PLoS Med. 2014 Jul 8;11(7): e1001673. https://doi.org/10.1371/journal.pmed.1001673. PMID: 25003901; PMCID: PMC4087039.
3. Andres A, Revilla Y, Ramos A, et al. Helical computed tomography angiography is the most efficient test to assess vascular calcifications in the iliac arterial sector in renal transplant candidates. Transplant. Proc. 2003;35:1682–3.
4. Pham PT, Pham PA, Pham PC, Parikh S, Danovitch G. Evaluation of adult kidney transplant candidates. Semin Dial. 2010;23(6):595–605. https://doi.org/10.1111/j.1525-139X.2010.00809.x. PMID: 21175834.
5. Segall L. Nistor I, Pascual J, Mucsi I, Guirado L, Higgins R, Van Laecke S, Oberbauer R, Van Biesen W, Abramowicz D, Gavrilovici C, Farrington K, Covic A. Criteria for and appropriateness of renal transplantation in elderly patients with end-stage renal disease. Transplantation. 2016;100(10):e55–e65. https://doi.org/10.1097/TP.0000000000001367.
6. The European Renal Best Practice (ERBP) Transplantation Guideline Development Group, Abramowicz D, Cochat P, Claas F, Dudley C, Harden P, Heeman U, Hourmant M, Maggiore U, Pascual J, Salvadori M, Spasovski G, Squifflet J-P, Steiger J, Torres A, Vanholder R, Van Biesen W, Viklicky O, Zeier M, Nagler E. ERBP guideline on the management and evaluation of the kidney donor and recipient. Nephrol Dial Transplant. 2013;28(Suppl 2): ii1–ii71. https://doi.org/10.1093/ndt/gft218, 01 August 2013.

# Chapter 8
# What a Safe and Successful Kidney Transplant Program Depends on?

## 8.1   Introduction

Patient safety culture is a debated issue worldwide; it is a fundamental principle and a prerequisite for quality of care in the health field, and to be properly proportioned, it is necessary to acquire a culture of safety in which professionals and services share practices, values, attitudes and behaviors that make it possible to replace the guilt and punishment with the opportunity to learn from their own failures, and improve health care, ensuring patient safety [1]. Patient safety culture is associated with the capacity of health institutions to adapt to the human and operational risks inherent in the work process [2, 3]. In this sense, patient safety meets quality care, which is the degree of compliance with established standards, as opposed to the norms and protocols that organize the practice actions as well as the current technical and scientific knowledge [4]. The success of the kidney transplantation program and the safety of the donor and recipient are thus guaranteed by the following.

1. Transplant Surgeon Training and Education

Very good knowledge of anatomy, and excellent surgical skills in the field of organ procurement, transplantation, vascular surgery and microsurgery. Based on the present findings, it is suggested that all transplant surgeons with experience of less than 25 transplants should perform their operations under close supervision (assistance) by an attending transplant surgeon. A donor age of more than 60 years and a recipient with cardiovascular disease (CVD) are also independent risk factors of post-kidney transplantation vascular and hemorrhagic complications, therefore it is suggested that these high risk patients should preferably be operated on by surgeons with experience of more than 26 transplantations [5]. The European Renal Best Practice (ERBP) Transplantation Guideline Development Group suggests that cold ischemia time (CIT) is kept as short as possible (strength of this recommendation is weak and the quality of evidence is very low). ERBP recommends also the

© The Author(s), under exclusive license to Springer Nature Switzerland AG 2023

A. Baranski, *Kidney Transplantation*,
https://doi.org/10.1007/978-3-030-75886-8_8

following rules: keeping CIT below 24 h when transplanting kidneys from donors after brain death (strength of this recommendation is strong and the quality of evidence is moderate), keeping CIT <2 h when using kidneys from donors after cardiac death (strength of this recommendation strong and the quality of evidence very low). ERBP recommends also that the decision to use donor kidneys with a CIT of >36 h should be made on a case by case basis [5, 6].

2. Creating the latest standards based on the latest knowledge

Based on the recent literature, your own experience and experience abroad, try to establish protocols for the management of patients presenting for kidney transplantation, operation protocols and postoperative management. Standards developed by the entire team should also take into account the capabilities of the transplant unit and operating theater. When qualifying patients for surgery, try to use the previously established standards, which will facilitate rapid and professional preparation of the patient for transplantation and the transplant itself, as well as easy management of the patient after transplantation. When qualifying a patient for a transplant think about their medical history, do not think that he or she can receive any kidney. Think of which kidney is not acceptable for him/her due to the condition of the iliac vessels on both sides, such as a third kidney transplant, advanced aortic and iliac artery atherosclerosis on both sides. Remember that for a difficult patient, e.g. with advanced aortic and iliac artery atherosclerosis, accepting a kidney with many vessels may not help him/her, but may become fatally dangerous for him/her (a very long time of warm ischemia, delayed function, loss of a kidney, loss of a leg, death of the patient). Before making a decision, it is necessary to consider whether the procured kidney can be transplanted in each recipient. This is not only about immunological aspects, but mainly about technical requirements that the kidney must meet, such as the condition of the recipient's iliac vessels, the number of kidney vessels in the retrieved kidney and the number of ureters. The final conclusion must also include a statement about the limitations, for example: for this patient, one can accept the left kidney with one vein, one artery and one ureter, any other kidney anatomy is associated with too high risk of complications after transplantation. If the recipient is young, slim and has no atherosclerotic changes in the iliac vessels, we are not limited in anything and can accept virtually any kidney for him or her without increasing the risk of complications after transplantation. Good cooperation with other specialists, collegiality, ensuring maximum safety for the patient during and after surgery as well as standardization of procedures in protocols and continuous improvement of one's knowledge and surgical skills through daily and continuous education of themselves and others create an environment in which you will enjoy working and be successful [6, 7].

3. Work, communication and productivity

The domain "working climate", which assesses the quality of the relationship and collaboration among professionals, is one of the variables that influences the performance of an organization of the proposed objectives. Honest permanent monitoring and analysis of complications are a big part of improving the quality of the operations and the safety of the patient. Job satisfaction, teamwork and good relationships with the team and managers is important. These aspects are fundamental and need to be managed by professionals who work in health institution administration, and in the units, in order to present a warm, humane and participative working environment, enabling safe and effective care contributing to favorable results for the patient undergoing transplantation. The most frequent results of job satisfaction are productivity, role activities, low absenteeism, low turnover, organizational citizenship, health and well-being, life satisfaction, and satisfaction of clients. Professional satisfaction favors positive attitudes towards oneself, and with others and contributes to greater professional participation in the work environment. This all improves professional performance and, consequently, strengthens the safety culture [1]. Safety at work also means trusting each other. In a hospital not only the patient has to feel safe but also the staff. Everyone in the hospital is working to achieve the best outcome for the patient. Sometimes during an operation there are difficult moments when the patient's life is in danger, and when it is necessary to help each other in dramatic moments to save the patient's life, everyone helps each other, because the common good of all is to save the patient's life. I give you one example: you or one of the team members during an operation has a problem or gets lost. He/she asks his/her closest colleague whom he/she trusts to help not only him or her but also the patient, because the most important person in the operating theater is the vulnerable patient who is suddenly in great danger and needs the help of everyone who can help him at this moment. These are the rules of the game and if they are overstepped then not only you as the operator but the whole team must and should do everything possible to save the patient if possible and in such a way that he suffers as little as possible [1].

Remember that this game is not about you but about the safety of the patient who has trusted you and whom you, as a surgeon, can never and under no circumstances put in any danger in the name of your own particular interests!

4. Work together with everyone, treat everyone fairly and with the same rights

Develop good cooperation with the Department of Vascular Surgery, Radiology, Infection Disease, Nephrology, Anesthesiology, Cardiology, Anatomopathology and Immunology.

5. Remember that your most important partner is the Nephrology Department

Together with the Department of Nephrology try to improve medication safety and monitoring in kidney transplant recipients. Use informatics and mobile health for that. Try to reduce as much as possible medication errors, medication nonadherence and adverse drug events [8, 9].

6. Surgical equipment

Use the best surgical equipment such as:

- Professional abdominal retractors: in kidney transplantation this is slowly becoming the rule, as it significantly contributes to the reduction of intraoperative and postoperative complications. Especially when performing difficult transplants, the operating field must be very well exposed and stable, because only such a field is in the full control of the operator. It is not pleasant when, for example, in the middle of the night a kidney is transplanted without the use of a professional abdominal retractor, it is the second or third transplant, the patient is "deep" or obese, the assistant is tired, and the iliac vessels consist of advanced types of atherosclerotic lesions.
- Headlamps with high power of cold light (which does not heat the organ)—it is perfect and safe—especially in "deep", obese recipients.
- Professional surgical magnifying loupes, or a surgical microscope.
- High quality surgical tools for transplantation and microsurgical reconstruction. There are more and more people on dialysis and we are therefore trying to do more transplants, taking organs from older and older living and deceased donors, but also transplanting them to older and older recipients who, because of their extensive medical history, cannot become kidney recipients overnight, as this would be too much of a burden on them in particular. This does not mean that these patients can never be transplanted, some of them certainly not, but some can be transplanted after multidisciplinary preparation of the potential kidney recipient for the transplant, which could be the implantation of a new heart valve, vessel unblocking or replacement with vascular prostheses. A commitment to the ability of the center to comprehensively prepare patients for transplantation and to transplant them in accordance with international guidelines for complications, organ and patient survival places such a center and its kidney transplantation program at the top of the pyramid of centers worldwide.

7. Read a lot, go to congresses, compare the results of your centre with the best in the world, be very flexible, make good changes, try to achieve the results of the best centres for kidney procurement and transplantation

Here you can check and compare your own center's results with the best kidney recipient survival results and the survival of the kidney itself after transplantation that have been achieved in the world in kidney transplant patients.

According to the national Organ Procurement and Transplantation Network, the success rate after a kidney transplant with a living-donor kidney was reported as 97% at one year and 86% at five years. The success rate after transplant with a deceased-donor kidney was 96% at one year and 79% at five years [5, 10]. A living donor kidney functions, on average, 12 to 20 years, and a deceased donor kidney from 8 to 12 years. Patients who get a kidney transplant before dialysis live an average of 10 to 15 years longer than if they stayed on dialysis. The mortality rate for related kidney recipients (who have not recieved a kidney) was 43 out of 128 (34%). The mortality rate for patients who received a primary graft and at least one retransplant during the study period (during 2.5 to 7.5 years of follow-up) was 12 out of 44 (27%). The mortality rate for diabetic patients on dialysis was 11 out of 22 (50%) [10].

## 8.2 First Do no Harm—*Primum Non Nocere*—The Hippocratic Oath

The Council of Europe bioethical principles of transplantation are laid down in the Convention of Human Rights and Biomedicine (1997) and reiterated in its Additional Protocol to the Convention on Human Rights and Biomedicine, on the Transplantation of Organs and Tissues of Human Origin, which was formally approved by the Committee of Ministers on 24 January 2002. The Council of Europe Committee of Experts on Organizational Aspects in Transplantation has produced under authorization of the European Health Committee several recommendations and guidelines dealing with the transplantation of organs and tissues. The most important regarding safety and quality aspects was the Guide to Safety and Quality Assurance for Organs, Tissues and Cells, whose seventh version was published in 2018 [6–8, 10]. The Guide provides useful information for transplantation centers, organ exchange organizations and tissue establishments and it goes through the whole transplantation process beginning with the identification of the potential donor and ending with the long-term follow-up of transplant recipients. The Guide is updated regularly according to the scientific and technical progress in the field. The essential spirit of all these documents is the same. National laws and international agreements should set the framework within which transplantation operates in each country. They should ensure the protection of donors and recipients against exploitation. The ethical rules must include protection of human integrity, avoidance of bodily harm and coercion, as well as exclusion of commercialism and financial gain from human material. The patients should have equitable access to transplantation, and thus the allocation rules must be fair and the system open and transparent. In order to guarantee a high level of quality, safety and efficacy of the transplantation program, all institutions involved should implement an effective quality assurance system. This includes well defined requirements not only for all human material to be removed and transplanted, but also all tests and methods of analysis, as well as materials, packaging, labeling, storage and transport. It also includes competence requirements for staff. An effective quality assurance also needs a good quality management system. The final measures of safety and quality of transplantation are the long-term results obtained from a life-long follow-up of all transplant recipients. In this follow-up, the data on the recipients, living donors and transplanted material including any adverse effects should be recorded, analyzed and reported [11–15].

## 8.3 Conclusion

Only mutual trust in each other, cooperation with each other and belief in each other, supported by daily continuing education, guarantees the lowest number of complications and the highest safety for the patient in the intra- and postoperative period. Based on the present findings, it is suggested that all transplant surgeons with experience of less than 25 transplants should perform their operations under close supervision (assistance) by an attending transplant surgeon literature [2, 5, 12–15].

## References


1. Pavan NFP, Magalhães ALP, Poncio DF, Ascari RA, Zanini PD, Da Silva KN, Silva OM. Patient safety culture in kidney transplant patients in western Santa Catarina. Acta Paul Enferm. 2019;32(4):398–405.
2. World Health Organization (WHO). WHO guidelines on hand hygiene in health care. First Global Patient Safety Challenge–Clean Care is Safer Care [Internet]. Geneva: WHO; 2004 [cited 2018 Mar 15]. https://apps.who.int/iris/bitstream/handle/10665/44102/978924159790 6_eng.pdf;jsessionid=E254EFFAA8CF30381ADC63F1E9DA3E4F?sequence=1.
3. Caldana G, Guirardello EB, Urbanetto JS, Peterlini MA, Gabriel CS. Brazilian network for nursing and patient safety: challenges and perspectives. Texto Contexto Enferm. 2015;24 (3):906–11.
4. Vituri DW, Matsuda LM. Content validation of quality indicators for nursing care evaluation. Rev Esc Enferm USP. 2009;43(2):429–37.
5. The European Renal Best Practice (ERBP) Transplantation Guideline Development Group, Abramowicz D, Cochat P, Claas F, Dudley C, Harden P, Heeman U, Hourmant M, Maggiore U, Pascual J, Salvadori M, Spasovski G, Squifflet J-P, Steiger J, Torres A, Vanholder R, Van Biesen W, Viklicky O, Zeier M, Nagler E. ERBP guideline on the management and evaluation of the kidney donor and recipient. Nephrol Dial Transplant. 2013;28(Suppl 2): ii1–ii71. https://doi.org/10.1093/ndt/gft218, 01 August 2013.
6. Guyatt GH, Oxman AD, Kunz R et al. Going from evidence to recommendations. Br Med J. 2008;336:1049–51.
7. Washer GF, Schröter GP, Starzl TE, Weil R. Causes of death after kidney transplantation. JAMA. 1983;250(1):49–54. PMID: 6343652; PMCID: PMC3091385.
8. Batabyal P, Chapman JR, Wong G, Craig JC, Tong A. Clinical practice guidelines on wait-listing for kidney transplantation: consistent and equitable? Transplantation. 2012;94 (7):703–13.
9. Salmela K. Quality and safety of organ transplantation. Ann Transplant. 2004;9(1):51–2.
10. Kulu Y, Fathi P, Golriz M, Khajeh E, Sabagh M, Ghamarnejad O, Mieth M, Ulrich A, Hackert T, Müller-Stich BP, Strobel O, Michalski C, Morath C, Zeier M, Büchler MW, Mehrabi A. Impact of surgeon's experience on vascular and haemorrhagic complications after kidney transplantation. Eur J Vasc Endovasc Surg. 2019;57(1):139–49. https://doi.org/10. 1016/j.ejvs.2018.07.041. Epub 2018 Sep 17. PMID: 30236441.
11. https://www.coe.int/en/web/conventions/full-list/-/conventions/treaty/164.
12. Council of Europe. Draft protocol on transplantation of organs and tissues of human origin. 2000;20(1):0–101.

13. https://rm.coe.int/168008371a; Additional protocol to the convention on human rights and biomedicine, concerning biomedical research.
14. https://www.edqm.eu/node/12729; 4th Edition of the Guide to the quality and safety of tissues and cells for human application; 2019.
15. https://www.edqm.eu/node/12729; Guide to the quality and safety of organs for transplantation; 2018.

# Index




© The Editor(s) (if applicable) and The Author(s), under exclusive license to
Springer Nature Switzerland AG 2023
A. Baranski, *Kidney Transplantation*,
https://doi.org/10.1007/978-3-030-75886-8

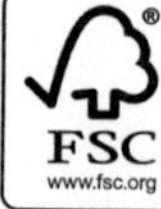MIX
Papier aus verantwortungsvollen Quellen
Paper from responsible sources
FSC® C105338

FSC
www.fsc.org

If you have any concerns about our products,
you can contact us on
ProductSafety@springernature.com

In case Publisher is established outside the EU,
the EU authorized representative is:
Springer Nature Customer Service Center GmbH
Europaplatz 3, 69115 Heidelberg, Germany

Printed by Libri Plureos GmbH
in Hamburg, Germany